A COMPREHENSIVE CURRICULUM FOR TRAUMA NURSING

The Jones and Bartlett Series in Nursing

Adult Emergency Nursing Procedures, Proehl

Basic Steps in Planning Nursing Research, Third Edition, Brink/Wood

Bone Marrow Transplantation, Whedon

Cancer Chemotherapy: A Nursing Process Approach, Barton Burke et al.

Cancer Nursing: Principles and Practice, Second Edition, Groenwald et al.

Chemotherapy Care Plans, Barton Burke

A Clinical Manual for Nursing Assistants, McClelland/Kaspar

Children's Nutrition, Lifshitz/Finch/Lifshitz

Chronic Illness: Impact and Intervention, Second Edition, Lubkin

Clinical Nursing Procedures, Belland/Wells

A Comprehensive Curriculum for Trauma Nursing, Bayley/Turcke

Comprehensive Maternity Nursing, Second Edition, Auvenshine/Enriquez

Concepts in Oxygenation, Ahrens/Rutherford

Critical Care Review, Wright/Shelton

Emergency Care of Children, Thompson

Essential Medical Terminology, Stanfield

Family Life: Process and Practice, Janosik/Green

Fundamentals of Nursing with Clinical Procedures, Second Edition, Sundberg

1991-1992 Handbook of Intravenous Medications, Nentwich

Handbook of Oncology Nursing, Johnson/Gross

Health Assessment in Nursing Practice, Third Edition, Grimes/Burns

Health and Wellness, Fourth Edition, Edlin/Golanty

Healthy People 2000, U.S. Department of Health & Human Services

Human Development: A Life-Span Approach, Fourth Edition, Freiberg

Instruments for Clinical Nursing Research, Oncology Nursing Society

Intravenous Therapy, Nentwich

Introduction to the Health Professions, Stanfield

Introduction to Human Disease, Third Edition, Crowley

Journal of Perinatal Education, ASPO

Management and Leadership for Nurse Managers, Swansburg

Management of Spinal Cord Injury, Second Edition, Zejdlik

Math for Health Professionals, Third Edition, Whisler

Medical Terminology, Stanfield

Memory Bank for Chemotherapy, Preston

Memory Bank for IVs, Second Edition, Weinstein

Memory Bank for Medications, Second Edition, Kostin/Evans

Mental Health and Psychiatric Nursing: A Caring Approach, Davies/Janosik

The Nation's Health, Third Edition, Lee/Estes

Nursing and the Disabled: Across the Lifespan, Fraley

Nursing Assessment: A Multidimensional Approach, Third Edition, Bellack/Edlund

Nursing Diagnosis Care Plans for Diagnosis-Related Groups, Neal/Paquette/Mirch

Nursing Management of Children, Servonsky/Opas

Nursing Pharmacology, Second Edition, Wallace

Nursing Research: A Quantitative and Qualitative Approach, Roberts/Burke

Nutrition and Diet Therapy: Self-Instructional Modules, Second Edition, Stanfield

Pediatric Emergency Nursing Procedures, Bernardo/Bove

Perioperative Nursing Care, Fairchild

Perioperative Patient Care, Second Edition, Kneedler/Dodge

A Practical Guide to Breastfeeding, Riordan

Psychiatric Mental Health Nursing, Second Edition, Janosik/Davies

Ready Reference of Common Emergency and Prehospital Drugs, Cummings

Ready Reference for Critical Care, Strawn

The Research Process in Nursing, Third Edition, Dempsey/Dempsey

Understanding/Responding, Second Edition, Long/Prophit

Writing a Succesful Grant Application, Second Edition, Reif-Lehrer

A COMPREHENSIVE CURRICULUM FOR TRAUMA NURSING

Edited by

Elizabeth W. Bayley, MS, PhD, RN
Associate Professor
Burn, Emergency, and Trauma Graduate Program
School of Nursing, Widener University
Chester, Pennsylvania

Susan Allyn Turcke, MSN, RN, CEN
Trauma Coordinator
The Children's Hospital of Philadelphia
Philadelphia, Pennsylvania

JONES AND BARTLETT PUBLISHERS
Boston London

Editorial, Sales, and Customer Service Offices

Jones and Bartlett Publishers
20 Park Plaza
Boston, MA 02116

Jones and Bartlett Publishers International
PO Box 1498
London W6 7RS
England

Library of Congress Cataloging-in-Publication Data

A Comprehensive curriculum for trauma nursing / edited by Elizabeth W. Bayley, Susan Allyn Turcke.
p. cm.
Includes bibliographical references and index.
ISBN 0-86720-628-4 (hc) 0-86720-331-5
1. Wounds and injuries—Nursing—Outlines, syllabi, etc.
2. Emergency nursing—Outlines, syllabi, etc. I. Bayley, Elizabeth W. II. Allyn Turcke, Susan.
[DNLM: 1. Curriculum—outlines. 2. Emergencies—nursing—outlines. 3. Wounds and Injuries—nursing—outlines. WY 18 C7393]
RD93.95.C66 1992
617.1—dc20
DNLM/DLC
for Library of Congress 92-10303
CIP

Production service: *Hoyt Publishing Services*
Typesetting: *Pine Tree Composition*
Cover design: *Lina Haddad*
Printing and binding: *Hamilton Printing Company*

The selection and dosage of drugs presented in this book are in accord with standards accepted at the time of publication. The authors and publisher have made every effort to provide accurate information. However, research, clinical practice, and government regulations often change the accepted standard in this field. Before administering any drug, the reader is advised to check the manufacturer's product information sheet for the most up-to-date recommendations on dosage, precautions, and contraindications. This is especially important in the case of drugs that are new or seldom used.

Printed in the United States of America
96 95 94 93 92 10 9 8 7 6 5 4 3 2 1

To the pioneers and present practitioners of trauma nursing

CONTENTS

Module 7
Trauma Nursing 65
Mary L. Beachley

Module 8
The Trauma Team 74
Mary L. Beachley and Mary Pat Erdner

Module 9
Trauma Transport 81
Elizabeth Blunt and Eileen M. Sweeney Crowther

Section III
Comprehensive Topics in Trauma Nursing

Module 10
Shock 98
Donna A. Gares

Section VI
Professional Perspectives in Trauma Nursing

PREFACE

Only in the past two decades has trauma been recognized as a significant health problem. Trauma systems are now in various stages of development throughout the United States. With this evolution has come the emergence of the specialty of trauma nursing.

With few exceptions, pioneers in this field have had no specific nursing curriculum to facilitate the development of a comprehensive knowledge base for the practice of trauma nursing. *A Comprehensive Curriculum for Trauma Nursing* fills that void by providing a framework and the essential content needed by trauma nurses throughout the trauma continuum. Using a modular format, this book addresses the care of the trauma patient in the prehospital, emergency, perioperative, critical care, acute, and rehabilitative phases. In addition, important information about the context of care, specific patient populations, and issues of concern to trauma nurses is included.

This book will be valuable to nurses who are new to the complexity and demands of trauma nursing, as well as those who have years of hands-on experience caring for the trauma patient. The former will find that it gives them a solid knowledge base and confidence as they enter the exciting realm of trauma care. Experienced nurses will validate their knowledge and gain a more comprehensive exposure to care at different phases of the trauma continuum. Nurse managers will use it to gain a broader perspective on trauma care development, to develop standards of care, and to guide nursing staff in the acquisition of skill and knowledge. Nurse educators will find *A Comprehensive Curriculum for Trauma Nursing* invaluable in planning orientation and inservice programs for nursing units that care for trauma patients and for developing trauma courses in various health care institutions and academic programs.

The book is divided into six sections. Section I, Trauma as a Health Care Problem, contains four modules covering the epidemiology of trauma, mechanisms of injury, recording and using trauma data, and prevention of trauma. The evolution of trauma systems and the nurse's role in emerging systems are covered in Section II, Trauma Nursing and the Health Care System. Teamwork and transport of the trauma patient by land and air are also discussed in this section.

Section III, Comprehensive Topics in Trauma Nursing, includes modules on nine patient problems or nursing challenges that may be presented by every patient, regardless of the specific organ(s) injured. Shock, nutrition, infection, wound healing, pain, psychological and social responses, major sequelae, and rehabilitation are addressed. Nursing care of the organ donor is also included.

The core of this book is found in Section IV, Systematic Approach to Trauma Nursing. The patterns of injury and related medical and surgical interventions for eight major body systems are described. Using the nursing process as an organizing framework, each module discusses nursing assessments related to injuries of a specific system, common nursing diagnoses, and nursing interventions, with expected patient outcomes and measurable criteria. Nursing care required at each phase of the trauma continuum is included.

Section V, Special Patient Populations, is intended to help the trauma nurse meet the unique needs of distinct patient populations. Separate modules address pediatric and obstetric patients, the elderly, trauma patients with a history of substance abuse, individuals with self-inflicted injury, and people of all ages who have been abused or battered. The book concludes with Section VI, Professional Perspectives in Trauma Nursing, which provides important information on legal and ethical issues, personal stress management, and professional development of trauma nurses.

An outline format is used throughout the book to facilitate its use as a study guide and to make information readily visible and succinct. Prerequisite knowledge is identified at the beginning of those modules for which specific prior learning or review is desirable. Behavioral objectives are listed for every module, to guide the reader and to provide a basis for self-assessment or teacher assessment of learning. References and Suggested Readings are listed at the end of each module, for those who wish more information on various aspects of trauma care.

This book reflects the experience of a variety of contributors, chosen for their high level of expertise and ability to identify the information of greatest relevance to patient care and to the nurse clinician. As trauma nursing develops in the future, it is anticipated that this curriculum will provide a foundation for formal recognition of the trauma nurse's knowledge and skills.

Elizabeth W. Bayley
Susan Allyn Turcke

ACKNOWLEDGMENTS

The development and completion of *A Comprehensive Curriculum for Trauma Nursing* has occurred only through the efforts and support of many individuals. We would like to express our gratitude here.

The William Penn Foundation, through a trauma education grant to Hahnemann University, provided funding for the initial design of the curriculum and honoraria for our contributors. A faculty development grant and sabbatical award from Widener University provided release time for work on the book.

Members of the Delaware Valley Trauma Nurse Consortium have contributed their expertise as authors of many modules in this book. In addition, they have provided much support and encouragement to us throughout the editing process. Mary L. Beachley (Trauma Nurse Coordinator, Maryland Institute for Emergency Medical Services Systems) reviewed early outlines of the book and extended the support of the Trauma Nurse Network (now the Society of Trauma Nurses). Carol Forrester Staz, Executive Director of the Pennsylvania Trauma Systems Foundation, promoted high standards for trauma nurse education and encouraged our pursuit of a book that would facilitate the educational process.

The administration, faculty, and staff of the School of Nursing of Widener University expressed frequent interest in and continuous belief in this project; their support is most appreciated. The Trauma Service at Hahnemann University saw the need for a trauma nursing curriculum and helped to bring it about.

Our students, past, present, and future, provided the stimulus to set down on paper the concepts that are essential for professional trauma nursing practice. We hope they will use this book to develop their knowledge further and provide the leadership to advance trauma nursing in the future.

We are grateful to Susan Glover, Margie Keating, and Linda Napora, whose enthusiasm for this book was essential to its completion. We also thank David Hoyt for his attention to the many details of production. The efforts of Joni Hopkins McDonald and Jim Keating of Jones and Bartlett are also greatly appreciated.

As always, our work was greatly enhanced by the love and extra encouragement of our families and friends, who believed in our ability to succeed. To them, we give our special thanks.

CONTRIBUTORS

Mary M. Bailey, RN, CEN
Trauma Education Coordinator
Albert Einstein Medical Center
Philadelphia, Pennsylvania

Elizabeth W. Bayley, MS, PhD, RN
Associate Professor
Burn, Emergency, and Trauma Graduate Program
School of Nursing, Widener University
Chester, Pennsylvania

Mary L. Beachley, MS, RN, CEN
Trauma Nurse Coordinator
Maryland Institute for Emergency Medical Services Systems
Department of EMS Nursing and Specialty Care
Baltimore, Maryland

Cynthia Gurdak Berry, MSN, RN, CCRN
Trauma Clinical Nurse Specialist
University of Alabama Hospital
Birmingham, Alabama

Elizabeth M. Blunt, MS, RN, CEN, EMT
Nursing Care Coordinator
Emergency and Trauma Center
Thomas Jefferson University Hospital
Philadelphia, Pennsylvania

Nancy Bucher, MSN, RN, CCRN
Clinical Coordinator, Intensive Care Unit
Crozer Chester Medical Center
Upland, Pennsylvania

Janet Marie Burns, MSN, RN, CEN
Nursing Instructor, Senior Level Critical Care
Frankford Hospital School of Nursing
Philadelphia, Pennsylvania

Susan Butler, MSN, RN, CCRN
Trauma Nurse Coordinator
The Reading Hospital and Medical Center
Reading, Pennsylvania

Jacqueline M. Carolan, RN, JD
Labrum and Doak Law Firm
Philadelphia, Pennsylvania

Rae L. Conley, MSN, RN, CCRN
Clinical Nurse Specialist
Thomas Jefferson University Hospital
Philadelphia, Pennsylvania

Eileen M. Sweeney Crowther, MSN, RN, CEN, HPRN
Chief Flight Nurse, University MedEvac
The Allentown Hospital—Lehigh Valley Hospital Center
Allentown, Pennsylvania

Donna Wivell Dorozinsky, MSN, RN
Nursing Consultant
Medco
Hatboro, Pennsylvania
Formerly, Trauma Nurse Coordinator
Brandywine Hospital and Trauma Center
Caln Township, Pennsylvania

Helen Noyes Downey, MSN, RN
Education Specialist
Hahnemann University Hospital
Philadelphia, Pennsylvania

Mary Pat Erdner, MSN, RN, CRRN
Clinical Coordinator, Day Treatment Program
ReMed Recovery Care Centers
Conshohocken, Pennsylvania

Barbara Esposito, RN, CEN
Manager, Trauma Program
Frankford Hospital—Torresdale Campus
Philadelphia, Pennsylvania

Steven Frantz, MSN, RN, CCRN
Staff Nurse, Surgical Intensive Care Unit
The Graduate Hospital
Philadelphia, Pennsylvania

Paula Crawford Gamble, MSN, RN
Clinical Nurse Specialist
University of Pennsylvania Medical Center
Philadelphia, Pennsylvania

Donna A. Gares, MSN, RN, CCRN
Trauma Program Coordinator
Abington Memorial Hospital
Abington, Pennsylvania

Karen A. Gilbert, MSN, RN, CNSN
Clinical Specialist, Nutrition Support Service
Albert Einstein Medical Center
Philadelphia, Pennsylvania

Laura Coates Hammond, MSN, RN, CCRN
Trauma Program Coordinator
Crozer Chester Medical Center
Upland, Pennsylvania

Barbara Mankey Henninger, BA, BSN, RN, C
Executive Staff Associate
Division of Trauma
Hospital of the University of Pennsylvania
Philadelphia, Pennsylvania

Lynn Kennedy-Ewing, MA
Director
Delaware County, PA Critical Incident Stress Management Program
Media, Pennsylvania

Cyndy Kraft-Fine, MSN, RN, CRRN
Nurse Educator
Magee Rehabilitation Hospital
Philadelphia, Pennsylvania

Julia C. Mahon, RN, CNRN, CCRN
Staff Nurse, Neurosurgical Intensive Care Unit
Wake Medical Center
Wake Forest, North Carolina

Joanne Michener, MSN, RN, CS
Nurse Consultant
Bates and Associates Health Care Management Consultants
Bala Cynwyd, Pennsylvania

Timothy O. Morgan, BSN, RN, CCRN
Division Administrator, Trauma and Critical Care
University of Pennsylvania Medical Center
Philadelphia, Pennsylvania

Betsy L. Musser, MSN, RN, CEN
Patient Care Coordinator
St. Joseph Hospital and Health Care Center
Lancaster, Pennsylvania

Mary Jean Osborne, MSN, RN, CCRN
Clinial Nurse Specialist in Trauma
The Allentown Hospital—Lehigh Valley Hospital Center
Allentown, Pennsylvania

Sally Boyle Quinn, MSN, RN, CEN
Critical Care Clinical Nurse Specialist
Temple Universiy Hospital
Philadelphia, Pennsylvania

Sharon G. Smith, MSN, RN
Trauma Coordinator
The Allentown Hospital—Lehigh Valley Hospital Center
Allentown, Pennsylvania

Susan W. Somerson, MSN, RN, CEN
Clinical Educator/Clinical Specialist, Emergency Department
Presbyterian Medical Center
Philadelphia, Pennsylvania

Denise C. Schleicher Stein, MSN, RN, CEN
Clinical Nurse Specialist
Emergency and Trauma Nursing
York Haven, Pennsylvania

Judith J. Stellar, MSN, RN, CPNP
Nursing Care Coordinator, Pediatric and Pediatric Intensive Care Units
Thomas Jefferson University Hospital
Philadelphia, Pennsylvania
Formerly, Surgery/Trauma Clinical Nurse Specialist
St. Christopher's Hospital for Children
Philadelphia, Pennsylvania

Susan Allyn Turcke, MSN, RN, CEN
Trauma Coordinator
The Children's Hospital of Philadelphia
Philadelphia, Pennsylvania

Marla Leyendecker Vanore, BSN, RN, CCRN
Director of Trauma Administration
Hahnemann University Hospital
Philadelphia, Pennsylvania

Nancy Vanore-Black, MSN, RN
Private Psychotherapy Practice
Bryn Mawr, Pennsylvania

Pat Walsh, MSN, RN, C
Trauma Education Coordinator
Thomas Jefferson University Hospital
Philadelphia, Pennsylvania

Jean Will, MSN, RN, CEN, EMT-P
Director, Regional Emergency Medical Services Training Center
Hahnemann University
Philadelphia, Pennsylvania

Linda M. Woodin, MSN, RN, CCRN
Clinical Nurse Specialist, Acute Pain Management
The Milton S. Hershey Medical Center
Hershey, Pennsylvania

Section I
Trauma as a Health Care Problem

MODULE 1
EPIDEMIOLOGY OF TRAUMA

Denise C. Schleicher Stein, MSN, RN, CEN

Prerequisite

Review major concepts related to epidemiology including host, agent, and environment.

Objectives

1.0 Describe the phases of an injury event.
1.1 Outline how interaction between host and environment impacts on the actual event.
1.2 Describe how the release of energy affects the injury severity.
1.3 Describe the interaction between phases of injury and the body's attempts to preserve homeostasis.
2.0 Describe human/host factors that contribute to injury occurrence.
2.1 Identify age groups at greatest risk of injury.
2.2 Recognize several preexisting biological factors that place someone at risk of injury.
3.0 Describe common agents/causes of injury.
3.1 List the most common methods of unintentional injury and/or death.
3.2 State two intentional methods of injury and/or death.
4.0 Describe the role of environment in the incidence of injury.

4.1 Identify the role that time variation plays in determining the incidence of injury.
4.2 Describe how seasonal variation impacts the incidence of injury.

A. PHASES OF INJURY EVENT

1. **Preinjury phase**
a. Precedes the moment of energy release
b. Describes interaction between human host and environment
c. Includes situations that determine if trauma-producing event will occur, e.g., crash
d. Examples of preinjury phase interaction
   (1) Observance of speed limit laws
   (2) Avoidance of alcohol consumption before or while driving
   (3) Preventive automobile maintenance
2. **Injury phase**
a. Describes the release and transmission of energy
b. Includes determinants regarding whether injury occurs
c. Homeostasis can be lost during this phase
d. Examples of injury phase interaction
   (1) Improved crashworthiness of auto
   (2) Improved highway engineering
      (a) Breakaway roadside sign poles
      (b) Antiskid and antihydroplane road surfaces
   (3) Use of safety belts
3. **Postinjury phase**
a. Describes actions taken to regain homeostasis
b. Examples of postinjury phase interaction
   (1) Development and implementation of trauma systems
   (2) Prompt emergency medical service response
   (3) Acute trauma resuscitation
   (4) Physical and emotional rehabilitation

B. COMPONENTS OF EPIDEMIOLOGY OF TRAUMA

1. **Host**
a. Factors affecting risk
   (1) Age
      (a) 0- to 5-year-olds
         i) Developmental changes
            a) Motor skills development—rolls over; begins to walk; progresses to running
            b) Object permanence

c) Intuition
d) Inquisitiveness
e) Increased independence
ii) Common mechanisms of injury
a) Motor vehicle crashes—occupant or pedestrian
b) Falls from one level to another
c) Abuse—children less than 3 years old at highest risk
d) Burns
(i) Scalds
(ii) Contact with stoves and ovens
(b) 6- to 14-year-olds
i) Developmental changes
a) Daring and adventuresome
b) Further development of gross and fine motor skills
c) Increased independence related to attending school
d) Increased peer pressure
e) Increased rule formation ability
ii) Common mechanisms of injury
a) Bicycle-related injuries frequent
b) Pedestrian injuries
(c) 15- to 24-year-olds
i) Developmental changes
a) Limited decision-making experience
b) Belief in self-immortality
c) Sexual maturity
d) Identity formation
e) Moral reasoning
ii) Common mechanisms of injury
a) Motor vehicle occupant injuries frequent
b) Sports-related injuries high
c) Homicide frequent in black urban population
(d) Adults
i) Developmental changes
a) Economic independence
b) More self-assured
c) Increased intellectual knowledge
d) Improved judgment
ii) Common mechanisms of injury
a) Occupation-related
b) Motor vehicle crashes—driver
(e) Elderly
i) Physiologic changes
a) Decreased visual and auditory perception
b) Gait and balance disturbances
c) Decreased tensile bone strength
d) Decreased cardiovascular adaptability
e) Decreased immune system responsiveness
ii) Greater likelihood of injury when subjected to force

iii) Poorer outcome following injury
iv) Common mechanisms of injury
a) Falling
b) Motor vehicle-pedestrian-related

(2) Sex
(a) Males are generally at greater risk of trauma than females
i) Males represent 70% of drivers in automobile crashes and 82% of drivers in fatal crashes (1) (all nonreferenced statistical information has been extracted from *The Injury Fact Book*)
ii) Male:female ratio is 17:1 for death by electrical current
(b) Females are at greater risk of injury from domestic violence

(3) Race
(a) Native Americans—highest unintentional injury death rate
(b) Blacks—highest homicide rate; leading cause of death for blacks age 15 to 34 (2)
(c) Suicide death rate
i) 14 per 100,000 for Caucasians and Native Americans
ii) 6 per 100,000 for Asians and blacks
iii) Asian Americans—lowest overall death rate

(4) Economic status
(a) Homicide rates 200% higher in low-income areas
(b) Death rates from clothing ignition several times higher in low-income areas

(5) Preexisting illnesses
(a) Diabetes mellitus
(b) Osteoporosis
(c) Cardiovascular disease
(d) Mental illness leading to:
i) Suicidal acts
ii) Altered sensorium secondary to medication
iii) Reality base changes
a) Schizophrenia
b) Flashbacks
(e) Alcoholism leading to
i) Coordination deficit
ii) Altered sensorium secondary to blood alcohol content
iii) Delirium tremens
iv) Hypoglycemia
v) Chronic subdural hematoma
(f) Mental retardation
(g) Physical limitations due to cerebral palsy, muscular dystrophy, multiple sclerosis, polio, or traumatic brain injury
(h) Carcinoma with bone and brain metastasis

b. Beliefs regarding one's risk of trauma
(1) Accident may be defined as uncontrollable, an act of God with a random chance of involvement
(2) Behaviors may be based on the belief that accidents are nonpreventable (fatalism)

(a) Mixing alcohol and driving
(b) Ignoring safety belt use
(c) Swimming unaccompanied
(d) Refusing to wear protective equipment
(3) Behaviors based on belief that accidents are preventable
(a) Avoiding dangerous sports
(b) Observing speed limit laws
(c) Reducing speed during hazardous weather conditions
(4) See Module 4 (Prevention) for the model of injury versus accident
c. Use of drugs that alter sensorium
(1) Alcohol
(2) Narcotic analgesics
(3) Hallucinogens
(4) Excitant-stimulants
(5) Antidepressants
(6) Tranquilizers

C. AGENT/CAUSE

1. Unintentional methods
a. Motor vehicle crashes (MVC)
(1) Leading cause of death for ages 1 to 34 (2)
(2) 40% of all deaths among 16 to 22 age group
(3) 52,000 deaths and 5,300,000 injuries annually
(4) Leading cause of work-related deaths
(5) Categories
(a) Occupant—death rates highest at ages 16 to 19
(b) Motorcycle crashes (MCC)
i) Death rates highest at ages 18 to 24 and in Western states (2)
ii) 10% of MVC deaths
(c) Pedestrian
i) Death rates highest after age 70 and in Southeast and Southwest
ii) Majority of motor vehicle-related deaths in 5 to 9 age group
(d) Bicyclist
i) Death rates highest at ages 11 to 15
ii) One-sixth of MVC-related deaths
b. Falls
(1) Most common cause of nonfatal injury in U.S.
(2) 13,000 deaths annually; second only to MVC as cause of fatal injury (2)
(a) 9% of occupation-related deaths
(b) Higher death rates in Northern states
(c) 20% of unintentional deaths among females; 10% among males
(3) Primary cause of approximately 200,000 hospital admissions annually
(4) Incidence
(a) Falls cause 150 deaths annually in children under 5 years of age

(b) Those 75 years and older make up 4% of population but sustain 50% of fall deaths

(c) Those 85 years and older make up 1% of population and sustain 30% of fall deaths for a death rate of 3800 per 100,000

c. Drowning

(1) Third most common cause of unintentional death in all age groups; second most common cause in 1 to 44 age group; more than 30,000 near-drownings per year (3)

(2) Categories

(a) Nonboat-related

i) 6000 deaths annually

ii) 500 deaths annually from MVCs

iii) 1000 deaths annually from suicide and undetermined intent

(b) Boat-related (small recreational crafts)

i) 1200 deaths annually

ii) 66% of deaths caused by capsizing or falling overboard

iii) 20% of deaths involve boats with inadequate number of personal flotation devices

d. Fires and burns

(1) 6000 deaths annually; fourth leading cause of death in 1987 (2)

(2) 90,000 hospital admissions annually

(3) Categories

(a) Housefires

i) Responsible for 75% of all burn deaths; most deaths occur due to smoke inhalation before medical treatment is provided

ii) Common causes are related to cigarette smoking or heating equipment

iii) Most deaths occur during winter months

(b) Clothing ignition

i) 5% of all burn deaths

ii) 75% occur among those 65 and older

iii) Second most common cause for hospitalization

iv) Nonflammable clothing legislation caused a significant decrease (71% among males to 82% among females) in death rate between 1968 and 1979

(c) Scalds and contact with hot substances

i) 200 deaths annually

ii) 3% of all burn deaths

iii) 30% of all hospital burn admissions

iv) Death rate dropped 75% among those ages 0 to 19 and almost 50% for all age groups between 1968 and 1979

v) Causes

a) 80% by hot liquids or steam

b) Hot water in tubs and showers most common source for all ages

c) High incidence of injury among 0 to 4 age group (hot coffee)

d) 20% by caustic or corrosive substances and hot objects

(d) Explosions

i) Most often involve explosive gases

ii) Death rate decreased 50% from 1968 to 1979

iii) 350 deaths annually at homes (32%), industrial sites (29%), and mines (2%)

(e) Electrical

i) 1100 deaths annually at homes (33%), and industrial sites and farms (25%)

ii) Deaths occur predominantly in the summer

iii) Lightning causes an additional 100 deaths annually

a) Highest death rate among males and the 10 to 19 age group

b) Most common during summer

2. Intentional methods

a. Suicide

(1) 27,000 deaths annually

(a) Eighth leading cause of death in U.S. (2)

(b) Second leading cause of death in 15 to 24 age group (2)

(c) Highest rate among elderly males

(2) Methods causing death

(a) Firearms—57%; used predominantly by males (64%)

(b) Hanging—14%; responsible for 48% of deaths among 10 to 14 age group

(c) Poisoning

i) Predominantly used by females 65 and older

ii) Ingestion of solid and liquid—11%; method of choice in females in early 40s

iii) Inhalation of carbon monoxide—7%

(d) Jumping—3%

(e) Drowning—2%

(f) Cutting with sharp instrument—1%

(g) Single vehicle accidents

(h) Self-immolation

(3) Methods of suicide attempt (parasuicide); eight times as common as suicide (2)

(a) Drug ingestion—70%

(b) Wrist cutting—15%

b. Homicide

(1) Eleventh leading cause of death in U.S.

(a) Firearms—66%

(b) Stabbing—18%

(c) Strangulation—4%

(d) Battery other than strangulation, e.g., baseball bats

(2) Incidence

(a) Leading cause of death among blacks ages 15 to 34 (2)

(b) Highest for males ages 25 to 29

(c) Death rate peaks for females at age 20 to 24

c. Legal intervention

(1) Lethal injection

(2) Poisonous gas

(3) Hanging

(4) Firearms

D. ENVIRONMENT

1. Physical

a. Geographic region
   (1) Urban areas have high rate of intentional, penetrating injuries
   (2) Rural areas have high rate of fatal motor vehicle crashes and drownings
   (3) Topography can delay crash or injury discovery and can make extrication and retrieval difficult
   (4) Availability and quality of emergency medical service in areas with varying skill levels, response times, and available resources, e.g., aeromedical evacuation, extrication, water and cave rescue
   (5) Presence of state laws governing
      (a) Safety belt usage
      (b) Drinking age
      (c) Driving age
      (d) Automobile inspection rate
      (e) Swimming pool safety
      (f) Transportation, handling, and storage of hazardous materials
      (g) Firearms
      (h) Class A explosives (firecrackers)
      (i) Amusement ride safety
      (j) Life safety codes
         i) Panic hardware
         ii) Access to exits
         iii) Handicap ramps
   (6) Municipal codes
      (a) Fire detection and suppression
         i) Smoke alarms
         ii) Sprinklers
         iii) Fire extinguishers
      (b) Building safety standards
      (c) Firearms
      (d) Explosives

b. Occupational risks
   (1) Vehicle crashes—delivery personnel, common carrier (public), and tractor-trailer drivers
   (2) Aircraft crashes—pilots and crew of fixed and rotary wing aircraft
   (3) Falls—linemen, construction workers, firefighters, window washers, and painters
   (4) Ballistic injuries—military, law enforcement, and construction trades
   (5) Burn injuries—firefighters, roofers, chemical workers, and paving contractors
   (6) Agricultural injuries—farmers, grain handlers, and meat processors
   (7) Industrial injuries—quarry workers, machinists, and foundry workers

c. Automobile design
   (1) Crashworthiness
      (a) Deformability
      (b) Integrity of passenger compartment

(c) Convertible vs hardtop—17% of deaths in passenger cars and 41% in heavy trucks involve rollovers

(2) Restraints

(a) Passive—air bags and automatic safety belts and shoulder harnesses (front)

(b) Active—safety belts and shoulder harnesses (front and rear) and child safety seats

(c) Shoulder harnesses in rear seats may prevent injuries from lap belts

d. Residence

(1) Proximity to other structures

(2) Fire wall protection decreases risk of death in attached dwellings, apartments, and condominiums

(3) Elevation above ground level increases risk of death, e.g., high-rise apartment vs ranch-style home

(4) Structural composition

(5) Location (geographic)

(a) Hillside slope

(b) Proximity to industry and transport, e.g., factories, highways, airports

(6) Weather—hurricanes, tornadoes, floods, lightning, hail and sleet, snow, and wind

(7) Geophysical—landslides, earthquakes, floods, tidal waves, volcanoes, and avalanches

2. Socioeconomic factors affecting risk

a. Social influences may result in riots, arson, and/or abuse

b. Income impacts on unintentional suicide and homicide risk

c. Influence of culture on acceptable risk—machismo, hunting, athletics, and gangs

3. Time variation

a. Day of week

(1) Unintentional

(a) Motor vehicle crash

i) 33% of deaths occur between Friday and Saturday nights

ii) Occupant death rate, per person per mile traveled, highest on Friday and Saturday, lowest on Tuesday and Wednesday

(b) Pedestrian crashes

i) Injury rates are highest on weekdays

ii) Death rates are highest on Saturday

(c) Occupational—highest on Monday and Friday

(d) Drowning—40% occur on weekend

(2) Intentional

(a) Suicide—highest on Monday

(b) Homicide

i) 50% occur Friday through Sunday

ii) 20% occur Saturday

b. Time of day

(1) Motor vehicle crashes

(a) 40% of death rate occurs between 2200 and 0400 hrs; injury rate is 17%

(b) Peak in multiple-vehicle crashes at 1700 hrs

(c) Peak in single-vehicle crashes from 0100 and 0259 hrs

(2) Pedestrian crashes

(a) Fatalities
i) 66% occur between 1800 and 0559 hrs
ii) Peak between 1800 and 2159 hrs
(b) Injuries—peak at 1600 hrs
(3) Motorcycle crashes
(a) Fatalities—peak from 1600 and 0200 hrs
(b) Injuries—30% occur between 1500 and 1859 hrs

4. Seasonal variation

a. Unintentional
(1) Motor vehicle crashes—death rate highest in summer and lowest in winter
(2) Drowning—66% of nonboating-related and 50% of boating-related occur during May through August
(3) Motorcycle crashes—deaths per month range from 100/month in January to 700/month during June through August

b. Intentional
(1) Homicide—death rate highest during July through December, with December the peak month
(2) Suicide frequently peaks during spring months, rises again in the fall, and is lowest in December (4)

References

1. Baker, S. P., O'Neill, B., & Karpf, R. S. (1984). *The injury fact book.* Lexington, MA: Lexington Books.
2. Rice, D. P., MacKenzie, E. J., and Associates. (1989). *Cost of injury in the United States: A report to Congress.* San Francisco: Institute for Health and Aging, University of California and Injury Prevention Center, the Johns Hopkins University.
3. The National Committee for Injury Prevention and Control. (1989). *Injury prevention: Meeting the challenge.* New York: Oxford University Press.
4. MacMahon, K. (1983). Short-term temporal cycles in the frequency of suicide in the United States, 1972–1978. *American Journal of Epidemiology, 117*(6), 744–750.

Suggested Readings

Cardona, V., Hurn, P., Mason, P., Scanlon-Schilpp, A., & Veise-Berry, S. (Eds.). (1988). *Trauma nursing: From resuscitation through rehabilitation.* Philadelphia: W. B. Saunders Co.

Committee on Trauma Research, Commission on Life Sciences, National Research Council and the Institute of Medicine. (1985). *Injury in America: A continuing public health problem.* Washington, DC: National Academy Press.

Joy, C. (Ed.). (1988). *Pediatric trauma nursing.* Rockville, MD: Aspen Publishers, Inc.

Waller, J. (1985). *Injury control: A guide to the causes and prevention of trauma.* Lexington, MA: Lexington Books.

MODULE 2
MECHANISMS OF INJURY

Marla Leyendecker Vanore, BSN, RN, CCRN

Prerequisite

Review of basic anatomy and physiology.

Objectives

1.0 Define certain terms and principles important to the study of mechanisms of injury.
1.1 Define kinematics and its importance in patient assessment.
1.2 Define basic principles of physics involving energy and motion.
1.3 Define characteristics of body tissue that affect vulnerability to injury.
2.0 Describe common patterns of injury in blunt trauma.
2.1 Identify three types of force that commonly occur in blunt trauma.
2.2 Given a common accident scenario, list injuries that might occur.
2.3 Given a common accident scenario, describe how the energy forces cause the expected injuries.
3.0 Identify injuries that might occur in specific body regions with blunt trauma.
3.1 List injuries that can occur in each body region.
3.2 Describe the type of force that can cause each of these injuries.
3.3 List extrinsic and intrinsic factors that determine the probability of a bone being fractured.

4.0 Describe the different types of penetrating trauma and the extent of injury that can be expected with each.
4.1 List ways to calculate the pathway of injury in stab wounds.
4.2 Relate several gun types to extent of injury expected with each.
4.3 Describe properties of tissue and missiles that increase the damage sustained by the victim.
4.4 Describe injuries that may occur in specific body areas from penetrating trauma.
5.0 Describe important properties of smoke inhalation and pulmonary burns.
5.1 List the types of gases that might be inhaled.
5.2 Describe factors related to smoke inhalation and pulmonary burns that increase injury severity.
5.3 List situations that would increase suspicion of smoke inhalation.
5.4 Identify effects of chemical irritants in smoke on the respiratory tract.
6.0 Describe the mechanisms of thermal injury.
6.1 List types of thermal injuries.
6.2 Describe variables that influence the amount of damage sustained in thermal injuries.
7.0 Describe the mechanisms of explosive blasts.
7.1 Describe the types of injuries that occur from explosive blasts.
7.2 Describe the forces that cause the above injuries in explosive blasts.
8.0 Describe the properties that affect the severity of radiation exposure.
9.0 Describe the mechanisms of near-drowning and drowning.
9.1 List the different types of drowning situations.
9.2 Describe the protective mechanisms of the body against drowning.

A. GENERAL DESCRIPTION OF TERMS AND PRINCIPLES

1. Kinematics

a. Process of evaluating the probability of injuries based on the forces and motion involved in the trauma

b. Accident information should be obtained or be available at the time of the initial patient assessment

c. A high index of suspicion should be maintained for certain injuries based on the mechanism of injury

2. Principles of physics

a. Newton's first law of motion—a body at rest will remain at rest, and a body in motion will remain in motion until acted upon by some outside force

b. Energy cannot be destroyed, only changed

c. Extent of injury is based on magnitude of the energy, speed or velocity, and duration of impact

d. Kinetic energy $= \dfrac{\text{mass} \times \text{velocity}^2}{2}$

3. Tissue response to energy

a. The body absorbs energy, but injury occurs when tissue limits are surpassed

b. Inertial resistance—ability of body to resist movement

c. Tensile strength—amount of tension a tissue can withstand and ability to resist stretching forces

d. Elasticity—ability to resume the original shape and size after being stretched

e. Compressive strength—ability to resist squeezing forces or inward pressure

B. BLUNT INJURY

1. Forces that commonly occur in blunt trauma

a. Acceleration/deceleration
   (1) An increase in the velocity of a moving body followed by a decrease in velocity
   (2) In a motor vehicle crash (MVC), three collisions generally occur
      (a) The vehicle hits an object
      (b) The occupant impacts the vehicle interior
      (c) Internal organs and tissues impact against rigid structures of the body
   (3) In an MVC, deceleration begins when the occupant contacts seat belt or the interior surfaces of car

b. Compression—squeezing together

c. Shearing—two oppositely directed parallel forces

2. Usual patterns of injury in motor vehicle crashes

a. Pedestrian vs car
   (1) Children or very short adults—Waddell's Triad
      (a) Usually frontal impact because children face the oncoming vehicle
      (b) Bumper and hood of car impact femur and/or chest
      (c) Victim is thrown upon impact, hitting the head or upper back
      (d) Contralateral skull is injured by the force of the impact with the ground
   (2) Adults
      (a) Lateral impact since adults try to protect themselves by turning sideways
      (b) Bumper and hood of car impact the lower and upper leg causing a bowing effect and fractures above and below the impacted joint
      (c) Strain on the opposite extremity causes ligament damage to knee
      (d) Fractured pelvis is common

b. Frontal impact of a motor vehicle with another object
   (1) Down and under motion
      (a) Frontal motion is stopped abruptly; occupant continues to travel downward into the seat and forward into the dashboard or steering column
      (b) Knees hit the dashboard
      (c) Upper leg absorbs most of the impact causing dislocation of patella, midshaft femur fractures, and posterior fracture/dislocation of femoral head or acetabulum; may be followed by an up and over motion

(2) Up and over motion
   (a) Frontal motion is stopped abruptly; upper body of the unrestrained driver travels forward
   (b) Victim's head hits the windshield causing head injuries, e.g., lacerations and contusions to the scalp, skull fractures and/or cerebral contusions and/or hemorrhage, or facial fractures
   (c) Cervical spine can be injured from impact to the head
   (d) Chest is compressed against steering wheel causing injuries, e.g., fractured sternum, fractured ribs with possible anterior flail chest, pulmonary contusion, and myocardial contusion
   (e) Abdomen is injured as it hits the steering wheel; can cause rupture of solid organs such as liver or spleen
   (f) As organs keep moving inside the person's body, aorta may be torn and liver lacerated
   (g) The thoracic vertebrae are well-protected, but energy can travel down or up and cause combination vertebral injuries
(3) If the passenger extends his/her lower extremities, fractures of the feet, ankles, and proximal portions of lower extremities may occur

c. Rear impact
   (1) Impact causes acceleration of the vehicle
   (2) Vehicle may then incur frontal collision
   (3) Whiplash may occur (hyperextension of neck over top of seat) if headrest is positioned too low
   (4) Injuries include torn and strained ligaments in the neck

d. Side impact
   (1) Injuries occur on the side of the impact
   (2) Possible chest injuries include fractured ribs, flail chest, and pulmonary contusions
   (3) Ruptured spleen may occur if impact on driver's side, and ruptured liver if on passenger's side
   (4) Musculoskeletal injuries may occur
      (a) Victim's arm may be pinned against car; energy can be transferred causing injury to the clavicle and chest wall
      (b) The head of the femur may be forced through the pelvis at the acetabulum causing a fractured acetabulum and/or pelvic fracture
      (c) Lateral neck strain may occur causing ligament tears or spine fractures

e. Other types of accidents
   (1) Rotational force—vehicle spins around; injuries are combinations of those seen in frontal and lateral impacts
   (2) Rollover of vehicle—victims are impacted from many different angles causing various combinations of injuries
   (3) Ejection from vehicle—victim is thrown through the air; injury occurs at point of impact, and energy is reflected to rest of the body
   (4) MVC with a seat belt in place
      (a) A shoulder harness with a lap belt fastened loosely or strapped above the anterior iliac crests can cause
         i) Compression to soft abdominal organs, such as spleen, liver, and pancreas

ii) Diaphragmatic rupture and herniation of abdominal organs from increased intraabdominal pressure and anterior compression fracture of lumbar spine may occur

(b) Lap belt worn alone can still allow head, neck, facial, and chest injuries

(c) Shoulder harness worn alone can cause severe neck injuries and even decapitation

(d) Other injuries associated with seat belts are cervical vertebral fractures caused by flexion, neck strains caused by hyperextension of the neck, rib and sternal fractures, cardiac contusions, and, from deceleration forces, shearing of organs attached by ligaments

3. Usual patterns of injury in motorcycle crashes (MCC)

a. Head-on impact

(1) Motorcycle tips forward and rider goes over the handlebars

(2) Direct contact with handlebars can cause chest and abdominal injuries and shearing fractures of ilia

(3) The head and neck may be injured if impacted; a helmet does not protect the neck, but nonuse increases the chance of head injury by 300%

(4) If rider's feet remain on foot pegs, bilateral femur fractures may occur

b. Angular impact

(1) Motorcycle is hit at an angle and bike collapses on rider

(2) Injuries may include a crushed lower leg, open tibia-fibula fracture, and dislocation of ankle

c. Ejection

(1) Rider is thrown off bike and flies through the air

(2) Injury occurs at point of impact and is reflected to the rest of the body

d. Laying the bike down

(1) Maneuver used by riders to separate themselves from the bike in an impending accident

(2) Rider turns bike sideways and drags the inside leg on ground causing the rider to slow down more than the bike, so that the bike moves out from under him or her

(3) Injuries are usually abrasions and minor fractures, but crush injuries to legs may occur

4. Types of bicycle accidents and usual patterns of injury

a. Common types of bicycle accidents

(1) Collision with a motor vehicle

(a) Most common type of accident

(b) 90% of bicycle deaths result from this type

(2) Losing control of bicycle and falling off

(a) Cause of most nonfatal bicycle accidents

(b) Frequently caused by lack of ability, hazardous ground surfaces, speeding, and/or stunts

(3) Pedestrians hit by bicycles

b. Common patterns of injury

(1) Spoke injuries

(a) Passenger's foot caught in spokes of wheel

(b) Injuries to the involved foot occur; possible associated injuries if person falls off bicycle

(c) Wheel guards decrease incidence of this type of injury

(2) Over the handlebars injuries
  (a) Occur with head-on impact or other incident that causes the bicycle to tip forward, e.g., hazardous road surfaces
  (b) Bicycle tips forward and rider goes over the handlebars
  (c) Chest and abdominal injuries may occur as handlebars are impacted
  (d) Head and neck may be injured if impacted; bicycle helmets decrease the incidence of head trauma
  (e) If the rider's feet remain on the pedals, bilateral femur fractures may occur
  (f) Both upper and lower extremities may be injured if impacted
(3) Straddle injuries
  (a) Caused by impact on the bicycle seat or bar
  (b) Can cause perineal contusions, vaginal tears, or scrotal injuries
(4) Injuries related to bicycle-mounted child seats
  (a) Causes of injury include
    i) Bicycle tipping over
    ii) Child falling out of seat
    ii) Seat detaching from the bicycle
    iv) Extremities catching in spokes
  (b) Most common and severe injuries are head and facial trauma since the seat offers no head protection, and the child has insufficient muscle development to break the fall; children in bicycle seats should wear bicycle helmets
  (c) Extremities, especially lower, may be injured
(5) Injuries from impact of extended rearview mirrors
  (a) Small trucks or vans frequently have rearview mirrors that extend from the vehicle
  (b) Head, neck, or facial injuries can occur
  (c) Fatal, deep lacerations to the head and neck have occurred from sharp edges on the mirrors

5. Usual patterns of injury in falls

a. Fall from height, e.g., balcony, onto heels (Don Juan syndrome)
  (1) Energy is displaced upward causing bilateral calcaneus fractures, femoral shaft fractures, hip dislocations, thoracolumbar vertebral compressions, and basilar skull fractures
  (2) Impact pushes victim into acute flexion and forces person to fall forward onto the arms and sustain wrist fractures
b. Landing on other body areas causes injury to occur at the point of impact and force to be reflected to the rest of the body

6. Usual patterns of injury in sports accidents

a. Caused by sudden deceleration or compressive forces
b. Spinal cord injuries commonly occur from gymnastics and football
c. Head injury frequently occurs in football and horseback-riding accidents
d. Fractures and knee injuries occur in skiing and football

7. Specific organ injuries

a. Head
  (1) Acceleration/deceleration injuries
    (a) Closed head injury with no direct impact

- (b) Contusion of the brain with contrecoup injury
- (c) Torn blood vessels causing subdural hematomas, epidural hematomas, and subarachnoid hemorrhages
- (d) Diffuse axonal injury
- (e) Brain stem injury

(2) Compression injuries
- (a) Skull fractures
- (b) Intracranial bleeding and/or contusion from fractures

b. Spinal injuries

(1) Axial loading
- (a) A force travels up or down the spine without neck bending
- (b) Usual injury is a burst fracture of vertebral body or disc extrusion

(2) Flexion
- (a) Neck injury when head is bent forward
- (b) Injury is worse when associated with rotation
- (c) Vertebral body moves forward and spinal cord can be compressed
- (d) A wedging force is placed on an adjacent vertebra and crushes it, driving fragments of bone into spinal canal

(3) Hyperextension
- (a) Head is bent backward
- (b) Causes whiplash from acceleration forces
- (c) Compression of vertebral bodies occurs with posterior dislocation of upper vertebrae onto lower ones

(4) Distraction
- (a) Separation of spinal column with cord transection
- (b) Occurs in hangings

(5) Rotation

(6) Lateral bending

c. Chest and thorax injuries

(1) Deceleration can cause aortic tears, which most commonly occur at the ligamentum arteriosum

(2) Compression forces cause
- (a) Fractured ribs; flail chest
- (b) Cardiac or pulmonary contusion
- (c) Cardiac rupture possible if heart compressed between sternum and vertebral column
- (d) Pneumothorax—victim takes a deep breath and holds it, closing off the glottis and sealing off the lungs (paper bag effect)

d. Abdominal injuries

(1) Deceleration
- (a) As the forward motion of the body stops and deceleration begins, the abdominal organs continue to move forward causing tears at the point of attachment to the mesentery
- (b) Organs usually injured in this manner—kidneys, small intestine, large intestine, and spleen
- (c) The liver may be lacerated as it impacts on the ligamentum teres

(2) Compression forces
- (a) Frontal forces compress organs, usually the pancreas, spleen, liver, and kidneys, against the vertebral column

(b) May cause pelvic fractures with injuries to bladder and blood vessels; full bladder more susceptible to compression forces
(c) A buildup of pressure in abdomen may cause
i) The diaphragm (weakest point in the abdomen) to tear or herniate
ii) Retrograde blood flow may cause the rupture of the aortic valve

e. Fractures of bony skeleton
(1) The probability of fracture depends on
(a) Extrinsic factors or properties of the force, such as magnitude, duration, direction, and speed or velocity
(b) Intrinsic factors or properties of bone, such as elasticity, density, fatigue in cumulative stress, and the energy-absorbing capacity
(2) Extremity fractures in blunt injuries can be caused by two types of trauma
(a) Direct trauma, such as direct blows, compression forces, or crushing
(b) Indirect trauma, such as traction injury, angulation fractures, rotational injury, vertical compression, and axial loading

C. PENETRATING INJURY

1. Stab wounds (SW)—description and considerations

a. Low-velocity weapons—damage caused by sharp cutting edge with very little secondary trauma
b. Pathway of injury can be calculated by knowing
(1) Victim's position
(2) Attacker's position
(3) Attacker's gender, since men usually stab with an upward motion and women stab downward
(4) Weapon used
c. Additional considerations
(1) More than one wound should be suspected
(2) Entrance wound may be small, but internal damage may be extensive from weapon movement

2. Impalements

a. Occur in MVCs, falls, and after being hit with a falling or flying object
b. Low-velocity injuries
c. Impaled objects should not be removed until the patient is in a controlled medical environment

3. Gunshot wounds (GSW)—description and considerations

a. General principles
(1) Cavitation—kinetic energy of missile compresses surrounding tissues and stretches attached tissue causing cellular structure damage; large, temporary cavity produced and smaller, permanent cavity left
(2) Kinetic energy—determined by bullet caliber, mass, and speed
(3) Yaw and tumbling—common movements of bullets that affect the velocity and amount of damage done

(4) Muzzle blast—cloud of hot gas and burning powder at the muzzle of a gun when it is fired; at close range, can cause burns and even an internal explosion

b. Types of guns
   (1) Low-velocity
      (a) Bullet travels 1000–3000 feet/second
      (b) Temporary cavity two to three times diameter of missile
      (c) Handguns and some rifles
   (2) High-velocity
      (a) Bullet travels over 3000 feet/second
      (b) Temporary cavity three to four times missile size
      (c) M-16s and other military assault rifles
   (3) Shotguns
      (a) Low-velocity pellets
      (b) Injury dramatically changes with changes in distance

c. The extent of damage to the victim depends on
   (1) Density and compressibility of the tissue damaged
      (a) The denser the tissue, the more damage that occurs
      (b) Bone is the most dense tissue, followed by solid organs (liver, spleen, kidney, and brain), followed by muscle and fat, and, lastly, fasciae, lung, and skin
   (2) Velocity of the missile
      (a) The higher the velocity, the more damage that occurs
      (b) Missile velocity depends on
         i) Muzzle velocity—bullet velocity as it leaves the muzzle of the gun; affected by rifling inside the barrel, the type of bullet, and gun used
         ii) Distance of weapon from target—air resistance slows the bullet
   (3) Amount of frontal area that comes in contact with tissue; frontal area is increased by
      (a) Modification of bullet profile—hollow-point, soft-nose, flat-nose, and dumdum bullets (expand on impact)
      (b) Tumble—bullet tumbles as it moves through the body
      (c) Fragmentation—bullets break apart on impact; common with soft-nose, hollow-point, and dumdum bullets; shotgun blasts act in a similar way when the pellets disperse inside the victim's body

d. Specific organ involvement in penetrating trauma
   (1) Gunshot wound to the head
      (a) Entails a large amount of energy in a closed space
      (b) Brain tissue is compressed against the skull, and the skull can explode from the inside out
   (2) Penetrating wound to the thorax
      (a) Lungs usually sustain little injury since they are compliant and filled with air
      (b) Small blood vessels may move aside, but aorta and venae cavae do not and can be lacerated
      (c) With any penetrating injury to the lower chest (nipples to costochrondral margin), suspect an abdominal injury; one in four people with penetrating abdominal injuries have associated thoracic injury

(3) Gunshot injury to the extremities
    (a) When bones are fractured, fragments become secondary missiles lacerating surrounding tissues
    (b) Muscles often expand away from the path of a bullet; however, the stretching causes hemorrhaging
    (c) Blood vessels can be penetrated or bruised; bruising can cause clotting and obstructing of vessels in minutes or hours

D. OTHER INJURIES

1. Smoke inhalation and pulmonary burns

a. Type and severity depend on
  (1) Type of gas inhaled
    (a) Forced hot air—may burn area above the vocal cords
    (b) Smoke—consists of soot and small particles suspended in hot air and gases
    (c) Steam—has 4000 times the heat capacity of air and can be inhaled causing thermal injury to the lower respiratory tract; rarely occurs due to protective closure of the glottis
    (d) Carbon monoxide—odorless and colorless gas; always generated during partial combustion
    (e) Toxic chemicals
      i) Cyanide/hydrogen cyanide
        a) Combustion products of silk, wool, polyurethane, and nylon
        b) Cyanide-containing ingredients are found in silver polish, fumigants, and metal cleaners
      ii) Hydrochloric acid
        a) Product of polyvinyl chloride
        b) Formed by combustion of electric or telephone wires, wall or floor coverings, synthetic fibers in furniture, carpets, draperies, appliances, records, toys, shower curtains, office equipment or furniture, and raincoats
        c) Causes chemical burns in lungs
      iii) Others—nitrogen oxide, benzene, aldehyde, ammonia
  (2) Concentration of gases
  (3) Duration of exposure

b. Chemical burns of the airway—location depends on
  (1) Duration of exposure
  (2) Size of particles
    (a) Large particles are usually trapped in nasopharynx
    (b) Smaller particles are carried to terminal bronchioles
  (3) Solubility of gases
    (a) Highly soluble gases, such as chlorine, sulfadioxide, ammonia, and hydrogen chloride, generally stay in the upper respiratory tract

(b) More insoluble gases, such as acrolein, phosgene, oxides of nitrogen, and other aldehydes, travel further down the respiratory tract

c. Inhalation injuries should be suspected in the following

(1) Fire in a closed space—common in house, auto, and airplane fires

(2) An unconscious or inebriated person who has been exposed to smoke

(3) Fires involving plastics

(4) Steam explosions

2. Burn injuries

a. Thermal burns

(1) Include flame burns, scalding by hot liquid, hot surface contact, or contact with hot substances such as tar, asphalt, and melted plastic

(2) Severity of injury depends on the following

(a) Intensity of heat

(b) Duration of exposure

(c) Tissues involved

b. Chemical burns

(1) Caused by

(a) Oxidizing agents, e.g., sodium nitrates

(b) Reducing agents, e.g., hydrochloric acid, nitric acid

(c) Corrosives, e.g., phenol, lye, white phosphorus

(d) Protoplasmic poisons, e.g., tannic acid, hydrofluoric acid

(e) Desiccants (drying agents), e.g., dry ice

(f) Vesicants (blistering agents), e.g., mustard gas, phosgene oxime, nitrogen mustard, arsenical vesicants

(2) Factors affecting severity

(a) Quantity

(b) Concentration

(c) Degree of penetration

(d) Mode of action

(e) Duration of contact

c. Electrical injuries

(1) Caused by

(a) Lightning—direct or near-strike; involves million of volts with 5000 to 200,000 amperes of current

(b) Arcing—result of electrical generation of heat outside the skin; can increase the atmospheric temperature to 3000°C and cause either direct burns or ignition of clothing

(c) Direct contact with electrical current—occurs with either defective electrical equipment, improperly installed devices, or contact with a circuit or high-tension power lines

(2) Severity of injury depends upon

(a) Strength (voltage) of current

i) Determines degree of burn

ii) Over 1000 volts is considered high voltage

(b) Current type—alternating (AC), or direct (DC)

i) AC causes tetanic muscle spasms, freezes victim to source, and results in increased duration of exposure

ii) DC throws victim to ground
iii) Skin is more resistant to DC
(c) Path of current through the body
i) Low voltage takes path of least resistance
ii) High voltage takes most direct path
iii) Lightning—near-strike, e.g., current enters one leg and exits the other
iv) Lightning flashover—passes around body
(d) Skin resistance
i) Increased by thickness of skin
ii) Decreased by moisture and vascularity
iii) Increased resistance causes larger entrance burn
(e) Tissue resistance (least to most)—nerve, blood, muscle, skin, tendon, fat, bone
(f) Relationship of victim to electrical field
(g) Duration of contact

3. Exposure to cold

a. Types of cold injuries
(1) Frostbite
(a) Tissue freezes with cellular disruption
(b) Ischemia and necrosis due to vasospasm, increased viscosity, and sludging
(c) Vessel wall damage with increased capillary permeability and edema
(2) Hypothermia—core body temperature below 35°C, which can occur with exposure to the cold or immersion in cold liquid

b. Degree of injury depends on
(1) Length of exposure
(2) Ambient temperature
(3) Tissue involved—ears, toes, fingers lack subcutaneous fat protection and are most susceptible

c. Conditions that increase susceptibility to cold injury
(1) Lack of adequate body tissue insulation, i.e., elderly, infants, and small children
(2) Certain disease states, e.g., diabetes, hypothyroidism, arteriosclerosis
(3) Inadequate nutrition
(4) Poverty, i.e, inability to afford heat, food, clothing, or shelter
(5) Recent ingestion of vasoactive agents, e.g., barbiturates, alcohol, or nicotine
(6) Immobilization from trauma while outside in the cold
(7) Wet clothing
(8) Wind chill factor
(9) Fatigue
(10) Refreezing
(11) Burns

4. Explosive blasts

a. Types of injuries
(1) Primary injuries—usually most severe but are frequently overlooked because they may occur without external signs
(a) Direct concussive effects of the pressure wave occur as explosives are converted to an expanding mass of heated gas

(b) Gas-containing organs may rupture, e.g., GI perforation, pneumothorax, alveolar rupture causing air embolism
(c) Small vessels and membranes may tear, e.g., pulmonary bleeding, ruptured tympanic membranes
(d) Central nervous system injury
(2) Secondary injuries
(a) Fragments become high-velocity projectiles
(b) Projectiles cause lacerations, fractures, burns, imbedded foreign materials, and traumatic amputations
(3) Tertiary injuries
(a) Victim becomes a missile and is thrown through the air
(b) Injury pattern is the same as that seen with falls from high places and ejections from automobiles

5. Radiation exposure—severity of injury depends on
a. Intensity of the ionizing radiation (more than 1000 rads is almost always fatal)
b. Type of radiation (least to most dangerous)—alpha particles, beta particles, and gamma rays
c. Distance of victim from radiation source
d. Length of exposure

6. Near-drowning or drowning
a. Etiology
(1) Wet (with aspiration) vs dry (with asphyxiation due to laryngospasm and nonaspiration)
(2) Saltwater vs freshwater submersion
(3) Secondary or delayed drowning—death in minutes to days after the incident
(4) Immersion syndrome—sudden death after submersion in very cold water probably from cardiac arrhythmias
b. Mechanisms protecting against drowning
(1) Immersion hypothermia, which decreases cerebral metabolic demands
(2) Dive reflex, which slows the heart rate and shunts blood to the brain and heart when a person's face is immersed in cold water

Suggested Readings

Andrews, J. F. (1987). Patterns in blunt trauma. *Trauma Quarterly*, 3(4), 1–5.

Barach, E., Tomlanovich, M., & Nowak, R. (1986). Ballistics: A pathophysiologic examination of the wounding mechanisms of firearms: Part 1. *The Journal of Trauma*, 26(3), 225–235.

Barach, E., Tomlanovich, M., & Nowak, R. (1986). Ballistics: A pathophysiologic examination of the wounding mechanisms of firearms: Part II. *The Journal of Trauma*, 26(4), 374–383.

Butman, A., Paturas, J., McSwain, N., & Dineen, J. (Eds.). (1986). *Prehospital trauma life support*. Akron, OH: Education Direction, Inc.

Cardona, V., Hurn, P., Mason, P., Scanlon-Schilpp, A., & Veise-Berry, S. (Eds.). (1988). *Trauma nursing: From resuscitation through rehabilitation*. Philadelphia: W. B. Saunders Co.

Committee on Trauma Research, Commission on Life Sciences, National Research Council and the Institute of Medicine. (1985). *Injury in America: A continuing public health problem.* Washington, DC: National Academy Press.

Feliciano, D. V. (1988). Patterns of injury. In K. M. Mattox, E. E. Moore & D. V. Feliciano (Eds.), *Trauma* (pp. 91–103). East Norwalk, CT: Appleton & Lange.

Orlando, R. (1985). Smoke inhalation injury. *Emergency Care Quarterly, 1*(3), 22–30.

Strange, J. (Ed.). (1987). *Shock trauma care plans.* Springhouse, PA: Springhouse Corp.

MODULE 3
RECORDING AND USING TRAUMA DATA

Susan Butler, MSN, RN, CCRN

Objectives

1.0 Describe common methods of injury scoring.
1.1 List major injury scoring systems used in trauma care.
1.2 Identify variables necessary for obtaining a score by each method.
1.3 State advantages and disadvantages of several injury scoring systems.
2.0 Discuss the nurse's responsibility for documentation in trauma care.
2.1 List rationale for accurate nursing records.
2.2 Identify advantages of using flowsheets in all aspects of trauma care.
2.3 State the types of information essential for documentation in specific phases of the trauma continuum.
3.0 Identify steps in developing a trauma registry.
3.1 List basic information required for setting up a trauma registry.
3.2 Identify three types of data collection.
3.3 Discuss method of data reporting.
3.4 List variables involved in hospital-based vs system-based registries.
3.5 State the specific kinds of data required for hospital-based vs system-based registries.
4.0 Describe components of a comprehensive quality assurance program for the trauma patient.
4.1 Define steps in assuring quality trauma care.

4.2 Define the role of the nursing and surgery departments and the trauma administrator in a trauma quality assurance program.
4.3 Discuss guidelines for videotaping as a quality assurance tool.
5.0 Discuss a situation in which use of collected data changed legislation and encouraged trauma prevention.

A. INJURY SCORING

1. Defining characteristics
a. Measures selected patient characteristics
b. Assesses severity of injury
c. Quantifies mortality and morbidity resulting from injury
d. Develops a common language for comparative studies

2. Purposes
a. Objective evaluation of patient outcome for quality assurance (QA)
b. Comparison of patient outcomes within an institution or between several systems
c. Collection of epidemiologic data on injury
d. Patient classification or triage in the prehospital setting or within an institution

3. Criteria
a. Validity
   (1) Predictive validity—high correlation with outcome measures such as death and disability
   (2) Construct validity—correlation with other severity indicators
   (3) Face validity—reasonable to all users
b. Reliability
   (1) Stability—repeated measurements give the same results
   (2) Interrater—similar measurements obtained when more than one individual collects data
c. Simple to use and can be used with accessible data
d. Independent of quality of medical care

4. Injury severity scales
a. For patient triage—Trauma Score, Revised Trauma Score, Pediatric Trauma Score, CRAMS (Circulation impairment, Respiratory disruption, Abdominal wall tenderness, Motor disruption, Speech impairment)
b. For patient evaluation and research—Abbreviated Injury Scale, Injury Severity Score

5. Trauma Score (TS) (1)
a. Developed by Howard Champion in 1981
b. Provides a rapid and simple method for assessment of patient severity
c. Provides accurate and predictive data on patient survival

d. Utilizes four physiologic parameters combined with the Glasgow Coma Scale (GCS)

(1)

Respiratory Rate	Points
10–24/min	4
25–35/min	3
>35/min	2
1–9/min	1
0	0

(2)

Respiratory Effort	Points
Normal	1
Retractive/ none	0

(3)

Systolic Blood Pressure	Points
>90 mmHg	4
70–90 mmHg	3
50–69 mmHg	2
<50 mmHg	1
0	0

(4)

Capillary Refill	Points
Normal	2
Delayed	1
None	0

(5) Glasgow Coma Scale—based on total points for eye opening, verbal response, motor response

Glasgow Coma Scale	Points
14–15	5
11–13	4
8–10	3
5–7	2
3–4	1

e. Total the points for sections 1, 2, 3, 4, and 5 to obtain Trauma Score; ranges from 0 to 16 with the lowest values indicating the worst prognosis

f. Utilization
   (1) Important field index indicating severity of injury
   (2) Trauma Score of 12 or less indicates greater than 10% probability of death; patient would benefit most from prompt diagnosis and definitive treatment in a trauma center
   (3) Review of prehospital care can be accomplished by monitoring TS in the field and at time of hospital entry; appropriate care would cause TS to improve

g. Limitations
   (1) 20% of patients with severe injuries will not be identified due to physiologic compensation causing undertriage
   (2) TS overtriages the severity of injury when physiologic parameters are altered due to factors other than hypovolemia, hypoxia, or cerebral injury

6. Revised Trauma Score for Triage (RTS-T) (2)

a. Utilizes three categories

Glasgow Coma Scale	Systolic Blood Pressure (mmHg)	Respiratory Rate/min	Coded Points
13–15	>89	10–29	4
9–12	76–89	>29	3
6–8	50–75	6–9	2
4–5	1–49	1–5	1
3	0	0	0

b. Elimination of respiratory expansion and capillary refill makes RTS-T easier to apply in prehospital settings
c. Allows more weight for the GCS which enables isolated head injuries to be better identified
d. An RTS-T-coded value of 11 or less represents a survival rate of less than 90% and indicates the need for evaluation at a trauma center
e. RTS-T is not yet universally accepted; therefore, data needs to be collected for both the TS and RTS-T

7. **Pediatric Trauma Score (PTS)** (3)

a. Developed as a triage tool for pediatric trauma victims
b. Provides rapid and accurate prediction of injury severity in children
c. Assesses severity of six components (see Table 3.1)

Table 3.1

Component	*Severity Category*		
	+2	*+1*	*−1*
Weight	>44 lbs (20 kg)	22–44 lbs (10–20 kg)	<22 lbs (10 kg)
Airway	Normal	Oral or nasal airway	Intubated or tracheostomy
Blood pressure*	>90 mmHg	50–90 mmHg	<50 mmHg
Level of consciousness	Completely awake	Obtunded	Comatose
Open wound	None	Minor	Major or penetrating
Skeletal (fractures)	None	Closed fracture	Open/multiple fractures

*If proper blood presure cuff is not available, blood pressure can be assessed by palpating pulses and assigning a score as follows:
+2—pulse palpable at wrist
+1—pulse palpable at groin
−1—no pulse palpable

d. Obtain total score by adding severity points for each component
   (1) Total points range from +12 indicating no injury, to −6 indicating fatal injury
   (2) A patient with a PTS range of 0 to 8 has increased chance of mortality and should be transported to highest level of trauma care available, preferably a pediatric trauma center
e. Utilization

(1) Important pediatric scoring mechanism for prehospital personnel and emergency care personnel to indicate severity of injury and triage to appropriate facility
(2) A decrease in PTS predicts an increased injury severity and mortality

f. Limitations
(1) The PTS needs to be tested on larger and more diverse populations
(2) An upper age limit group has yet to be defined

8. **CRAMS Scale (4)**

a. Devised specifically for field triage of trauma patients

b. Five categories with 0 to 2 points given in each area
(1) Circulation impairment
(2) Respiratory disruption
(3) Abdominal wall tenderness
(4) Motor disruption
(5) Speech impairment

c. Separates trauma patients into categories of major trauma (scores of 8 or below) or minor trauma (scores of 9 or 10)

d. Advantages
(1) Easy to use in prehospital setting
(2) Accurate predictor of major or minor trauma

e. Disadvantages
(1) Less precise than Trauma Score
(2) Determination of inter- and intrarater reliability for abdominal and thoracic categories not definitive

9. **Abbreviated Injury Scale (AIS) (5)**

a. Introduced in 1971 by the Committee on Injury Scaling; composed of members from the American Association for Automotive Medicine (AAAM), American Medical Association, and Society of Automotive Engineers; revised in 1976, 1980, 1985, and 1990

b. Established a standard language and systematic format to describe severity of injuries from automobile accidents

c. Describes anatomic injury and severity
(1) Severity ranked on a numerical scale from 1 (minor injury) to 6 (critical, survival uncertain)
(2) Injuries are grouped into six body regions
(a) Head/neck—cranium, brain, neck, throat, cervical spine
(b) Face—eyes, nose, mouth, facial structures
(c) Thorax—thoracic organs, ribs, thoracic spine
(d) Abdomen—abdominal pelvic organs, lumbar spine
(e) Extremities—upper and lower limbs, bony pelvis
(f) External—any body surface, integumentary

d. Current edition (AIS-90) contains more than 1200 injury descriptions including blunt and penetrating trauma; has been refined to provide more detailed descriptions of head/neck, thoracic, and abdominal injuries

e. Limitations of current AIS tables
(1) Establishes severity of single system injuries, without accounting for multiple system injuries that can occur
(2) Does not correlate well with outcome measures, e.g., disability, mortality, morbidity

(3) Entire medical record must be reviewed retrospectively for accurate scoring

10. **Injury Severity Score (ISS) (6)**
  a. An extension of AIS developed by Susan Baker and others
  b. Accounts for variations in death rate associated with both severity of trauma and the number of body areas involved (7)
  c. To determine the ISS, take the highest AIS score in each of the three most severely injured body regions, square each one, and total them, e.g.,

AIS Region	Patient Injuries	AIS Score
Head	Fracture base of skull	3
Thorax	Flail chest	4
	Unilateral pneumothorax	3
Extremities	Fractured humerus	2

$$ISS = 3^2 + 4^2 + 2^2 = 29$$

  d. Scores range from 0 to 75 with higher scores indicating an increase in severity of injury and mortality (10% mortality occurs with an ISS of 15)
  e. Advantages/utilization
    (1) Powerful predictor of mortality
    (2) Reflects multiple injuries
    (3) Useful to control case mix in patient populations for evaluation of care, triage, and quality assurance indicators
  f. Disadvantages
    (1) Only provides one score per body region
    (2) Used retrospectively, though current research is being obtained on prospective use

11. **TRISS methodology (2)**
  a. Estimates probability of patient survival
  b. Based on ISS, TS, RTS-T, and patient age
  c. Two techniques
    (1) PRE approach
      (a) Graph with TS plotted against ISS indicating isobar at 50% survival probability
      (b) Unexpected deaths or survivors are indicated, facilitating peer review for quality assurance
    (2) DEF method
      (a) Specific to Major Trauma Outcome Study (MTOS)
      (b) Uses Z and M statistics to compare outcomes between baselines (i.e., national) and study populations

B. NURSING DOCUMENTATION

1. **Provides essential information needed for patient care and provides continuity in care**
2. **Enables health professionals to communicate with each other**

3. **Provides a method for evaluation of care and demonstrates that professional and regulatory standards have been met**
4. **Vital to provide information required for reimbursement**
5. **Provides data for education and research**
6. **Provides a legal justification of actions**
7. **Flowsheets are very advantageous in trauma care**
a. Concise, thorough data reporting on one sheet
b. Specific for each nursing area, i.e., flight, emergency department, operating room
c. May combine areas such as ED or OR when continuing resuscitation
   (1) Allows for easy review of interventions
   (2) Enables continuity of patient care to be followed
d. Can be filled out quickly during an emergent situation
e. Provides data required for trauma registry
8. **Documentation for specialized areas**
a. Prehospital—ground or air transport (also see Module 9—Trauma Transport)
   (1) Single page flowsheet offers rapid, concise documentation
      (a) History of injury and nature of emergency
      (b) Status of patient on arrival and TS
      (c) Brief patient assessment including care given prior to team arrival
      (d) Referring physician or medic
      (e) Receiving physician and facility
      (f) Crew identification
      (g) Travel and on-scene times, mileage
b. Initial receiving facility—prior to transfer of patient to trauma center
   (1) Referring and receiving physicians
   (2) Origin/destination of transfer
   (3) Mode of transportation with estimated departure and arrival times
   (4) Mechanism of injury
   (5) Demographic data
   (6) Trauma protocols initiated
      (a) Primary interventions
      (b) X-rays performed
      (c) Laboratory results
      (d) Wound interventions
c. Trauma center resuscitation area
   (1) Mechanism of injury
   (2) Past medical history, medications, tetanus immunization
   (3) Trauma team members and times of arrival
   (4) Initial assessment—vital signs, GCS, TS
   (5) Primary and secondary interventions
   (6) Intake and output
   (7) Medications
   (8) Diagnostic procedures
   (9) Patient disposition
d. Rehabilitation and patient follow-up
   (1) Follow-up form completed by discharge planning nurse, trauma nurse coordinator, rehabilitation personnel, and/or physician or clinic staff responsible for continuing care

(2) Information for follow-up
   (a) Injury description and severity
   (b) Rehabilitation assessment score, e.g., Rancho Los Amigos, Functional Independence Measure
   (c) Admission/discharge dates
   (d) Past medical history
   (e) Current treatments, medications
   (f) Complications due to injury
   (g) Employment status
   (h) Financial status, assistance, need
   (i) Dwelling place and household composition
(3) Periodic follow-up should occur at discretion of rehabilitation team and/or in accordance with established protocols
(4) If in rehabilitation facility, discharge summary should be requested

C. TRAUMA REGISTRY

1. Definition
a. Data base integrating medical and trauma systems information
b. A comprehensive and accessible means of collecting and reviewing data
c. Provides a method of evaluation
d. Enables storage and analysis of data for future study

2. Register organization
a. Identify goals of register
   (1) Quality assurance
   (2) Injury epidemiology
   (3) Trauma system verification
   (4) Trauma system management
b. Institution-based vs system-based (e.g., EMS council or region)
c. Explore work done by others and what is currently in place
d. Tailor system to meet institution/system needs
e. Structure register for easy integration with other systems or data sources

3. Data collection
a. Concurrent
   (1) Information acquired from patients and their charts via daily rounds
   (2) Accurate and reliable method
   (3) Lengthy time involvement for data collector
   (4) Lapses occur during data collector's time off causing inconsistencies with data
b. Retrospective
   (1) Information collected after discharge when medical record is complete
   (2) Conserves resources and time
   (3) May be difficult to acquire some aspects of data
c. Combination
   (1) Most effective for a thorough collection

(2) Concurrent collection of data acquired daily while patient is in acute phase of care (ED, OR, ICU), followed by less frequent checks throughout remainder of hospitalization
(3) Retrospective review of chart to locate missed information, disabilities, codings, and charges

4. Data reporting

a. Design based on register objectives
   (1) Patient log
      (a) Quick reference of trauma activity updated on a daily basis
      (b) Contains demographic data and/or billing information
      (c) Allows for a quick look at selected data
   (2) Patient abstract/record
      (a) In-depth data collection on a patient
      (b) Includes demographic data, prehospital care, information from emergency department and hospitalization
      (c) Lists procedures and complications
      (d) Includes discharge data, disposition, and follow-up
   (3) Administrative summaries
      (a) Monitor trauma service activity
      (b) Report patient acuity and outcome
      (c) Examine system of care
      (d) Report utilization and costs of resources expended for care
   (4) Quality assurance (process) reports
      (a) Evaluate quality of patient care
      (b) Evaluate functioning of trauma system
      (c) Evaluate specific cases and provide peer review
      (d) Identify expected deaths and/or survivors
   (5) Outcome reports
      (a) Examine patient outcomes based on severity of injury
      (b) Evaluate overall care in system
      (c) Research
         i) Investigates nature of trauma and correlation with injuries
         ii) Establishes standards of care based on specific results achieved
         iii) Compares methods and results of trauma systems over large populations

5. Evaluation of register

a. Reliability
   (1) Sensitivity of register—picks up all cases that should be included
   (2) Specificity of register—contains intended cases that are correctly included, and excludes unintended cases
   (3) Monitor for frequency of missing data
   (4) Monitor data fields with a low completion rate; determine whether rate can be corrected or field eliminated
   (5) Interrater agreement upon random comparison
b. Validity—monitor appropriateness and accuracy of data by having another reviewer reabstract a certain percentage of patient records; compare with registrar's data
c. Utility

(1) Is the current register meeting intended goals?
(2) Does data contribute to changes in policies, procedures, quality assurance, staff education, and prevention activities?

d. Cost effectiveness

6. Hospital-based registry

a. Responsibility shared by trauma program director, trauma program coordinator, registrar, and abstracting personnel

b. Population
(1) All hospitalized patients with injuries classified by ICD-9-CMN coding from 800.00 through 959.90 (8)
(2) Trauma patients requiring activation of trauma system
(3) Transfer patients from another facility
(4) All trauma deaths

c. Limitations
(1) There is not a concise definition of a trauma patient in any system
(2) Registry may not identify
(a) Undertriaged patients
i) Those who should have received trauma care but were not classified appropriately
ii) Those treated at nontrauma center facilities
(b) Overtriaged patients—inappropriately identified as having major injuries, thus consuming system resources inefficiently
(c) Appropriately triaged patients—do not meet any stated criteria

d. Data collection
(1) Patient log—identified by name, medical record number, trauma number
(2) Patient report—all recorded data for a specific patient (see 6e., Minimum data sets)
(3) Administrative summaries
(a) Patient access to trauma center
(b) Flow of patients within hospital
(c) Financial data including charges, collections, and sources of reimbursement
(4) Quality assurance
(a) Availability of resources within hospital
(b) Monitors quality of care given by physicians, nurses, other services
(c) All deaths
(5) Patient outcome reports examine patient outcomes

e. Minimum data sets
(1) Most common type of hospital-based trauma registers
(2) Usually contain 65 to 150 data elements
(3) Described by the MTOS
(a) Demographic—identification (linkage) numbers, incident date and time, injury mechanism, preexisting disease, protective equipment
(b) Prehospital—mode of transport, response times, facility
(c) Emergency—resuscitation initiated, ED time, physician notification, disposition
(d) Clinical data (at scene and on admission)—vital signs, GCS, TS, drug screen

(e) Surgery—operation date and time, procedures, unexpected operations
(f) Intensive care—number of days
(g) Outcome—total hospital days, complications, disposition, functional status, AIS/ISS scores

f. Specialized data sets—more descriptive for particular injuries and populations, e.g., burns, spinal cord, pediatric

7. **System-based registry**

a. Responsibility
(1) Regional trauma system
(2) Emergency Medical Services Council
(3) System register personnel

b. Population
(1) All patients triaged to trauma centers
(2) All patients treated by a trauma response team
(3) All patients transferred from nondesignated hospitals to trauma centers
(4) All patients hospitalized in trauma centers with injuries classified by ICD-9-CMN codes from 800.00 through 959.90 (8)

c. Data collection
(1) Patient log—identified by crash report number, prehospital report number, date of birth
(2) Patient record—contains selected data only
(3) Administrative summaries—report patient flow within overall system
(4) Quality assurance
(a) Monitors system access and prehospital care
(b) Monitors patient population in nondesignated hospitals and trauma centers
(c) Identifies all deaths for review
(5) Outcome reports
(a) Examine patient outcomes and severity of injury on a system basis
(b) Can evaluate institutions within the system

d. Limited data sets
(1) Usually fewer than 30 data elements per case
(a) Demographic—identification (linkage) numbers, incident date and time, injury mechanism, protective equipment
(b) Prehospital—response times, mode of transport, trauma score, facility
(c) Disposition

D. QUALITY ASSURANCE (QA)

1. **Definition**

a. An ongoing systematic evaluation of care
b. A plan to ensure that an agreed upon level of excellence is maintained

2. **Objectives**

a. Measure care and compare to written standards
b. Introduce changes based on information acquired

c. Monitor for improvement of care given

3. JCAHO ten-step QA process (9)

a. Assign responsibility
b. Identify scope of care—types of patients or diagnoses, treatments performed, site of care provided
c. Identify important aspects of care to be monitored and evaluated
   (1) High volume—seen often
   (2) High risk to patient
   (3) Problem-prone, e.g., causing patient infection; staff unfamiliar with equipment
d. Identify indicators—measurable variables of care
   (1) Structural—includes framework, environment
   (2) Process—addresses methods and activities related to patient
   (3) Outcome—patient response to care, functional status, end result
e. Establish threshold for evaluation—should be a preestablished level of performance based on literature and institutional standards of care
f. Collect and organize data
g. Analyze data
h. Take action—specify appropriate activities, time frame, and responsible person
i. Continue reviews to assess effectiveness of actions and document improvement
j. Communicate findings

4. Trauma system quality assurance program

a. Follows continuum from prehospital care through rehabilitation
b. Involves multidisciplinary services
c. Integral part of hospital medical and nursing quality assurance programs
d. Responsibility of trauma nurse coordinator, trauma director, and program administrator
e. Based on institution and trauma program philosophy and values

5. Trauma nursing quality assurance program

a. Integral part of institution's nursing QA program
   (1) Chaired by nursing representative of trauma program, trauma nurse coordinator, or nursing QA coordinator
   (2) Committee membership representative of all units involved in care of trauma patients
   (3) Standards of care are written stating appropriate care of trauma patients
b. Unit representatives assist staff in ongoing evaluation of indicators specific to their units and report findings to QA committee
c. Chair of trauma nursing QA program collects and evaluates results of monitoring
d. A corrective plan of action is developed and implemented with input from committee members
e. Action plan is evaluated through focused review, and problem is determined to be resolved or to require further investigation
f. Trauma system in nursing department is evaluated by specific indicators reflecting appropriate standards of care
   (1) Indicators can be structural, process, or outcome; may be applied at various phases of the trauma continuum
   (2) Example—an indicator examining appropriate cervical spine immobilization can be evaluated in flight nursing, emergency department, operating room, intensive care unit, and medical-surgical unit

g. All information is communicated to the nursing QA committee and trauma program QA committee

6. **Trauma surgical quality assurance committee**

a. Integral part of medical-surgical department QA program
   (1) Chaired by surgical representative of trauma program, trauma director, surgical director, or department QA coordinator
   (2) Committee membership representative of all surgeons involved in care of trauma patients

b. Standards of care are based on national standards, e.g., American College of Surgeons Committee on Trauma, Joint Commission on the Accreditation of Health Care Organizations, or state and institutional norms

c. Cases are examined through peer review for process and outcome of patient care
   (1) Examine probability of survival vs actual outcome of patient
   (2) Review, in depth, unexpected survivals and unexpected deaths focusing on treatment protocols, time of treatment, preexisting factors in patients, functioning of trauma system in institution

d. Based on results obtained from review, a corrective plan of action is developed and implemented to improve surgical management of trauma patient

e. Evaluation of action plan is continued

f. Information is communicated to the hospital QA committee and trauma program QA committee

7. **Trauma program (system) quality assurance committee**

a. Cochaired by a surgeon and a trauma nurse
   (1) Committee membership includes medical and nursing QA coordinators, medical records representative or trauma registrar, and all physicians (e.g., anesthesia, neurosurgery, orthopaedics) involved in trauma program
   (2) Nurses from trauma units may also be represented
   (3) A representative from major departments involved in trauma care may be invited, i.e., emergency department, radiology, blood bank, laboratory

b. Aspects of care are identified based on
   (1) National standards, e.g., American College of Surgeons
   (2) State and institutional norms
   (3) Areas of concern that may encompass several clinical disciplines

c. Medical records representative or trauma registrar reports findings of pertinent data to the QA committee based on charts abstracted

d. Representative from trauma nursing and trauma surgeons QA committees report findings and action plans

e. When program problems are identified, the chairman develops and implements a corrective plan of action with input from all committee members

f. Evaluation of action plan is accomplished and determines whether problem is resolved or further investigation is necessary

8. **Administrative support**

a. Trauma administrator must see QA program as valid and essential

b. Support is manifested by providing financial resources for personnel, overtime, and education, and through demonstrated commitment to program

9. **Videotaping resuscitations as a QA tool**

a. Used to evaluate compliance with standards of resuscitation specific to the institution

(1) Timeliness of team member arrivals
(2) Adherence to dress code in trauma room
(3) Identifiable team leader
(4) Appropriate sequence of resuscitation

b. Must maintain anonymity of patient
(1) Place camera high and at foot of stretcher
(2) Do not identify by time or patient record numbers

c. Must have written policy and procedure, reviewed by institution's legal representative
(1) Erase tape within 24 hours
(2) Limit tape reviewers
(3) Store tapes in locked cabinet, accessible only to appropriate QA personnel

d. Options for using tapes
(1) Tape all resuscitations and view all tapes
(a) Advantageous for a new program
(b) Excellent educational opportunity for new trauma team
(2) Randomize taping of resuscitations and view all tapes
(3) Tape all resuscitations and randomly view 25%

E. RELATING TRAUMA REGISTER TO TRAUMA PREVENTION

1. **Almost half of all trauma deaths occur upon impact or shortly after injury: therefore, prevention is the most effective intervention to reduce trauma deaths**
2. **Traumatic injuries can be reduced if increased attention is given to prevention modalities**
3. **Data acquired via trauma scoring systems, data registries, and QA programs can be used on a local, regional, or national level to promote prevention**

a. Data will define populations at greatest risk of injury
b. Prevention programs can then be aimed at those identified groups
c. Traumatic events can be tracked and prevention programs initiated
d. Data can impact legislation and establish new standards
(1) Data from the National Burn Information Exchange indicated devastating injuries in young children when clothing ignited (10)
(2) Analysis and communication of this data led to the establishment of flammability standards for children's sleepwear and other fabrics
(3) In young children, mortality and morbidity from burns due to flammable fabrics decreased approximately 75% between 1968 and 1979 (11)

References

1. Champion, H. R., Sacco, W. J., Carnazzo, A. J., Copes, W. S., & Fouty, W. J. (1981). Trauma score. *Critical Care Medicine,* 9(9), 672–676.
2. Boyd, C. R., Tolson, M. A., & Copes, W. S. (1987). Evaluating trauma care: The TRISS method. *The Journal of Trauma,* 27(4), 370–378.

3. Tepas, J., Romanenofsky, M., Mollitt, D., Ganz, B., & DiScala, C. (1988). The pediatric trauma score as a predictor of injury severity: An objective assessment. *The Journal of Trauma, 28*(4), 425–429.
4. Gormican, S. P. (1982). CRAMS scale: Field triage of trauma victims. *Annals of Emergency Medicine, 11*(3), 132–135.
5. Association for the Advancement of Automotive Medicine. (1990). *Abbreviated injury scale, 1990 revision.* Des Plaines, IL: Author.
6. Baker, S. P., O'Neill, B., Haddon, W., Jr., & Long, W. B. (1974). The injury severity score: A method for describing patients with multiple injuries and evaluating emergency care. *The Journal of Trauma, 14*(3), 187–196.
7. Greenspan, L., McLellan, B. A., & Greig, H. (1985). Abbreviated injury scale and injury severity score: A scoring chart. *The Journal of Trauma, 25*(1), 60–64.
8. U.S. Department of Health and Human Services. (1989). *International classification of diseases, 9th revision* (DHHS Publication No. PHS 89-1260, Vol. 1, 3rd ed).
9. Joint Commission on the Accreditation of Healthcare Organizations. (1988). *Guide to quality assurance.* Chicago: Author.
10. Feller, I., & Jones, C. (1987). The national burn information exchange. *Surgical Clinics of North America, 67*(1), 167–189.
11. Baker, S. P., O'Neill, B., & Karpf, R. S. (1984). *The injury fact book.* Lexington, MA: Lexington Books.

Suggested Readings

Cales, R. H., Bietz, D. S., & Heilig, R. W. (1985). The trauma registry: A method of providing regional system audit using the microcomputer. *The Journal of Trauma, 25*(3), 181–187.

Cales, R. H., & Kearns, S. T. (1989). Concepts. *Trauma Quarterly, 5*(3), 1–8.

Cales, R. H. (1989). Reports. *Trauma Quarterly, 5*(3), 9–16.

Hoyt, D., Shackford, S., Hollingsworth-Fridlund, P., Mackersie, R., Hansbrough, J., Wachtel, T., & Fortune, J. (1988). Video recording trauma resuscitations: An effective teaching technique. *The Journal of Trauma, 26*(4), 435–440.

Mattox, K. L., Moore E. E., Feliciano, D. V., (1988). *Trauma.* East Norwalk, CT: Appleton & Lange.

Mayer, T. A., & Keaton, B. F. (1989). Data sets. *Trauma Quarterly, 5*(3), 17–24.

Patterson, C. H. (1988). Standards of patient care: The Joint Commission focus on nursing quality assurance. *Nursing Clinics of North America, 23*(3), 625–637.

Shackford, S. R., Hollingsworth-Fridlund, P., McArdle, M., & Eastman, A. B. (1987). Assuring quality in a trauma system—the medical audit committee: Composition, cost, and results. *The Journal of Trauma, 27*(8), 866–875.

Thompson, J., & Dains, J. (1986). Indices of injury: Development and status. *Nursing Clinics of North America, 21*(4), 655–671.

MODULE 4
PREVENTION OF TRAUMA

Pat Walsh, MSN, RN, C

Objectives

1.0 **Recognize trauma as a preventable disease.**
1.1 List the types of energy that cause physical injury.
1.2 Describe the difference between intentional and unintentional injuries.
2.0 **Relate injury theories with regard to occurrence and intervention.**
2.1 Review the five postulates of injury occurrence.
2.2 Describe the three phases of an injury event.
2.3 List several strategies for injury control.
2.4 Define and relate an example of a countermeasure, stating the advantages and problems associated with that strategy.
3.0 **Briefly describe the role of the nurse in trauma prevention education.**
3.1 Define health education in relation to trauma.
3.2 Review the health belief model with regard to injury prevention.
3.3 State the three levels of prevention intervention applied to trauma care.
4.0 **Evaluate the potential for nursing education in trauma prevention.**
4.1 Discuss the expanded role for nurses in trauma prevention education.
4.2 Relate opportunities that exist to promote trauma prevention education.

A. CONCEPTS RELATED TO TRAUMA PREVENTION

1. Introduction

a. Trauma—leading cause of death in people ages 1 to 44
   (1) Injuries occur throughout the life spectrum
   (2) Population most at risk remains young males
b. Major cure for trauma is prevention
   (1) Sophisticated technology and rapid emergency response cannot substitute for preventive action
   (2) Prevention educators must address diverse audiences with complex attitudes, beliefs, and behaviors
      (a) Concepts of youth and immortality are embedded in our psyche
      (b) Various strategies are needed to challenge risk-taking behavior and heighten safety awareness
      (c) All trauma education efforts require basic knowledge of prevention concepts and health education theories to effectively promote safety and reduce injury
c. Trauma nursing is holistic
   (1) Nurses are key health professionals to make people cognizant of the potential for harm
   (2) Nurses carry out trauma prevention efforts in diverse settings including classrooms, community halls, and retirement homes

2. Trauma as a disease

a. Trauma means bodily injury
b. Trauma is caused by applied physical energy
   (1) Kinetic—mechanical energy related to moving objects
   (2) Chemical energy
   (3) Thermal energy
   (4) Electrical energy
   (5) Radiation
c. The application of energy is
   (1) Intentional or
   (2) Unintentional
   (3) Rarely random

B. INJURY OCCURRENCE AND CONTROL

1. Models to explain injury occurrence (1)

a. Single-cause theory, e.g., car crash caused by excessive speed
b. Random interaction of multiple factors, e.g., driver suffers a heart attack and loses control of vehicle, which then plunges into a crowd of people
c. Specific human-environment interactions occurring in
   (1) Preinjury phase—time immediately prior to the release of energy
   (2) Injury phase—the released energy is applied to people and property

(3) Postinjury phase—the final outcome is determined by various homeostatic mechanisms

d. Systems analysis of technologic design, e.g., motor vehicles, roadways
e. Extended epidemiologic review of probable causation

2. **Injury control strategies (2)**

a. Preventing the creation of hazards, e.g., draining swimming pools in the off-season
b. Reducing the number of hazards, e.g., limiting speeds of vehicles
c. Preventing the release of hazards, e.g., improved gasoline tank designs in cars and trucks
d. Modifying the rate or spatial distribution of hazards, e.g., seat belts
e. Separating potential hazards in terms of time or space, e.g., restriction of time for spraying fields with poisons; maintaining electric power lines that are unreachable
f. Separating hosts from hazards using material barriers, e.g., helmets
g. Modifying the characteristics of hazards by surface or structure, e.g., rounded dashboard edges; air bags
h. Increasing the resistance of hosts to damage, e.g., reducing sports injuries by stronger musculature
i. Countering the damage that has already occurred, e.g., emergency medical services
j. Stabilizing, repairing, and restoring function to the damaged host, e.g., trauma centers

C. EDUCATIONAL AND LEGISLATED INJURY CONTROL APPROACHES

1. **Educational-persuasive strategy**

a. Voluntary behavior alteration, which requires
   (1) Perception of self to be at risk for injury
   (2) Belief that behavior change will reduce risk of personal injury
   (3) Consistent performance of countermeasures to reduce risk, e.g., always wearing a seat belt; never driving while intoxicated
b. Problems encountered with educational strategy include
   (1) Lack of scientific evaluation to document effectiveness
   (2) Costly to incorporate for diverse population
   (3) Mass media provide counterinfluence by continued repetition of violent and risk-taking behaviors
   (4) Retrospective review of injury events reveals that lack of knowledge is not the problem; failure to apply the knowledge is more prevalent

2. **Legal regulation of behavior**

a. Federal regulations for motor vehicles
   (1) Federal Motor Vehicle Safety Standard 208 requires the introduction of automatic occupant protection systems, such as safety belts that are automatic, or air bags, in automobiles manufactured for sale in the U.S., beginning with model year 1990

   (2) National Traffic and Motor Vehicle Safety Act and the Highway Safety Act of 1966 promote safe roadways and standardize safety features in automobiles
b. State regulations for motor vehicles
   (1) Speed limit compliance on most highways at 55–65 mph
   (2) Increased enforcement of laws against drinking and driving
   (3) Mandatory child safety seat and seat belt usage in all 50 states and the District of Columbia
   (4) Mandatory helmet usage for drivers of all-terrain vehicles, dirt bikes, and motorcycles
c. Building and housing codes
   (1) Installation of smoke detector and automatic sprinkler systems
   (2) Floor covering standards to protect against falls
   (3) Access for handicapped
   (4) Physical barriers for swimming pools
   (5) Mandatory nonscald settings for hot water heaters
d. Violence
   (1) Uniform laws to license and control the purchase and possession of handguns
   (2) Uniform laws to license and control the purchase and possession of alcohol and medically prescribed drugs
e. Problems encountered with legislative regulation of behavior include
   (1) Detection and conviction not consistently probable
   (2) Punishment varies; severity is a factor for deterrence
   (3) Complex societal attitudes regarding personal pleasure, convenience, and comfort; the rights of the individual vs the good of the society

3. Automatic environmental protection

a. Motor vehicles
   (1) Federal safety standards by Department of Transportation (DOT) for the manufacture of new cars include
      (a) Crash avoidance, e.g., glare reduction; braking systems
      (b) Injury severity reduction, e.g., seat belts, air bags, headrests
      (c) Postcrash safety, e.g., stronger gas tanks
   (2) Biomechanical engineering for improved vehicular design
      (a) Automatic safety restraints
      (b) Air bags—front seats
      (c) Energy-absorbing steering columns and dashboards
      (d) Refinement of windshield design
b. Roads and highways
   (1) Improved highway design to remove obstacles
   (2) Increased use of impact attenuators on highways, e.g., sand-filled barrels
   (3) Appropriate time delays for street crossings in neighborhoods with many elderly or children
   (4) Creation of bike paths
c. Consumer products
   (1) Development of flame-retardant clothing and furnishings
   (2) Improved safety design of toys and playground equipment
   (3) Safety packaging of medications and foods to prevent poisoning
   (4) Helmets and impact-absorbing equipment for sports injury reduction

D. INTRODUCTION OF HEALTH EDUCATION CONCEPTS

1. **Definition of health education—"Any combination of learning experiences designed to facilitate voluntary adaptations of behavior conductive to health" (3, p. 95)**
2. **Identification of key words (3)**
   a. Belief—statement of sense, declared or implied, intellectually and/or emotionally accepted as true by a person or group
   b. Attitude—relatively constant feeling or set of beliefs directed toward an object, person, or situation
   c. Value—preference shared within a community
   d. Behavior—action that has a specific frequency, duration, and purpose, whether conscious or unconscious
3. **Incorporation of the health belief model in trauma prevention education (4)**
   a. Health-related action on the part of the individual depends on the simultaneous occurrence of the following factors
      (1) Personal concern or motivation that makes the health issue relevant
      (2) Belief that personal susceptibility to threat exists
      (3) Belief that following particular health recommendations will reduce the perceived threat
   b. Specific trauma programming for the community should include
      (1) Increasing awareness of the problem thereby raising personal concern
      (2) Realistic depiction of the physical effects for unsuspecting/unbelieving population
      (3) Providing convincing evidence that safety measures are effective in reducing morbidity and mortality
4. **Review of social learning theory**
   a. Behavior is determined by expectancies
      (1) About environmental cues—what leads to what
      (2) About the consequences of one's own actions—otherwise termed outcome expectation
      (3) About one's own competence to perform the behaviors needed to influence outcomes—otherwise termed efficacy expectation
   b. Behavior is determined by incentives
5. **Other educational theories influencing trauma prevention programs**
   a. Rational model—facts and information will ultimately shape attitudes and consequently behavior
   b. Social norms—affect educational content and methods of presenting educational information
   c. Developmental theory—determines appropriate learning objectives for age-specific education
6. **Trauma prevention education should occur on three levels:**
   a. Primary—consumer health education that intends to prevent an injury event
   b. Secondary—patient health education that explains the injury event and intends to prevent subsequent injuries
   c. Tertiary—client health education that intends to prevent injury as sequelae to a handicapped state

E. PROFESSIONAL IMPLEMENTATION OF TRAUMA PREVENTION

1. **Review of practice standards**
a. Governmental recommendations by the Department of Health and Human Services include assessment of community resources and needs for health care, with participation in the development of resources to meet those needs
b. Professional standards determined by nursing organizations
   (1) American Nurses' Association
      (a) Nursing actions that provide for client or patient participation in health promotion, maintenance, and restoration
      (b) Nursing actions that assist client or patient participation to maximize his/her health capabilities
   (2) Society of Trauma Nurses
   (3) Trauma-related nursing specialty organizations, e.g.,
      (a) Emergency Nurses' Association
      (b) American Association of Critical Care Nurses
      (c) Association of Operating Room Nurses
c. Professional standards determined by related professional organizations
   (1) American College of Surgeons
   (2) American College of Emergency Physicians
   (3) American Academy of Pediatrics
2. **Opportunities for involvement**
a. Community-based programs, e.g., "Buckle Up" project (DOT); the "Safe Kids" campaign; the National Head and Spinal Cord Injury Prevention Program
b. Hospital-based programs, e.g., "Life Is Fragile: Handle with Care"; "Staying Alive"; "Trauma of Drinking, Drugs, and Driving"
c. Professional programs, e.g., American Trauma Society—"Tommy Trauma"; Emergency Nurses' Association—"We Care"
3. **Future trends in trauma prevention**
a. Secondary prevention for trauma patients to minimize recidivism—recurrence of injury
b. Tertiary prevention for handicapped clients, with environmental emphasis
c. Multidisciplinary research efforts to measure behavioral responses to prevention education
d. Increased interaction with legislators and biomechanical engineers to combine efforts in minimizing overall incidence of injury

References

1. Benner, L., Jr. (1985). Accident theory and accident investigators. In J. M. Last (Ed.), *Maxcy Rosenau public health and preventive medicine* (12th ed., pp. 1550–1551). New York: Appleton-Century-Crofts.
2. Haddon, W., Jr., & Baker, S. P. (1981). Injury control. In D. Clark & B.

MacMahon (Eds.), *Preventive and community medicine* (pp. 111–113). Boston: Little, Brown & Co.
3. Green, L. W., & Lewis, F. M. (1980). *Health education planning: A diagnostic approach* (pp. 95–97). Palo Alto, CA: Mayfield Publishing Co.
4. Rosenstock, I. M., Stretcher, V., & Becker, M. (1988). Social learning theory and the health belief model. *Health Education Quarterly, 15*(2), 175–183.

Suggested Readings

Baker, S. P., O'Neill, B., & Karpf, R. S. (1984). *The injury fact book.* Lexington, MA: Lexington Books.

Committee on Trauma Research, Commission on Life Sciences, National Research Council, and the Institute of Medicine. (1985). *Injury in America: A continuing public health problem.* Washington, DC: National Academy Press.

Edwards, L. (1986). Health education. In C. Edelman & C. L. Mandle (Eds.), *Health promotion throughout the lifespan* (pp. 94–112). St. Louis: C. V. Mosby Co.

Fontaine, D. K. (1989). Physical, personal, and cognitive responses to trauma. *Critical Care Nursing Clinics of North America, 1*(1), 11–22.

Jacobs, L. M., Jr., & Jacobs, B. B. (1988). Injuries: Statistics, preventions, and costs. In K. Mattox, E. Moore, & D. Feliciano (Eds.), *Trauma.* East Norwalk, CT: Appleton & Lange.

Murray, R. B., & Zentner, J. P. (1985). *Nursing concepts for health promotion* (3rd ed.). Englewood Cliffs, NJ: Prentice-Hall.

Nahum, A. M., & Melvin, J. (Eds.). (1985). *The biomechanics of trauma.* Norwalk, CT: Appleton-Century-Crofts.

Promoting health/preventing disease: Objectives for the nation. (1980, Fall). Washington, DC: U.S. Department of Health and Human Services, Public Health Service.

United States Public Health Service, Office of the Surgeon General. (1979). *Healthy people: The surgeon general's report on health promotion and disease prevention.* (USDHEW Publication No. PHS 79-55071A, pp. 53–80). Washington, DC: U.S. Government Printing Office.

Waller, J. A. (1986). Prevention of premature death and disability due to injury. In J. M. Last (Ed.), *Maxcy Rosenau public health and preventive medicine* (12th ed.). New York: Appleton-Century-Crofts.

Section II
Trauma Nursing and the Health Care System

MODULE 5
EMERGENCY MEDICAL SERVICES SYSTEMS

Jean Will, MSN, RN, CEN, EMT-P

Objectives

1.0 Define emergency medical services systems.
2.0 Briefly describe the historical background and highlights of EMS systems development.
2.1 Discuss the effects of various wars regarding actual care, transportation, and system organization.
2.2 Recognize the differences between cardiac care and trauma care.
2.3 Describe the impact of the National Academy of Sciences–National Research Council paper, "Accidental Death and Disability: The Neglected Disease of Modern Society."
2.4 Discuss the impact of the federal EMS legislation of 1973.
3.0 Describe the major components of the EMS system.
4.0 Discuss the prehospital providers' roles and responsibilities.
4.1 First responder.
4.2 Emergency medical technician (EMT).
4.3 Emergency medical technician paramedic (EMT-P).
4.4 Mobile intensive care nurse (MICN) or health professional nurse.
4.5 Physician.
4.6 Dispatcher.
5.0 Discuss current EMS legislation on the federal and state levels.
6.0 Identify and discuss four major current issues affecting the development of EMS today.

A. EMERGENCY MEDICAL SERVICES (EMS) DEFINED

1. **Began as a method of transportation of the sick and injured**
2. **Evolved into a comprehensive system that responds to an individual's actual or perceived need for immediate intervention in order to prevent loss of life or aggravation of physiological or psychological illness or injury**
3. **Integration of all components includes the following steps in a chain of events scenario**
   a. Event occurs—medical, traumatic, psychological
   b. Detection—includes recognition of the problem and the need for assistance
   c. Notification and temporary action
      (1) Centralized access through 911 is *not* available nationwide
      (2) The public must know how to access the local system for emergency services
      (3) Temporary action provides immediate basic life support until an ambulance arrives
      (4) Ideally performed by someone trained as a first responder
   d. Dispatch of the appropriate resources occurs in a predetermined fashion
   e. Response often occurs in a tiered manner including
      (1) Police
      (2) First responders
      (3) Basic life support ambulance
      (4) Advanced life support ambulance
      (5) Other specialized units as needed
         (a) Hazardous materials units
         (b) Electric/gas companies
   f. Care at the scene is dependent on
      (1) Levels of personnel (training)
      (2) Patient needs
      (3) Medical protocols
   g. Communications—essential for coordination and medical command, especially between
      (1) On-scene units
      (2) Base station medical command
      (3) Receiving facilities
      (4) Specialty units
   h. Transport of the patient to the most appropriate facility occurs next
   i. Inhospital care continues through the
      (1) Emergency department
      (2) Operating room
      (3) Postanesthesia recovery unit
      (4) Intensive care units
      (5) Medical-surgical units
   j. Rehabilitation—essential to return the persons to their maximum potential
4. **Prevention**
   a. Major component often overlooked
   b. Epidemiologic model useful for illness and injury prevention
   c. Reduces the need for EMS services

B. EMS HISTORICAL DEVELOPMENT

1. **Early development and military impact**
a. Earliest mention of EMS in Homer's *Iliad*
b. Documentation of care to the injured continues through the Roman Empire
c. 19th-century improvements included lightweight horse-drawn carriage to transport the injured to definitive care facility close to the battle line; developed by Baron Dominique Jean Larrey, chief surgeon for Napoleon
d. Aeromedical transport utilizing hot air balloons began in the 1870s, during the Franco-Prussian War (Siege of Paris)
e. From World War I, 1914 to 1918, to more recent conflicts, evacuation time from the battlefield to definitive care has progressively decreased, with subsequent decreases in mortality rate (1)
f. Major improvements in technology and system of care have occurred with each conflict
   (1) WW I—technology improved; Thomas ring splint reduced mortality rate from fractured femur from 80% to 20%
   (2) WW II—universal draft forced physicians into field evacuation and care
   (3) Korea—patients were transported directly to a MASH unit via helicopter for definitive care
   (4) Vietnam—rapid evacuation and medical corpsmen trained in more advanced techniques
2. **Civilian developments**
a. Before World War II
   (1) Hospital-based ambulances
   (2) Attendants received little or no training
   (3) Transport only—care initiated at hospital, not in ambulance
b. During and after World War II
   (1) Fire companies, volunteers, and others provided ambulance service
   (2) Hearses operated by mortuaries were often used as ambulances through the 1970s
c. Classic 1942 study by Trueta suggested survival was greater with early care
d. Belfast, 1966—John Pantridge, M.D., successfully demonstrated the efficacy of using physicians to correct ventricular fibrillation outside of the hospital
e. Miami, late 1960s—Eugene Nagel, M.D., began training nonprofessional rescue personnel in treatment and stabilization techniques similar to Pantridge
f. National Academy of Sciences released the National Research Council report, "Accidental Death and Disability: The Neglected Disease of Modern Society" (2)
   (1) Identified weaknesses in prehospital care and the inadequate EMS system
   (2) Outlined goals and implementation strategies for EMS system development
g. Resultant presidential and congressional interest led to
   (1) Highway Safety Act
   (2) National Traffic and Motor Vehicle Safety Act of 1966
   (3) New role for federal involvement leading to
      (a) Training programs
      (b) Improved equipment design standards for ambulances

(c) Improved communications
(d) Guidelines and standards for EMS operations

h. U.S. Department of Transportation—National Highway Traffic Safety Administration began research and demonstration projects and introduced the role of a new health care provider, the emergency medical technician
i. Robert Wood Johnson Foundation projects funded the development of EMS communications in 45 locales with the goal of integrating an area's EMS resources into a comprehensive network
j. Emergency Medical Services Act of 1973 (Public Law 93-154, amended 1976, 1979) was signed into law
   (1) Provided the mechanisms and funds for communities to develop effective coordination and delivery of regional EMS systems
   (2) Included 15 mandatory components; each EMS system must address
      (a) Manpower—provides an adequate number of appropriately trained and experienced personnel, available 24 hours a day, 7 days a week
      (b) Training—provides appropriate programs for all levels of personnel, from lay public to physician
      (c) Communications—develops system to interconnect personnel, facilities, and equipment with appropriate components
         i) Centralized dispatch utilizing call screening
         ii) 911
      (d) Transportation—provides an adequate number of ground, air, and water vehicles meeting standards of location, design, performance, and equipment; staffed with appropriate personnel
      (e) Facilities—categorizes to identify readiness and capability of each hospital in the region
         i) Limits duplication of services
         ii) Ensures adequate number of appropriate, easily accessible facilities 24 hours a day
      (f) Critical care units—ensures access either directly or through interhospital transfer to appropriate specialty unit
         i) Trauma
         ii) Burns
         iii) Spinal cord injury
         iv) Cardiac care
         v) Poisonings
         vi) High-risk infants and mothers
         vii) Behavioral/psychiatric emergencies
      (g) Public safety agencies—provides for coordination and mutual aid plans between agencies for day-to-day operations, as well as disasters
      (h) Consumer participation—provides opportunities for lay public to participate in policymaking
      (i) Accessibility to care—provides access to emergency services regardless of ability to pay
      (j) Transfer of patients—develops formalized agreements to provide definitive care and follow-up to allow maximum recovery
      (k) Coordinated recordkeeping—standardizes recordkeeping system that traces patient from entry at prehospital phases through hospitalization and rehabilitation

(l) Public information and education—disseminates information on access to the system, appropriate use, cost, and first aid training
(m) Review and evaluation—provides periodic, comprehensive, and independent review of the extent and quality of the EMS system
(n) Disaster linkages—plans for multiagency function during a mass casualty incident
(o) Mutual aid—arranges for reciprocal services where access would be more effective in response, distance, and resources

(3) Provided $185 million for systems that addressed the 15 components in four phases
(a) Feasibility and planning
(b) Establishment and operations
(c) Improvement and expansion
(d) Training

k. Early prehospital care successful for the cardiac patient but not for the trauma patient
(1) Myocardial infarction (MI) patients survived with intervention at the scene
(2) Trauma patients died with similar interventions
(3) Changes are occurring in prehospital trauma care as the study of trauma gains momentum
(4) American College of Surgeons developed educational programs such as Advanced Trauma Life Support (1979)

l. Emergency residency programs began to develop, especially after 1976; emergency medicine became the 23rd medical specialty in 1979

m. With the end of federal categorical funding in 1981, the Preventive Health and Human Services block grant program was implemented allowing states to divide monies among
(1) EMS
(2) Health incentive grants
(3) Hypertension control
(4) Rodent control
(5) School-based fluoridation
(6) Health education/risk reduction
(7) Home health
(8) Rape crisis centers

n. Individual states have enacted specific legislation to meet their own needs

C. PREHOSPITAL PROVIDERS

NOTE: There are more than 30 variations designating emergency medical services personnel levels nationwide. The following reflect the most common designations.

1. First responder

a. Nonmedical person readily available in the community
b. 45 hrs of training based on U.S. Department of Transportation (DOT) guidelines
c. Supports life until ambulance arrives

d. Must recertify every three years

2. Emergency Medical Technician (EMT)

a. Minimum recommended level of training for ambulance personnel
b. 81 to 160 hrs based on DOT guidelines
c. Includes training in patient assessment, cardiopulmonary resuscitation (CPR), basic oxygen administration, management of bleeding, soft tissue injuries, shock, fractures, medical emergencies, childbirth, environmental emergencies, vehicle rescue, and behavioral emergencies
d. 10 hrs clinical experience in emergency department required
e. May use pneumatic antishock garment (PASG) or military antishock trousers (MAST) upon medical command
f. All EMT skills are noninvasive
g. Must recertify every three years

3. Emergency Medical Technician-Paramedic (EMT-P; Paramedic)

a. Capable of performing advanced life support in addition to basic life support
b. Prerequisite—EMT certification
c. 600 to 1500 hours of didactic, clinical, and field preceptorship, based on DOT guidelines
d. Functions under medical control either through direct voice communication, protocol, or standing orders from a physician or authorized nurse, i.e., mobile intensive care nurse (MICN)
e. Skills include venipuncture, administration of intravenous (I.V.) fluids, administration of medications, advanced airway management, electrocardiograph (ECG) monitoring, defibrillation, and cardioversion
f. Additional skills at the discretion of state legislation and medical command
g. Must recertify every three years

4. Emergency Medical Technician—Intermediate

a. Role varies state to state
b. Usually allows for I.V. fluids, defibrillation, and, possibly, additional airway management skills

5. Nurses

a. Depending on the state, utilization in prehospital care varies
b. Mobile intensive care nurses designation may allow clinical prehospital practice or provision of radio instruction to field paramedics
c. State recognition may be required for nurses to function in the prehospital setting
d. Flight nursing provides another arena for prehospital nursing involvement since most flight programs provide on-scene services, as well as interfacility services (see Module 9—Trauma Transport)
e. The nursing role in prehospital care is under scrutiny regarding cost-effectiveness, the shortage of nurses, and appropriate role functions

6. Physicians

a. Few provide direct clinical care in the prehospital setting
b. Some states require "recognition" as a health professional physician
c. Provide medical command and quality assurance (QA)
    (1) Prospective—guide protocol development
    (2) Immediate—direct command to field personnel
    (3) Retrospective—review patient records and audit actual calls via tape review for QA

7. **Dispatchers**
   a. Receive technical training on communications equipment to effect rapid, accurate dispatch
   b. Many now receive emergency medical dispatch training that includes prearrival instructions for first aid and BLS

D. FEDERAL LEGISLATION

1. **Senate Bill 15—The Emergency Medical Services and Trauma Care Improvement Act (1989) requires development of state trauma plans and criteria for trauma center designation in order to receive funding**
2. **House Bill 1602—The Trauma Care Systems Planning and Development Act (1989)**
3. **House Bill 1587—The Rural Emergency Medical Services Improvement Act (1989) establishes state grants to improve the availability and quality of rural EMS**
4. **Above initiatives reconciled to P.L. 101-590 in 1990, with limited funding ($5 million in FY92; 10% to rural development)**

E. CURRENT STATUS AND ISSUES IN EMS DEVELOPMENT

1. **The U.S. is divided into 304 federal EMS regions**
2. **There is a trend toward paid prehospital care, but majority of care is provided by volunteers**
3. **Manpower shortages are common in both volunteer and paid organizations due to recruitment and retention issues**
4. **Public education and information**
   a. An uninformed public remains a problem
   b. System access, personnel, and identification of emergency are ongoing targets for public education
5. **Prevention activities require research, funding, and increased emphasis on the national health agenda**
6. **System evaluation needs refinement, funding, and priority**
7. **Training and education is haphazard, with variations state to state; research is needed in this area**
8. **Funding for system administration is limited**
9. **Research direction and funding lacking**
10. **Positive trends in EMS**
    a. Nursing has a more active role in direct provision and coordination of prehospital care
       (1) There is controversy about proper education to function in prehospital setting; varies by state
       (2) Specific certification and recognition may be required

(3) Clinical specialization in emergency nursing provides leadership in EMS system development and evaluation
(4) Nurses have had long-standing roles in the prehospital realm including educator, volunteer or paid provider, and/or supervisor

b. Advanced education for EMS personnel
(1) Increased preparation for management, administration, education, and information systems positions is available
(2) Bachelor's and master's degree programs are increasing
(3) Salary differential for educational credentials is just beginning

F. CLINICAL ISSUES IN EMS

1. Controversies in field care

a. I.V. therapy
(1) Accepted for most medical problems on-scene
(2) Unacceptable for trauma patients if therapy causes delay in transport, unless entrapment present
(3) Insert I.V. enroute

b. MAST or PASG—questionable effectiveness according to recent studies; still used especially with extended transport times

c. Intubation vs esophageal obturator airway; preference is intubation, although training is more difficult

d. Time delay at scene is basis for most technique controversies; delay of the trauma patient reaching definitive facility is considered negligence

2. Factors influencing prehospital care

a. Uncontrolled environment
(1) Weather
(2) Bystanders
(3) Natural or man-made disaster
(4) Confined space
(5) Hazardous materials
(6) Weapons
(7) Infectious diseases

b. Lack of control

c. Lack of resources

d. High-stress occupation leading to high turnover

e. Communication difficulties with emergency department staff

f. Varying skill levels among providers

3. Critical incident stress management (see Module 36—Stress Management)

References

1. Stewart, R. (1985). Prehospital care of trauma. *Trauma Quarterly, 1*(3), 1–13.
2. National Academy of Sciences, National Research Council. (1966). *Accidental death and disability: The neglected disease of modern society.* Washington, DC: U.S. Government Printing Office.

Suggested Readings

Boyd, D., Edlich, R., & Micik, S. (Eds.). (1983). *Systems approach to emergency medical care.* Norwalk, CT: Appleton-Century-Crofts.

Cales, R., & Heilig, R. (Eds.). (1986). *Trauma care systems.* Rockville, MD: Aspen Publishers.

Cleary, V., Wilson, P., & Super, G. (Eds.). (1987). *Prehospital care: Administrative and clinical management.* Rockville, MD: Aspen Publishers.

Mustalish, A. (1986). Emergency medical services: Twenty years of growth and development. *New York State Journal of Medicine, 86*(8), 414–420.

Van de Leuv, J. (Ed.). (1987). *Management of emergency services.* Rockville, MD: Aspen Publishers.

Section II
Trauma Nursing and the Health Care System

MODULE 6
TRAUMA CARE SYSTEMS

Timothy O. Morgan, RN, CCRN, BSN

Objectives

1.0 Identify reasons why trauma is considered a major public health problem.
1.1 List the demographics related to trauma death.
1.2 Describe the impact of trauma on the health care system.
1.3 State the cost of trauma to our society in disability and economic loss.
2.0 Describe the evolution of a systems approach to trauma care.
2.1 List the three time periods identified for traumatic death.
2.2 List two strategies for mortality reduction related to each time period.
2.3 List three early advances in battlefield care, from the *Iliad* to the Civil War.
2.4 Identify trends in delay of treatment and mortality, as battlefield trauma care progressed.
2.5 List three advances in medical knowledge that came about as a result of the Vietnam conflict.
2.6 Identify two important publications that were instrumental in forwarding the cause of civilian trauma care.
3.0 Describe the process of trauma center designation.
3.1 Distinguish between accreditation, designation, and verification.
3.2 Discuss the roles in trauma system development of specific organizations such as the American College of Surgeons, Joint Commission on the Accreditation of Healthcare Organizations, American College of Emergency Physicians, etc.
3.3 Discuss the importance of the document "Hospital Resources for Optimal Care of the Injured Patient" to trauma system development.
3.4 Describe the current status of trauma center designation across the United States.

A. TRAUMA AS A HEALTH CARE PROBLEM

1. 70 million people a year suffer injury

2. Death from trauma

a. In ages 1 to 44, number-one killer

b. Kills approximately 140,000 per year (1)
   (1) Road crash—48,700 (2)
   (2) Gunshot wound—30,842 (2)
   (3) Knife stab wound—15,000 (2)
   (4) Falls—11,564 (2)
   (5) Other—34,300 (3)

c. More years of potential life lost, per year, than cancer and heart disease combined

d. Estimated that between 30 and 40% of deaths are preventable with trauma systems (3)

3. Leading cause of short- and long-term disabilities in 1985 (4)

a. Short-term—8,700,000 temporary disabilities

b. Long-term—340,000 permanent disabilities

4. Impact on health care systems

a. Medical expenses—more than $17 billion per year (4)
   (1) Physician fees
   (2) Hospital charges
   (3) Medication costs
   (4) Ambulance and emergency medical service fees

b. Trauma is responsible for the majority of physician contacts (1)

c. Trauma is the most common cause of hospitalization under age 45

d. Trauma patients occupy one of every eight hospital beds (1)
   (1) Trauma patients occupy four times the number of hospital beds occupied by cancer patients (5)
   (2) Trauma patients occupy more hospital-bed-days than all heart patients (5)

5. Economic impact of trauma on society

a. Estimated to cost over $100 billion per year, $227 million per day (6)
   (1) Lost wages
   (2) Medical expenses
   (3) Insurance administration
   (4) Property damage
   (5) Indirect work loss, i.e., costs to replace injured workers and losses in productivity
   (6) Cost of rehabilitation

b. Additional lifelong costs are associated with numerous permanent disabilities that occur each year
   (1) Custodial care for patient
   (2) Societal responsibility for family care of those permanently disabled (Social Security benefits)

6. Research in trauma

a. Although injuries are responsible for the loss of more economically productive years of life than heart disease and cancer combined, the federal expenditure for research in injury control is relatively small

b. Total federal expenditures in trauma are approximately $112 million per year (1)
   (1) Two percent of the total National Institutes of Health (NIH) research budget (1)
   (2) One-tenth the amount spent on cancer research (1)
   (3) One-fifth the amount spent on heart disease (1)

B. THE EVOLUTION OF A SYSTEMS APPROACH TO CARE

1. **Foundations for a systems approach to reduce death and disability from trauma**
   a. Trauma care must be addressed before injury, during rehabilitation, and upon return to society
   b. Numerous studies show that preventable deaths have been reduced in areas with comprehensive trauma care systems (3)
   c. A trimodal distribution of death can be used as a model to "target" components of the system for reduction in deaths
2. **Immediate death (over 50% of deaths) (7)—"at the scene"; reduction must occur through prevention**
   a. Drunk driving prevention
   b. Seat belt/motorcycle helmet usage
   c. Gun control
   d. Burn prevention
3. **Early death (approximately 30%) mostly from central nervous system injury and hemorrhage (7); reduction in mortality is best achieved with a systems approach**
   a. Immediate identification of the injured patient and transport to the appropriate level trauma care hospital
   b. Immediate evaluation of all trauma victims in the emergency department by trained emergency or surgical personnel
   c. Resuscitation and comprehensive intervention for major unisystem and all multisystem trauma patients by experienced surgeons
   d. Utilization of a team approach
   e. Priority availability of all related hospital resources for the care of the injured patient, e.g., x-ray, laboratory, blood bank, etc.
4. **Late death (approximately 15%)—days or weeks after injury (7); most die from sepsis or multiple organ failure; reduction involves high-quality medical and nursing care**
   a. Establishment of an integral intensive care unit dedicated to the needs of the critically injured
   b. Specially trained nurses and staff support throughout the trauma continuum
   c. Ongoing, continuing education for all professionals and paraprofessionals working in trauma care
   d. Ongoing, continuous research, both basic and clinical, into trauma prevention, pathophysiology, treatment, and outcome
5. **Problems in rehabilitation**

a. Trauma as a disease had not been included as part of rehabilitation planning and development
b. High technology and sophisticated medical care cause increased numbers of survivors with disabilities, etc.
c. Insurance system, legal system, etc., provide disincentives to return to work
d. Return to work, i.e., job retraining, needs to be emphasized

6. **Impact of war on trauma system organization**

a. The *Iliad* first documented organized battlefield care with soldiers taken to barracks or waiting ships; 147 different types of wounds documented with 77% mortality (7)
b. During the Roman Empire, 25 special field hospitals were strategically placed near battlefields (7)
c. French–Napoleonic Era (1800s)
   (1) Baron Dominique Jean Larrey, surgeon, implemented horse-drawn ambulances to reduce the time from injury to definitive care, triage (sorting wounded), field hospitals, and placed surgeons near the front lines
   (2) Delay to treatment—24 to 36 hrs
d. Crimean War (1854)—Florence Nightingale implemented improved sanitary conditions, more efficient design of hospitals, and the services of female nurses
e. The Civil War (1860 to 1865)—demonstrated need for formal training of nurses, physicians, and surgeons
   (1) Nightingale's ideas on sanitation applied
   (2) Continued improvements in care
      (a) Field hospitals
      (b) American Red Cross established and carried out large-scale war relief operations; furnished supplies to the Union Army and hospitals
      (c) Use of drugs such as morphine, chloroform
   (3) Mortality rate—33%; more deaths from infection and disease than wounds themselves (8)
f. World War I (1914 to 1918)
   (1) Motorized ambulances and evacuation trains
   (2) Systems of care
      (a) Aid stations on the battlefield
      (b) Evacuation hospitals 4 to 10 miles from battle line
      (c) Base hospitals back in U.S.
   (3) Advances in care
      (a) Antisepsis concepts—use of Dakin's solution
      (b) Improved debridement—decreased amputation
      (c) Improved fracture management
      (d) Research teams in hospitals
   (4) Delay to treatment— 12 to 18 hrs
   (5) Mortality rate—8.5% (7)
g. World War II (1939 to 1945)
   (1) Systems of care
      (a) Aid stations on the battlefield used triage-trained medics
      (b) Evacuation hospitals 5 to 50 miles from battlefield
      (c) Use of fixed-wing transport and flight nurses
   (2) Advances in care

        (a) Complete surgical care at evacuation hospital
        (b) Resuscitation and surgery linked—Advanced Trauma Life Support (ATLS) concepts
    (3) Delay to treatment—6 to 12 hrs
    (4) Mortality rate—5.8% (7)

h. Korea (1950 to 1952)
    (1) First use of helicopters to transport the injured
    (2) Mobile army surgical hospitals (MASH)—patients went directly to surgery then were transferred to other hospitals
    (3) Delay to treatment—2 to 4 hrs
    (4) Mortality rate—2.4% (7)

i. Vietnam (1966 to 1974)
    (1) Improved systems
        (a) Rapid evacuation by improved (faster, larger) helicopters
        (b) Specialized training for corpsmen and evacuation hospital trauma teams
        (c) Improved communications resulting in more accurate triage of patients to facilities that could handle their injuries, e.g., serious head injury to a facility with complete neurosurgical care
    (2) Improved care
        (a) Antibiotics continued to be developed and were more effective with the increased applicability and knowledge of wound bacteriology
        (b) Whole blood and packed red blood cells were used and were more widely available
    (3) Research/advances in care and knowledge
        (a) Discovery of "Da Nang Lung"—adult respiratory distress syndrome (ARDS) was extensively studied in search of improved ventilatory and treatment modalities
        (b) Military antishock trousers (MAST) introduced and used on soldiers suffering from hemorrhagic shock
        (c) Improved understanding of the process of coagulopathy and disseminated intravascular coagulation (DIC) in the trauma patient
        (d) Blood gas analyzers developed and introduced
        (e) Vascular techniques such as arterial anastomosis and vein grafting became firmly established and routine
        (f) Neurosurgical advances in care of serious head and spinal cord injuries, as well as rehabilitation of the neurosurgical patient
    (4) Delay to treatment—65 min
    (5) Mortality rate—1.7% (7)

C. DEVELOPMENT OF CIVILIAN TRAUMA SYSTEMS

1. **In wartime, rapid evacuation from the battlefield to MASH units, equipped with needed supplies and staffed with highly skilled personnel, saved lives**
2. **However, the care of civilians injured in America was less organized and less successful in ameliorating the suffering of trauma victims than the care of the injured in Vietnam**

3. **Landmark publication—"Accidental Death and Disability: The Neglected Disease of Modern Society" (National Academy of Sciences, 1966)**
 a. Acknowledged trauma as a major public health problem
 b. Recommendations submitted regarding
  (1) Accident prevention
  (2) Emergency first aid and medical care
   (a) Ambulance services
   (b) Communications
   (c) Emergency departments
   (d) Intensive care units
  (3) Development of trauma registries
  (4) Hospital trauma committees
  (5) Convalescence, disability, rehabilitation
  (6) Medicolegal concerns
  (7) Autopsy of all victims
  (8) Disaster management
  (9) Research in trauma
4. **Passage of Highway Safety Act (1966)**
 a. Provided for development of highway safety standards
 b. Specified equipment and manpower requirements on ambulances
 c. Provided funding to states to upgrade prehospital care
 d. Provided funding to develop training programs for EMTs and paramedics, purchase new rescue vehicles, improve communications equipment, and purchase new patient care equipment
5. **Passage of Emergency Medical Services Systems Act (1973)**
 a. Established guidelines for specific technical measures to support a nationally coordinated and comprehensive system of emergency health care accessible to all citizens
 b. Included provisions for manpower, training of personnel, communications, transportation, facilities, critical care units, use of public safety agencies, consumer participation, accessibility to care, transfer of patients, standard medical recordkeeping, consumer education, independent review/evaluation, disaster linkage, and mutual aid agreements (see Emergency Medical Services module)
6. **Credentialing/accrediting**
 a. 1976—American College of Surgeons, by publishing "Optimal Resources for Care of the Seriously Injured," provided leadership and guidance in matching the needs of the traumatized patient with a facility that has the appropriate capabilities
 b. 1979 (revised in 1983, 1986, 1989)—American College of Surgeons published standards for categorization of trauma facilities entitled "Hospital Resources for Optimal Care of the Injured Patient"; expanded and refined the 1976 document and identified three levels of care
 c. 1989—Joint Commission on the Accreditation of Healthcare Organizations has developed quality assurance standards for trauma patients; the standards are in the process of evaluation and implementation
 d. Three professional organizations also have been involved in the recent development of standards for trauma care facilities and treatment—American Society of Testing and Materials, American College of Emergency Physicians, and the American Academy of Pediatrics

e. However, the 1979 document (Hospital Resources for the Optimal Care of the Injured Patient, and subsequent revisions) by the American College of Surgeons remains the "gold standard" in categorizing trauma centers

7. **Methods of trauma center determination**

a. Voluntary accreditation—if a hospital meets criteria, it can be a trauma center
   (1) No determination of optimal number of centers
   (2) May result in too many trauma centers
   (3) May dilute volume of patients treated and, therefore, reduce efficiency

b. Verification
   (1) In areas that lack voluntary accreditation standards
      (a) The American College of Surgeons sends a team of experts (at the request of the individual institution) to review, consult, and comment on that institution's capabilities for trauma care, i.e., level I, II, or III (1)
      (b) Consultation review may aid in the "self-designation" common in areas without organized trauma systems
   (2) In areas with formally designated or accredited trauma centers, verification refers to the process of rereviewing those centers for continued adequacy of quality trauma care and outcome (1)

c. Current status of trauma center designation
   (1) There is no national policy on trauma care—systems are state-based
   (2) In 1986, 20 states claimed to have a designation process in place; all 20 conducted designation of Level I and Level II hospitals (9)
   (3) All 20 states used the American College of Surgeons Hospital Resource Document (1983) as the guideline; 8 modified it (9)
   (4) Thirteen of the 20 states allowed for individual hospitals to initiate the process; EMS councils and states performed the task in 3 and 4 states respectively (9)
   (5) Fundamental problems of system design, including overdesignation, lack of triage criteria, and inadequate monitoring, exist in remaining states

8. **Challenges to trauma system survival**

a. Financial—by far the greatest challenge facing trauma system survival
   (1) Reimbursement under DRGs and many third-party payors is often inadequate (10, 11, 12)
   (2) The number of uninsured in America continues to rise at alarming rates; from 28.4 million people in 1979 to 36.8 million in 1986 (13)
   (3) Currently, uncompensated trauma care costs $1.69 billion per year (14)
   (4) Regionalization and triage guidelines burden trauma hospitals by directing a larger proportion of severe and costly injuries to fewer hospitals

b. Internal barriers (institutional)
   (1) Commitment for the "wrong" reasons—institution becomes a trauma center for prestige rather than true commitment to caring for the critically injured in a community
   (2) "High profile" nature of trauma cases may overshadow other departments that are carrying out equally important work; may decrease interdepartmental cooperation
   (3) Increased numbers of severely injured patients put increased stress on resources and may overwhelm an institution's capacity

c. External barriers

(1) Political opposition from other hospitals that do not want to lose strategic marketing advantages or patients
(2) EMS system resistance and "parochial" attitudes against bypassing closest hospital and proceeding to a trauma center
(3) Lack of understanding by the public regarding trauma centers/systems and why they are needed

References

1. Committee on Trauma Research, Commission on Life Sciences, National Research Council, and The Institute of Medicine. (1985). *Injury in America: A continuing public health problem.* Washington, DC: National Academy Press.
2. The National Safety Council. (1988). *Accident facts.* Chicago: Author.
3. Cales, R. H., & Trunkey, D. D. (1985). Preventable trauma deaths: A review of trauma care systems development. *Journal of the American Medical Association, 254*(8), 1059–1063.
4. The National Safety Council. (1986). *Accident facts.* Chicago: Author.
5. Zuidema, G. D., Rutherford, R. B., & Ballinger, W. F. (Eds.). (1979). *The management of trauma* (3rd ed.). Philadelphia: W. B. Saunders Co.
6. Trunkey, D. D. (1982). 1981 A.A.S.T. presidential address: On the nature of things that go bump in the night. *Surgery,* 92(2), 123–132.
7. Trunkey, D. D. (1983). Trauma. *Scientific American, 249*(2), 28–35.
8. Howell, E., Widra, L., & Hill, M. G. (Eds.). (1988). *Comprehensive trauma nursing: Theory and practice.* Glenview, IL: Scott, Foresman & Co.
9. Aprahamian, C., Wolferth, C., Daren, J. C., McMahon, J., & Weitzel-DeVeas, C. (1989). Status of trauma center designation. *Journal of Trauma, 29*(5), 566–570.
10. Jacobs, L. M., & Schwartz, R. J. (1986). The impact of prospective reimbursement on trauma centers: An alternative payment plan. *Archives of Surgery, 121*(4), 479–483.
11. Jacobs, L. M. (1985). The effect of prospective reimbursement on trauma patients. *Bulletin of the American College of Surgeons, 70*(2), 17–22.
12. Schwab, C. W., Young, G., Civil, I., Ross, S. E., Talucci, R., Rosenberg, L., Shaikh, K., O'Malley, K., & Camishion, R. C. (1988). DRG reimbursement for trauma care: The demise of the trauma center. *The Journal of Trauma, 28*(7), 939–946.
13. Green, C. (1990, February 4). The steep premium on health. *Philadelphia Inquirer,* p. C–1.
14. Champion, H., & Mabee, M. (1989, August). *An American crisis in trauma care reimbursement.* Paper presented at the September 1989 Scientific Assembly of the Emergency Nurses' Association, Washington, DC.

Suggested Readings

Beachley, M., Snow, S., & Trimble, P. (1988). Developing trauma care systems: A nursing perspective. *Journal of Nursing Administration, 18*(4), 22–29.

Boyd, D. R. (1980). Trauma: A controllable disease in the 1980s. *The Journal of Trauma, 29*(1), 14–23.

Cardona, V., Hurn, P., Mason, P., Scanlon-Schilpp, A., & Veise-Berry, S. (Eds.). (1988). *Trauma nursing: From resuscitation through rehabilitation.* Philadelphia: W. B. Saunders Co.

National Academy of Sciences, National Research Council. (1966). *Accidental death and disability: The neglected disease of modern society.* Washington, DC: U.S. Government Printing Office.

Trunkey, D. D. (1990). What's wrong with trauma. *Bulletin of the American College of Surgeons,* 75(3), 10–15.

West, J., Williams, M. J., Trunkey, D. D., & Wolferth, C. C. (1988). Trauma systems: Current status—future challenges. *Journal of the American Medical Association,* 259(24), 3597–3600.

Section II
Trauma Nursing and the Health Care System

MODULE 7
TRAUMA NURSING

Mary L. Beachley, MS, RN, CEN

Prerequisite

Review Module 6 (Trauma Care Systems).

Objectives

1.0 Define trauma nursing.
1.1 Relate the scope of trauma nursing to the trauma care system.
1.2 Discuss a philosophy of trauma nursing including the elements of optimal functioning which impact the health of an individual.
2.0 Describe the critical functions of trauma nursing through the cycle of trauma.
2.1. Discuss the different levels of functioning, in the prehospital cycle, of a nurse with training as (1) first responder, (2) mobile intensive care nurse, and (3) flight nurse.
2.2 List the priorities of nursing assessment during the resuscitation cycle.
2.3 Identify nursing role priorities in the emergency department.
2.4 Explain the nurse's role during the resuscitation cycle.
2.5 List three critical nursing functions during the perioperative cycle.
2.6 Discuss the nurse's role in "trending" vital functions and patient responses during the critical care cycle.

2.7 Describe the major nursing responsibilities during the medical-surgical supportive care cycle.
2.8 Discuss the critical nursing functions during the rehabilitation cycle of care.
3.0 List certifications, based on standard continuing education programs, which are desirable for specific trauma nursing roles.
4.0 Relate the specific skill needs for trauma nursing.
4.1 Discuss the need for specialty skills and expertise during each phase of the trauma cycle.
4.2 Define various approaches to patient assessment in trauma nursing during various phases of the trauma care continuum.
4.3 List five major skills needed to support respiratory function.
4.4 List five major skills needed to support circulation in the resuscitation phase of trauma care.
4.5 List three skills specifically needed for burn care.

A. DEFINITION OF TRAUMA NURSING

"Trauma nursing is a specialty area of nursing practice which encompasses all aspects of nursing care for the injured or those at risk for injury. The practice of trauma nursing is a holistic endeavor to provide a continuum of care beginning with prevention and encompassing prehospital, resuscitation, stabilization, supportive care, rehabilitation and reintegration into society." (1)

From *Trauma Nurse Network Newsletter* (1988), 2(2), p. 2.

B. PHILOSOPHY OF TRAUMA NURSING

"Trauma nursing is an integral part of the emergency medical care system. Its nursing philosophy is based on a series of assumptions about people and health. In this philosophy statement, a person is defined as an individual, as well as part of a family and/or the community. Health is defined as optimal functioning of all elements, including the behavioral, cultural, emotional/psychological, physical, and spiritual dimensions of an individual." (1)

From *Trauma Nurse Network Newsletter* (1988), 2(2), p. 2.

C. ROLES OF NURSES THROUGH THE TRAUMA CONTINUUM

1. Major prehospital nurse functions

a. First responder

(1) Recognize event and identify mechanism of injury

(2) Alert emergency medical services—call 911 if available
(3) Assess and support airway and breathing
(4) Maintain spinal immobilization
(5) Assess and support circulation
(6) Stop bleeding

b. Mobile intensive care nurse (MICN)—role expectations vary widely throughout the United States; generally, advanced cardiac life support (ACLS) certification plus basic trauma life support (BTLS) or prehospital life support (PHTLS) certifications are needed; essential role functions include
  (1) Recognize event and identify mechanism of injury
  (2) Support and maintain airway, breathing, and circulation
  (3) Provide special immobilization
  (4) Control obvious bleeding
  (5) Arrange for rapid transportation to trauma center
  (6) Package patient for transport
  (7) Document assessment, time of treatment and event, and mechanism of injury
  (8) Triage according to specific protocols
  (9) Scene management
  (10) Personal safety
  (11) Extrication procedures
  (12) Hazardous materials management
  (13) Vehicle safety
  (14) Use of communication equipment
  (15) Use and care of specialized mobile equipment
  (16) Additional certifications are desirable
    (a) Advanced trauma life support (ATLS)
    (b) Pediatric advanced life support (PALS)
    (c) Advanced burn life support (ABLS)
    (d) Neonatal advanced life support (NALS)

c. Flight nurse—role expectations may vary; generally, ACLS certification plus BLTS or PHTLS certifications are needed; other functions are similar to those listed above for MICNs; additional functions are
  (1) Assessments based on knowledge of effects of altitude and appropriate adaptation of techniques
  (2) Provision of care based on effects of altitude and modification or use of specialized equipment
  (3) Personal safety in and around the aircraft

2. **Essential emergency nurse critical role functions**

a. Perform primary and secondary survey of patient on arrival at emergency department
b. Assure priority of care
c. Maintain high index of suspicion of possible life-threatening injury
d. Initiate resuscitation protocols
e. Monitor patient's response to treatment
f. Frequently reassess vital signs and mental status
g. Communicate with other health team members, family, and external agencies, including the media

h. Provide instruction to patient and family regarding self-care for minor injuries
i. Document assessment, critical times, treatments, and information from patient/family regarding past medical history

3. Critical perioperative nurse role functions

a. Obtain information from resuscitation team regarding injuries and treatment
b. Obtain baseline vital signs and perform a preoperative assessment
c. Assure immediate access to operating room
d. Anticipate multiple procedure needs; provide equipment and supplies
e. Provide support for continued resuscitation efforts in operating room, including ventilation, and fluid and blood replacement
f. Protect airway and closely monitor postoperative vital functions
g. Coordinate the participation of various specialty surgical teams
h. Document assessment, patient response, and perioperative care

4. Important critical care nurse functions

a. Coordinate efforts of all members of the health care team
b. Assure availability of life-support equipment and supplies
c. Assure priority of critical care beds with adequate nursing care
d. Assess for intact vital physiologic functions; monitor and interpret trends
e. Review initial assessment and resuscitation measures
f. Repeat systems assessment at regular intervals; be alert to concomitant or evolving injuries not identified initially
g. Provide timely notification of changes in patient's condition to physicians
h. Provide frequent feedback to family regarding patient's condition and progress
i. Develop a holistic plan of care which addresses the patient's physiological, psychosocial, and family needs
j. Collaborate with support services to develop a discharge/rehabilitation plan for patient and family
k. Monitor patient specifically for signs of infection and predicted complications of trauma; institute appropriate preventive and treatment protocols
l. Provide adequate pain control
m. Begin planning for rehabilitation needs
n. Provide appropriate nutritional support
o. Provide ongoing documentation of assessment, treatment, and patient response

5. Major medical-surgical nurse functions

a. Provide ongoing systems assessment
b. Observe for subtle changes in physiologic, cognitive, and emotional status
c. Support patients through stages of loss and grieving
d. Promote self-care activities
e. Initiate discharge teaching for patient and family
f. Help patient adapt to altered body functions and body image; assist in relearning activities of daily living
g. Maintain adequate nutritional support
h. Promote patient mobility

6. Essential rehabilitation nurse functions (see Module 17—Rehabilitation)

a. Promote healing
b. Assess process of recovery in patient and family
c. Integrate therapy gains into 24-hr daily routine
d. Teach patient and family

e. Assess functions and screen for areas of difficulty in adaptation
f. Act as case manager—coordinate the interdisciplinary rehabilitation team
g. Develop rehabilitation program plan and make referrals to appropriate community services for ongoing health care needs

Reference

1. Staff. (1988). Trauma nurse network standards. *Trauma Nurse Network Newsletter,* 2(2), 2.

Suggested Readings

Adams, H. R. (1984). Trauma nursing: A collaborative model. *Topics in Emergency Medicine,* 6(1), 60–71.

Beachley, M., Snow, S., & Trimble, P. (1988). Developing trauma care systems: A nursing perspective. *Journal of Nursing Administration,* 18(4), 22–29.

Butler, V., & Campbell, S. (1988). Resuscitation in the operating room. *Trauma Quarterly,* 5(1), 57–61.

Cardona, V. D., Hurn, P. D., Mason, P. J. B., Scanlon-Schilpp, A. M., & Veise-Berry, S. W. (Eds.). (1988). *Trauma nursing from resuscitation through rehabilitation.* Philadelphia: W. B. Saunders Co.

Freeman, M. C., Flanagan, M. E., & Champion, H. R. (1989). Perioperative nursing care of the multiple trauma patient: When seconds count. *AORN Journal,* 50(1), 40–50.

Morgan, T., Berger, P., Land, S., & Schwab, C. W. (1986). Trauma center and the OR: A cooperative approach to caring for the massively injured. *AORN Journal,* 44(3), 416–426.

Saufl, N., & Garmon, J. (1988). Assessment and management of the multiple trauma patient in the PACU. *Journal of Post-Anesthesia Nursing,* 3(5), 305–312.

Table 7.1

Trauma nursing skills. Specific skills, specialized equipment, and procedures that trauma nurses may commonly be expected to perform, use, or assist with during various phases of the trauma continuum.

	Prehospital Cycle	*ED Resuscitation Cycle*	*Operative Cycle*	*Stabilization ICU Cycle*	*Supportive Care Rehabilitation Cycle*
Assessment Skills					
1. Primary/secondary survey	×	×	×	×	
2. Vital signs	×	×	×	×	×
3. Fetal heart tones	×	×	×	×	×
4. Systems assessment	×	×	×	×	×
5. Neurosensory assessment	×	×	×	×	×
6. Psychosocial assessment		×		×	×
7. Nutritional assessment		×		×	×
8. Trend monitoring	×	×	×	×	×
9. Data analysis		×	×	×	×
Airway/Breathing					
1. C-spine immobilization	×	×	×	×	
2. Airway maneuvers—jaw thrust, chin lift	×	×	×	×	
3. Helmet removal	×	×			
4. Insertion of oral airway	×	×	×		
5. EOA insertion and removal	×	×			
6. Endotracheal intubation and care	×	×	×	×	×
7. Cricothyroidotomy	×	×	×		
8. Tracheostomy tube care		×	×	×	×
9. Oxygen administration	×	×	×	×	×
a. Face mask	×	×		×	×
b. T-piece or "blow-by"		×		×	×
c. Aerosol mask		×		×	×
d. Nasal cannula	×	×	×	×	×
e. Nonrebreathing mask	×	×		×	
f. Bag-valve mask	×	×	×	×	
10. Portable O_2 tanks	×	×	×	×	×
11. Tracheal suction	×	×	×	×	×
12. Mechanical ventilation					
a. Modes of ventilation					
(1) AC, CMV, IMV, SIMV		×	×	×	×
(2) High frequency			×	×	
(3) Independent lung			×	×	
b. Positive airway pressure management—CPAP and PEEP		×	×	×	
c. Monitoring airway and pulmonary parameters	×	×	×	×	×
d. Weaning techniques and protocols			×	×	×
13. Drawing and interpretation of ABGs		×	×	×	

	Prehospital Cycle	ED Resuscitation Cycle	Operative Cycle	Stabilization ICU Cycle	Supportive Care Rehabilitation Cycle
14. Chest tube insertion and management		×	×	×	×
15. Chest decompression	×	×			
16. Chest physiotherapy				×	×
17. Incentive spirometry				×	×
18. Diaphragmatic pacemaker		×	×		×
19. Cardiopulmonary resuscitation	×	×	×	×	×
Circulation					
1. High-volume infusion		×	×		
2. Blood product administration		×	×	×	×
3. I.V. insertion and management	×	×	×	×	×
4. Apply and remove PASG	×	×	×		
5. Pericardiocentesis		×			
6. Peritoneal lavage		×			
7. Emergency thoracotomy		×	×		
8. Emergency laparotomy		×	×		
9. Autotransfusion		×	×		
10. Piggyback I.V. medications		×	×	×	×
11. I.V. push (bolus) medications	×	×	×	×	
12. Total parenteral nutrition				×	×
13. Fluid warmer		×	×		
14. Infusion controllers and pumps	×	×	×	×	×
15. Cardioversion	×	×	×	×	
16. Defibrillation	×	×	×	×	
17. Catheter insertion and monitoring					
a. Central venous pressure		×	×	×	×
b. Direct arterial pressure		×	×	×	
c. Pulmonary artery pressure			×	×	
d. Left atrial pressure			×	×	
e. Intracranial pressure		×	×	×	
18. Monitoring					
a. Cardiac monitoring	×	×	×	×	
b. Holter monitoring				×	×
c. Cardiac output			×	×	
19. Twelve-lead ECG		×	×	×	
20. Pacemaker insertion and use					
a. Transvenous	×	×	×	×	
b. External	×	×	×	×	
c. Atrial			×	×	×
d. AV sequential			×	×	×
e. Ventricular			×	×	×
21. Oximetry/SVO			×	×	
22. Transcutaneous O_2 monitor	×	×	×	×	×
23. Tissue pressure measurement		×	×	×	
24. Use of Doppler	×	×	×	×	×

Table 7.1 continued

	Prehospital Cycle	*ED Resuscitation Cycle*	*Operative Cycle*	*Stabilization ICU Cycle*	*Supportive Care Rehabilitation Cycle*
25. Application of sequential compression boots			×	×	×
Miscellaneous					
1. Notification of trauma team	×	×			
2. Helicopter loading and off-loading	×	×			
3. Organ procurement procedures		×	×	×	×
4. Evidence collection and preservation	×	×	×		
5. Pain management	×	×	×	×	×
6. Crisis intervention	×	×	×	×	×
7. Nutritional assessment				×	×
8. Venipuncture for specimen collection	×	×	×	×	×
9. Hematocrit (spun)		×	×	×	
10. Blood glucose—finger-stick method		×	×	×	×
11. Specimen collection		×	×	×	×
12. Specific gravity		×	×	×	×
13. Guiaic for occult bleeding		×	×	×	×
14. Gastric pH determination		×		×	×
15. Feeding tube insertion				×	×
16. Enteral feeding			×	×	×
17. Peritoneal dialysis				×	×
18. Continuous arteriovenous hemodialysis				×	×
19. Application of traction devices	×	×	×	×	×
20. External fixator care		×	×	×	×
21. Cast management		×	×	×	×
22. Application of splints	×	×		×	×
23. Range of motion exercise				×	×
24. Wound care					
a. Debridement		×	×	×	
b. Cleansing	×	×	×	×	×
c. Irrigation		×	×	×	×
d. Dressing	×	×	×	×	×
e. Graft care			×	×	×
f. Donor site care			×	×	×
g. Escharotomy care	×	×	×	×	×
h. Fasciotomy care			×	×	×
i. Topical therapy (burns)		×	×	×	×
25. Preservation of amputated parts for replantation	×	×	×		
26. External temperature control					
a. Hypo/hyperthermia blanket		×	×	×	×
b. Radiant heat shield		×	×	×	
c. Infrared lights		×			

	Prehospital Cycle	ED Resuscitation Cycle	Operative Cycle	Stabilization ICU Cycle	Supportive Care Rehabilitation Cycle
27. Special beds					
a. Frames (Stryker, Foster)			×	×	×
b. Oscillating support surface, e.g., RotoRest			×	×	×
c. Air-fluidized			×	×	×
d. Low air loss				×	×
Insertion and/or Maintenance of Drainage Systems					
1. Suprapubic		×	×	×	×
2. Urethral catheter		×	×	×	×
3. Nasogastric tube	×	×	×	×	×
4. Abdominal drainage tubes			×	×	×
5. Feeding tubes			×	×	×
6. Wound drains			×	×	×
7. Ostomy care			×	×	×
8. Water-sealed drainage		×	×	×	×
9. Ventricular catheter			×	×	

Section II
Trauma Nursing and the Health Care System

MODULE 8
THE TRAUMA TEAM

Mary L. Beachley, MS, RN, CEN
Mary Pat Erdner, MSN, RN, CRRN

Prerequisite

Review Module 7 (Trauma Nursing).

Objectives

1.0 Define teamwork as it relates to trauma care.
1.1 List at least four critical elements of teamwork.
1.2 Discuss the importance of leadership and coaching in teamwork.
1.3 Discuss collective action as a process of teamwork.
2.0 Define the roles of the trauma team members.
2.1 Describe the primary role and functions of the trauma surgeon.
2.2 List at least three major roles of the truama nurse coordinator.
2.3 Discuss the role of the staff nurse as a team member throughout the continuum of trauma care.
2.4 Relate the primary role and functions of the anesthesiologist on the trauma team.
2.5 Describe the role of the respiratory therapist in airway management.
2.6 Explain the roles of laboratory and radiology personnel during the resuscitation phase of trauma care.
2.7 Compare and contrast the roles of psychological support personnel.
2.8 Explain the roles of the physiatrist, physical therapist, occupational therapist, recreational therapist, and vocational counselor in trauma care.

A. TEAMWORK

1. Critical elements

a. Communication
   (1) Essential for teamwork among the trauma team, the patient, and the family
   (2) Team members must communicate regularly with the team leader and other team members regarding their roles and the impact of their care on the patient
   (3) Communication is critical in evaluating the team's effectiveness and making appropriate changes in protocols

b. Competence
   (1) Each team member must be able to perform his/her role independently
   (2) Each member contributes to the team's overall competence in caring for the trauma patient
   (3) Competence in trauma care is obtained by acquiring knowledge and skills and ongoing practice that is continually evaluated and refined

c. Collaboration
   (1) The trauma team is a multidisciplinary group of health care providers
   (2) Each member brings special knowledge and expertise to the team and provides a broad range of skills to meet the complex needs of trauma patients
   (3) All members must collaborate with one another to integrate skills and knowledge that provide optimal support for the trauma patient

d. Leadership
   (1) There must be an identified leader for the trauma team
   (2) Usually the trauma surgeon directs the immediate team functions and defines the patient's plan of care

e. Coaching
   (1) Helps trauma team members develop their roles, skills, and protocols
   (2) Feedback, encouragement, teaching, and promoting high standards make optimal teamwork possible

2. Collective action

a. Most effective and efficient when based on predetermined protocols
b. Assumes that well-defined functions are known and performed by individual team members
c. Promotes best use of individual expertise and skills

B. ROLES AND MAJOR FUNCTIONS OF TRAUMA TEAM MEMBERS

1. Trauma surgeon

a. Team leader and coach
b. Provides resuscitative medical interventions
c. Provides definitive surgical care
d. Provides direction for the trauma care team through the cycles of trauma care

e. Adjusts treatment plan based on patient's response to therapy
f. Evaluates team performance and patient care outcomes

2. **Trauma nurse coordinator**
a. Coach
b. Coordinates the various team functions
c. Directs or provides nursing care interventions through the continuum of care
d. Collaborates with administrators, department heads, medical and nursing staff to define protocols and team functions
e. Monitors and evaluates team care through the continuum of care in conjunction with the trauma director
f. Provides education to the public and professionals regarding trauma care
g. May have responsibility for budget, data collection and analysis, and other management functions

3. **Trauma nurse**
a. Provides holistic nursing care, based on the nursing process, to patients and families throughout the continuum of trauma care
b. Monitors vital functions and responds immediately to a potential life-threatening change
c. Identifies actual and potential patient problems and states these as nursing diagnoses
d. Provides nursing interventions based on priorities directed by protocols, primary physicians, nursing assessments, and nursing diagnoses
e. Evaluates and documents patient response to injury, and medical and nursing care
f. Participates in, coordinates, and facilitates communications with all health care providers who are involved in the care of the patient and family
g. Analyzes trends in patient status, assumes responsibility for notifying appropriate team members and initiating actions and referrals that are within the scope of nursing practice
h. Consults with appropriate clinical nurse specialists to solve complex nursing care problems

4. **Anesthesiologist**
a. Assures adequate airway; provides artificial airway when appropriate or needed as an emergency intervention
b. Provides or prescribes oxygen therapy
c. Monitors vital functions related to ventilation and perfusion
d. Assures cervical spine stabilization during airway management
e. Consults with other physicians and health care providers on appropriate airway management and oxygen treatment
f. Provides and maintains anesthesia during operative procedures
g. Manages patient's critical functions during immediate postoperative period
h. May prescribe or provide regional anesthesia and analgesia for pain control in selected patients

5. **Consulting physicians**
a. Collaborate with trauma team on specialized needs of trauma patient
b. Communicate with trauma surgeon and primary nurse regarding modifications to treatment plan and medical-surgical interventions
c. Provide ongoing input to the treatment plan based on specialty expertise

6. **Respiratory therapist**
   a. Under direction of an anesthesiologist or trauma surgeon, may manage airway during initial resuscitation
   b. Collaborates with trauma team to provide airway support and oxygen therapy as needed
   c. Monitors emergency airway support
   d. Supports effective airway clearance through physical techniques of percussion, vibration, and postural drainage
   e. Monitors patient's respiratory status by obtaining and analyzing blood gases and through pulmonary function testing
   f. Maintains appropriate ventilator settings and assures proper functioning of ventilator equipment
7. **Laboratory personnel**
   a. Assure priority of necessary laboratory tests during resuscitation phase
   b. Collaborate with trauma team to provide immediate availability of blood and blood products
   c. Collaborate with the trauma team to develop protocols for admission baseline tests for trauma patients
8. **Radiology personnel**
   a. Collaborate with trauma team to establish protocols for initial baseline radiologic studies
   b. Assure priority of necessary radiologic studies during the resuscitation phase
   c. Assure immediate response at all times
   d. Consult with trauma surgeon to assure accurate views of film
9. **Psychologist**
   a. Uses crises intervention techniques to assist patient and family in decisionmaking during crises
   b. Assesses and treats behavioral, emotional, and family dynamics/issues through counseling and assisting the patient and family in adapting to physical disability
   c. Evaluates patient's cognition, providing strategies and techniques aimed at facilitating adjustment to disability
   d. Counsels to foster realistic adaptive adjustment to work and employment plans
   e. Assists the trauma team with assessment of different stages of loss and grief exhibited by patient and family
   f. Provides information and counsels patients about sexuality and sexual function
   g. Provides patients and families with information, counseling, and referrals for drug and alcohol rehabilitation
10. **Social worker**
   a. Assesses family dynamics and coping strategies related to disability or illness, and facilitates the grief process and role adjustments immediately after the injury
   b. Prepares the family to face the ill or disabled family member, both emotionally and physically
   c. Begins education process with an initial family team conference to discuss the reality of the illness or disability, and provides a balance of hope and realism
   d. Assists the family in making alternative plans for the worst outcome, if recovery does not progress
   e. Initiates short- and long-term plans regarding finances and family support

f. Anticipates the course and outcome of the patient's rehabilitation process
g. Helps the family initiate plans for discharge

11. **Pastoral counselor**
a. Supports spiritual needs of patient and family
b. Assists family with crises decisionmaking
c. Counsels family members with shifting roles and responsibilities
d. Counsels family members and patients through stages of loss; supports grieving

12. **Physiatrist**
a. Consults with trauma surgeon to design comprehensive rehabilitation plan, individualized to patient's injuries and expected optimum performance
b. Collaborates with trauma team members to facilitate congruent rehabilitation goals and consistent approaches to care
c. Using functional assessment tools and specialized knowledge of physical medicine, provides medical leadership during the rehabilitation cycle of trauma care to improve functions and minimize complications related to disability

13. **Physical therapist**
a. Assesses functions and potential complications related to disability, immobility, and neuromuscular function including
(1) Quality of patient's movements
(2) Spontaneous initiation of movement
(3) Incorporation of involved extremities, head and trunk, into functional activities
(4) Coordination of movements
(5) Position of body and extremities during movement
(6) Types of movements of the involved muscle groups, e.g., absent, reflexive, synergistic, automatic, or under selective control
b. Develops a treatment plan with the patient to
(1) Maintain mobility, gait, joint range of motion, limb length, and muscle tone
(2) Promote sensorimotor activities, daily living skills, and pulmonary function
(3) Limit pain
c. Consults with trauma team to prevent hazards of immobility through positioning, exercise, splinting, and ambulation
d. Treats with heat, ultrasound, electrical stimulation, and cold modalities
e. Evaluates and recommends equipment, including wheelchairs, braces, prostheses, ambulation aids, shower chairs, and transfer aids

14. **Occupational therapist**
a. Assesses functions and potential complications related to movement of the upper extremities, daily living skills, cognition, and perception
b. Assesses daily living skills and equipment needs for eating, dressing, bathing, community reintegration, and prevocational skills
c. Assesses visual acuity, and cognitive and perceptual strengths and weaknesses
d. Assesses and recommends treatment and equipment related to maintaining normal movement of the upper extremities
e. Recommends and/or designs adaptive equipment and splints
f. Collaborates with trauma team to establish functional goals for patient
g. Facilitates community reentry through treatment and discharge planning in numerous settings, including work, school, home, and recreational activities

15. **Speech pathologist/therapist**
    a. Assesses and evaluates speech, including articulation, muscle strength, coordination, and apraxia
    b. Assesses and develops a treatment plan for disorders of language including aphasia, reading, writing, verbal comprehension, and anomia
    c. Assesses and develops a treatment plan for swallowing disorders related to mechanical and neurological impairments
    d. Evaluates and recommends communication devices including speech boards, tracheostomy devices, and speech assisting devices
    e. Provides information to trauma team on a variety of techniques to promote stimulation from coma—frequently implemented by nurses and occupational therapists
16. **Recreation therapist**
    a. Assesses and plans treatment to assist in resocialization skills and physical activities
    b. Assesses and makes recommendations related to leisure time, avocation, and community reintegration
    c. Considers developmental age, interests, cognitive and functional abilities in developing play activities for pediatric trauma patients
    d. May assist children with schoolwork and plans for tutoring and school reentry
17. **Vocational counselor**
    a. Assesses and evaluates vocational potential of disabled trauma patient, considering patient's goals, interests, experiences, and actual and potential skills
    b. Assesses and counsels the patient to explore new occupations after a disability
    c. Prepares treatment plan with the patient and employer that facilitates smooth reintegration
18. **Additional roles that support the trauma program**
    a. Trauma director
    b. Trauma registrar
    c. Trauma clinical nurse specialist
    d. Trauma prevention/outreach coordinator
    e. Trauma quality assurance coordinator
    f. Trauma educator
    g. Trauma research nurse
    h. Clinical pharmacist

Suggested Readings

American College of Surgeons. (1990). *Resources for optimal care of the patient.* Chicago: Author.

Beachley, M., Snow, S., & Trimble, P. (1988). Developing trauma care systems: The trauma nurse coordinator. *Journal of Nursing Administration, 18*(7,8), 34–42.

Boyd, D., Edlich, R., & Micik, S. (1983). *Systems approach to emergency medical care.* Norwalk, CT: Appleton-Century-Crofts.

Brent, R. J., & Poltorak, I. (1987). The pharmacist as a trauma team member. *Hospital Pharmacy, 22*(2), 152–155.

Cardona, V. D., Hurn, P. D., Mason, P. J. B., Scanlon-Schilpp, A. M., & Veise-Berry, S. W. (Eds.). (1988). *Trauma nursing: From resuscitation through rehabilitation.* Philadelphia: W. B. Saunders Co.

Carraway, R. P., Brewer, M. E., Lewis, B. R., Shaw, R. A., Berry, R. W., & Watson, L. (1984). Life saver: A complete team approach incorporated into a hospital-based program. *American Surgeon, 50*(4), 173–182.

Staff. (1988). Trauma nurse network standards. *Trauma Nurse Network Newsletter, 2*(2), 2–3.

MODULE 9
TRAUMA TRANSPORT

Elizabeth M. Blunt, MS, RN, CEN, EMT
Eileen M. Sweeney Crowther, MSN, RN, CEN, HPRN

Objectives

1.0 Outline responsibilities of the trauma transport team during each stage of a prehospital or interhospital transport mission.
1.1 Identify the components of pretransport planning.
1.2 Discuss communication and notification methods related to trauma patient transport.
1.3 Describe the responsibilities of land and air transport team members in prehospital and interhospital trauma care.
1.4 Discuss prehospital triage protocols for single incident and mass casualty situations.
1.5 Describe the focus of patient assessment and preparation for transport for on-scene and interhospital calls.
1.6 Discuss nursing care responsibilities during and immediately after transport of the trauma patient.
1.7 Identify the role of medical command in prehospital and interhospital transport.
1.8 Discuss the importance of mechanism of injury in establishing patient care priorities.
2.0 Discuss general considerations in utilizing transport services.
2.1 Identify common transport vehicles and their use in terms of availability, response time, size, patient access, patient capacity, and equipment.
2.2 Consider environmental factors of terrain and weather in transport selection.
2.3 Recognize federal and state regulations governing transport of trauma patients.

2.4 Recognize hazards associated with land and air transport modalities and the corresponding safety requirements.

3.0 Discuss the effects of altitude on specific physiologic parameters.

3.1 Define major gas laws that account for the expansion of gases with altitude.

3.2 Describe the hypoxic effects of altitude on major body systems.

3.3 For the following stresses of flight, list the clinical implications, preventive measures, and treatment modalities for each, i.e., barometric pressure changes, vibration, dehydration, hypoxia, fatigue, G-forces, noise, thermal effects, third spacing.

3.4 Describe rapid decompression and list the emergency procedures to be implemented in the event of its occurrence.

4.0 Describe aspects of the nursing process that are unique to prehospital transport.

4.1 Identify the types of information obtained from the prehospital setting and referring hospital that govern the focus of in-transport assessment and intervention.

4.2 Describe the essential parameters that will be monitored during transport.

4.3 Given the limitations of weather, space, noise, vibration, patient access, and number of caregivers, discuss the special equipment and procedures that assist the transport team in performing ongoing assessment during the transport process.

5.0 List nursing diagnoses specific to the transport experience; include etiologic factors and manifestations.

6.0 Anticipate and provide the appropriate in-transit nursing interventions.

6.1 Given specific patient data, recognize and prioritize the nursing interventions that may be required.

6.2 Given the limitations of the prehospital environment, list equipment and skills particular to nursing care during transport.

7.0 Evaluate patient response to medical and nursing interventions.

7.1 List nursing activities required for continuous monitoring and evaluation of patient status.

7.2 Cite trends in patient status which may require priority interventions from the transport team.

7.3 Describe desirable outcomes with measurable criteria for specific nursing interventions.

8.0 Discuss communications guidelines as applied to medical transport.

8.1 Discuss the functions of the Federal Communications Commission (FCC) as they pertain to radio usage in the transport process.

8.2 Describe radio equipment by type, frequency, and range.

8.3 Discuss communication priorities and proper radio technique and terminology.

8.4 List the required dispatch information for prehospital and interfacility transport.

8.5 Explore general communication techniques that foster effective communication between transport staff, the patient and family, and the staff of the referring facility.

8.6 Identify pertinent patient data obtained from the referring agency.

8.7 Identify patient data to be included in written documentation of the mission.

9.0 Identify specialized equipment encountered and used in prehospital care and transport.

A. GENERAL CONCEPTS IN PATIENT TRANSPORT

1. Overview of stages of a transport mission

a. Planning stage
   (1) General planning for trauma patient transport includes establishing protocols and procedures, providing initial and recurrent training, and routine checking and restocking of equipment and supplies
   (2) Mission-specific responsibilities include determining the role of each transport team member, preparing equipment, and verifying dispatch information

b. Notification/communication stage
   (1) Transport team may be notified by telephone, radio, scanner, or pager
   (2) Dispatch and en-route information for prehospital transports
      (a) Name and location of caller with callback information
      (b) Exact location of patient(s)
      (c) Nature of call
      (d) Number of patients
      (e) Special equipment needed
      (f) Hazards at scene
      (g) Age, sex, suspected injuries of patient
      (h) Entrapment; time until extrication
      (i) Treatment in progress
      (j) Preplanned route of travel
      (k) For air transport, also determine
         i) Whether ground transport is required to move patient to landing zone (LZ)
         ii) Ground contact's radio frequency and call sign
         iii) Landing zone description
   (3) Dispatch and en-route information for interhospital transports
      (a) Hospital name and location
      (b) Patient's location; unit
      (c) Diagnosis
      (d) Reason for transfer
      (e) History of present illness or injury
      (f) Clinical findings
      (g) Pertinent diagnostic test results
      (h) Current treatment and patient's response
      (i) Patient's expected needs during transport
      (j) For air transport, also determine whether ground transport is required to landing zone and obtain LZ information

c. Transport team responsibilities during travel from base to patient
   (1) Securely fasten seat belts
   (2) Secure all loose equipment
   (3) Limit use of intercom and radios
   (4) Check supplies and equipment
   (5) Assist in observing for and reporting hazards en route and at scene
   (6) For ground transport, obey speed laws en route; safety has a higher priority than speed

d. Transport team responsibilities during initial patient care stage
   (1) Prehospital
      (a) For air transport, secure the LZ by preventing unauthorized approaches to the aircraft; remain with the aircraft until released by pilot
      (b) For all transports, ensure scene is safe; observe for hazards, including fire, traffic, power lines, hazardous materials, unstable persons
      (c) Park as close to scene as safely possible
      (d) Rapidly assess overall scene
      (e) Communicate with scene commander to determine location and number of patients to be transported
      (f) Establish triage area and call for additional transport if required
      (g) Divide personnel into triage teams if multiple victims
      (h) Obtain pertinent patient and scene data from other prehospital personnel and from patient, if possible
      (i) Ensure that rapid primary survey of each person has occurred and that life-threatening conditions are corrected
      (j) Ensure stabilization of C-spine
      (k) Contact medical command with patient data and obtain treatment instructions as necessary
      (l) If air transport, notify pilot of estimated time of arrival (ETA) at LZ and number of patients to be transported
      (m) Prepare patient(s) for transport based on mechanism of injury, patient's response, and environmental conditions
      (n) Provide analgesia and/or sedation to promote safety, comfort, and initiation of treatment measures
      (o) Direct transfer of patient(s) to aircraft or ambulance
      (p) Direct loading of patient to effect proper placement and treatment
      (q) Determine if patient has been identified and if patient's family has been notified
      (r) Collect any available copy of written records from referring agency as applicable
      (s) Confirm on-load and departure with medical command and receiving agency; give update on patient status and ETA to receiving agency
   (2) Interhospital
      (a) Ensure necessary equipment and supplies are present and pertinent data about the transfer is available prior to leaving base
      (b) For air transport, ensure LZ is secure
      (c) Communicate with staff from referring hospital, family, and patient to obtain pertinent patient data
      (d) Brief patient and family about transport procedures and obtain necessary consent for transport
      (e) Obtain pertinent patient report from present caregivers, and copies of chart and diagnostic studies
      (f) Prepare patient for transport—patient should have a secure airway and intravenous (I.V.) line established prior to transport
         i) Check vital signs; assess breath sounds and adequacy of ventilation
         ii) Consider elective endotracheal (ET) tube for airway maintenance
         iii) Place patient on portable oxygen source

iv) Ensure presence of portable suction unit
v) Attach cardiac and hemodynamic monitors as indicated
vi) Ensure all I.V. lines are patent and secure; change glass I.V.s to plastic bags as appropriate
vii) Label I.V. drips and place on infusion pumps, if needed
viii) For air transport, remove air from I.V. bag and pressurize to ensure adequate flow rate
ix) Heparin flush arterial and pulmonary artery (PA) pressure lines prior to capping or maintain with pressure infusion line
x) Maintain intracranial pressure lines
xi) Attach chest tubes to Pleurovac; for air transport, may attach one-way flutter valve to chest tube(s)
xii) Consider the need for nasogastric (NG) tube and/or urinary catheter if not already in place
xiii) Empty drainage bags; for air transport, attach vented collection bag to drainage tubes as indicated
xiv) Provide analgesia and/or sedation to promote comfort and safety
xv) Restrain patient appropriately
xvi) Direct transfer of patient onto transport litter
xvii) Secure patient, pumps, and other ancillary equipment
xviii) Recheck vital signs with special attention to ventilatory status prior to leaving referring hospital
xix) Brief the patient on what to expect throughout the transport process
xx) Direct loading of patient into transport vehicle
xxi) Recheck ventilatory status after each move
xxii) Provide headsets for conscious patients transported by helicopter; instruct regarding use
xxiii) Ensure all equipment, personnel, and patient are securely restrained
xxiv) Ensure LZ is secured prior to the start of helicopter engines

(g) Transport team responsibilities for patient care during transport stage
i) Anticipate and prepare for potential patient complications
ii) Communicate with patient as indicated to provide emotional support and allay anxieties
iii) Update medical command physician and give ETA
iv) Ensure adequate monitoring of patient's status
v) Monitor ventilation for adequacy and adjust ventilatory support as indicated by patient's condition
vi) Adjust treatment measures and interventions as patient's condition warrants, based on established protocols and/or medical command

(h) Transport team responsibilities during posttransport stage
i) Direct transfer at receiving facility
ii) Provide accurate, concise report of patient's history and current medical status to include in-transit treatment and patient response
iii) Deliver copy of patient's records
iv) Complete transport documentation and leave one copy at the receiving facility
v) Inform receiving staff of status of patient's family, if known

vi) Notify other prehospital caregivers and/or referring facility's primary nurse and physician, of patient's outcome

2. Personnel and training for prehospital care—common configurations

a. Ground transport
   (1) Basic life support—EMT, advanced first aid provider
   (2) Advanced life support—paramedics, prehospital nurses, and/or physicians

b. Air transport—at least one paramedic or one prehospital nurse (usually both are utilized); physicians are utilized in some programs

c. Scope and training—see Module 5—Emergency Medical Services—and Module 7—Trauma Nursing

3. Equipment unique to prehospital care and transport

a. General equipment guidelines (**NOTE:** asterisked items may not necessarily be carried by all transport programs)
   (1) Provides capability for advanced life support during transport
   (2) Is self-contained, lightweight, portable
   (3) Has portable, self-contained power for twice the expected transport duration
   (4) Has AC power capability
   (5) Is packaged to allow continuous critical care monitoring and intervention while entering and exiting transport vehicles
   (6) Is easily cleaned and maintained
   (7) Does not interfere with electromagnetic navigation devices and communication systems
   (8) Is durable to withstand severe mechanical, thermal, and electrical stress, and repeated use

b. Extrication equipment*—Jaws of Life, air bags, center punch, Stokes' basket

c. Spinal immobilization devices—long spine board, short spine board,* cervical immobiling device (CID), cervical collars, sandbags*

d. Splinting devices
   (1) Traction splints*—Hare, Klippel, Thomas, etc.
   (2) Rigid splints*—ladder, premolded, board, etc.
   (3) Soft splints*—sling and swathe, triangular bandage, etc.
   (4) Air splints*—should not be used on air transports

e. Pneumatic antishock garments (PASG), also called military antishock trousers (MAST)

f. Airway maintenance
   (1) Bag-valve mask
   (2) Supplemental oxygen—nasal cannula, pocket mask,* partial rebreather mask, nonrebreather mask
   (3) Oxygen-powered breathing devices*
   (4) Esophageal obturator airway*
   (5) Endotracheal tubes
   (6) Nasal and oral airways
   (7) Equipment for needle cricothyroidotomy and oxygen adapter

g. Cardiac compression unit (Thumper)*

h. I.V. and intraosseous infusion fluids and catheters

i. I.V. pump infusion devices*

j. Low-tone Doppler*

4. Special procedures performed during prehospital care and transport

a. Intubation
b. Needle cricothyroidotomy
c. Needle decompression for tension pneumothorax
d. Intraosseous I.V. access
e. Helmet removal
f. Tourniquet placement and monitoring

5. Mass casualty triage

a. Mass casualty is defined as a medical emergency, i.e., event, series of events, or act of God, that overwhelms local capabilities and resources; the actual number of injured patients may vary depending upon local resources, medical personnel, and prehospital systems (1)
b. General principles
   (1) Those who are most seriously injured but salvageable are evacuated first
   (2) The most dramatic injuries may not be the most serious—assess airway breathing and circulation (ABCs)
   (3) Only initial assessment and ABCs are done at the scene—initiate care en route
   (4) Assume any patient with significant head or facial injuries also has a spinal injury
   (5) If tourniquet is used, write "T" and time applied on patient's forehead
c. Guidelines for mass casualty situation
   (1) Team leader establishes a triage area
      (a) Safe distance from known hazards
      (b) Located between casualties and access route to ensure an orderly system of triage, treatment, evacuation
   (2) Deploy personnel in teams
   (3) Assess every victim rapidly (ABCs) and assign a priority level
   (4) Identify each victim with a prenumbered tag; include identification number, information about the scene, brief physical examination for major injuries, treatment, priority level
   (5) Initiate ABCs
   (6) Report to team leader the number of victims and the priority levels
   (7) Team leader assigns evacuation number
   (8) Team leader assigns bystanders tasks according to their capabilities
d. Priority levels for evacuation
   (1) Class I—first priority
      (a) Airway compromise—actual or potential (e.g., person with tracheal or facial injuries)
      (b) Hemorrhagic shock
      (c) Severe head injury with unequal pupils
      (d) Ventilatory compromise—tension pneumothorax, flail chest, hemo/pneumothorax
      (e) Psychologic distress with uncontrolled behavior
   (2) Class II
      (a) Multiple long bone fractures
      (b) Stable patients at risk for occult injury—head, chest, abdomen, extremity

(c) Head injury with altered level of consciousness
(d) Large surface area burns
(3) Class III
(a) Lower extremity fractures
(b) Large muscle or tissue damage—avulsion, burns, degloving
(c) Amputation
(d) Hand injuries
(e) Eye injuries
(4) Class IV
(a) Upper extremity fractures
(b) Soft tissue injuries
(c) Walking wounded
(5) Class V—victims with psychological manifestations

6. Limitations for transport vehicles

a. All vehicle types are subject to limitations including availability, configuration, capability, and capacity
b. Considerations that affect care include
(1) Interior size
(2) Patient capacity
(3) Patient position and access
(4) Ease of loading and unloading
(5) Access to equipment
(6) Temperature control
(7) Speed
c. Operational limitations include weather, terrain, maintenance schedules, and environmental factors
d. Department of Transportation regulations address such factors as ambulance equipment, lights, maintenance schedules, vehicle safety, and personnel
e. Prehospital guidelines are also published in state EMS legislation, by the American College of Surgeons, and by the American Academy of Pediatrics
f. Safety considerations for all transports
(1) Hazards
(a) Unsecured equipment and personnel
(b) Other vehicles
(c) Untrained personnel
(d) Environmental factors
(e) Hazardous material
(f) Power lines and other obstructions
(g) "Sightseeing" by bystanders
(2) Safety measures
(a) Ensure personal safety
(b) Observe for visible hazards at the scene
(c) Ensure scene is secured by police or fire personnel
(d) Provide initial and recurrent training in safety and emergency procedures
(e) Properly secure equipment and personnel
(f) Limit intercom and radio transmissions
(g) Insist on adequate rest, sleep, and eating patterns for team members
(h) Provide safety orientation and regular drills

B. CONCEPTS SPECIFIC TO AIR TRANSPORT

1. Physiologic concepts related to altitude

a. Gas laws

(1) Boyle's—at a constant temperature, the volume of a given gas is inversely proportional to the pressure to which it is subjected (2); as altitude increases, barometric pressure decreases and gas expands

(2) Dalton's—the pressure of a gaseous mixture is equal to the sum of the partial pressure of the gases in that mixture (2); as altitude increases, gas molecules move farther apart, causing a decrease in the amount of available oxygen

(3) Henry's—the weight of a gas dissolved in a liquid is directly proportional to the weight of the gas above the liquid (2); decompression sickness, the "bends," occurs when a scuba diver ascends too rapidly and gas bubbles form in the blood

b. Systemic effects of altitude changes

(1) The physiologic zone is sea level to 8000 feet

(2) Barotrauma

(a) Barosinusitis—trapped gas in the sinuses, due to infection or edema, results in jaw or facial pain

(b) Barodentalgia—trapped gas in abscessed teeth, crowns, or fillings causes pain in the jaw or teeth

(c) Barobariatrauma—occurs in the presence of obesity when pressure changes cause the cell membranes of adipose tissue to weaken, resulting in a release of nitrogen and lipids (fat emboli) into the blood stream

(d) Barotitis media—occurs as a result of a blocked eustachian tube from infection or edema that, with pressure changes, prevents the escape of gas from the middle ear; rupture of the tympanic membrane may occur

(3) Respiratory conditions

(a) Pneumothoraces should be treated prior to transport to prevent air expansion at altitude

(b) In chronic obstructive pulmonary disease, trapped gas behind a mucus plug expands at altitude and may produce a pneumothorax

(4) High-altitude pulmonary edema (HAPE)

(a) Seen in people who are acclimated to an altitude above 9000 feet who move to a lower altitude, and then return to a higher altitude while exerting themselves with strenuous activities, such as skiing or hiking (3); may occur at any age

(b) Manifested by cerebral and pulmonary interstitial edema, causing confusion, restlessness, and symptoms of a myocardial infarction or pneumonia

(c) Prevent and treat by decreasing altitude and providing supplemental oxygen

(5) Rapid decompression—sudden loss of cabin pressurization

(a) Time of useful consciousness is limited by the flight altitude at which the decompression occurred

(b) Supplemental oxygen is immediately required for all persons on board the aircraft

(6) Decompression sickness
  (a) May be precipitated by loss of cabin pressurization while at an altitude of 30,000 feet or more for more than 5 to 10 min
  (b) Manifested by air embolus or "the chokes"—paroxysmal involuntary dry coughs, with associated chest pain and a feeling of suffocation (3)
  (c) Treatment includes rapid descent, 100% oxygen, and hyperbaric therapy (3)

c. Principles of cabin pressurization
  (1) Defined as a method of creating an artificial atmospheric pressure or "cabin altitude" inside the aircraft (2)
  (2) Each aircraft has a maximum pressure differential, the maximum limit of pressurization specified by the manufacturer

d. Oxygen requirements
  (1) Altitude oxygen requirement equation determines the amount of oxygen needed at any given altitude (3), i.e.,

$$\frac{\text{Current } FIO_2 \times \text{current barometric pressure}}{\text{Destination barometric pressure}} = FIO_2 \text{ required}$$

  (2) Calculation of alveolar-arterial difference of oxygen is useful in determining the presence of a shunt, i.e.,

$$PAO_2 - PaO_2 = AaDO_2$$

e. Stresses of flight
  (1) Hypoxia
    (a) As altitude increases, available oxygen decreases
    (b) Prevention
      i) Recognize the four categories of hypoxia, i.e., hypoxic hypoxia, anemic hypoxia, stagnant hypoxia, and histotoxic hypoxia (4)
      ii) Identify patients at risk and treat underlying conditions
      iii) Recognize the signs and symptoms of hypoxia and the stage at which they occur
  (2) Vibration
    (a) Vibration from the aircraft can cause circulatory constriction and override the body's cooling mechanism, thereby decreasing the ability to sweat (3)
    (b) Prevention and treatment
      i) Identify patients at risk, i.e., hypo- or hyperthermic
      ii) Monitor closely and institute cooling or warming measures as indicated
  (3) Thermal
    (a) As altitude increases, temperature decreases (3)
    (b) Prevent by providing a controlled ambient temperature and adequate thermal attire
  (4) Noise
    (a) Prolonged exposure can result in hearing loss; prevent by providing hearing protection
    (b) Makes auscultation of breath sounds and blood pressure difficult; use alternate methods not dependent on auscultation
  (5) Dehydration

(a) Ambient cabin environment is dry
(b) Provide humidified oxygen and adequate fluid
(6) G-forces
(a) Gravitational forces are applied to the body on ascent and descent; the gravitational pull and centrifugal forces may cause blood pooling
(b) Prevent by positioning patients to minimize the potential G-force effects
(7) Third spacing of fluids
(a) May occur or worsen due to vibration effects, or changes in temperature or G-forces
(b) Prevent by recognizing and minimizing the effects of the potential cause
(8) Fatigue
(a) Develops as a result of the body adapting to the other stresses of flight; affects patients and caregivers
(b) Minimize by adequate rest, proper diet, and avoiding alcohol and cigarettes

2. General concepts related to rotor-wing (helicopter) use in aeromedicine

a. Types of helicopters and configurations
(1) Single-engine, e.g., Aerospatiale Alouette and A-Star, Bell 206 Jet Ranger and Long Ranger
(2) Twin-engine, e.g., MMB BK-117 and BO-105, Bell 412 and 222, Aerospatiale Dauphin and Twin Star, Augusta 109, and Sikorsky S76

b. Capabilities and limitations
(1) Cabin size
(2) Patient position and access
(3) Ease of loading and unloading
(4) Airspeed
(5) Weight and balance considerations

c. Operational limitations
(1) Weather and environmental factors
(a) Ceiling and visibility
(b) Icing conditions
(c) Wind
(d) Temperature
(e) Thunderstorms
(2) Altitude limitations
(a) Supplemental oxygen required above 10,000 feet
(b) Aircraft performance hindered at higher altitudes
(c) Service ceiling—highest altitude at which flight characteristics and handling for an aircraft have been satisfactorily demonstrated (3)
(3) Airspeed limitations
(a) Velocity never exceed (VNE)—maximum allowable airspeed for an aircraft (3)
(b) VNE varies depending on type of aircraft, weight, altitude (3)
(4) Terrain
(a) Confined landing areas
(b) Surface considerations such as mud, light snow, ground slope, open water
(c) Obstacles such as antennas, mountains, high-tension wires

d. Federal Aviation Regulations (FAR) (3)

(1) FAR Part 91 details the general operating and flight rules for aircraft flying within U.S. airspace
(2) FAR Part 135 specifies rules for air taxi and commercial operators

e. Prehospital application
(1) State and local regulations may address staffing requirements, minimum equipment specifications, triage criteria, destination hospitals for specific patient conditions, licensure issues
(2) American College of Surgeons guidelines detail criteria to be utilized in determining the need for rapid transport of a trauma patient to a trauma center (5)
(3) Multiple victims tax available resources; aeromedical helicopters may be utilized to provide additional personnel and rapid transport capability

f. Interhospital application
(1) For patients with time-critical conditions, e.g., those requiring immediate operative intervention such as epidural bleeding or multiple trauma with internal bleeding
(2) No ground ALS available within a suitable time frame
(3) Critical care services required are not available from ground ALS
(4) Ground transport may aggravate or worsen patient's condition, e.g., unstable fractures

g. Safety considerations
(1) Hazards
(a) Other aircraft
(b) Wires and other obstructions
(c) Unsecured equipment and/or personnel
(d) Fire
(e) Mechanical problem with aircraft
(f) Untrained personnel
(g) Unsecured and/or unprepared LZ
(h) Rotor wash—strong winds produced by the aircraft during takeoffs and landings
(i) Noise
(j) "Hot" loading—loading the aircraft while engines are running and the blades are turning
(k) Main and tail rotor considerations
(2) Safety measures
(a) Observe for hazards in flight
(b) Participate in initial and recurrent training in safety and emergency procedures
(c) Secure equipment and personnel properly
(d) Keep intercom transmissions to a minimum
(e) Get adequate rest and adhere to duty time restrictions
(f) Provide safety orientations and drills for individuals and organizations that use the aircraft
(g) Assist the pilot in directing the activities of the ground personnel in and around the aircraft

3. General concepts related to fixed-wing use in aeromedicine

a. Types and configurations

(1) Dedicated, medically configured fixed-wing aircraft
(2) Chartered fixed-wing
(3) Commercial fixed-wing

b. Capabilities and limitations
(1) Cabin size
(2) Patient position and access
(3) Ease of loading and unloading
(4) Weight and balance considerations
(5) Airspeed
(6) Cabin pressurization capabilities
(7) Availability of fixed-wing aircraft
(8) Availability and location of medical equipment and supplies in aircraft

c. Operational limitations
(1) Weather and environmental factors
(2) Altitude limitations
(3) Intermediate ground or rotor-wing transport required

d. Federal Aviation Regulations

e. Safety considerations
(1) Hazards
(a) Untrained personnel
(b) Unsecured equipment and/or personnel
(c) Fire
(d) Mechanical problem with aircraft
(e) Noise
(f) Moving propellers, high exhaust temperatures, and fumes
(g) "Hot" loading
(2) Safety measures
(a) Equipment and personnel are secured properly
(b) Initial and recurrent training for air crew members in emergency procedures and basic fixed-wing aircraft safety
(c) Adequate rest and adherence to duty time restrictions

C. NURSING PROCESS DURING TRANSPORT

1. Assessment

a. Assess adequacy of ABCs
b. Determine chief complaint, obtain history of present illness, and perform secondary survey

2. Limitations to adequate assessment

a. Patient access
b. Motion, vibration
c. Minimal light
d. High noise level
e. Limited number of caregivers
f. Lack of privacy for patient

g. In air transport, G-forces/barometric pressure

3. Monitoring patient status during transport

a. Airway and ventilation
   (1) Respiratory excursion—depth, effort, symmetry, rate, and rhythm
   (2) Vital signs, level of consciousness
   (3) Tracheal shift
   (4) Assess breath sounds by low-tone Doppler
   (5) Presence of condensate in ET tube
   (6) Skin color
   (7) Pulse oximetry
   (8) Airway pressure assessment with gauges or through lung compliance with bagging
   (9) Capnometry—disposable carbon dioxide indicators to verify placement of ET tube

b. Circulatory
   (1) Skin color and temperature
   (2) Vital signs
      (a) Blood pressures measured by palpation, Doppler, and/or Dinemapp
      (b) Pulse—presence, amplitude, rhythm, and rate
   (3) Capillary refill
   (4) Urinary output
   (5) Level of consciousness

c. Neurologic response
   (1) Glasgow Coma Scale
   (2) Pupillary response

d. Neurovascular status distal to injury site

4. Nursing diagnoses commonly encountered during transport

a. Anxiety
b. Fear
c. Pain
d. Impaired communication
e. Impaired gas exchange
f. Sensory-perception alteration
   (1) Visual
   (2) Auditory
   (3) Kinesthetic
g. Impaired physical mobility
h. Alteration in tissue perfusion
   (1) Cerebral
   (2) Cardiopulmonary
   (3) Renal
   (4) Gastrointestinal
   (5) Peripheral
i. Potential change in body temperature
j. Potential for injury related to violent behavior

5. Priority nursing interventions during transport

a. Maintain airway
   (1) Suctioning

(2) Oral, nasopharyngeal airway
(3) Intubation
(4) Cricothyroidotomy

b. Maintain ventilation
(1) Manual ventilation
(2) Mechanical ventilator
(3) PEEP, CPAP
(4) Chest decompression
(5) Sedation and paralysis as needed

c. Maintain circulation
(1) I.V. fluid therapy with crystalloid, colloid, and volume expanders
(2) MAST (if indicated)
(3) Chest decompression
(4) Hemorrhage control

d. Prevention of secondary disabilities
(1) Spinal immobilization
(2) Stabilization of fractures
(3) Chemical restraints and sedation as needed
(4) Hyperventilation for suspected head injury

6. Communication

a. Radio usage
(1) Function of the Federal Communications Commission (FCC)
(2) Operational aspects
(a) Description and range of frequency bands
i) Ultrahigh frequency (UHF)
ii) Very high frequency (VHF)
(b) Types of frequencies
i) Simplex
ii) Duplex
(c) Functions of repeaters
(d) Function of continuous tone controlled subaudible squelch (CTCSS)
(e) Power output, range
(3) Types of radios and range
(a) Base station
(b) Mobile
(c) Portable
(d) Cellular phone
(e) Biotelemetry
(4) Guidelines for use
(a) Communication priorities
(b) Terminology

b. Communication with medical command
(1) Identify yourself, training level, and transport unit
(2) Obtain the same information from medical command
(3) Report should be brief, concise, and accurate

c. Utilize a standardized report format (**NOTE:** asterisked data may be omitted unless time permits)
(1) Age and sex of patient

(2) Pertinent brief history of mechanism of injury
(3) Chief complaint or major injury
(4) Time of extrication*
(5) Departure time from scene or facility*
(6) Arrival time at destination
(7) Vital signs and level of consciousness
(8) Glasgow Coma Score and Trauma Score*
(9) Pertinent physical findings
(10) Interventions performed, including medications administered
(11) Patient response

d. Review instructions given by medical command
   (1) Treatment interventions
   (2) Travel destination
e. Give medical command ETA to destination
f. Communications with the staff from referring and receiving facilities, family, and patient
   (1) Establish favorable rapport
   (2) Obtain/provide pertinent patient information
   (3) Provide explanations and reassurance to family and patient
   (4) Provide family with directions to the receiving facility
   (5) Inform staff at the receiving hospital of the whereabouts of the patient's family
g. Written documentation
   (1) Description of call
      (a) Prehospital scene
      (b) Interhospital transport
   (2) Information received prior to dispatch and/or while en route
   (3) Mechanism of injury and description of scene
   (4) Location of patient in reference to accident scene
   (5) Pertinent times
      (a) Dispatch
      (b) En route
      (c) Arrival at scene, landing zone, and/or hospital
      (d) Extrication
      (e) Departure from scene or referring hospital
      (f) Arrival at destination
   (6) Vital signs taken
   (7) Medication administered
   (8) Procedures performed
   (9) Treatment in progress by prehospital or hospital staff upon arrival of transport team
   (10) History of present injury, illness
   (11) Pertinent assessment findings
   (12) Pertinent diagnostic findings
   (13) Interventions rendered by team
   (14) Intake, output, and vital signs
   (15) Consent for transport
   (16) Summary of discussion with patient and family

(17) Report given to medical command physician and staff at receiving hospital
(18) Status of patient on arrival at destination

References

1. Cowley, R. A., & Dunham, C. M. (1982). *Shock trauma/critical care manual: Initial assessment and management.* Baltimore: University Park Press.
2. Sharp, G. R. (1978). The earth's atmosphere. In G. Dhenin (Ed.), *Aviation medicine I* (pp. 1–14). London: Tri–Med Books Ltd.
3. U.S. Department of Transportation, National Highway Traffic Safety Administration. (1986). *Air medical crew national standard curriculum: Advanced student manual.* Pasadena, CA: American Society of Hospital-Based Emergency Air Medical Services.
4. Sredl, D. (1983). *Airborne patient care management: A multidisciplinary approach* (pp. 45–52). St. Louis: Medical Research Associated Publications.
5. American College of Surgeons, Committee on Trauma. (1987). *Hospital and prehospital resources for optimal care of the injured patient (Appendices A–J).* Chicago: Author.

Suggested Readings

American Academy of Pediatrics Committee on Hospital Care. (1986). Guidelines for air and ground transportation of pediatric patients. *Pediatrics, 78*(5), 943–949.

Campbell, J. E. (Ed.). (1985). *Basic trauma life support.* Bowie, MD: Brady Communications.

Caroline, N. (1986). *Emergency care in the streets.* Boston: Little, Brown, & Co.

Hodges, J. B. (1989). Aeromedical transport. *Emergency Care Quarterly, 4*(4), 40–47.

Lee, G. (Ed.). (1991). *Flight nursing: Principles and practice.* St. Louis: Mosby-Year Book.

National Flight Nurses' Association. (1986). *Practice standards for flight nursing.* Columbia, MO: Waters Printing Co.

Stohler, S., & Jacobs, B. B. (1989). Interhospital transfer of the critical patient. *Emergency Care Quarterly, 4*(4), 66–78.

Zucker, L. (1989). Transport of the neurologically injured patient. *Emergency Care Quarterly, 4*(4), 40–47.

Section III
Comprehensive Topics in Trauma Nursing

MODULE 10
SHOCK

Donna A. Gares, MSN, RN, CCRN

Prerequisite

Review cardiovascular anatomy and physiology.

Objectives

1.0 Define shock and the mechanisms of compensatory, noncompensatory, and irreversible shock.
2.0 Describe the various types of shock.
2.1 List the five types of shock.
2.2 Identify the primary abnormality for each type of shock.
2.3 List diagnostic indicators for each type of shock.
2.4 List identifying signs and symptoms for the various shock states.
3.0 Discuss the medical management of the patient in shock.
3.1 List items/equipment that may be utilized to manage the patient in shock.
3.2 Identify parenteral agents used for the patient in shock.
3.3 List radiologic/laboratory studies used in the assessment of shock.
4.0 Describe the nursing management of the patient in shock.
4.1 Identify assessment data, including mechanism of injury and prehospital care, that may contribute to the shock state.
4.2 List common nursing diagnoses for the patient in shock.

4.3 Describe and prioritize nursing interventions for the patient in specific types of shock.
4.4 List expected outcomes and indicators of patient response to treatment of shock.

A. OVERVIEW OF THE PATHOPHYSIOLOGY OF SHOCK

1. Shock is a condition in which oxygen delivery or uptake at the tissue level is compromised, resulting in decreased cellular oxygenation and subsequent cellular ischemia and death

a. Adequate blood flow through the vascular bed is diminished secondary to
  (1) Decreased blood volume—hypovolemic shock
  (2) Increased peripheral vasodilation—septic, neurogenic, anaphylactic shock
  (3) Poor pumping ability of the heart—cardiogenic shock
b. Diminished blood flow results in decreased venous return to the heart
c. Decreased venous return results in a reduced cardiac output, low blood flow state, and decreased oxygen delivery or consumption by the cell
d. Decreased output by the left ventricle results in a low blood flow state and a reduction in cellular oxygenation

2. Nonprogressive or compensated shock

a. Body attempts to maintain hemodynamic stability
b. Cardiac output is reduced and blood pressure declines
  (1) Baroreceptors, triggered by a decline in blood pressure, stimulate the sympathetic nervous system to release catecholamines
  (2) Catecholamine release results in increased total peripheral resistance, heart rate, and myocardial contractility; leads to a rise in cardiac output (CO) and blood pressure (BP), and improved tissue perfusion
  (3) Decreased renal blood flow, due to renal arteriolar vasoconstriction, stimulates the renin-angiotensin system
    (a) Increases BP by vasoconstriction
    (b) Stimulates release of aldosterone to increase sodium reabsorption and water retention, causing an increase in the volume of extracellular fluid
  (4) Increased secretion of antidiuretic hormone, stimulated by decreased CO, causes retention of water and constriction of arterioles; restores fluid volume and elevates BP
  (5) Constricted arterioles reduce capillary hydrostatic pressure, causing translocation of fluid from the interstitial space into the intravascular space; increases circulating blood volume

3. Progressive or uncompensated shock

a. Occurs when the body is unable to compensate for the underlying failure
  (1) Blood vessels are unable to sustain vasoconstriction; vasodilation results in decreased total peripheral resistance and BP
  (2) Decreased tissue perfusion results in anaerobic metabolism and buildup of metabolic waste

(3) Acids and waste products act as potent vasodilators, further decreasing venous return and diminishing blood flow to vital organs and tissue
(4) Hypoxia and acidosis cause histamine and lysosomal enzyme release into the extracellular space, resulting in weakening of capillary membranes and increased capillary permeability
(5) Fluid shifts from the intravascular space to the interstitial space, further decreasing blood volume and venous return to the heart
(6) Decreased venous return causes sluggish blood flow and pooling in vessels; leads to agglutination and formation of microclots
(7) Myocardial depressant factor (MDF) is released from the ischemic pancreas; MDF depresses pumping ability of the heart and further decreases CO
(8) Ischemic changes begin to occur
(a) Kidneys—leads to acute renal failure
(b) Lungs—leads to adult respiratory distress syndrome
(c) Liver—leads to altered metabolic function and coagulopathies
(d) Gastrointestinal tract—leads to the release of vasodilating endotoxins, which contribute to shock progression
(e) Central nervous system—leads to confusion, lethargy, and coma

b. Uncompensated shock is a vicious cycle that must be aggressively managed and treated to prevent progression to irreversible shock

4. Irreversible shock—point at which patient is refractory to therapeutic management

a. Tissue damage extensive and incompatible with life
b. Multisystem organ failure becomes evident

B. HYPOVOLEMIC SHOCK

1. Pathophysiology

a. A decrease or loss of circulating fluid volume, i.e., blood, plasma, water, resulting in inadequate tissue perfusion
(1) Causes decreased venous return to the heart and reduced CO
(2) BP falls, resulting in inadequate tissue perfusion

b. Precipitating factors
(1) Acute whole blood loss (hemorrhage)—most prevalent type of shock in the trauma patient
(a) Blunt or penetrating injury to the vessels and organs
(b) Long bone or pelvic fractures
(c) Major vascular injury including traumatic amputation
(d) Multisystem injury
(2) Plasma loss—plasma shifts from intravascular space to interstitial space as a result of increased capillary permeability, e.g., crush, burn injuries
(3) Body fluid loss
(a) Dehydration
(b) Excess gastrointestinal drainage
(c) Diarrhea

(d) Ascites
(e) Diabetes insipidus
(f) Excess wound drainage
(g) Acute renal failure—high output phase
(h) Insensible loss through skin and lungs
(i) Osmotic diuresis secondary to hyperosmolar parenteral/enteral nutrition

c. Diagnostic indicators
(1) Evidence of bleeding via radiologic studies
(2) Evidence of bleeding via diagnostic procedures, e.g., peritoneal lavage, thoracostomy, thoracotomy
(3) Clinical findings (see 2b., physical examination)

2. Assessment

a. Interview (as outlined in Module 19—Nursing Assessment)
(1) Prehospital information including mechanism of injury
(2) Patient history

b. Physical examination—signs and symptoms depend on the amount of volume lost, the age of the patient, preexisting disease, and shock phase
(1) Phase I
(a) Loss of up to 15% of circulating blood volume
(b) Associated with most fractures and minor injuries to solid intraabdominal organs
(c) Clinical manifestations minimal if compensatory mechanisms intact
i) Anxiety—from stimulation of the sympathetic nervous system and release of catecholamines
ii) Prolonged capillary refill (slight)—occurs secondary to peripheral vasoconstriction
iii) Pallor of skin—secondary to peripheral vasoconstriction
iv) Heart rate, BP, pulse pressure, respiratory rate, and urine output are within normal limits (WNL)
(2) Phase II
(a) Loss of 15% to 30% of circulating blood volume
(b) Associated with hepatic and splenic injury, long bone fractures, pelvic injury, controlled vessel injuries
(c) Clinical manifestations become more evident
i) Altered sensorium—secondary to catecholamine release
ii) Delayed capillary refill
iii) Cool, pale, dry skin—occurs as blood from periphery is shunted to viscera
iv) Tachycardia (slight)—due to sympathetic vasoconstriction
v) Elevated diastolic blood pressure (slight)—secondary to increased peripheral resistance
vi) Decreased pulse pressure—due to increased peripheral resistance, which increases diastolic pressure
vii) Systolic blood pressure—normal or decreased if total blood volume decreased by 20%
viii) Decreased urine output (slight)—secondary to decreased renal perfusion
(3) Phase III

(a) Loss of 30% to 40% of circulating blood volume
(b) Associated with chest and vascular injuries, hepatic and splenic rupture, and multisystem injury
(c) Compensatory mechanisms ineffective, and signs and symptoms more apparent
i) Restlessness and apprehension occur with decreased blood flow to brain
ii) Cyanotic nailbeds
iii) Moist, cold skin—secondary to diminished tissue perfusion
iv) Tachycardia—120 to 130 beats/min
v) Hypotension—secondary to decreased venous return
vi) Decreased pulse pressure
vii) Oliguria—secondary to reduced blood flow to kidneys
viii) Tachypnea—secondary to metabolic acidosis and buildup of metabolic waste products

(4) Phase IV
(a) Loss of more than 40% of circulating volume
(b) Associated with uncontrolled chest injuries, severe injury to solid intraabdominal organs, and multisystem injury
(c) Compensatory mechanisms inactive—classic shock symptoms evident
i) Lethargy, unconsciousness—secondary to diminished cerebral perfusion
ii) Cyanotic nailbeds, lips
iii) Cyanotic or ashen gray skin
iv) Severe tachycardia
v) Severe hypotension
vi) Rapid, shallow respirations
vii) Anuria
viii) Cardiac arrhythmias—secondary to decreased myocardial oxygenation and lactic acidosis

c. Laboratory studies
(1) Trauma profile (see Module 19—Nursing Assessment)
(2) Other blood studies
(a) Serum lactate
(b) Type and cross-match for six units
(c) Serum osmolality
(d) Mixed venous gases
(3) Peritoneal lavage fluid analysis
(4) Radiologic studies
(1) Chest, pelvic, and spinal x-rays
(2) Computerized axial tomography
(3) Arteriograms

3. Medical management

a. Maintain patent airway; provide high flow humidified oxygen
b. Intubate and mechanically ventilate, if necessary
c. Perform needle or tube thoracostomy for tension pneumothorax
d. Insert two large bore vascular lines—protocols may vary
(1) Additional lines are inserted if patient is exhibiting signs of Phase III/IV shock

(2) Peripheral venous access is usually obtained via cannulation of upper extremity sites, i.e., antecubital fossa, with 14- or 16-gauge catheter
(3) Central venous access can be obtained via cannulation of large veins with an 8 Fr or larger catheter introducer, if peripheral access is unobtainable
(4) Venous cutdown can be accomplished via the femoral, saphenous, or basilic/cephalic veins
(5) Catheter sizes and types vary depending on site; use those that administer large volumes of fluid in a short period of time

e. Fluid management
(1) Patient's injuries, clinical presentation, and hemodynamic profile dictate which type(s) of fluid therapy will be used
(2) Crystalloids
(a) Used in early shock to increase plasma volume, replete interstitial fluid losses, and replace electrolyte deficits
(b) If blood loss is suspected, administer fluid in a 3:1 ratio, i.e., 3 liters of crystalloid for every 1 liter of blood loss
(c) Types
i) Lactated Ringer's solution—isotonic and similar in composition to serum plasma
a) Contains NaCl, KCl, CaCl, and sodium lactate
b) Normal liver converts lactate to bicarbonate; aids in buffering acidosis
ii) Sodium chloride injection (0.9%)—isotonic; contains sodium and chloride in excess of plasma levels
a) May cause fluid retention/overload and marked electrolyte imbalance due to high sodium content
b) Careful monitoring of serum electrolytes and hemodynamic parameters is essential
iii) Hypertonic saline is being used in clinical trials
iv) 5% dextrose in water (generally not used)
a) Though isotonic in solution, becomes hypotonic when infused and causes expansion of both intracellular and extracellular compartments
b) Massive amounts required to restore circulating volume
c) Contains no electrolytes
d) Incompatible with blood transfusions
e) Limited usefulness in hemorrhaging trauma patient
(3) Colloid solutions
(a) Used for plasma volume expansion
(b) Remain in intravascular compartment longer than crystalloids
(c) May be used with crystalloids
(d) Common types
i) Albumin
a) Isotonic (5%), or hypertonic (25%)
b) Chemically processed fraction of pooled plasma that is heat treated
c) Contains no preservatives; must be used immediately or discarded if opened

ii) Plasma
a) Separated from uncoagulated whole blood; fresh or fresh frozen
b) Contains clotting factors and plasma proteins but no platelets
c) Restores clotting factors and supplies plasma proteins

iii) Plasma protein fraction
a) 5% solution of selected plasma proteins diluted with buffered saline
b) Deficient in most clotting factors

iv) Hetastarch
a) Chemical colloid that approximates human albumin
b) May prolong bleeding times

(4) Blood and blood component therapy

(a) Whole blood
i) Complete, undivided blood; contains red and white blood cells, platelets, plasma, and coagulation factors
ii) Coagulation factors are inactivated as blood ages (storage time increases)
iii) If available, fresh whole blood is ideal
iv) Restores volume and improves oxygen-carrying capacity of red cells

(b) Packed red blood cells (PRBCs)
i) Remnants of whole blood after the removal of plasma
ii) Oxygen-carrying capacity of one unit of PRBCs equals one unit of whole blood
iii) Contains minimal platelets/clotting factors
iv) Used to restore a red blood cell deficiency

(c) Platelets
i) Thrombocytes extracted from plasma and resuspended in plasma
ii) Used to control bleeding in the individual with thrombocytopenia
iii) Used when massive transfusion of stored blood has caused dilutional thrombocytopenia

(d) Cryoprecipitate
i) A concentrate removed from cold-thawed plasma which contains Factor I (fibrinogen), Factor VIII (antihemophilic factor), and Factor XIII (fibrin stabilizing factor)
ii) Used to restore fibrinogen when massive transfusion of stored blood has caused a dilutional coagulopathy

(e) Complications of massive transfusion therapy must be considered when managing the hemorrhaging trauma patient
i) Dilutional (washout) coagulopathy—develops from transfusion of large amounts of stored blood with minimal platelets/clotting factors
ii) Hypothermia—from transfusion of large amounts of cold blood
iii) Hypocalcemia—stored blood contains calcium citrate, which binds with ionized serum calcium and causes a calcium deficit
iv) Early acidosis followed by alkalosis
a) Stored blood has a pH of 7.0; pH decreases over storage life
b) Citrate in stored blood is broken down by the liver to become bicarbonate, causing metabolic alkalosis

(5) Additional considerations

(a) Warm fluids to maintain normothermia; crystalloid solutions may be kept in a fluid warmer or given via rapid infusion warming devices

(b) Immediate transfusion needed for exsanguination or unstable vital signs despite infusion of crystalloids/colloids
  i) Use O-negative blood for females of childbearing age and O-positive for all others
  ii) Use type-specific and/or cross-matched blood when available
(c) Administer blood using a high volume, rapid infusion warmer; if not available, add warm saline to increase blood temperature and decrease viscosity
(d) Eliminate extension sets and stopcocks from I.V. setups as they may inhibit fluid flow
(e) Pressure bags may be used on I.V. solutions and blood products to increase flow rate
(f) The minimum I.V. tubing setup for the trauma patient should be standard blood tubing with a "Y" spike (larger diameter than standard I.V. tubing)
(g) Large bore I.V. tubing (8 Fr or larger) is also available

f. Control bleeding by pressure and elevation
g. Apply pneumatic antishock garment (PASG)
  (1) Increases BP by increasing peripheral vascular resistance through compression of the lower extremities and abdomen
  (2) Tamponades bleeding from fractures and wounds
  (3) Stabilizes/immobilizes pelvic and extremity fractures
  (4) Contraindicated in
    (a) Pulmonary edema (absolute)
    (b) Congestive heart failure (absolute)
    (c) Pregnancy (relative)—leg compartments may be inflated
    (d) Abdominal evisceration or impalement (relative)
    (e) Impalement of lower extremity (relative)—the abdominal compartment and remaining extremity may be inflated
    (f) Spinal trauma (relative)
    (g) Intrathoracic trauma (relative)
    (h) Head injury with increased intracranial pressure (relative); in the presence of hypotension, application of the PASG may actually improve cerebral perfusion pressure by increasing mean arterial pressure
  (5) Complications of use of PASG include compartment syndrome, respiratory embarrassment, skin breakdown, and metabolic acidosis
  (6) Other considerations in use of PASG
    (a) Systolic BP should be maintained between 90 and 100 mm Hg
    (b) Monitor patient's blood pressure during inflation to determine appropriate inflation level
    (c) Inflate leg compartments first, then abdominal compartment until desired, optimal blood pressure is obtained
    (d) Keep PASG inflated until bleeding controlled, fluid therapy underway, and blood pressure adequate
    (e) Rapid deflation of the PASG can cause profound hypotension
      i) Deflate slowly and check BP immediately after each deflation
      ii) If the systolic pressure begins to fall more than 5 mm Hg, discontinue deflation

iii) Administer fluids as needed to return blood pressure to previous state
iv) Restart deflation process as prescribed
(f) Use of PASG in controlled settings, i.e., hospital, is controversial

h. Insert pulmonary artery catheter and central venous catheter
i. Insert arterial line for monitoring arterial blood gases (ABGs) and BP
j. Monitor mixed venous oxygen saturation via fiberoptic Swan–Ganz catheter
k. Perform pericardiocentesis if indicated; diagnose and treat cardiac tamponade
l. Perform emergency thoracotomy
m. Perform diagnostic peritoneal lavage; if positive, perform exploratory laparotomy (see Module 23–Abdominal Injury)
n. Perform surgical procedures as needed

C. SEPTIC SHOCK

1. Pathophysiology

a. Hemodynamic instability, metabolic derangement, and coagulation disturbances resulting from overwhelming systemic infection
 (1) Most commonly due to Gram-negative bacteremia
 (2) Also caused by Gram-positive bacteria, fungi, viruses, and rickettsiae
b. Endotoxins, found in cell walls of Gram-negative organisms, are released into the systemic circulation; results in activation of various hormonal and chemical mediators
c. Mediators have numerous effects; ultimately decrease tissue perfusion
 (1) Massive arterial and venous vasodilation—causes decreased total peripheral resistance, decreased venous return to the heart, and reduced CO
 (2) Increased capillary permeability—fluid shifts from vascular compartment to interstitial space; leads to loss of circulating volume, reducing CO
 (3) Activation of clotting factors and platelet aggregation—results in microcirculatory coagulation and impedes capillary blood flow
d. Precipitating factors associated with septic shock
 (1) Preexisting chronic disease
 (2) Age
 (3) Debilitation
 (4) Immunosuppression
 (5) Intravascular lines
 (6) Indwelling urinary catheter
 (7) Ventriculostomy catheter
 (8) Endotracheal intubation, tracheostomy
 (9) Peritonitis
 (10) Open wounds, soft tissue trauma, burns
 (11) Retained foreign bodies, inadequate debridement
 (12) Surgical procedures
 (13) Hypovolemic shock
e. Diagnostic indicators
 (1) Positive blood cultures

(2) Fever
(3) Elevated WBC with shift to the left
(4) Elevated liver and pancreatic enzymes
(5) Clinical findings (see 2b., physical examination)

2. Assessment

a. Interview (see Module 19–Nursing Assessment)
   (1) Prehospital information including scene contaminants; evidence of placement of invasive lines under less than ideal conditions
   (2) Recent surgical or diagnostic procedures

b. Physical examination
   (1) Evidence of traumatic wounds
   (2) Evidence of any infection processes, e.g., urinary tract or wound infection
   (3) Findings vary—patient may be in hyperdynamic shock (early, warm phase), or hypodynamic shock (late, cold phase)
      (a) Hyperdynamic shock—characterized by a normal or increased cardiac index (CO ÷ body surface area), decreased peripheral vascular resistance, and increased pulmonary vascular resistance
         i) Hypotension—from massive vasodilation
         ii) Tachycardia—due to decreased BP
         iii) Tachypnea and hyperventilation
         iv) Oliguria—results from decreased BP and renal vasoconstriction; occasionally a brief period of altered renal blood flow may cause a transient increase in urine output
         v) Altered sensorium (confusion, anxiety, restlessness)—from decreased cerebral perfusion
         vi) Warm, dry, pink skin with possible mottling of lower extremities
         vii) Fever
      (b) Hypodynamic shock—characterized by decreased cardiac index and increased systemic vascular resistance
         i) Severe hypotension
         ii) Persistent, extreme tachycardia with arrhythmias
         iii) Rapid, shallow respirations
         iv) Anuria and azotemia
         v) Obtunded or unresponsive to verbal or painful stimuli
         vi) Cold, pale, clammy skin with diffuse mottling
         vii) Hypothermia

c. Laboratory studies
   (1) Trauma profile (see Module 19—Nursing Assessment)
   (2) Arterial and mixed venous blood gases
   (3) Cultures of blood, urine, sputum, wounds, catheter tips, suspicious sites
   (4) Liver and pancreatic enzymes

d. Radiologic studies
   (1) Facial x-rays (for possible covert sinusitis)
   (2) Chest x-rays (for possible pneumonia)
   (3) Abdominal x-rays (for possible abscesses)

3. Medical management

a. Insert central and pulmonary artery catheters
b. Support circulation and provide fluids, e.g., crystalloids, colloids, and/or blood products

c. Initiate broad spectrum antibiotics for Gram-negative and Gram-positive organisms, until septic focus is determined
d. Initiate vasopressor/inotropic agents; steroids as necessary
e. Surgical intervention—debride necrotic tissue; drain infected fluid collections, e.g., abscesses

D. NEUROGENIC SHOCK

1. **Pathophysiology**
a. A loss of vasomotor tone, secondary to interruption of sympathetic outflow, resulting in generalized vasodilation
   (1) Usually occurs following spinal cord injury above T_6 level
   (2) May occur from insult to medullary area of brain
b. Transection or severe injury to the spinal cord results in complete loss of reflexes below the level of injury, and interruption of sympathetic pathways from the medullary vasomotor center to peripheral blood vessels
c. Interruption of sympathetic outflow blocks vasoconstrictive response, and results in vasodilation of the vascular bed below the level of injury
d. Vasodilation causes decreased systemic vascular resistance and peripheral pooling of blood
e. Venous return to the heart is diminished, reducing CO
f. Precipitating factors
   (1) Spinal trauma as a result of motor vehicle crashes, falls, gunshot wounds, stabbing, diving, motorcycle crashes, and sports injuries
   (2) High spinal anesthesia and epidural block
   (3) Depression of medullary brain stem function from head injury, overdose of barbiturates, tranquilizers, and general anesthesia
g. Diagnostic indicators
   (1) Evidence of spinal cord injury and reflex loss through neurologic examination (see 2b., physical examination)
   (2) Evidence of spinal cord injury on radiologic films
2. **Assessment (see Module 19—Nursing Assessment—and Module 21—Spinal Cord Injury)**
a. Interview
   (1) Prehospital information including field assessment of neurologic status
   (2) Past medical history including recent drug intake
b. Physical examination—neurologic shock can result in altered cardiovascular status and loss of sensory, motor, and reflex functions
   (1) Cardiovascular changes
      (a) Hypotension—secondary to decreased venous return
      (b) Bradycardia—secondary to loss of sympathetic control
      (c) Loss of temperature control—poikilothermia
      (d) Inability to sweat below injury level—secondary to lack of innervation of sweat glands
   (2) Loss of motor function

(a) Absence of voluntary motor activity below the level of injury
(b) Flaccid paralysis below level of lesion
(3) Loss of sensory function—pain, temperature, touch, pressure, proprioception
(4) Areflexia
(5) Warm, dry skin
(6) Priapism
c. Laboratory studies
(1) Trauma profile
(2) Arterial blood gases
(3) Alcohol level
(4) Toxicology profile
d. Radiologic studies
(1) Spinal x-rays
(2) Computerized axial tomography (CAT scan) of head, neck, and/or abdomen
(3) Myelogram

3. Medical management

a. Maintain airway and breathing
b. Insert central catheters
c. Support circulation and provide fluids, i.e., crystalloids, colloids, and/or blood products
d. Initiate vasopressor agents

E. ANAPHYLACTIC SHOCK

1. Pathophysiology

a. Severe allergic reaction that results from exposure to an antigen to which an individual was previously sensitized; culminates in profound vasodilation
b. Antigen is introduced into previously sensitized body tissues
c. Antigen-antibody reaction occurs and results in the activation of various mediators with numerous effects, including
(1) Vasodilation and increased capillary permeability
(a) Results in peripheral blood pooling and translocation of intravascular fluid into interstitial space
(b) Circulating blood volume, venous return, and CO are decreased
(2) Contraction of nonvascular, smooth muscle, i.e., bronchospasm
(3) Laryngeal and pulmonary edema secondary to fluid shifting from vascular to interstitial compartment
d. Precipitating factors
(1) Drugs
(2) Contrast media, especially those with iodine
(3) Anesthetics
(4) Blood products
(5) Foods
(6) Snake and insect venom
e. Diagnostic indicators
(1) Evidence of prior allergic reaction

(2) Previous exposure to the antigen
(3) Laryngeal edema via bronchoscopy
(4) Clinical findings (see 2b., physical examination)

2. **Assessment**

a. Interview
(1) Past medical history
(2) Detailed information on allergies to foods, drugs, or other substances; describe reaction
(3) Recent exposures to potential causative agents; include time of exposure, ingestion, injection, onset of symptoms
(4) Current medications

b. Physical examination—findings
(1) Cardiovascular system—hypotension (secondary to decreased circulating volume), tachycardia (secondary to hypotension), arrhythmias/arrest, decreased CO, cyanosis
(2) Respiratory system—dyspnea, hoarseness, stridor, wheezing, rales, rhonchi, respiratory arrest
(3) Severe anxiety, apprehension
(4) Syncope
(5) Unconsciousness
(6) Urticaria, pruritus, diffuse erythema
(7) Angioedema
(8) Abdominal pain, nausea, vomiting, diarrhea

c. Laboratory and radiologic studies
(1) Trauma profile
(2) ABGs
(3) Coagulation profile
(4) Chest x-ray

3. **Medical management**

a. Establish airway via endotracheal intubation, tracheostomy, or cricothroidotomy
b. Insert central I.V. line and/or pulmonary artery line
c. Insert arterial line to monitor blood pressure
d. Administer medications to counteract shock state
(1) Epinephrine—vasoconstricts blood vessels and increases cardiac contractility; relaxes bronchial smooth muscle and relieves bronchospasm
(2) Antihistamines—block histamine effects on vascular bed and bronchioles; help relieve pruritus and erythema
(3) Steroids—may stabilize the capillary membrane and minimize intravascular volume loss
(4) Aminophylline—relaxes bronchial smooth muscle

F. CARDIOGENIC SHOCK

1. **Pathophysiology**

a. Pumping ability of heart is altered secondary to left ventricular failure, myocardial cell degeneration, mechanical obstruction, obstruction of venous return, and/or cardiac arrhythmias

b. Cardiac muscle is unable to contract effectively, resulting in increased ventricular filling pressures
c. Stroke volume decreases and cardiac output falls
d. Tissue hypoperfusion ensues secondary to decreased BP and circulating volume
e. Precipitating factors
  (1) Acute myocardial infarction—most common
  (2) Cardiomyopathies
  (3) Ventricular wall or papillary muscle rupture
  (4) Severe cardiac contusion
  (5) Cardiac tamponade
  (6) Tension pneumothorax
  (7) Pulmonary embolus
  (8) Myocarditis
  (9) Atherosclerotic heart disease
  (10) Hypovolemic, septic, neurogenic, anaphylactic shock states
f. Diagnostic indicators
  (1) Suspicion or evidence of cardiac trauma
  (2) Clinical findings (see 2b., physical examination)
  (3) Evaluation of hemodynamic parameters
  (4) Other tests utilized to diagnose the underlying event

2. Assessment

a. Interview (see Module 19—Nursing Assessment)
b. Physical examination—findings and hemodynamic parameters
  (1) Hypotension
  (2) Weak, thready pulses
  (3) Abnormal heart sounds—S_3, S_4, or murmur
  (4) Dyspnea or tachypnea
  (5) Pulmonary edema, congestion, and rales
  (6) Delayed capillary refill
  (7) Cool, pale, clammy skin with possible mottling
  (8) Dependent edema
  (9) Oliguria
  (10) Lethargy, agitation
  (11) Hypoxemia
  (12) Metabolic acidosis
  (13) Cardiac arrhythmias
  (14) Evidence of acute myocardial infarction—chest pain, ECG changes, positive cardiac isoenzymes
  (15) Increased systemic vascular resistance and pulmonary artery diastolic pressures
  (16) Decreased cardiac output/cardiac index
c. Laboratory studies
  (1) Trauma profile
  (2) Arterial and mixed venous blood gases
  (3) Cardiac isoenzymes
  (4) Electrocardiogram/echocardiogram
d. Radiologic studies
  (1) Chest x-ray

(2) Ventilation/perfusion scan
(3) Multiple gate acquisition (MUGA) scan
(4) Technetium/thallium scan

3. **Medical management**

a. Ensure patent airway; endotracheal intubation
b. Maintain breathing; mechanical ventilation
b. Insert central, arterial, and pulmonary artery catheters
c. Provide fluids as indicated, i.e., crystalloids, colloids, and/or blood products; use caution—patient is frequently overloaded
d. Evaluate hemodynamic profile—CO, cardiac index, pulmonary end diastolic pressure and/or pulmonary capillary wedge pressure, systemic vascular resistance
e. Initiate appropriate drug therapy
   (1) Inotropic agents—to increase cardiac output, e.g., Dopamine, Dobutamine, Isuprel, Amrinone
   (2) Vasopressors—to increase BP through vasoconstriction; may cause increased oxygen consumption, e.g., epinephrine, norepinephrine, Aramine
   (3) Vasodilators—to decrease afterload and reduce oxygen consumption; do not use if hypotension is present, e.g., sodium nitroprusside, nitroglycerin
   (4) Diuretics—to reduce preload and improve CO, e.g., furosemide
f. Intraaortic balloon pump to reduce afterload
g. Pericardiocentesis, if indicated; diagnose and treat cardiac tamponade
h. Formal pericardial window/exploration in operating room for tamponade
i. Rotating tourniquets

G. NURSING DIAGNOSES, EXPECTED OUTCOMES, AND INTERVENTIONS

1. **Potential or actual impaired gas exchange related to decreased blood flow, obstructed airway, or pulmonary edema**

a. Expected outcome—adequate gas exchange as evidenced by
   (1) Normal respiratory rate and rhythm
   (2) Clear and equal breath sounds
   (3) Adequate ABGs—pH 7.35 to 7.45; PaO_2 more than 80 mm Hg; O_2 saturation more than 95%
   (4) Normal chest x-ray
b. Nursing interventions
   (1) Maintain patent airway
   (2) Administer high flow humidified oxygen
   (3) Assist with intubation and mechanical ventilation as needed; monitor peak inspiratory pressure
   (4) Suction pro re nata (prn); preoxygenate and limit actual suctioning time (prevents vasovagal reflex and subsequent bradycardia)
   (5) Monitor respiratory rate, rhythm, chest excursion, and use of accessory muscle
   (6) Assess breath sounds for rales, rhonchi, wheezes

(7) Obtain ABGs and monitor for signs of hypoxemia and/or hypercapnia
(8) Monitor arterial oxygenation via pulse oximeter
(9) Assist with thoracostomy tube placement and monitor functioning of system and drainage
(10) Position patient for optimal perfusion of lungs and lung function
(11) Administer chest physiotherapy and encourage use of incentive spirometry
(12) Prevent aspiration by inserting nasoorogastric tube and connecting to straight drainage or suction

2. **Fluid volume deficit related to loss of fluid from the intravascular compartment**

a. Expected outcome—hemodynamic stability as evidenced by
(1) Heart rate 60 to 100 beats/min
(2) Normal sinus rhythm
(3) Systolic BP more than 90 mm Hg
(4) Peripheral pulses normal (+2)
(5) CO 4 to 6 liters/min
(6) Cardiac index 2.8 to 4.2 liters/min/m^2
(7) Pulmonary artery diastolic pressure 8 to 15 mm Hg
(8) Systemic vascular resistance 900 to 1400 dynes/sec/cm^2
(9) Central venous pressure 5 to 8 mm H_2O
(10) Mixed venous oxygen saturation 60 to 80%
(11) Normal serum electrolytes

b. Nursing interventions
(1) Control bleeding with direct pressure or PASG
(2) Observe for early signs of shock
(3) Insert large bore peripheral I.V. catheters
(4) Assist with insertion of arterial and central venous catheters
(5) Administer warmed crystalloids and colloids for Phase I/II shock via large bore administration set
(6) Administer warmed crystalloids, colloids, and blood components for Phase III/IV shock via large bore administration set; provide calcium supplements as prescribed
(7) Prepare for autotransfusion; monitor blood loss and reinfuse autologous blood as needed
(8) Obtain and monitor initial and serial blood studies, including hemoglobin and hematocrit, platelets, coagulation factors, and serum calcium
(8) Monitor vital signs and hemodynamic parameters, including pulmonary artery pressure (PAP), pulmonary capillary wedge pressure (PCWP), CO, cardiac index, and mixed venous oxygen saturation
(9) Insert urinary catheter; measure intake and output
(10) Anticipate need and assist with emergency thoracotomy and diagnostic peritoneal lavage

3. **Inadequate tissue perfusion related to hypovolemia, vasoconstriction, peripheral pooling of blood, and/or decreased venous return to the heart**

a. Expected outcome—adequate perfusion of vital organs as evidenced by
(1) Orientation to person, place, and time
(2) Pupils equal, reactive to light
(3) Urine output more than 30 cc/hr

(4) Skin warm, dry, pink
(5) Capillary refill less than 3 sec

b. Nursing interventions
(1) Apply PASG if indicated
(2) Monitor neurologic status frequently; observe for signs of cerebral hypoperfusion
(3) Monitor temperature, capillary refill, appearance of skin; regulate ambient temperature
(4) Monitor pulse and BP, PAP, PCWP, CO, and cardiac index
(5) Provide warmed fluid (I.V. and lavage) and warmed, humidified oxygen to prevent hypothermia
(6) Insert urinary catheter and monitor urine output and specific gravity
(7) Administer medications to counteract shock state, e.g., epinephrine, antihistamines, steroids, aminophylline
(8) Administer and titrate vasopressors as prescribed; avoid use of vasopressors if patient is vasoconstricted
(9) Monitor liver enzymes, coagulation profile
(10) Monitor blood pH for signs of acidosis or alkalosis
(11) Auscultate bowel sounds every (q) 4 hrs; maintain naso/orogastric tube to suction, if needed
(12) In neurogenic shock, monitor heart rate for bradycardia (parasympathetic innervation is unopposed secondary to impaired sympathetic nervous system); keep Atropine at bedside and administer for heart rate less than 40 or as prescribed
(13) Observe for signs of deep vein thrombosis; measure thigh/calf circumference daily and note serial changes (see Module 16—Medical Sequelae—for interventions)

4. Alteration in cardiac output; decreased, secondary to hypovolemia, massive vasodilation, and/or increased capillary permeability

a. Expected outcome—hemodynamic stability (see 2a., expected outcome criteria)

b. Nursing interventions
(1) Establish large bore peripheral catheters
(2) Administer crystalloids, colloids, and blood products as prescribed
(3) Assist with insertion, and maintain pulmonary artery and peripheral arterial catheters
(4) Monitor heart rate, rhythm, BP, PAP, PCWP, CO, cardiac index, and mixed venous oxygen saturation
(5) Assess frequently for signs of circulatory overload and pulmonary edema
(6) Administer vasopressor and inotropic agents; titrate and monitor for patient response
(7) Manage patient on intraaortic balloon pump

5. Ineffective airway clearance related to bronchospasm or pulmonary edema

a. Expected outcome—patent airway as evidenced by
(1) Normal character and rate of respirations
(2) PaO_2 greater than 80 mm Hg
(3) Clear breath sounds

b. Nursing interventions
(1) Administer antihistamines, bronchodilators, and diuretics as prescribed

(2) Suction airway as needed
(3) Anticipate need for/assist with intubation
(4) Administer high flow humidified oxygen
(5) Assess respiratory rate, rhythm, breath sounds, chest excursion; monitor for signs of distress
(6) Monitor ABGs for hypoxemia/hypercapnia
(7) Auscultate for rales, S_3, S_4 heart sounds
(8) Provide pulmonary hygiene
(9) Apply rotating tourniquets for severe pulmonary edema

6. **Additional nursing diagnoses**

a. Potential for infection related to presence of invasive catheters (see Module 12—Infection)
b. Potential for further injury to spinal cord related to loss of sensory, motor, and reflex functions in neurogenic shock
c. Potential for injury in the unconscious patient related to administration of potential allergens, e.g., penicillin, radiopaque dyes
d. Fluid volume excess related to cardiac failure, renal failure, and/or excessive, rapid I.V. infusion

Suggested Readings

Balk, R., & Bone, R. (1989). The septic syndrome: Definition and clinical implications. *Critical Care Clinics, 5*(1), 1–6.

Beckwith, N., & Carriere, S. R. (1985). Fluid resuscitation in trauma: An update. *Journal of Emergency Nursing, 11*(6), 293–299.

Bressnack, M., & Raffin, T. (1987). Physiology and management of shock. *Chest,* 92(5), 906–912.

Cardona, V., Hurn, P., Mason, P., Scanlon-Schilpp, A., & Veise-Berry, S. (Eds.). (1988). *Trauma nursing: From resuscitation through rehabilitation.* Philadelphia: W. B. Saunders Co.

Conn, A. (1985). Hypovolemic shock. *Emergency Care Quarterly, 1*(2), 37–46.

Cowley, R. A. (Ed.). (1987). *Trauma care: Vol. I. Surgical management.* Philadelphia: J. B. Lippincott Co.

Dickerson, M. (1988). Anaphylaxis and anaphylactic shock. *Critical Care Nursing Quarterly, 11*(1), 68–74.

Jeffries, P., & Whelan, S. (1988). Cardiogenic shock: Current management. *Critical Care Nursing Quarterly, 11*(1), 48–56.

McCormac, M. (1990). Managing hemorrhagic shock. *American Journal of Nursing, 90*(8), 22–27.

Myers, K., & Hickey, M. (1988). Nursing management of hypovolemic shock. *Critical Care Nursing Quarterly, 11*(1), 57–67.

Nikas, D. (1988). Pathophysiology and nursing interventions in acute spinal cord injury. *Trauma Quarterly, 4*(3), 23–44.

Olsen, J., & Larson, E. (1985). Cardiogenic shock. *Emergency Care Quarterly, 1*(2), 19–27.

Reed, M. (1987). Nursing considerations in acute spinal cord injury. *Critical Care Clinics, 3*(3), 679.

Rice, V. (Ed.). (1990). Shock. *Critical Care Nursing Clinics of North America,* 2(2), entire issue.

Rice, V. (1984). The clinical continuum of septic shock. *Critical Care Nurse,* 4(5), 86–109.

Strange, J. (1987). *Shock trauma care plans.* Springhouse, PA: Springhouse Corp.

Swearingen, P. L., Sommers, M. S., & Miller, K. (Eds.). (1988). *Manual of critical care: Applying nursing diagnoses to adult critical illness.* St. Louis: C. V. Mosby Co.

Wahl, S. (1989). Septic shock: How to detect it early. *Nursing,* 19(1), 52–60.

Walt, A. (Ed.). (1982). *Early care of the injured patient.* Philadelphia: W. B. Saunders Co.

Section III
Comprehensive Topics in Trauma Nursing

MODULE 11
NUTRITION

Karen A. Gilbert, MSN, RN, CNSN

Prerequisite

Review anatomy and physiology of gastrointestinal and metabolic systems.

Objectives

1.0 Describe the metabolic effects of trauma and their impact on nutritional status.
1.1 List major catabolic hormones stimulated during stress response.
1.2 Explain alterations in carbohydrate, protein, and fat metabolism in trauma; compare them to alterations in unstressed starvation.
1.3 Describe the impact of stressed starvation on patient outcome.
2.0 Identify common medical and surgical interventions used during initiation and maintenance of nutritional support.
3.0 Describe nutritional assessment of the trauma patient.
3.1 Explain aspects of medical and dietary history needed to evaluate nutritional status.
3.2 Identify key components of physical and clinical nutritional assessment.
3.3 State three categories used to classify malnourished patients.
3.4 Recognize the need for early nutritional assessment in the trauma population.

4.0 Develop nursing diagnoses, including etiologies, based on nutritional assessment data.
5.0 Identify nursing interventions related to nutritional support.
6.0 Define desirable nutritional outcomes for the trauma patient including measurable criteria for evaluation of nutritional progress.
7.0 Given a specific case history, anticipate the plan for nutritional support of a patient at various phases of the trauma continuum.

A. EFFECT OF TRAUMA ON METABOLISM

1. **Anabolic and catabolic equilibrium is disrupted during acute phase of injury; favors protein utilization and negative nitrogen balance**
2. **Sympathetic nervous system generates a neuroendocrine response resulting in**
   a. Hypermetabolism
   b. Increased protein catabolism
   c. Increased secretion of catecholamines (epinephrine), glucocorticoids (cortisol), and glucagon, which increase metabolism
   d. Increased insulin secretion with insulin resistance and hyperglycemia
   e. Increased excretion of urinary nitrogen
   f. Stimulation of gluconeogenesis (conversion of protein to carbohydrate by the liver) to provide energy
   g. Aldosterone (adrenal cortex) and antidiuretic hormone secretion (posterior pituitary) lead to water and sodium retention with potassium secretion; patient may become oliguric, hypervolemic, hyponatremic, alkalotic, and edematous
3. **Alterations in substrate metabolism**
   a. Carbohydrate
      (1) Glucagon stimulates utilization of liver glycogen to produce glucose; glucose stores last less than one day
      (2) Glycogen is the first substrate to be used by the body for energy under stress
      (3) Epinephrine and norepinephrine enhance gluconeogenesis; gluconeogenesis is difficult to suppress due to increased epinephrine and norepinephrine
      (4) Although serum glucose levels increase, glucose is less available to the cells
      (5) Note: brain, RBCs, WBCs, bone marrow, and heart are very glucose dependent
   b. Protein
      (1) All body proteins are functional; none exist in storage form
      (2) Amino acids (AA) are a preferred energy source during stress and trauma, and are broken down simultaneously with fat during periods of stress
      (3) Moderate increase in protein synthesis with large amount of protein breakdown and excretion
      (4) Muscle protein breakdown occurs via gluconeogenesis; alanine, leucine, isoleucine, and valine are especially significant

(5) Major organs are broken down and used for energy as skeletal muscle is depleted
(6) Negative nitrogen balance adversely affects wound healing, resistance to infection, and other protein-related functions

c. Fat
(1) Triglyceride breaks down to glycerol and free fatty acids
(2) Catecholamines increase the rate of fat mobilization
(3) Exogenous fat supply is necessary to prevent essential fatty acid deficiency

4. Effect of stress and malnutrition on patient outcomes

a. Impaired wound healing, wound dehiscence
b. Weight loss, primarily lean body mass
c. Increased incidence of infection and sepsis
d. Decreased function of major organs
e. Contributes to major organ failure and death
f. Due to above, length of hospital stay is increased

B. MEDICAL AND SURGICAL NUTRITIONAL SUPPORT INTERVENTIONS

1. **Limit hypermetabolic state by surgically repairing tissue injury, grafting burns, treating infection, debriding necrotic tissue, and draining abscesses**
2. **Replace fluids and electrolytes and maintain balance**
3. **Determine if gastrointestinal tract is functional or dysfunctional**
4. **Initiate appropriate nutritional therapy no later than two to three days postinjury**
5. **Insert appropriate enteral feeding devices: nasogastric, nasoenteric, esophagostomy, percutaneous endoscopic gastrostomy (PEG), percutaneous endoscopic jejunostomy (PEJ), surgical gastrostomy, or surgical jejunostomy**
6. **Insert central venous catheter, either percutaneous or indwelling, for total parenteral nutrition (TPN)**
7. **Prescribe appropriate enteral feeding products and/or total parenteral nutrition (TPN) solution**
8. **Prescribe and read necessary x-rays to evaluate nutrition support access**
9. **Monitor serum electrolytes frequently to aid ongoing nutritional assessment**
10. **Monitor for complications of enternal/parenteral nutritional support therapy**
11. **Initiate nutrition support consult**

C. NURSING ASSESSMENT

1. Nutritional history

a. Present weight, usual weight, recent weight, and weight change over defined time period; consider hydration status in evaluating weight changes
b. Percent of ideal body weight

(1) Standard tables, e.g., Metropolitan height/weight charts
(2) Rule of thumb (+/− 10% for body frame size)
(a) Males—106 lbs for first 5 feet of height; add 6 lbs for every inch above 5 feet
(b) Females—100 lbs for first 5 feet of height; add 5 lbs for every inch above 5 feet

c. Number of days without food
d. 24-hr recall of usual day's food intake
e. Food preferences, intolerances, appetite
f. Concurrent medical problems—chronic conditions may affect preinjury nutritional status, e.g., diabetes, COPD, cardiac dysfunction, cancer; chewing, swallowing, and GI dysfunction, alcohol/drug abuse, renal/liver dysfunction, medications

2. Clinical assessment

a. Physical examination
(1) Signs of deficiencies can be noted in hair, skin, mouth, and eyes; many are late signs of vitamin deficiencies
(2) Examination should concentrate on indicators of protein and calorie loss, e.g., easily pluckable hair, *edema,* subcutaneous fat and muscle wastage, decreased muscle strength, nonhealing wounds, depressed respiratory and cardiac function, and lethargy
(3) Head to toe assessment to establish other factors that influence type of nutrition needed—*is GI tract functional?*
(a) Mechanical difficulties—oral or esophageal surgery/trauma; surgery/trauma of the stomach, intestine, or other area of GI tract, fistulas, obstructions, abdominal abscesses, GI bleeding
(b) Malabsorption—diarrhea, short gut syndrome, pancreatitis, biliary disease, vomiting
(c) Neuropsychiatric—inability to take food, chew, or swallow; refusal to eat or depressed appetite due to altered mental status
(4) Anthropometrics uses linear and caliper measurements to make judgments as to whether body mass will influence morbidity
(a) Accurately measured height and weight
(b) Compare skinfold thickness and mid-upper arm circumference to standard measurements; affected by edema
(5) Classification to describe malnourishment
(a) Marasmus—slow wasting of body fat and muscle with preservation of visceral proteins, e.g., starvation without stress, anorexia, chronic illness
(b) Kwashiorkor—visceral protein depletion with preservation or increase in body weight
(i) Seen in low protein and/or calorie intake under increased stress
(ii) Hallmark is edema, common in trauma patients
(c) Mixed—combination of above two conditions has high morbidity and mortality

3. Visceral protein measurements (reflect functional protein status)

a. Serum albumin—carrier protein that maintains oncotic pressure
(1) Long half-life; slow to reflect acute changes

(2) Easily affected by hydration status
(3) Levels below 3.5 gm/dl reflect protein depletion

b. Serum transferrin—iron transport protein
(1) Shorter half-life than albumin; better reflects acute changes
(2) Values altered by patient's total iron, blood loss, and transfusions
(3) Values below 200 mg/dl reflect depletion

c. Prealbumin—carries retinol-binding protein
(1) Most sensitive visceral protein; clinical usefulness questionable
(2) Levels below 20 mg/dl reflect depletion

4. Creatinine height index (CHI)

a. Used to calculate muscle mass from 24-hr urine collection for creatinine
b. Ideal excretion = 23 mg/kg/day for males and 18 mg/kg/day for females
c. Clinical usefulness limited as results are affected by alterations in renal function, fever, amputations, some medications, and small errors in urine collection

5. Measuring immune function

a. Total lymphocyte count $= \frac{\% \text{ lymphocytes} \times \text{WBC}}{100}$

(1) Count below 2000 mm^3 suggests impaired immune function
(2) Clinical usefulness limited because tissue necrosis, infection, and stress raise the lymphocyte count

b. Skin tests measure anergy—delayed hypersensitivity
(1) Intradermal injection of common antigens is given and observed for reaction at 48 hrs; no response indicates depressed immune function
(2) Clinical usefulness controversial as many nonnutritional factors affect results

6. Nitrogen balance (difference between nitrogen intake and nitrogen output)

a. Evaluates adequacy of protein intake (6.25 gm protein provides 1 gm nitrogen)
b. Clinical method of choice to measure short-term changes in body protein stores
c. Nitrogen output is measured with a 24-hr urine collection for total nitrogen and then compared to nitrogen intake
d. Positive nitrogen balance indicates anabolism; negative balance indicates catabolism
e. Difficult to assess during renal failure

7. Nutritional requirements

a. Calorie and protein requirements are directly related to degree of injury and duration of hypermetabolism
b. Estimation of calorie needs
(1) Harris-Benedict Equation for basal energy expenditure (BEE)
(a) Males: BEE = 66 + (13.75 × W) + (5.0 × H) − (6.75 × A)
(b) Females: BEE = 655 + (9.56 × W) + (1.85 × H) − (4.68 × A)
(c) W = weight in kg; H = height in cm; A = age in years
(2) Stress and activity factors must be added to the above result to obtain total kcals/24 hrs (see Figure 11.1)
(a) BEE × 1.3 for low stress, low to moderate activity
(b) BEE × 1.75 for severe stress, multiple trauma, confined to bed
(c) BEE × 2.0 for major burns

Figure 11.1

Estimate of energy requirements for critically ill patients. From D. W. Wilmore, *The metabolic management of the critically ill.* New York: Plenum Medical, 1977, p. 36. Reprinted with permission.

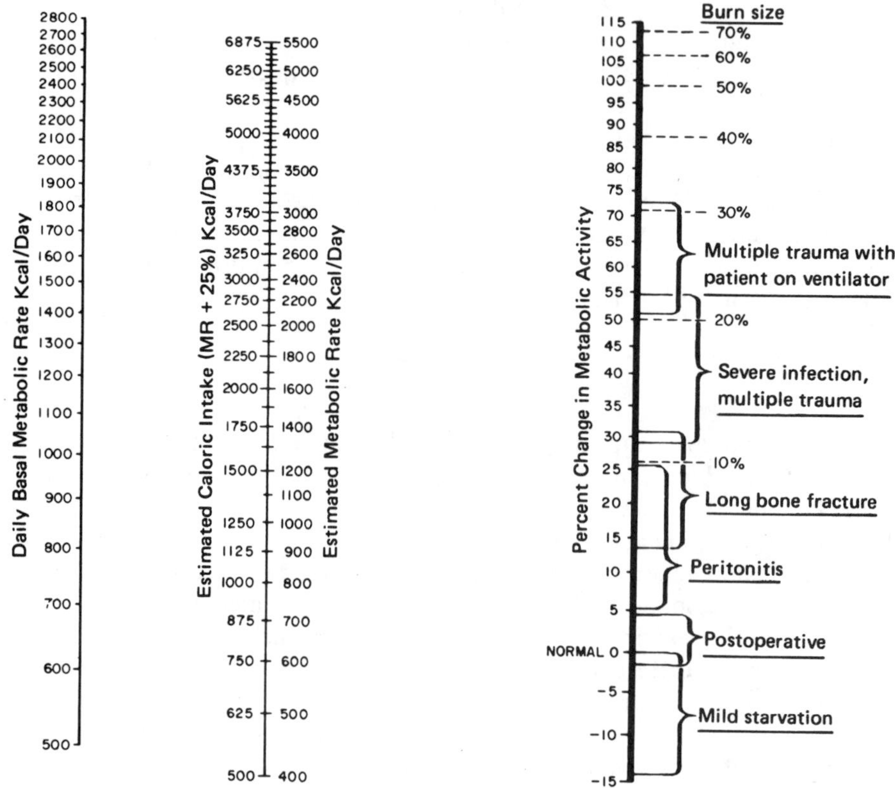

(3) A shortcut approximation of calorie needs is 35 to 45 kcals/kg/day dependent on stress level
(4) Curreri formula for burns: (25 kcal × kg preburn weight) + (40 × % total body surface area burned)

c. Indirect colorimetry—measured with metabolic cart
   (1) Caloric needs determined by measuring oxygen consumption and carbon dioxide production
   (2) Values obtained can help decrease problems with underfeeding and overfeeding patient
   (3) Equipment is expensive and not widely available

d. Estimation of protein requirements
   (1) Depends on degree of stress, serum albumin, grams of nitrogen lost each 24 hrs in urine, tolerance by renal and hepatic systems
   (2) Goal—1.3 to 2.0 gms protein/kg/day
   (3) Severely burned patient may require more than 2.5 gm/kg/day
   (4) Patients with hepatic and renal failure may need protein restriction

D. NURSING DIAGNOSES, EXPECTED OUTCOMES, AND INTERVENTIONS

1. Alteration in nutrition: less than body requirements related to

a. Insufficient intake secondary to
   (1) Inability to chew, swallow, or obtain food
   (2) Anorexia, depression
   (3) Altered consciousness
   (4) Nothing by mouth (NPO) for testing
b. Increased metabolic needs secondary to
   (1) Trauma/burns, stress of surgery, sepsis
   (2) Increased physical activity
   (3) Pregnancy, growth, hyperthyroidism
   (4) Cancer
c. Increased losses secondary to
   (1) Vomiting, diarrhea, draining fistulas, NGT, diaphoresis
   (2) Open burns, wound
   (3) Dialysis
d. Decreased ability to digest and metabolize food
   (1) Malabsorption
   (2) GI obstruction or ileus
   (3) Inflammatory bowel disease
   (4) Pancreatitis
   (5) NPO for surgical healing
e. Expected outcomes
   (1) Patient maintains or improves nutritional status by delivery and absorption of adequate nutrients as manifested by
      (a) Weight maintenance or gain of 1 to 2 lbs/week
      (b) Fluid intake will equal fluid output, after initial fluid resuscitation phase
      (c) Normal skin turgor
      (d) Increased serum albumin (more than 3.5 gm/dl)
      (e) Positive nitrogen balance
      (f) Progressive wound healing
   (2) Patient demonstrates appropriate absorption and utilization without untoward effects from nutritional support or its delivery methods
      (a) Serum electrolytes, glucose, liver enzymes, BUN, creatinine, magnesium, phosphorus, calcium, and other lab studies remain within normal limits
      (b) No side effects from enteral delivery systems occur
      (c) No complications from parenteral nutritional systems occur
   (3) Enteral nutrition used in preference to parenteral nutrition when GI tract is functional and can be accessed; enteral nutrition is safer, cheaper, and more physiologic than parenteral
f. Nursing interventions
   (1) General
      (a) Identify patients at risk for malnutrition early
      (b) Collaborate with nutrition support professionals

(c) Ensure that patient has gag reflex and can eat safely; obtain speech therapy consult for dysphagia if needed
(d) Provide assistance with eating
(e) Measure caloric and protein intake and compare with calculated requirements
(f) Monitor function of GI tract
i) Assess bowel sounds
ii) Document stools and drainage
iii) Assess for distension
(g) Weigh and monitor serial trends
(h) Monitor serum electrolytes, glucose, albumin, minerals, and other appropriate lab values
(i) Obtain and monitor results of 24-hr urine for total nitrogen
(j) Measure intake and output; compare results and note trends
(k) Closely monitor wound healing and recovery of major organ systems

(2) Enteral nutrition
(a) Assess appropriateness of delivery route; *enteral nutrition is preferred when GI tract is functional*
(b) Assist physician with placement of small bore feeding tube and obtain abdominal x-ray
(c) Do not administer feeding until tube placement has been confirmed radiologically by physician
(d) Give gastric feedings intermittently, generally; give small bowel or duodenal feedings continuously
(e) To guard against aspiration of intragastric feedings
i) Keep head of bed elevated more than 30°
ii) Check gastric residuals before each feeding
iii) Assess abdomen before and after each feeding
iv) Auscultate tube placement
v) Administer feeding slowly and *intermittently* by gravity infusion
(f) Keep small bowel feedings on enteral pump; run continuously
(g) Start all feedings with low volumes/rates; gradually increase to estimated requirements
(h) Start hypertonic feedings (more than 1.0 kcal/cc) at half strength
(i) Monitor for stool output and volume; collect stool for analysis if needed
(j) Monitor skin integrity surrounding feeding tube insertion site
(k) Prevent complications from enteral delivery systems such as aspiration, malpositioning of feeding tube, skin breakdown/infection at tube insertion site, diarrhea, constipation, nausea, vomiting, and dehydration (see Figure 11.2)

(3) Total parenteral nutrition (TPN)
(a) Assess appropriateness of delivery route; enteral route should be nonfunctional
(b) Assist physician with placement of central venous access and obtain chest x-ray
(c) Do not administer TPN until central venous catheter (CVC) placement confirmed radiologically

Figure 11.2

Enteral feedings. Adapted from M. Koruda, P. Guenter & J. Rombeau, Enteral nutrition in the critically ill. *Critical Care Clinics, 3*(1) (1987), p. 138. Adapted with permission.

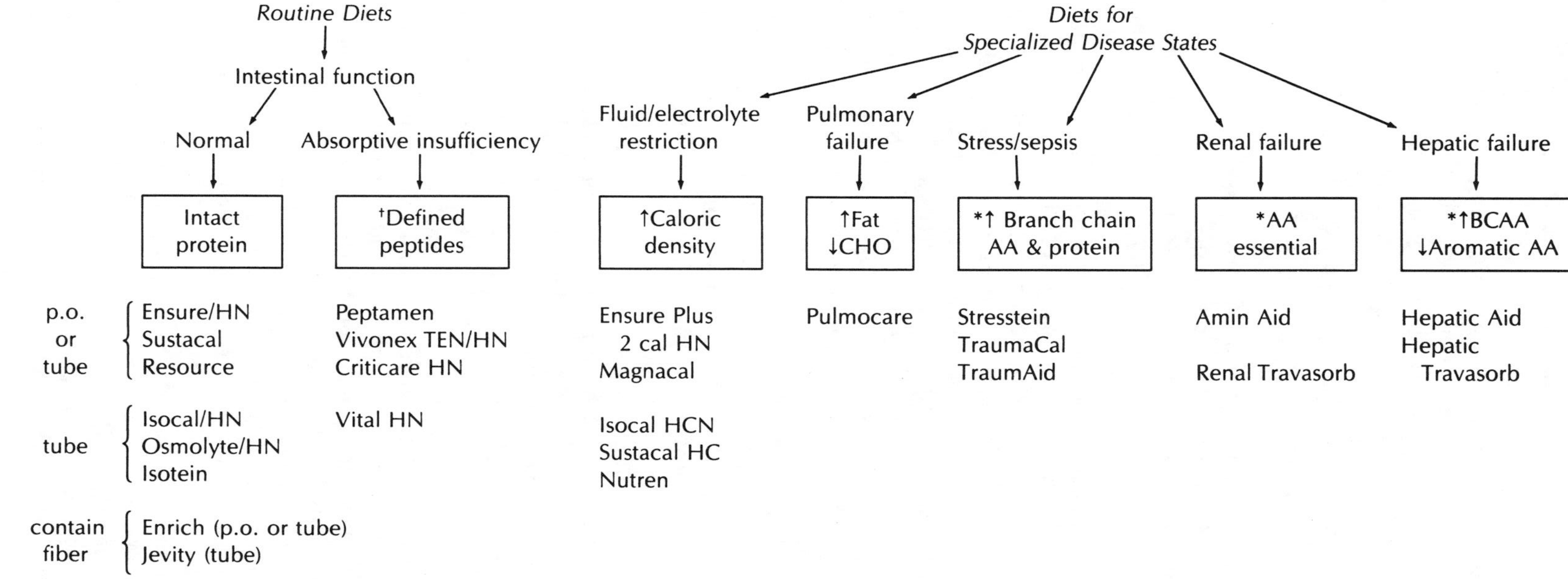

†Most of these diets may also be used in stress and sepsis.
*The use of specialized amino acids for these disease states remains controversial; the efficacy remains under investigation.

(d) Assess for complications of CVC insertion, including line sepsis, pneumothorax, hemothorax, air embolism, brachial/phrenic nerve injury, catheter malposition, and catheter thrombosis
(e) Start TPN at slow rate, usually one liter on day one, and gradually increase to estimated requirements over 24 to 48 hrs
(f) Run TPN on volume controller I.V. infusion pump
(g) Monitor glucose by finger-stick every six hours until stable; urine sugar and acetone tests may be used
(h) Maintain sterile, waterproof dressing over CVC; change dressing per hospital policy; assess insertion site
(i) Maintain sterility of infusion system by ensuring placement of a new CVC prior to initiation of TPN, running TPN only in the TPN line or multilumen catheter port
  i) Generally, do not piggyback other drugs, push medications, monitor CVP, or draw blood using TPN line
  ii) Ensure all line connections are direct, without needles or stopcocks
  iii) Wash hands and wear gloves for any manipulation of TPN line
(j) TPN additives should be injected into infusion bag only by pharmacist
(k) Administer lipid solutions as prescribed; use peripheral vein if available
  i) If piggybacked into TPN, prepare injection port with iodine
  ii) Lipid solutions may be infused over 4 to 12 hrs, or may be directly mixed with TPN and infused over 24 hrs according to pharmacy protocol
(l) Guard against accidental disconnection of CVC line; use Luer-Lok device
(m) Wean patient from TPN over several hours or several days; reduction of rate should be in conjunction with increases in enteral intake
(n) Hang 10% dextrose in water if abrupt cessation of TPN occurs
(o) CVC may be left in for a few days after TPN discontinued to ensure adequate enteral intake
(p) Continually assess for catheter infection and sepsis while CVC is in place
(q) When peripheral parenteral nutrition is used
  i) Final dextrose concentration should not exceed 10%
  ii) Monitor for phlebitis as solutions cause sclerosis
  iii) Monitor for fluid overload; large volumes are needed to supply adequate calories
(r) Assess for complications, including hypo/hyperglycemia, hyperosmolar, hyperglycemic nonketotic dehydration (HHNK), essential fatty acid deficiency, fat overload, electrolyte imbalances, mineral imbalances, hepatic dysfunction, hypercapnia, azotemia, and acid-base imbalances

2. **Alteration in nutrition: more than body requirements related to**

a. Excessive intake secondary to overestimating caloric expenditure, compulsive eating, or infusion of enteral or parenteral nutrients greater than bodily expenditure
b. Decreased metabolic needs secondary to decreasing caloric and protein needs as healing occurs, "yo-yo" dieting, or hypothyroidism
c. Expected outcomes
  (1) Infused kilocalories and protein within recommended limits for patient's calculated basal energy expenditure with appropriate stress adjustments

(2) Liver enzymes/function within normal limits
(3) Hypercapnia does not occur and is not exacerbated by nutritional support therapy

d. Nursing interventions
(1) Assess obese patients carefully for protein malnutrition; this may be overlooked due to their size
(2) Assess for hepatic failure, hypercapnia and renal failure; may indicate overinfusion of kilocalories or protein, especially with TPN
(3) Compare amount of infused kilocalories and protein to estimated needs to avoid complications of overfeeding
(4) Decrease kilocalories as patient's stress level decreases, after acute phase of injury has passed

3. Knowledge deficit related to lack of information regarding

a. Nature of illness and ability to eat normally
b. Amount of nutrients necessary to improve and/or maintain nutritional status
c. Operation of complex devices necessary for safe delivery of enteral and parenteral nutrition
d. Self-monitoring for complications
e. Expected outcomes
(1) Patient and caregivers demonstrate knowledge and utilize nutritional support methods to meet requirements
(a) Patient demonstrates adequate oral intake by calorie count or food diary
(b) Patient or caregiver demonstrates satisfactory use of enteral/parenteral equipment and products
(2) Patients unable to take adequate oral intake meet their nutritional needs safely at home, without complications and independent of professional care providers

f. Nursing interventions
(1) Provide patient education necessary to cover entire spectrum of patient's needs; involve family as much as possible
(2) Use principles of adult learning theory
(3) Consult dietitian for diet counseling, if needed
(4) Coordinate activities with patient's home care company to provide continuity of care; bring home equipment into the hospital so patient may receive supervised instruction before discharge
(5) Obtain psychological consult, if needed
(6) Refer to home TPN support groups, if available

E. NURSING SKILLS

1. **Skinfold measurements**
2. **Calculation of energy and protein needs**
3. **Administration of intradermal injections for anergy testing**
4. **Assist with metabolic cart measurements**

5. **Auscultation for feeding tube placement**
6. **Maintain indwelling feeding systems**
7. **Sterile CVC dressing change**

Suggested Readings

Byone, R., & Kudsk, K. (1988). Nutrition in trauma patients. *Nutrition in Clinical Practice,* 3(4), 137–143.

Forlaw, L. (1983). The critically ill patient: Nutritional implications. *Nursing Clinics of North America, 18*(1) 111–117.

Grant, J., & Kennedy-Caldwell, C. (Eds.). (1988). *Nutritional support nursing.* Philadelphia: Grune and Stratton.

Keithly, J. K. (Ed.). (1989). Advances in nutritional support. *Nursing Clinics of North America, 24*(2).

Kennedy-Caldwell, C., & Guenter, P. (Eds.). (1988). *Nutrition support nursing core curriculum.* Silver Spring, MD: American Society for Parenteral and Enteral Nutrition.

Luterman, A., Adams, M., & Curreri, P. W. (1984). Nutritional management of the burn patient. *Critical Care Quarterly,* (December), 34–43.

Majories, T. C., & Lyons-Patterson, J. (1988). Nutrition and trauma. *Trauma Quarterly,* 4(4).

Rombeau, J., & Caldwell, M. (Eds.). (1984). *Clinical nutrition: Vol. 1. Enteral and tube feeding.* Philadelphia: W. B. Saunders Co.

Rombeau, J., & Caldwell, M. (Eds.). (1986). *Clinical nutrition: Vol 2. Parenteral nutrition.* Philadelphia: W. B. Saunders Co.

Rosequist, C., & Shepp, P. (1985). The nutrition factor. *American Journal of Nursing,* 85(1), 45–47.

Section III
Comprehensive Topics in Trauma Nursing

MODULE 12
INFECTION

Cynthia Gurdak Berry, MSN, RN, CCRN

Prerequisite

Review major components of the immune system and their functions.

Objectives

1.0 Describe the normal immune system.
1.1 Describe the primary mechanical defenses of the body.
1.2 Describe the chemical defenses of the body.
1.3 Describe the role of cellular defenses in the immune response.
2.0 Describe the immunological response to trauma.
2.1 State the vascular component of the acute inflammatory response.
2.2 List two chemical mediators involved in the vascular response to acute inflammation.
2.3 Differentiate four common types of inflammatory exudates.
2.4 Describe local and systemic indicators of acute inflammation.
2.5 Discuss the characteristics of chronic inflammation.
2.6 Identify components of trauma-related immunosuppression.
3.0 Identify strategies to prevent infection in the trauma patient.
3.1 State the importance of maintaining normal host physiology.
3.2 Differentiate two types of skin flora and ways to control their spread.

3.3 List four categories of wounds with respect to potential for infection.
3.4 Describe nosocomial infections with relation to common sites.
4.0 Describe infections common to trauma patients.
4.1 Describe staphylococcal infections.
4.2 List signs and symptoms and treatment of streptococcal infections.
4.3 Discuss pneumococcal infections.
4.4 State types of Gram-negative enteric rod infections.
4.5 Discuss *Candida* infections.
4.6 Briefly describe clostridial infections.
5.0 Describe unusual, but serious, infections evident in trauma patients.
5.1 Discuss necrotizing anorectal and perineal infections.
5.2 List characteristics of necrotizing fasciitis.
5.3 Identify characteristics of wound botulism.
5.4 State causes and treatment of tetanus.
5.5 Describe rabies and its prophylaxis.
6.0 Develop and evaluate a plan of nursing care for patients with infection, or potential for infection, in various body systems.

A. THE IMMUNE SYSTEM—HOST DEFENSE MECHANISMS

1. **Mechanical defenses—first line of defense**
   a. Skin provides an impermeable barrier and also produces lipids with antimicrobial activity
   b. Skin commonly harbors bacteria with low virulence in sweat glands and hair follicles
   c. Mucous membranes have antimicrobial properties, i.e., production of IgA in the gut, pH changes in the stomach and vagina, and the mucociliary elevator in the respiratory tract
2. **Chemical defenses—second line of defense**
   a. Despite mechanical barriers, pathogens do invade the host and initiate the second line of defense
   b. Activation of the complement, coagulation, fibrinolytic and kinikallikrein, and bradykinin systems causes
      (1) Increased local vascular permeability
      (2) Inflow of plasma, clotting factors, and immunoglobulins (IgG, IgM), which activate the complement system, leading to the activation of cellular defenses
      (3) Leukocytes to undergo margination (sticking to vessel wall) and migration through walls of small venules and capillaries into injured tissue
      (4) Enkephalin release from the adrenal medulla at the time of injury, producing stress analgesia
3. **Cellular defenses—third line of defense**
   a. Mononuclear phagocytic system (formerly called reticuloendothelial system)
      (1) Fixed components

(a) Phagocytic cells located mainly in the hepatosplenic circulation and lymphatics; responsible for removing invading pathogens
  i) Polymorphonuclear leukocytes (PMNs) are the first cells to attack and phagocytize an invading pathogen
  ii) Macrophages destroy invading pathogens and large particles, including RBCs, necrotic tissue, and dead neutrophils
    a) Histiocytes—found in skin and subcutaneous tissue
    b) Lymph node macrophages—line the sinuses in large numbers
    c) Alveolar—in lungs
    d) Kupffer—in liver sinuses
    e) Spleen and bone marrow—in red pulp and venous sinuses
  iii) Phagocytosis is the most important function of neutrophils and macrophages
    a) Phagocytosis increases if the pathogen's surface is rough
    b) Most body surfaces have protein coats that repel phagocytes
    c) Chance of phagocytosis increases when antibodies adhere to pathogen
  iv) Opsonization, the coating of invading pathogens with complement products, increases the chance of phagocytosis
  v) When the mononuclear phagocytic system is overwhelmed or impaired, a clinically significant bacteremia occurs

(2) Wandering components (B and T lymphocytes)
  (a) B lymphocytes—from beta cells, they are the memory cells of the immunologic system
    i) Produce immunoglobulins that are bacteriocidal and active in the acute inflammatory response
    ii) Constitute humoral immunity or the antibody system
  (b) T lymphocytes—active in certain bacterial and viral infections; cell mediated rather than humoral
    i) Cytotoxic or T killer cells—bind to invading pathogen and destroy it if they have previously been sensitized to that pathogen; e.g., can destroy cancer cells and transplanted organs
    ii) T helper cells—most numerous type
      a) Enhance immune response by increasing activation of B lymphocytes, T killer, and T suppressor cells
      b) Release interleukin-2, a lymphokine that increases T cell activity
      c) Activate the macrophage system
    iii) T suppressor cells—regulate activities of the other types of T cells; play a role in immune tolerance, preventing the body from attacking its own tissue

(3) Two types of immunity
  (a) Innate—species-specific and nontransferable
    i) The tissue macrophage system
    ii) Acid secretion and digestive enzymes in the stomach
    iii) Skin immunoglobulins
    iv) Lysozymes, basic polypeptides, and complement
  (b) Acquired

i) Active—either postinfection or from administration of killed or attenuated toxoid, e.g., tetanus
ii) Passive—from injection with gamma globulin, e.g., Hyper-Tet

B. IMMUNOLOGIC RESPONSE TO TRAUMA

1. Acute inflammatory response—the body's initial response to injury

a. Vascular changes
  (1) Initially blood flow is decreased to the injured tissue due to transient arteriolar constriction; may not always occur
  (2) Vasodilation in response to chemical mediators; arterioles dilate, and previously constricted capillaries and venous beds open, increasing blood flow to the injured area, which produces redness and heat (hyperemic response)
  (3) Increased hydrostatic pressure leads to transudation of protein-poor fluid into the injured area
  (4) Increased microvascular endothelial permeability allows protein-rich fluid to escape into the extravascular space, causing edema
  (5) Excessive fibrinogen leaking from capillaries causes clotting in the extravascular space
b. Chemical mediators
  (1) Vasoactive amines produce venule dilation and increased vascular permeability
    (a) Histamine
      i) Stored in mast cells, basophils, and platelets
      ii) Stimulates release of serotonin
      iii) Released in response to trauma, cationic proteins, derived from neutrophil lysosomes, and certain complement fragments
    (b) Serotonin
      i) Found in platelets and cells of the GI tract
      ii) Released in response to trauma, cationic proteins, and certain complement fragments
c. Exudates—usually include serous, fibrinous, and suppurative matter
  (1) Significant exudate is usually seen only during the acute inflammatory response, but may be seen in some chronic reactions
  (2) Composition depends on cause of injury and severity of inflammatory response
    (a) Serous—typical of mild injuries; low protein content; often seen early in inflammatory reaction, e.g., blister fluid
    (b) Fibrinous—contains large amounts of plasma proteins, mostly fibrinogen, and fibrin precipitate
      i) Removal by fibrinolytic enzymes must occur before the area can begin the healing process
      ii) If this exudate is not removed, fibroblasts will grow into it, resulting in the formation of scar tissue and adhesions
    (c) Suppurative—purulent
      i) Contains large amounts of pus rich in leukocytes, cell debris, and living bacteria

ii) Pus is produced in the presence of the following organisms: staphylococci, pnemococci, meningococci, gonococci, coliform bacilli, and some streptococci

(d) Hemorrhagic—not a distinctive type of exudate, but a fibrinous or purulent exudate accompanied by a large number of red blood cells

d. Clinical indicators of acute inflammation

(1) Local response

(a) Redness—produced by microcirculatory dilation

(b) Heat—produced by microcirculatory dilation

(c) Edema—secondary to fluid shifting from the vascular to the extravascular space

(d) Pain—may be related to increased tissue tension secondary to edema or prostaglandin release (may be combined with bradykinin or serotonin)

(e) Loss of function—early in acute inflammation; this is directly related to edema and pain

(2) Systemic response

(a) Fever—associated with severe inflammatory response, particularly an infection that has overwhelmed the mononuclear phagocytic system; bacteremia usually results in wide swings in body temperature accompanied by shaking chills

i) Endogenous pyrogen (interleukin-1)—resets the thermoregulatory centers of the hypothalamus to higher levels; is apparently released with infectious, immunologic, or toxic reactions

ii) Prostaglandins—role is in fever production; aspirin may reduce fever by blocking prostaglandin production

(b) Leukocytosis

i) Often accompanies bacterial but not viral infections

ii) Shift to the left in a white blood count (WBC) differential indicates an increase in the number of immature neutrophils and bands, due to bacterial infection or effects of acute stress on the bone marrow

2. Chronic inflammation is characterized by

a. Infiltration of lymphocytes and cells of the mononuclear phagocytic system and proliferation of fibroblasts and small blood vessels

b. Scarring or adhesions may form at this point due to excessive production of fibrinous tissue

c. Acute and chronic responses often occur simultaneously with manifestations of both apparent

3. Trauma-related immunosuppression

a. Potential causes

(1) Products of injury released into the systemic circulation

(2) Prostaglandin release

(3) Release of bacterial endotoxins

(4) Immune depression

b. A functional loss of immune competence results; a dramatic rise in septic episodes and complications occurs with a high incidence of late posttrauma mortality

c. Patients with major traumatic injuries have been noted to be anergic, and have decreased neutrophil function and abnormal polymorphonuclear monocyte (PMN) function

d. Iatrogenic immunosuppression is potentiated by antibiotics, blood products, anesthesia, and massive fluid resuscitation; mechanism is unknown (1)

C. PREVENTION OF INFECTION

1. **Maintenance of normal host physiology**
a. Normal central blood pressure maintains renal, cardiac, and central nervous system function
b. Normal local tissue perfusion prevents hypoxia, acidosis, and electrolyte disturbances
c. Adequate ventilatory support
d. Optimal nutritional status
2. **Prevention of entrance of skin flora**
a. Two categories of skin flora
   (1) Resident—resides deep in skin glands and hair follicles; generally of low pathogenicity
   (2) Transient—acquired from the environment and often highly pathogenic
b. Hand washing eradicates resident and transient flora
c. Shaving causes trauma to the skin, allowing bacterial growth within hours
d. Mechanical barriers, e.g., gloves, drapes, masks, head covers, separate sterile from nonsterile environment
e. Autoclaving sterilizes operative instruments
3. **Wound types related to infection risk** (2)
a. Clean
   (1) Nontraumatic (elective)
   (2) No break in technique
   (3) Respiratory, GI, or GU tracts not entered
   (4) Infection rate less than 5%
b. Clean-contaminated (nontraumatic)
   (1) GI or respiratory tract entered without significant spillage
   (2) Minor break in technique
   (3) Entry into a prepared oropharynx or vagina
   (4) GU or biliary tract entered in the absence of infection
   (5) Infection rate 10%
c. Contaminated
   (1) Gross spillage from GI tract
   (2) Major break in technique
   (3) Traumatic wound (fresh)
   (4) Infection rate 16%
d. Dirty, infected
   (1) Perforated viscus encountered
   (2) Acute bacterial inflammation encountered (pus)
   (3) Transection of clean tissue to gain access to a pus collection
   (4) Traumatic wound with retained devitalized tissue, foreign body, fecal contamination, and/or delayed treatment, or a wound from a dirty source

(5) Infection rate 28%

4. Nosocomial infections

a. Usually wound, urinary tract, bloodstream, or respiratory-tract-related
b. Incidence correlates with length of stay; frequently related to invasive devices
c. Difficult to eradicate due to increased virulence of highly resistant organisms
d. The best preventive measure is removing all tubes and similar devices as soon as possible; use aseptic technique during manipulation of such devices and/or wounds

D. COMMON INFECTIONS IN TRAUMA VICTIMS

1. Staphylococcal

a. Characterized by local redness, pain, and purulent discharge
b. Extreme tenderness may develop
c. Pus is thick and creamy
d. Local wound margins may become necrotic and slough
e. Use Gram stain and culture to diagnose
f. Treat with wound drainage, irrigation, and systemic antibiotics
g. *Staphylococcus aureus* most common wound pathogen; most staphylococci are coagulase-positive, making them resistant to phagocytosis
h. Methicillin-resistant S. *aureus* (MRSA)
   (1) May be found in blood, sputum, and wounds
   (2) Almost always nosocomial
   (3) Generally resistant to all penicillins, cephalosporins, aminoglycosides, tetracycline, erythromycin, and clindamycin
   (4) Vancomycin is the drug of choice
   (5) Immunosuppressed patients are at risk for acquiring MRSA; health care providers and the general public are not

2. Streptococcal

a. Manifested by diffuse cellulitis, redness, edema
b. On extremity, red lymphangitic streaks extend proximally and precede diffuse edematous erythema
c. Wound discharge is thin, yellow-green, purulent
d. Symptoms may include malaise, myalgia, headache, rigors, sweats, and high fever
e. Responds rapidly to intravenous penicillin
f. β-hemolytic or Group A streptococci are most commonly implicated in soft tissue trauma

3. Pneumococcal

a. Encapsulated; retards phagocytosis
b. Normal flora of respiratory tract
c. Not of great concern in surgical patients, except those with splenectomy; spleen stores opsonins, which prevent the retardation of phagocytosis
d. Postsplenectomy pneumococcal sepsis is unusually aggressive, virulent, with death ensuing rapidly

4. Gram-negative rods

a. Usually colonize GI tract but also implicated in peritoneal, urinary tract, pressure ulcer, and nosocomial pulmonary infections

b. *Pseudomonas* and *Serratia* are primarily nosocomial and usually found in a moist environment, e.g., ventilator tubing

c. *E. coli, Klebsiella,* and *Enterobacter* are commonly cultured out of intraabdominal infections in patients after colon injury; thrive in both aerobic and anaerobic environments (facultative)

d. *E. coli* proliferates in community-acquired urinary tract infections

e. *Pseudomonas, Klebsiella,* and *Serratia* are most common in nosocomial urinary tract infections

f. *Pseudomonas* is most common burn wound pathogen

g. Enteric coliform and enterococcal wound infections cause fever, local wound redness, tenderness, and purulent drainage

h. Infections from Gram-negative rods are often polymicrobial due to contamination from dirt, clothes, or spilled bowel contents

i. Septicemia with shock, adult respiratory distress syndrome (ARDS), and disseminated intravascular coagulation (DIC) often follow these infections

j. Treatment of infected wounds requires probing and draining; antibiotics effective against aerobic and anaerobic organisms are used

5. Enteric anaerobes

a. *Bacteroides fragilis* occurs in wounds originally contaminated from colon

b. Surgical drainage usually required

c. Antibiotics recommended but controversial

6. Candidiasis

a. *Candida albicans* normally inhabits GI tract

b. Proliferates in patients on long-term, broad spectrum antibiotics

c. Indwelling central venous and urinary catheters are significant ports of entry

d. Diagnosis requires a high index of suspicion when patient exhibits clinical signs and symptoms of sepsis of unexplained origin

e. Use blood cultures to diagnose

f. Treatment includes discontinuing or changing all indwelling devices, discontinuing systemic antibiotics to allow gastrointestinal bacterial regrowth, oral nystatin, systemic antifungal therapy

7. Clostridial infection—gas gangrene

a. Gram-positive rod, anaerobe

b. Increased suspicion in patients with history of shock, hypotension, vascular impairment, or with edema, tight casts, or bandages

c. Signs and symptoms include

(1) Wound tightness and fullness

(2) Mild to severe local pain; progressive or disproportionately painful wound or incision

(3) Edema in wound and adjacent area

(4) Hemorrhagic bullae develop near wound; drain brown, watery fluid; surrounding skin becomes dusky and gray

(5) Wound edge becomes white and shiny, and progresses to bronze/copper-colored, gray, or purplish within hours; spreads rapidly peripherally

(6) Serous or serosanguineous wound drainage

(7) Wound odor ranges from sweet and putrid to none
(8) Necrotic muscle may herniate through wound
(9) Crepitus
(10) Malaise, myalgia, apprehension turning to apathy and/or combativeness
(11) Sensorium and orientation usually unaffected early, but may progress to delirium and stupor
(12) Fever not always present
(13) Sinus tachycardia disproportionate to fever
(14) Systemic toxicity occurs within 12 hrs; hypotension, jaundice, respiratory failure, and anemia; patients in coma unlikely to survive

d. Diagnosis difficult due to occurrence of other gas-producing infections; 80%—*C. perfringens*
(1) Gram stains supportive, but not diagnostic
(2) Tissue gas on x-ray inconclusive, especially in early hours postinjury
(3) Incubation period is 6 to 72 hrs; most cases occur 2 to 3 days postinjury

e. Treat with exploration and wide debridement of all necrotic tissue, fasciotomy, intravenous penicillin, fluid replacement, and hyperbaric oxygen

E. RARE WOUND INFECTIONS

1. Necrotizing anorectal and perineal infections

a. Severe pain is first sign
b. Obvious local edema and crepitus
c. Painful black spot on scrotum or posterior labia
d. Black area, skin gangrene, spreads to penis, thighs, buttocks, and anterior abdominal wall in 12 to 24 hrs
e. Toxicity may be severe with high fever, stupor, septic coma; renal failure and jaundice may occur
f. Usually caused by clostridia with an anaerobic streptococcus, *E. coli,* or staphylococcus; indistinguishable from nonclostridial causes, which are common in diabetics and leukemics
g. Treat with extensive, repeated debridement, high dose penicillin, and hyperbaric oxygen (limited success)

2. Necrotizing fasciitis

a. Usually develops outside the hospital secondary to minor trauma, particularly in persons with diabetes or peripheral vascular disease
b. Manifested as a red, warm, tender edematous area that enlarges and becomes purple-blue or black-gray; may become anesthetic indicating necrosis
c. Vesicles and blebs may drain serosanguineous fluid
d. Crepitus may occur
e. Cause is polymicrobial—streptococci, staphylococci, facultative anaerobes, enterobacteria, and anaerobic bacilli may be causative agents
f. Culture and Gram stain aspirated inflammatory fluid
g. Treat with extensive debridement beyond the zone of viable tissue, triple antibiotics, and heparin

h. Associated with high incidence of renal failure, DIC, limb amputation, venous thrombosis, ARDS, multiple organ failure, and death

3. Wound botulism

a. A very rare complication of penetrating or perforating wounds of the extremities
b. Diplopia, dry mouth, sore throat, dysphagia, blurred vision, dyspnea, and generalized weakness occur 4 to 14 days postinjury; bilateral ptosis, dysphonia develop; loss of speech may occur
c. Major danger is respiratory failure
d. Diagnose by wound culture and mouse neutralization test using patient's serum
e. Treat with intubation/tracheostomy and mechanical ventilation
f. Guarded prognosis; 20 to 25% mortality

4. Tetanus

a. Has 2- to 21-day incubation period
b. First manifested by irritability, restlessness, fever, and headache
c. Tight jaw muscles with rapid development of severe trismus is early symptom
d. Risus sardonicus, a wry, mask-like grin, follows facial muscle spasm
e. Local wound pain and muscle spasm occur
f. Paroxysmal seizures triggered by suctioning, noise, light, or movement may involve one or both sides of the body; respiratory arrest may result
g. Aspiration, profuse sweating, and rapid weight loss may occur
h. Hyperactive reflexes and fever appear
i. Cultures not useful; diagnosis based on clinical signs and symptoms
j. Treat with curare-like drugs (Pavulon), diazepam, low dose heparin, human tetanus immune globulin, and initial dose of tetanus toxoid; open and thoroughly debride wound; penicillin of little use

5. Rabies

a. Harbored in mouth and on teeth of pets and wild animals
   (1) Skunks, raccoons, foxes, and bats often culprits
   (2) Unprovoked attacks or abnormal behavior by family pets increases the suspicion of rabies
b. Cleansing of a bite from an animal suspected of rabies is critically important to prevent infection
c. The actual development of rabies is almost always fatal
d. Treatment includes human rabies immune globulin for immediate passive immunity, and human diploid cell rabies vaccine to stimulate active immunity

F. NURSING ASSESSMENT

1. Assess general immunocompetence

a. Skin integrity
b. Serum protein, albumin, prealbumin, urea nitrogen, transferrin
c. Serum immunoglobulin levels
d. Skin reactivity

2. Assess for signs and symptoms of local infection

a. Note character of wounds and surrounding skin; note color, temperature, edema, drainage, pain

b. Observe suture and staple lines for signs and symptoms of inflammation
c. Note culture and sensitivity results for blood, wound, and other body fluids
d. Measure rectal or core temperature
e. Report unusual fatigue, malaise, mental changes

3. Assess for signs and symptoms of systemic sepsis (see Module 10—Shock (septic) for more information)

a. Tachycardia
b. Increased cardiac output
c. Decreased blood pressure
d. Mental changes
e. Tachypnea

4. Assess body systems for specific sources of infection

a. Pulmonary
  (1) Color and quantity of sputum
  (2) Decreased breath sounds indicating atelectasis, effusion, or pneumonia
  (3) Increased respiratory rate indicating sepsis
b. Gastrointestinal
  (1) Decrease in bowel sounds could indicate abdominal infection or sepsis
  (2) Girth and tenderness of abdomen
  (3) Color, quantity, and quality of stool; large quantities of watery, brown stool could indicate *Clostridium difficile*
c. Genitourinary—assess voiding patterns and color and quantity of urine

G. NURSING DIAGNOSES, EXPECTED OUTCOMES, AND INTERVENTIONS

1. Potential for infection related to interruption of normal host defenses

a. Expected outcomes
  (1) Normothermic
  (2) Intact skin
  (3) Normal WBC
  (4) Body fluid cultures negative
b. Nursing interventions
  (1) Good hand washing is essential to prevent transmission of infection
  (2) Use aseptic technique for insertion and maintenance of all drainage systems
    (a) Maintain patency and integrity of closed and open drainage systems, e.g., urine, cerebral spinal fluid, wound drainage
    (b) If bag drainage system is used, maintain bag below level of drainage site to prevent reflux
    (c) Document quantity and quality of drainage
    (d) Provide catheter care according to protocol
  (3) Maintain sterile, occlusive dressings over invasive lines
    (a) Assess insertion sites for signs of infection
    (b) Follow Centers for Disease Control (CDC) recommendations for changing I.V. tubing

(4) Provide effective pulmonary toilet
  (a) Position to allow maximal lung expansion and drainage of secretions
  (b) Implement chest physical therapy as needed
  (c) Maintain sterile technique when suctioning or caring for endotracheal or tracheostomy tube
(5) Administer tetanus prophylaxis if indicated
(6) Discourage friends and families with community acquired infection, e.g., varicella, influenza, from visiting
(7) Initiate isolation precautions according to CDC guidelines
  (a) Purposes
    i) To contain infectious agents
    ii) To contain or limit reservoirs of infection
    iii) To interrupt transmission of infectious agents
    iv) To protect patients, staff, and visitors from acquiring hospital infections
  (b) The type and extent of isolation depends on the mode of transmission of the infectious agent; ensure compliance with infection control procedures by all persons coming in contact with the isolated patient

2. Alteration in nutrition, less than body requirements, related to increased metabolic demand

a. Expected outcomes
  (1) Patient is in positive nitrogen balance
  (2) Wounds heal
  (3) Minimal weight loss
  (4) Fluid and electrolyte balance normal
b. Nursing interventions
  (1) Assess nutritional status daily, including calorie intake and weight (see Module 11—Nutrition—for additional information)
  (2) Begin enteral and supplementary feeding as soon as possible
  (3) Infuse parenteral nutrients through sterile central access only; parenteral nutrition increases risk of septicemia
  (4) Monitor serum glucose and liver function studies; administer insulin, potassium, and other nutritional adjuncts as prescribed

3. Hyperthermia related to circulating pyrogens

a. Expected outcome—normothermia
b. Nursing interventions
  (1) Monitor core temperature frequently
  (2) Assess for overt and occult sources of infection
  (3) Administer antipyretics as prescribed
  (4) Implement cooling techniques
    (a) Ice packs
    (b) Hypothermia blanket for temperature greater than 39°C (102 to 103°F)

References

1. Ninneman, J. L. (1987). Trauma, sepsis, and the immune response. *The Journal of Burn Care and Rehabilitation,* 8(6), 462–468.
2. American College of Surgeons. (1984). *Manual on control of infection in surgical patients* (2nd ed.). Philadelphia: J. B. Lippincott.

Suggested Readings

Goodenough, R. N., Molnar, J. A., & Burke, J. F. (1988). Surgical infections. In J. D. Hardy (Ed.), *Hardy's textbook of surgery* (2nd ed., pp. 123–143). Philadelphia: J. B. Lippincott.

Guyton, A. C. (1986). *Textbook of medical physiology* (7th ed.). Philadelphia: W. B. Saunders Co.

Hoyt, N. J. (1989). Host defense mechanisms and compromises in the trauma patient. *Critical Care Nursing Clinics of North America, 1*(4), 753–765.

Larson, E. (1985). Infection control in critical care: An update. *Heart and Lung, 14*(2), 149–155.

Robins, E. V., (1989). Immunosuppression of the burned patient. *Critical Care Nursing Clinics of North America, 1*(4), 767–774.

Rosenthal, C. H. (1989). Immunosuppression in pediatric critical care patients. *Critical Care Nursing Clinics of North America, 1*(4), 775–785.

Wiener, S. L., & Barrett, J. (1986). *Trauma management for civilian and military physicians.* Philadelphia: W. B. Saunders Co.

Wilkerson, E. (1988). Inflammation, infection, and wound healing. In E. Howell, L. Widra, & M. G. Hill (Eds.), *Comprehensive trauma nursing: Theory and practice* (pp. 326–362). Glenview, IL: Scott, Foresman, & Co.

Wilmore, D. W., Souba, W. W., Bessey, P. Q., Aoki, T. T., & Smith, R. J. (1985). Physiology of trauma. *Acta Chirurgica Scandinavica,* 522(Supplement), 25–43.

Section III
Comprehensive Topics in Trauma Nursing

MODULE 13
WOUND HEALING

Cynthia Gurdak Berry, MSN, RN, CCRN

Objectives

1.0 Describe the anatomy, physiology, and function of the integumentary system.
1.1 Identify the skin appendages and the function of each.
1.2 Differentiate the structure and function of the layers of the skin.
2.0 Describe the three phases of wound healing.
2.1 Describe the characteristics of inflammation.
2.2 Describe the characteristics of the fibroblastic phase.
2.3 Describe the characteristics of maturation.
3.0 Differentiate types of wound healing.
3.1 Describe the healing process in primary, secondary, and tertiary intention.
3.2 Discuss the relationship between wound type and appropriate mechanism of wound healing.
4.0 Discuss categories of aberrant healing.
4.1 Define the following: hypertrophic scars, keloid scars, adhesions, and dehiscence.
4.2 Differentiate contracture and contraction.
4.3 Describe which wound types have potential for specific types of aberrant healing.
5.0 List inhibitors of wound healing.
5.1 Discuss the effect of tissue specificity on wound healing.
5.2 Describe the effect of factors such as malnutrition, anemia, cytotoxic agents, diabetes, jaundice, age, and radiation on wound healing.

5.3 Identify vitamins and minerals essential to wound healing.
5.4 Describe the role of oxygenation in wound healing.
5.5 Discuss the effect of steroids and nonsteroidal antiinflammatory drugs (NSAIDs) on wound healing.
6.0 Describe the characteristics of various types of wounds, including lacerations, abrasions, avulsions, amputations, punctures, crush, and missile injuries.
7.0 Indicate common sites of pressure ulcer formation.
8.0 Describe the Red-Yellow-Black (RYB) method of wound assessment.
9.0 Describe common approaches to wound care and closure.
9.1 Describe procedures for wound cleansing.
9.2 Describe techniques of wound irrigation.
9.3 List two methods of wound debridement.
9.4 State common methods of wound closure.
9.5 Differentiate free, mesh, and flap grafts.
9.6 Describe the types and purposes of commonly used wound dressings.
9.7 Describe techniques used to enhance wound healing.
10.0 Evaluate the status of wound healing.

A. THE SKIN

1. Functions
a. Senses heat, cold, pressure, and touch
b. Regulates body temperature
c. Protects body from noxious stimuli
d. Conserves body fluids
e. Excretes waste products
f. Absorbs and stores metabolic substances, e.g., vitamin D, fat
g. Contributes to body image

2. Anatomy and physiology
a. Epidermis
(1) Outermost layer is nonviable stratum corneum (portion that is shed)
(2) Innermost layer composed of basal cells
(a) Contain melanocytes, which produce melanin and protect dermis from sunlight and overproduction of vitamin D
(b) Germinates epithelial cells, which migrate across wound surface to close wound
b. Dermis
(1) Adheres tightly to underside of epidermis
(2) Contains rich supply of blood vessels and lymphatics
(3) Contains sensory receptors for touch, pain, pressure, heat, and cold which may project into epidermis
(4) Composed primarily of collagen and ground substances with elastic and reticular fibers
(5) Hyaluronic acid and other mucopolysaccharides are present

B. NORMAL WOUND HEALING

1. Phases

a. Inflammatory phase
   (1) Occurs in the first few days postinjury
   (2) Fibrin stops bleeding and a clot forms
   (3) Dilated vessels at the site of injury deliver debris-cleaning leukocytes within six hours of injury
   (4) Macrophages arrive, ingest debris, and release healing agents
   (5) Reepithelialization occurs with epithelial cells growing inward from the wound edges, until they meet in the middle; occurs within 24 to 48 hrs in closely approximated wounds (1)

b. Fibroblastic phase
   (1) Begins four to five days postinjury and continues for several weeks
   (2) Granulation tissue forms as does the stronger scar tissue, i.e., connective tissue and collagen
   (3) Called replacement healing or healing with scar tissue

c. Maturation phase
   (1) Takes six months to one year to complete
   (2) Collagen is replaced with a stronger type of collagen
   (3) Wound reaches full tensile strength after one year

2. Types of wound healing

a. Primary intention
   (1) Refers to the healing of a wound such as an incision or laceration in which wound edges are approximated with sutures, staples, or tape
      (a) Narrow spaces between the wound edges fill with scant amounts of clotted blood
      (b) The clot dehydrates and forms a protective crust
      (c) Within 24 hrs, neutrophils enter the wound and begin removing debris
      (d) Within 48 hrs, a thin, continuous epithelial layer forms
      (e) At 72 hrs postinjury, fibroblasts start to divide and enlarge, and neovascularization begins
      (f) By five days postinjury, the wound is filled and vascularization reaches its maximum
      (g) Suturing returns wound to 70% of its premorbid tensile strength; once sutures are removed, strength decreases to 10% (2)
      (h) The maturation or remodeling phase may continue for months to years
      (i) A small wound may also heal primarily without intervention

b. Secondary intention
   (1) Open or infected wounds, e.g., ulcers, abscesses, burns, traumatic wounds with extensive soft tissue injury, or any incised wound with separated edges
      (a) Inflammatory reaction is intense as wounds contain more bacteria, necrotic tissue, and exudate than do wounds closed by primary intention
      (b) The repair process cannot continue until the inflammatory response controls the invading pathogens
   (2) Granulation tissue begins to form, growing inward from the wound margins and outward from the dermis
      (a) Granulation tissue is highly vascular, pinkish-red, proliferative fibrous tissue

(b) It is edematous due to the leakiness of fragile new vessels; both RBCs and protein leak into the extravascular space

(3) Wounds healing by secondary intention take longer to heal because of large tissue defects

(a) Larger scars are produced due to large tissue defects and disruption in the deposition of collagen fibers

(b) Contraction can decrease scar size but may cause deformities or limit function

(4) Healing by secondary intention results in scars composed of fibroblasts, collagen, fragments of elastic tissue, blood vessels, and extracellular matrix

(5) The wound is fragile for about two weeks; at three weeks postinjury, it has approximately 70 to 80% of the tissue's original strength

c. Tertiary intention—delayed primary closure

(1) The wound is initially left open due to gross contamination

(2) The wound is debrided, irrigated, and packed with sterile gauze; daily evaluations continue until all layers of tissue appear viable and surgical wound closure can proceed, usually at 3 to 10 days postinjury

C. ABERRANT HEALING

1. Hypertrophic scars

a. Caused by excessive formation of granulation tissue and collagen fibers

(1) Configuration of collagen is disorganized

(2) Formation occurs above and between margins of unopposed wounds

(3) This tissue blocks the growth of epithelial cells and may need surgical removal before healing can occur

b. Occur in wounds deep enough to involve the reticular dermis; scar stays within wound margins

c. May result from increased tension on the wound

d. Occur most often around joints

e. Described as red, rigid, and raised

f. Scar size peaks and regression occurs over months to years; ultimate scar is usually flat, soft, and pink

g. Mechanical pressure, e.g., from elastic pressure garments or splints, prevents/treats hypertrophic scars by decreasing and altering collagen formation, and fostering a mature scar that is flat, soft, and cosmetically acceptable

2. Keloid scars

a. The balance between collagen synthesis and lysis is disturbed; may be due to increased tension on wound

b. There is an overgrowth of fibrous scar tissue, and abnormal deposition of collagen within a scar with little to no malignant potential

c. A bulging mass of hyperpigmented skin results beyond the wound margins and invades surrounding tissue

d. Occur most frequently about the shoulders, head, and neck but can be found on trunk and arms above the elbows

e. Most commonly occurs in blacks and persons of Mediterranean descent; is familial

f. Tend to recur even after surgical removal; pressure or steroid injections may help to deter

3. Adhesions

a. Scar formed between serous surfaces; common cause of intestinal obstruction
b. Associated with normal repair
c. Mature adhesions have vessels that parasitize from surrounding tissues
d. Causes of adhesions
   (1) Glove talc—the most potent macrophage stimulator; starch is a better alternative, but not free of problems
   (2) Gauze, suture material, and digestive products have been found in adhesions
e. Attempts at preventing adhesion formation have been ineffective as normal repair is also prevented
f. Adhesion formation peaks in about two to four weeks and then tends to decrease over time

4. Contraction

a. A normal and benign process by which an open wound shrinks
b. Occurs optimally in loose, pliable skin
c. Contracture, loss of motion of tissue or joint, may occur as a result of contraction
   (1) Results from excess collagen deposited in wound; collagen molecules cross-link and fix in a shortened, resting position
   (2) Patient protects wound by holding a body part in the most comfortable position, avoiding stretching, which causes pain
   (3) Stretching, pressure, and splinting may decrease contracture formation; surgical revision and release may be needed

5. Dehiscence

a. The separation of wound margins in a previously closed wound
b. Usually occurs in surgical wounds closed by primary intention when the fibrous bridge is not strong enough to hold the edges in approximation
c. Most common causes are infection or hematoma, inadequate nutrition, or inadequate blood supply
d. Typically occurs six to eight days postoperatively and is signaled by leakage of a pink, serous fluid from the wound
e. Common occurrence in stumps with inadequate blood supply, in obese patients and in smokers
f. May be precipitated by a sudden increase in intraabdominal pressure, e.g., cough, sneeze
g. If all layers of an abdominal wound are involved, evisceration, the protrusion of bowel contents, occurs; immediate surgical closure is indicated

D. INHIBITORS OF WOUND HEALING

1. Tissue specificity

a. Visceral healing occurs earlier than dermal healing since visceral cells are more metabolically active than skin

b. Bladder, stomach, colon, and vagina heal quickly
c. By three months postinjury, healed visceral tissues are 75 to 120% as strong as preinjury; at this time, the dermis has gained only 50% of its premorbid strength

2. **Nutrition**
a. Malnutrition adversely affects wound healing
(1) Ascorbic acid (vitamin C) deficiency interferes with collagen formation, neovascularization, and resistance to infection
(2) Wound healing requires increased amounts of protein and amino acids; decreased protein and albumin delay wound healing as the body taps its own protein stores for energy to survive, leaving less protein to synthesize collagen
b. Obesity predisposes patients to wound infection, incisional hernias, wound dehiscence, and seroma formation since adipose tissue is relatively avascular, and is difficult to manipulate and approximate
c. Chronic alcoholics are typically malnourished and, subsequently, have decreased neutrophil activity
d. Vitamin A helps strengthen wound and counteracts the deleterious effects of steroids; it does not accelerate healing
e. Vitamin E inhibits inflammation, as a free radical scavenger, and can actually slow the repair process
f. Zinc is essential to cell regeneration and is carried by albumin; since serum albumin frequently decreases posttrauma, zinc also transiently decreases

3. **Oxygenation**
a. Decreased oxygen tension impedes collagen synthesis, interfering with both soft tissue and bony regeneration
b. Oxygen utilization exceeds oxygen supply in injured tissues, due to inability of oxygen to diffuse into granulation tissue or areas of inadequate vascular supply

4. **Anemia associated with hypovolemia and decreased tissue perfusion**

5. **Steroids**
a. Delay inflammatory response when administered during the initial postinjury phase
b. Granulation tissue, fibroblast proliferation, and neovascularization are delayed, especially with cortisone administration
c. Vitamin A administration, topical or parenteral, will reverse this

6. **Nonsteroidal antiinflammatory drugs (NSAIDs)**
a. Are prostaglandin inhibitors which reduce the inflammatory response
b. Normal daily doses do not interfere with wound healing

7. **Radiation**
a. Causes local fibrosis, vascular sclerosis, and endarteritis, which delay wound healing
b. Causes bone marrow depression, which prevents an effective inflammatory response
c. May result in progressive necrosis, involving dermis, viscera, and bone, leading to sepsis, fistulae formation, or vessel rupture
d. Complications may occur months to years postradiation

8. **Cytotoxic agents**
a. Methotrexate

(1) Decreases tensile strength up to 50%
(2) Effect is more pronounced when given after wounding
(3) Leucovorin given within four hours of injury helps tensile strength approach normal

b. Alkylating agents
(1) Depress the formation rate of granulation tissue and, therefore, wound contraction
(2) Depress the rate of gain of tensile strength
(3) Effects are dose dependent
(4) Cytoxan (cyclophosphamide) does not impede wound healing

c. Doxorubicin (Adriamycin)
(1) Significantly impedes wound healing at dose 6 mg/kg
(2) Decreases collagen production and delays maturation
(3) Skin grafts slough, epithelialization stops, and full-thickness wound loss progresses
(4) Do not use until several weeks postinjury

9. Diabetes

a. Associated with a fivefold increase in risk of infections in clean wounds
b. Large and small vessel occlusive disease impairs circulation
c. Decreased inflammatory response and decreased sensation leave broken skin unnoticed; treatment may be delayed until infection is rampant
d. Decreased collagen synthesis and retarded neovascularization result in decreased tensile strength of wound

10. Jaundice

a. Associated with a higher incidence of abnormal wound infection and dehiscence
b. May be related to hypoproteinemia, increased bilirubin, and other hepatic metabolic alterations

11. Age

a. Age decreases wound healing due to diminished functional ability of the cells
b. The balance between synthesis and turnover of connective tissue varies with age
c. Age-related changes are believed to be a combination of interrelated factors of tissue regeneration and repair

E. WOUND ASSESSMENT

1. Types of wounds

a. Laceration—a cut in the skin by a sharp object or a tear due to blunt trauma; edges may be smooth or jagged
(1) Smooth, approximated wound edges heal by primary intention, while jagged-edged wounds may heal primarily or secondarily
(2) Wound surface may not be indicative of internal damage as penetrating injuries often seal over

b. Abrasion—a superficial wound caused by friction; depth may be uneven; removal of imbedded debris may further damage tissue
c. Avulsion—occurs when soft tissue is torn from the body resulting in significant blood and tissue loss
   (1) Degloving occurs secondary to shearing, which separates the skin from the fascia; vascular and nerve injuries often accompany this type of injury
   (2) Skin grafting required for closure, usually flap or free grafts
d. Amputation—a severe type of avulsion injury involving dermal, vascular, nerve, and bone loss
   (1) Usually caused by industrial, farm, or motorcycle accidents
   (2) Clean severed limbs/digits have the best chance of successful replantation (see Module 24—Musculoskeletal Injury—for care of amputated part)
e. Crush injury
   (1) Range in severity from contusions with ruptured small vessels to massive blood loss and edema in crushed limbs
   (2) Massive crush injuries release large amounts of myoglobin and hemoglobin, which predispose patient to acute renal failure
f. Missile injuries
   (1) The severity of missile injuries depends on the shape, caliber, and velocity of the missile, as well as the structures involved
   (2) Handgun bullets are usually of low velocity; they damage tissue in their direct path and anywhere the bullet ricochets
   (3) Rifle bullets are of higher velocity and can cause tissue damage to surrounding areas
g. Stab/puncture wounds
   (1) Stab wounds are those inflicted by a sharp object that is usually longer than it is wide, e.g., knife, ice pick
      (a) Wound edges are relatively well-defined and can be clean or dirty
      (b) Underlying injury, including neurovascular damage, cannot be predicted by mere observation of the wound and/or wounding instrument
      (c) Blood loss may not be externally apparent
      (d) Impaled objects should not be removed until the patient is in a controlled medical environment
      (e) Closure may be primary or secondary
   (2) Puncture wounds are caused by a sharp, narrow object, e.g., nail, glass fragment, penetrating the skin
      (a) The wound may be clean or dirty
      (b) A clean and/or superficial puncture usually seals rapidly with minimal blood loss and chance of infection
      (c) If the penetrating object was dirty, the wound must be opened, debrided, meticulously cleaned, and closed by secondary intention; tetanus prophylaxis is required
h. Pressure sores—interruption of the skin integrity due to prolonged pressure, causing insufficient capillary flow to skin and underlying tissue
   (1) Occurrence depends on skin thickness, site of localized pressure, hemodynamic status, and tissue perfusion
   (2) Epidermal cell necrosis occurs late in pressure sore development as avascular epidermal cells can tolerate anoxia longer than deeper tissues

(3) Most common sites of pressure sore formation are sacral area, greater trochanter, ischial tuberosity, tuberosity of the calcaneus, and lateral malleolus (see Module 16—Medical Sequelae (Pressure Sores)—for classification and care)

2. Wound classification

a. Red-Yellow-Black (3)
  (1) Can be used on any wound
  (2) Based on the color of the wound rather than the depth of tissue involvement
    (a) Red
      i) Acute traumatic or surgical injury with frank bleeding or recent hemostasis
      ii) Chronic wounds with pink or red granulation tissue
      iii) Goal—protect the wound from potential harm, and keep it moist as it is ready to heal and has defined edges
    (b) Yellow
      i) Soft, necrotic tissue with exudate ranging from ivory to yellow-green
      ii) May require cleaning and minor debridement with wet-to-damp saline dressings to promote growth of granulation tissue
      iii) Goal—keep wound clean and moist
    (c) Black
      i) Black, gray, or brown necrotic eschar
      ii) If soft and mushy, there may be pus underneath
      iii) If dry and without redness, leave alone until mechanical, surgical, or chemical debridement can occur
      iv) Goal—debride and heal
  (3) Always treat most severe wounds first, if they are in combination
  (4) This classification is based on, as yet, limited research data

b. American College of Surgeons (see Module 12—Infection—for classification according to level of wound contamination)

F. WOUND CARE

1. Cleansing

a. Removes debris, bacteria, foreign bodies, and necrotic tissue
  (1) Gently wash from the inside out, using gauze or swabs
  (2) Antimicrobial solutions may be used
    (a) Povidone-iodine scrub solution has questionable antiseptic action and has been shown to cause damage to new granulation tissue (4)
    (b) Hydrogen peroxide has also been shown to damage new granulation tissue (4)
    (c) Hibiclens (chlorhexidine gluconate) offers a wide range of bactericidal activity; few studies on tissue effects

b. Irrigation
  (1) Syringe or mechanical pulsing devices are recommended as low-pressure irrigation; gravity or bulb syringe may not clean wound adequately

(2) Saline is the best irrigant; antimicrobials may damage new granulation tissue and efficacy in decreasing wound infection is unproven
(3) Large volumes of irrigant are necessary for adequate cleansing

c. Debridement
(1) Removes nonviable tissue and debris by one of several methods (see Module 26—Integumentary Injury—for specific information)
(2) Necrotic tissue must be removed for wound healing to occur
(3) Wound must be excised to healthy, viable tissue
(4) Viable tissue bleeds; viable muscle is red and contracts when stimulated

2. Wound closure methods

a. Simple or superficial wounds can be sutured or approximated with tape or staples immediately after injury, if they are fresh and clean, e.g., lacerations

b. Suturing is used for many types of wound repairs
(1) Eliminates the space between margins and gives artificial strength to wound
(2) Many different types of sutures exist, each with specific uses
(3) Retention sutures are indicated when a wound is under a great deal of stress (abdomen); sutures go through all dermal layers, stretch across the wound, and may be covered to prevent erosion into the wound
(4) With wounds that are deep, contaminated, or older than six hours, the wound is left open, and closed after four or five days of cleansing (delayed primary closure)

c. Grafting
(1) Skin grafts
(a) Thickness varies, but a split-thickness graft usually includes epidermis and part of dermis
(b) Types
i) Autograft (from self)—surgical transplantation of skin from one area of a patient's body to another, e.g., split-thickness skin graft
ii) Homograft or allograft (from a donor of the same species)—usually from a cadaver; used temporarily until autograft is available
iii) Heterograft or xenograft (from a donor of another species, e.g., pigskin)—used only as a temporary, biological dressing
(c) Grafts may be applied in sheets or meshed to expand coverage area and permit drainage; mesh grafts conform well to irregular areas but are less desirable cosmetically
(d) Cultured epithelial autografts may be used when donor skin is inadequate; durability is unproved
(e) Skin grafts are nourished from underlying tissues, initially, and develop their blood supply through angiogenesis in granulation tissue recipient bed
(f) Graft take is usually assured within 6 to 10 days
(2) Skin flaps
(a) Composed of full thickness of skin and some subcutaneous fat
(b) Are left attached at one end and swung around to close the defective area
(c) Must be immobilized immediately postsurgery and kept free of stress until healing has begun (4 to 10 days)
(3) Myocutaneous flaps
(a) Contains muscle with its blood supply and skin attached

(b) Used to close complex wounds, e.g., sternum, lower extremity defects
(c) Advantages over skin grafts include
i) Substitute for unavailable local skin grafts
ii) Capable of providing large amount of bulk and coverage to achieve desired cosmetic effect
iii) Have a constant vascular anatomy, increasing likelihood of healing
iv) Less susceptible to infection
(4) Free flaps
(a) Contain various types of tissue, muscle and cutaneous; thickness varies
(b) Flap is disconnected from donor site; blood supply is reestablished directly at recipient site using microvascular techniques
(c) Donor site is hidden with no functional deformity (5)
d. Surgical repairs of amputation
(1) Closed amputation (usually nontraumatic in origin)—two large flaps of muscle and soft tissue remain to form a cover over exposed bone; closed primarily
(2) Open amputation—a blunt cut is made leaving no flaps; often performed for actual or potential infection and left open for daily observation and cleansing; closed by tertiary intention
(3) Primary amputation—performed after traumatic injury as soon as the patient is hemodynamically stable; closed primarily or secondarily
(4) Secondary amputation—performed after badly traumatized limb has become irreversibly nonviable or infected; usually left open and later closed by secondary or tertiary intention
3. Wound dressings
a. Purposes
(1) Protects wound from the environment, e.g., contaminants, further injury, extremes in temperature
(2) Lessens tension on suture line
(3) Immobilizes affected area
(4) Absorbs drainage
(5) Promotes hemostasis (pressure dressing)
(6) Provides moist environment, which promotes healing
(7) Promotes patient comfort
b. Match purpose of dressing with selection from the many types available
(1) A sterile dressing is recommended for all wounds for the first 24 hrs postinjury, or until wound surface is sealed
(2) Coarse mesh gauze is used for wounds that require debridement; using a wet-to-damp saline technique, necrotic tissue and exudate will adhere to the loosely woven gauze interstices and will be debrided when the dressing is removed
(3) Fine mesh gauze is used for clean, healing wounds; due to the closely woven fibers in this dressing, granulation tissue is unlikely to be disturbed when the dressing is gently removed
(4) Semipermeable dressings
(a) A moist surface environment has been found to enhance wound healing
(b) Polyurethane composition allows the exchange of water vapor and oxygen while preventing bacterial entry

(c) Synthetic types include Op-Site, Tegaderm, and Epilock; fluid collection beneath dressing may make wound inspection difficult; should only be used with clean wounds

(d) Biobrane is a biosynthetic type composed of nylon mesh bonded to silicone; adheres well to clean wounds and can be left intact until reepithelialization occurs; may be combined with topical antimicrobials for care of some contaminated wounds

G. TECHNIQUES TO ENHANCE WOUND HEALING

1. **Low-intensity electrotherapy**
   a. Proven useful only with indolent ulcers
   b. Decreases necessary debridement
   c. Increases scar length and minimizes risk of infection
2. **Low-energy laser therapy**
   a. Stimulates healing in ulcers without circulatory compromise
   b. May be related to prostaglandin release
3. **Hyperbaric oxygen (HBO)**
   a. Increases available oxygen to compromised tissues and enhances healing
   b. Wounds with delayed healing secondary to infection or compromised circulation have responded well to HBO
   c. HBO causes vasoconstriction in crush injuries, limiting exsanguination but not compromising oxygen delivery
   d. HBO has a bacteriostatic effect on the anaerobic bacteria that cause gas gangrene, necrotizing fasciitis, and myositis
4. **Skin respiratory factor**
   a. Stimulates oxygen utilization by fibroblasts, which increases epithelialization
   b. Increases collagen synthesis
   c. Found in Preparation H, which also contains vitamin A in the form of shark liver oil
5. **Growth hormone—clinical trials indicate this may have promise is some patient populations**
6. **Pressure garments**
   a. Constant pressure at 25 mm Hg induces alignment of collagen fibers and reduces vascularity of hypertrophic scar tissue
   b. Should be individually fitted for all scar-prone areas and worn continuously, except for bathing, for approximately one year post initial healing

H. WOUND EVALUATION

1. **Successful wound healing requires the collaboration of all the health care disciplines**
2. **Evaluation of the success of wound healing addresses the criteria of skin integrity, optimal function, and cosmetic appearance**

References

1. Robbins, S. L., Cotran, R. S., & Kumar, V. (1984). *Pathologic basis of disease* (3rd ed.). Philadelphia: W. B. Saunders Co.
2. Warden, G. (1987). Outpatient management of thermal injuries. In J. A. Boswick (Ed.), *The art and science of burn care* (pp. 45–51). Rockville, MD: Aspen Publishers, Inc.
3. Cuzzell, J. (1988). The new RYB color code. *American Journal of Nursing, 88*(10), 1342–1346.
4. Drug Information Bulletin (1987, March) *21*(3). Birmingham, AL: University of Alabama.
5. Reese, J. L. (1990). Nursing interventions for wound healing in plastic and reconstructive surgery. *Nursing Clinics of North America, 25*(1), 223–233.

Suggested Readings

Cooper, D. M. (Ed.). (1990). Wound healing. *Nursing Clinics of North America, 25*(1).

Guyton, A. C. (1986). *Textbook of medical physiology* (7th ed.). Philadelphia: W. B. Saunders Co.

Jackson, D. S., & Rovee, D. T. (1988). Current concepts in wound healing: Research and theory. *Journal of Enterostomal Therapy, 15*(3), 133–137.

Neuberger, G. B. (1985). A new look at wound care. *Nursing, 15*(2), 34–42.

Seiler, W. O., & Stahelin, H. B. (1986). Recent findings on decubitus ulcer pathology: Implications for care. *Geriatrics, 41*(1), 47–60.

Sieggreen, M. Y. (1987). Healing of physical wounds. *Nursing Clinics of North America, 22*(2), 439–447.

Vorosmarti, J. (1981). Hyperbaric oxygen therapy. *American Family Physician, 23*(1), 167–173.

Wilkerson, E. (1988). Inflammation, infection, and wound healing. In E. Howell, L. Widra & M. G. Hill (Eds.), *Comprehensive trauma nursing: Theory and practice* (pp. 326–362). Glenview, IL: Scott, Foresman & Co.

Section III
Comprehensive Topics in Trauma Nursing

MODULE 14
PAIN

Linda M. Woodin, MSN, RN, CCRN

Prerequisite

Review basic neuroanatomy and physiology, and basic analgesic pharmacology.

Objectives

1.0 **Discuss mechanisms of pain generation and transmission.**
1.1 Differentiate between two types of peripheral nerve nociceptive fibers and the types of sensations they transmit.
1.2 List and discuss the role of chemical peripheral pain mediators in pain generation.
1.3 Identify central pain pathways.
1.4 Define endogenous pain relief mechanisms.
1.5 Describe three mechanisms of endogenous pain relief with examples of each.
1.6 Discuss the gate control theory of pain.
2.0 **Identify the causes, with examples, of acute and chronic pain in trauma patients.**
3.0 **Identify the clinical physiological and psychological consequences of pain in trauma patients.**
4.0 **Describe assessment of the patient in pain.**
4.1 Define pain using at least two definitions.
4.2 Differentiate characteristics and assessment findings in acute and chronic pain.
4.3 List factors that influence the patient's perception of pain.

4.4 List factors that influence health care providers' perceptions of patients' pain.
4.5 Discuss questions used in the interview of a patient in pain.
4.6 Describe three pain assessment tools and their uses.
5.0 List three goals of pain management in trauma care.
6.0 Discuss the pharmacological management of pain in the trauma patient.
6.1 Discuss at least five factors affecting the choice of appropriate analgesic drugs.
6.2 Discuss at least two factors affecting the choice of appropriate drug administration routes.
6.3 Describe the uses of combination and adjuvant analgesic therapies in trauma patients experiencing pain.
6.4 Define at least three different drug delivery systems and their uses in trauma pain management.
6.5 Define the term "placebo" and describe its role in pain management.
6.6 Define the terms "tolerance," "dependence," "addiction," and "withdrawal."
6.7 Recognize signs of each of the above terms and propose strategies to manage each in the trauma patient.
7.0 Describe and give examples of five physical techniques for pain management.
8.0 Describe and give examples of six psychological techniques for pain management.
9.0 Given patient assessment data for trauma patients experiencing pain, develop appropriate nursing diagnoses.
10.0 Identify nursing interventions related to each nursing diagnosis presented by trauma patients in pain.
11.0 List expected outcomes with measurable criteria associated with each nursing diagnosis.

A. MECHANISMS OF NOCICEPTION

Nociception: the perception of pain through transmission of mechanical, chemical, or thermal stimuli

1. Peripheral nociception

a. Pain transmission occurs via two main nerve fibers
   (1) A-delta fibers—small diameter, myelinated; fast transmission of sharp, well-localized pain
   (2) C fibers—larger diameter, unmyelinated; slow transmission of dull, burning, poorly localized pain

b. Chemical pain mediators released in response to tissue injury increase the responsiveness of peripheral pain nerve fibers to pain stimuli, e.g., prostaglandins, prostacyclines, histamines, bradykinin, thromboxanes

2. Central pain stimulus transmission

a. Spinal nerves—enter through vertebral spaces and attach to spinal cord; composed of
   (1) Dorsal roots—contain ascending pathways
   (2) Ventral roots—contain both ascending and descending pathways

b. Spinal cord
   (1) Consists of several ascending (afferent) and descending (efferent) pathways
   (2) Pain stimuli thought to be transmitted by a neurotransmitter (substance P)
c. Brain—transmits and perceives stimulus via three areas
   (1) Brain stem reticular formation—transmits information to thalamus and cerebral cortex
   (2) Thalamus—relays ascending information to cerebral cortex
   (3) Cerebral cortex—integrates information; influences behavior based on cognitive-evaluative responses

B. MECHANISMS OF PAIN RELIEF

1. Endogenous (within the body) mechanisms

a. Inhibitory neurotransmitters in spinal cord and brain, e.g., norepinephrine, serotonin, dopamine, stop pain transmission through unknown mechanisms
b. Endogenous narcotic-like neuromodulators bind at opiate receptor sites to stop transmission of pain stimuli; composed of peptides found in the central and peripheral nervous systems and gastrointestinal system, e.g., endorphins, enkephalins, dynorphins
c. Gate control theory of pain—substantia gelatinosa, in laminae II and III of dorsal horn gray matter of spinal cord, acts upon central T cells to either open or close the pathway or "gate" for central pain transmission
   (1) Influenced by psychological and perceptual factors
   (2) Also may be influenced by therapeutics such as transcutaneous electronic nerve stimulation (TENS) or massage

2. Exogenous (outside of the body) mechanisms

a. Peripheral mechanical or chemical stimulus reduction by TENS, massage, or nonsteroidal inflammatory drugs (NSAIDs)
b. Peripheral transmission interruption along nerves through local or regional anesthesia
c. Central transmission interruption in spinal cord through means such as
   (1) Epidural or spinal local anesthetics
   (2) Neuromodulator and inhibitory transmitter enhancement, e.g., spinal cord stimulators or amino acids thought to increase serotonin
   (3) Surgical interventions, e.g., cordotomy, rhizotomy
d. Central perception alteration in spinal cord or brain through means such as opiates

C. CAUSES OF PAIN AND ITS CONSEQUENCES IN TRAUMA PATIENTS

1. Acute pain—indicates actual or potential tissue damage due to

a. Anatomic disruption—stretching, tearing, cutting, external or internal compression due to hemorrhage or edema, burns, tissue necrosis

b. Physiologic disruption—cramping, anoxia, ischemia, decreased muscle activity, e.g., in ileus
c. Inflammatory process—infection, edema
d. Coincidental pain—due to treatments (catheters), medication side effects (constipation from narcotics), or coincidental problems (headache, acute cholecystitis)

2. Chronic pain—beyond the expected course of an illness or injury, or lasting for six months or more due to

a. Neurogenic pain syndromes—myofascial pain syndrome, causalgia, reflex sympathetic dystrophy, phantom limb pain
b. Anatomic disruptions—nonunion of bone fractures, gastrointestinal adhesions, fistulae

3. Consequences may be physiological or psychological as described in Table 14.1

D. PAIN ASSESSMENT

1. Pain defined

a. "An unpleasant sensory and emotional experience associated with actual or potential tissue damage, or described in terms of such damage" (1)
b. "Whatever the experiencing person says it is, existing whenever he says it does" (2)

2. Characteristics of acute and chronic pain (Table 14.2)

3. Factors that influence pain perception

a. Degree of tissue injury
b. Culture and demographics, e.g., age, sex
c. Meaning of the pain
d. Prior pain experience
e. Insomnia
f. Anxiety
g. Perception of control over pain and situation

4. Factors that influence health care workers' perceptions of patients' pain

a. Patient demographics, e.g., age, sex, circumstances of injury
b. Presence or absence of pathology for the pain complaints
c. Patient credibility
d. Duration of the pain complaint
e. Identifying with the patient
f. Personal beliefs about pain tolerance, expression, and relief
g. Fears, myths, traditions surrounding narcotic analgesia

5. Pain assessment

a. Patient interview
   (1) Where is the pain located?
   (2) How intense is the pain? (describe quantity)
   (3) What does the pain feel like? (describe quality of pain sensations)
   (4) What makes the pain worse and what relieves it?
   (5) What does patient believe is causing the pain?

Table 14.1

Consequences of pain in trauma patients

Category	*Process*	*Clinical Consequences*
Cardiovascular	Venoconstriction, arteriole constriction; increased peripheral resistance, heart rate, and myocardial contractility	Increased cardiac work load, myocardial oxygen consumptions; decreased regional blood flow
Endocrine/metabolic	Stress response: increased epinephrine and norepinephrine release; renin and angiotension II production; ACTH release; ADH release; aldosterone secretion; cortisol production; glucagon release	Hypertension; hyperglycemia; fluid and electrolyte imbalances
Respiratory	Depressed medullary respiratory center neurons; decreased respiratory rate, tidal volume, minute ventilation; shift of CO_2 response curve	Hypoventilation; inadequate pulmonary toilet; atelectasis; retained secretions; respiratory infections
Musculoskeletal	Segmental/suprasegmental reflex motor activity (spasm at or above the area of pain brought on by nerve stimulation)	Muscle spasm
Gastrointestinal	Increased sympathetic activity resulting in increased intestinal secretions; decreased peristalsis	Gastric stasis and dilation; anorexia, nausea, vomiting
Urinary	Increased smooth muscle sphincter tone	Urinary retention; decreased urinary output (secondary to ADH and aldosterone secretion)
Immobility	Patient seeks to avoid painful movements	Venous stasis; respiratory (as above); musculoskeletal (as above); stiffness; contractures
Insomnia	Unable to fall asleep; awakened by pain, unable to return to sleep	Sleeping during day; sleeping after analgesic interpreted as excess sedation
Psychological	Anxiety	Crying, irritability; inability to concentrate or participate in treatment plan
	Depression (more common in chronic pain) leading to physical, psychological, or social/vocational disturbances	Weight gain, inactivity; anger, low self-esteem; estrangement from spouse and friends, social withdrawal; impairment in work performance, disability

Table 14.2

Characteristics of acute and chronic pain

Characteristic	*Acute*	*Chronic*
Purpose	Indicates actual or potential tissue damage; protects the organism from harm	Rarely, if ever, indicates new actual or potential tissue damage
Onset	Sudden	Gradual
Duration	Temporary	Beyond the expected time or usual course of an illness or injury, or lasting for a period of six months or more
	Usually subsides with time but may, and often does, progress to a chronic pain state if not effectively treated	Persists or recurs over indefinite periods of time
Location	Well localized and described	Poorly localized and described; characteristics change over time

(6) How is pain affecting the patient physically, emotionally, and socially?
(7) How is patient's pain affecting the patient's family?

b. Physical assessment
 (1) Vital sign changes, e.g., increased respirations, altered heart rate and/or blood pressure may indicate acute pain or other pathology
 (2) Other signs include pallor, diaphoresis, and pupil dilation
 (3) Behavioral cues—may indicate acute pain or other pathology
  (a) Grimacing
  (b) Moaning or crying
  (c) Rubbing the affected area or extremity
  (d) Restlessness, irritability
  (e) Drug-seeking behaviors—most commonly indicate unrelieved pain, however, may indicate actual or potential substance abuse
   i) Clock-watching
   ii) Manipulation of caregivers
   iii) Requests for other medications
   iv) Affective behaviors—anger, crying, refusal to participate in prescribed plan of care, etc.

c. Pain assessment tools
 (1) Intensity rating scales—patient's report is most reliable factor; can measure pain intensity and/or relief intensity
  (a) Visual Analog Scale (see Figure 14.1)
  (b) Wong-Baker Faces Rating Scale—used with children (see Figure 14.2)
  (c) Verbal Descriptor Scale (see Table 14.3)
 (2) Multidimensional scales, such as the McGill Pain Questionnaire, represent sensory and affective dimensions of pain (see Figure 14.3)

Figure 14.1

Visual Analog or Graphic Rating Scale. The patient is asked to place a mark at some point on the line to indicate pain intensity. The pain score is the distance from the left end, measured in millimeters. From A. Jacox, *Pain: A sourcebook for nurses and other health professionals.* Boston: Little, Brown, & Co., 1977, pp. 111, 113. Reprinted with permission.

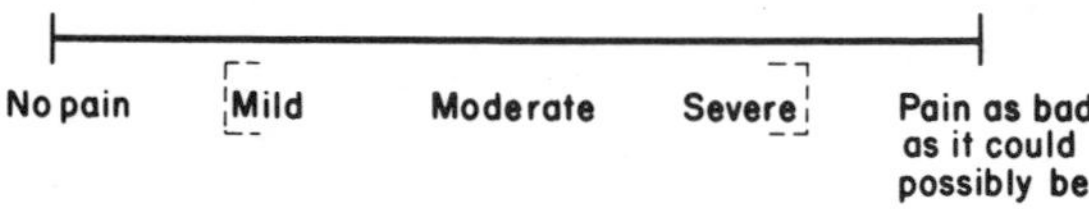

Figure 14.2

Wong-Baker Faces Scale. Can be used with children as young as 3 years. Explain to child that each face is for a person who feels happy because there is no pain (hurt) or sad because there is some or a lot of pain. Face 0 is very happy because there is no hurt. Face 1 hurts just a little bit. Face 2 hurts a little more. Face 3 hurts even more. Face 4 hurts a whole lot, but Face 5 hurts as much as you can imagine, although you don't have to be crying to feel this bad. Ask child to choose face that best describes how the pain feels.
Reproduced by permission from Wong, Donna L., and Whaley, Lucille F.: *Clinical manual of pediatric nursing,* ed. 3, St. Louis, 1990, The C. V. Mosby Co.

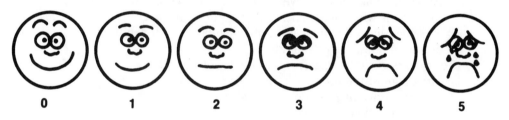

E. GOALS OF PAIN MANAGEMENT IN TRAUMA CARE

1. Reduce pain to tolerable level
2. Restore function
3. Prevent delayed sequelae
a. Chronic pain syndromes
b. Physiologic alterations, e.g., atelectasis, joint contractures

F. PHARMACOLOGIC PAIN MANAGEMENT

(See reference (3))
1. Factors influencing choice of correct analgesic drug
a. Severity of pain—"analgesic ladder" concept
(1) Nonnarcotics for mild to moderate pain; prototype is aspirin

Table 14.3

Verbal Descriptor Scale

Example A	*Example B*
None	Mild
Mild	Discomforting
Moderate	Distressing
Severe	Horrible
Worst ever	Excruciating

(2) "Weak" narcotics for moderate pain; prototype is codeine
(3) "Strong" narcotics for moderate to severe pain; prototype is morphine

b. Nature of pain
  (1) Cause of the pain—anatomic or physiologic disruption, inflammation, infection, coincidental pain
    (a) Combination compounds that combine peripheral stimulus reduction effect of nonnarcotics with central analgesic action of narcotics, e.g., Tylenol with codeine, Tylox, Percocet, Percodan
    (b) Combination regimens—narcotic, NSAID, antianxiety agent, muscle relaxant, hypnotic, etc.
    (c) Adjuvant analgesics—a diverse group of drug classes with other indications which may have analgesic effects in specific circumstances, e.g., tricyclic antidepressants, anticonvulsants, neuroleptics, antihistamines, corticosteroids
  (2) Pattern of occurrence, e.g., continuous vs only with activity
    (a) Drug administration modes—timing
      i) Preventive mode—around-the-clock
        a) Traditional chronic pain management mode
        b) Principle—treat pain before it occurs
        c) Advantages—takes less medication to prevent pain than to treat pain; increased patient physical comfort; decreased patient anxiety
        d) Example—continuous morphine sulfate I.V. drip; run at 4 mg/hr
      ii) Rescue mode—as needed (p.r.n.)
        a) Traditional acute management mode
        b) Principle—treat pain once it has occurred
        c) Disadvantages—takes more medication to treat pain than to prevent pain; patients sometimes reluctant to report pain; generally slow onset
        d) Example—morphine sulfate, 10 mg, I.M., q 4 hrs p.r.n. pain
      iii) Combined mode
        a) Used for continuous pain of injury plus episodic pain of treatments
        b) Example—morphine sulfate I.V. drip; run at 4 mg/hr; may give additional morphine sulfate, 2 mg I.V. push, p.r.n. for turning, dressing change

c. Status of vital organ systems

Figure 14.3

Short-form McGill Pain Questionnaire (SF-MPQ). Descriptors 1–11 represent the sensory dimension of pain experience, and 12–15 represent the affective dimension. Each descriptor is ranked on an intensity scale of 0 = none, 1 = mild, 2 = moderate, 3 = severe. The Present Pain Intensity (PPI) of the standard long-form McGill Pain Questionnaire (LF-MPQ) and the Visual Analog Scale (VAS) are also included to provide overall intensity scores.
From R. Melzack, The short form McGill pain questionnaire. *Pain, 30*(2) (1987), p. 193.

SHORT-FORM McGILL PAIN QUESTIONNAIRE

RONALD MELZACK

PATIENT'S NAME: ____________________ **DATE:** __________

	NONE	MILD	MODERATE	SEVERE
THROBBING	0) ____	1) ____	2) ____	3) ____
SHOOTING	0) ____	1) ____	2) ____	3) ____
STABBING	0) ____	1) ____	2) ____	3) ____
SHARP	0) ____	1) ____	2) ____	3) ____
CRAMPING	0) ____	1) ____	2) ____	3) ____
GNAWING	0) ____	1) ____	2) ____	3) ____
HOT-BURNING	0) ____	1) ____	2) ____	3) ____
ACHING	0) ____	1) ____	2) ____	3) ____
HEAVY	0) ____	1) ____	2) ____	3) ____
TENDER	0) ____	1) ____	2) ____	3) ____
SPLITTING	0) ____	1) ____	2) ____	3) ____
TIRING-EXHAUSTING	0) ____	1) ____	2) ____	3) ____
SICKENING	0) ____	1) ____	2) ____	3) ____
FEARFUL	0) ____	1) ____	2) ____	3) ____
PUNISHING-CRUEL	0) ____	1) ____	2) ____	3) ____

NO PAIN |————————————————| WORST POSSIBLE PAIN

PPI

0	NO PAIN	____
1	MILD	____
2	DISCOMFORTING	____
3	DISTRESSING	____
4	HORRIBLE	____
5	EXCRUCIATING	____

(1) Hypovolemia, cardiovascular decompensation, and impaired organ perfusion or muscle blood flow usually require reduced drug dosage and systemic administration of medications
(2) Hypoventilation and compromised oxygenation require caution with therapies or drugs that interfere with mechanics of respiration or central control
(3) Altered consciousness or intracranial pathology are contraindications for drugs that mask or imitate signs of increased intracranial pressure, e.g., sedation, vomiting, or pupillary dysfunction
(4) Alcohol or other substances in system
(a) Treat effects
(b) Adjust analgesic dosage based on effects, side effects, and tolerance to other drugs

d. Principles of narcotic use
(1) Physiologic effects of narcotic drugs are listed in Table 14.4
(2) Equianalgesics—defined as the dose that provides the same analgesic potency as another analgesic dose or route
(a) Equianalgesics are approximate values subject to individual patient and situational differences
(b) Morphine, 10 mg, I.M. is the "gold standard" against which all other analgesics are measured
(c) Useful concept for required analgesic changes due to tolerance, allergies, unacceptable side effects, route changes, or excess dilutional volume situations

e. Phase in trauma and recovery continuum
(1) Resuscitative/stabilization phase (acute pain)—parenteral and regional analgesics and anesthetics most common
(2) Recovery phase (acute and chronic pain)—parenteral and enteral narcotics, nonnarcotics, adjuvant medications, regional anesthetics, physical and psychological modalities most common
(3) Rehabilitative phase (chronic pain)—nonnarcotics, adjuvant medications, physical and psychological modalities most common

2. Factors influencing choice of drug administration route (see Table 14.5)

3. Alternative drug delivery systems

a. Patient-controlled analgesia (PCA)
(1) Computerized infusion pump that allows selected patients to administer ordered parenteral doses of narcotic analgesics within ordered time frames
(2) Advantages
(a) Rapid onset of analgesia
(b) Potential for less medication and fewer side effects
(c) Potential for decreased patient anxiety and increased sense of control and well-being
(3) Indications—patient candidate criteria
(a) Need for parenteral narcotic analgesia
(b) No contraindications to parenteral analgesia, e.g., allergy to prescribed nacrotic, severe pulmonary or metabolic dysfunction, etc.
(c) Oriented, cooperative patient capable of learning and using device
(d) Significant past or active substance abuse is not necessarily a contraindication to PCA, since patient is unable to receive more than the prescribed amount

Table 14.4

Physiologic effects of narcotic drugs

System	*Effect*	*Manifestation*	*Treatment*
Respiratory	Depresses medullary respiratory center neurons	Decreased respiratory rate, tidal volume, minute ventilation; shift of the CO_2 response curve	Adequate hydration, appropriate analgesic doses; encourage pulmonary toilet; if severe, arousal, airway maintenance, narcotic antagonist (naloxone)
Circulatory	Arterial and venous dilation, due either to direct alpha receptor-blocking activity, or histamine release	Postural hypotension	Adequate hydration, appropriate analgesic doses; if severe, arousal and pain stimulation
CNS	CNS excitation or depression; metabolite of meperidine (normeperidine), cumulative and neurotoxic	Drowsiness, lethargy, respiratory depression, convulsions, nausea, emesis, pupillary miosis	Appropriate drugs (codeine drug of choice) and doses in head injury, neurological checks
Gastrointestinal	Delayed gastric emptying; decreased intestinal motility; morphine may cause spasm of sphincter of Oddi	Constipation, decreased secretion of digestive fluids; anorexia, nausea, biliary spasm pain	Prophylactic bowel regimens (fiber foods, fluids, mobility, stool softeners, laxatives); small feedings, antiemetics as needed
Genitourinary	Increased muscle and sphincter tone	Urinary retention	Catheterization as needed; urinary antispasmodics as needed

b. Time-controlled analgesia
   (1) Continuous parenteral narcotic infusions via infusion controller, e.g., morphine, hydromorphone, meperidine drips, or sustained-release oral preparations, e.g., MS Contin, Roxanol SR
   (2) Advantages
      (a) Consistent release and action
      (b) Consistent analgesia—less peak and trough effects

Table 14.5

Considerations in drug administration routes

Route	*Relative Onset*	*Relative Duration*	*Relative Doses*	*Other Considerations*
I.V.	Rapid onset	Short duration	Small doses	Need available access; compatibility with solutions and other ordered medications; infection potential
S.C.	Moderately rapid onset	Moderate duration	Moderate but concentrated doses	Need available tissue and absorption
Epidural/ spinal	Rapid or slow onset (depending on agents)	Short or long duration (depending on agents)	Very small doses	Need trained physician; infection, nerve damage, respiratory depression potential
I.M.	Slower onset	Longer duration	Large doses	Often unpredictable absorption; painful; need available muscle mass; not in coagulopathies
P.O.	Slow onset	Long duration	Large doses	Large doses due to metabolism in liver; least invasive route; sometimes unpredictable absorption; need functional GI tract; need low risk for pulmonary aspiration and GI upset
Rectal	Slow onset	Long duration	Equal doses to P.O.	Predictable absorption if retained; need absence of diarrhea; Note: lower GI stoma can function as rectal route
Regional local, nerve block, intrapleural	Slow or rapid onset (depending on agents)	Short or long duration (depending on agents)	Local anesthetics (no narcotics)	Provides limited area of relief; need trained physician or staff

(c) Potential for less medication and side effects
(3) Indications
(a) Constant or severe pain uncontrolled by p.r.n. doses
(b) Need to avoid peak and trough effects of p.r.n. dosing

c. Regional analgesia—provides analgesia for distinct body area, not generalized pain
(1) Local infiltration—anesthetizes cutaneous area with local anesthetic injection
(2) Nerve block—blocks peripheral or visceral area supplied by nerve using local anesthetic injection
(3) Conduction (epidural/spinal) analgesia
(a) Medication administration requires trained physician for single injection via epidural or spinal needle, or placement of indwelling catheter for intermittent bolus injection, continuous infusion, or patient-controlled administration
(b) Drug choice
i) Opioids—short-acting fentanyl or meperidine or longer-acting morphine or hydromorphone; should be preservative-free to avoid neural damage
ii) Anesthetics—short-acting type, e.g., bupivacaine, or anesthetic plus epinephrine for longer action
iii) Combination therapies—combine opioid and local anesthetic, e.g., fentanyl and bupivacaine
iv) Chronic pain—ablative medications destroy peripheral or central pain transmission pathways, e.g., alcohol or phenol
(4) Interpleural analgesia
(a) Blocks transmission of peripheral pain stimuli
(b) Administered via chest tube or indwelling pleural catheter

4. Other considerations in pharmacologic pain management

a. Use of a placebo
(1) Defined as "any medical treatment (medication or procedure, including surgery or nursing care) that produces an effect in a patient because of its implicit or explicit intent and not because of its specific nature or therapeutic properties" (4)
(2) A minimum of one-third of all people with obvious physical stimuli for pain, e.g., abdominal surgery, report adequate relief from a placebo
(3) Physiological basis may involve release of endogenous opioids in response to psychological stimuli
(4) The deceptive use of placebos and the misinterpretation of the placebo response to distinguish "psychogenic" from "real" pain should be avoided (5)

b. Tolerance—as a result of prior administration, a larger dose of narcotic analgesic is required to maintain the original effect
(1) Can occur within one to two weeks of regular administration of a narcotic
(2) Manifested clinically as, first, a decrease in duration of analgesia, and then a decrease in the degree of analgesia
(3) Incomplete cross-tolerance—means that tolerance to one narcotic does not necessarily indicate same degree of tolerance to all narcotics
(4) Treatment of tolerance requires increase in dose to obtain same analgesic effect, or equianalgesic change to another narcotic (incomplete cross-tolerance between narcotics)

c. Physical dependence—"a state of biochemical or physiological adaptation of tissues characterized by withdrawal symptoms if treatment is stopped abruptly" (6)
  (1) Can occur as soon as one or two weeks after consistent narcotic administration
  (2) Prevention—judicious, appropriate courses of narcotics, combination pharmacologic and physical modalities, rapid correction of pain pathologies
d. Addiction (psychological dependence)—a behavior pattern of compulsive drug use characterized by craving a drug for other than pain relief, and becoming overwhelmingly concerned with using and obtaining a drug; high tendency to return to this behavior after withdrawal
  (1) Incidence of hospitalized patients who receive narcotics for pain and become addicted is less than 1% (7)
  (2) Treatment includes providing adequate pain relief with emphasis on nonnarcotic and physical analgesic modalities, goal-setting and behavioral contracting, and psychological support
e. Narcotic withdrawal—a syndrome that occurs upon discontinuation of a narcotic once physical dependence has occurred
  (1) Symptoms include yawning, dilated pupils, myalgia, rhinorrhea, restlessness, insomnia, elevated heart rate, respiratory rate, and blood pressure, perspiration, tremor, "gooseflesh," vomiting, and diarrhea
  (2) Systematic withdrawal can be accomplished by
    (a) Slow tapering of dosage
    (b) Conversion to a long-acting narcotic, e.g., methadone
    (c) Tapering with symptom management, e.g., antiemetics, antianxiety agents, and psychological support
    (d) Clonidine hydrochloride (8)

G. PHYSICAL MODALITIES IN PAIN MANAGEMENT

1. **Positioning**
a. Decreases muscle spasm, strain, fatigue, and coincidental pain
b. Includes body alignment and positioning of invasive equipment
2. **Immobilization/stabilization of body parts, e.g., fractured limbs**
a. Decreases anatomic and physiologic disruption
b. Includes use of splints, casts, traction, internal or external fixation devices, pillows for splinting incisions, etc.
3. **Cutaneous stimulation**
a. Reduces cause of pain, e.g., inflammation, edema
b. Interrupts peripheral pain stimulus transmission
c. May inhibit central transmission, i.e., close the "gate"
d. May enhance endogenous analgesia, e.g., endorphins
e. Techniques include application of heat or cold, massage, counterstimulation (massage on extremity or body side opposite affected painful area)
4. **Electrical or mechanical stimulation**

a. Affects large-diameter central transmission fibers
b. Modalities include TENS, acupuncture, or acupressure and are thought to close the "gate"

5. Biofeedback

a. Reduces peripheral or central stimulus transmission and enhances central endogenous opioids
b. Is aimed at either decreasing muscle tension, reducing cephalic or temporal artery blood flow, or increasing skin temperature
c. Requires trained practitioner and intense patient concentration

H. PSYCHOLOGICAL TECHNIQUES IN PAIN MANAGEMENT

1. Preparatory information

a. Reduces the fear of the unknown and anxiety
b. Should include descriptions of sensations as well as procedures to be expected

2. Relaxation

a. Reduces anxiety and muscle tension
b. Techniques include for rhythmic breathing, extremity relaxation, back rubs, and providing a quiet environment

3. Distraction

a. Focuses on stimuli other than the pain sensation
b. Enhanced by visitors, diversional activities, and/or humor

4. Guided imagery

5. Hypnosis

a. Aimed at blocking awareness of pain, substituting another feeling, moving or altering the pain perception, increasing tolerance, or dissociating perception of the painful body part
b. Requires a trained practitioner and intense patient concentration

6. Reassurance and support

a. Reduces anxiety, promotes a positive mood and outlook
b. Staying with patient, providing photographs of familiar persons, telephone calls, letters, and tape recordings may be supportive

7. Provide a sense of control over pain and environment

a. Offer patient-controlled analgesia if medically and psychologically indicated
b. Allow patient to participate in activity decisions as able

I. MULTIDISCIPLINARY APPROACH TO PAIN MANAGEMENT

1. **Coordinated team approach addresses the multidimensional nature of pain**
2. **Team members include trained individuals from specialties such as anesthesiology, nursing, psychiatry, psychology, physical and occupational therapy, social service, and vocational rehabilitation**

J. NURSING DIAGNOSES, EXPECTED OUTCOMES, AND INTERVENTIONS

1. **Acute pain related to injury or complications of injury, surgery/treatment, and/or coincidental causes**

a. Expected outcomes
   (1) Patient verbalizes or otherwise indicates pain state
   (2) Following specific interventions, patient rates pain as reduced on visual analog, verbal descriptor, other pain assessment scale
   (3) Patient and family participate in pain management strategies

b. Nursing interventions
   (1) Perform pain assessment
   (2) Administer pharmacologic agents as prescribed
      (a) Use preventive mode rather than p.r.n. mode whenever possible; premedicate prior to painful procedures
      (b) Use appropriate route, medication, and delivery system for pain severity, source, patient status
      (c) Utilize combination therapies and adjuvant agents for multiple sources and episodes of pain
      (d) Assess patient for prior dependency or substance abuse states
      (e) Consider the development of narcotic tolerance and the need for increased doses in prolonged use
      (f) Allow patient some control over analgesia, if possible
      (g) Assess effectiveness of medications
   (3) Provide physical modalities, including positioning, immobilization, and stimulation as indicated in section G., above
   (4) Coordinate schedule to provide for adequate rest and sleep, especially following analgesic administration
   (5) Use psychological techniques described in section H., above

2. **Chronic benign pain related to prolonged or permanent anatomic or physiologic disruption, or prolonged or permanent altered pain transmission**

a. Expected outcomes
   (1) Patient and family focus attention away from pain complaints and treatments
   (2) Patient and family address pain complaints and treatments through unified medical source
   (3) Patient uses appropriate and minimal pharmacological agents for pain management
   (4) Patient uses nonpharmacological pain management strategies as needed
   (5) Patient maximizes activities and productivity
   (6) Patient and family verbalize feelings and use adequate coping strategies

b. Nursing interventions
   (1) Validate, but do not focus on, pain complaints
   (2) Teach patient and family physiological and psychological facts about pain and its management
   (3) Promote appropriate nonpharmacological pain management modalities
   (4) Negotiate a specific treatment plan, for optimal patient activity, with patient and family

(5) Promote a unified, multidisciplinary approach to management of pain and consistency among caregivers
(6) Promote patient participation in decisionmaking related to pain therapies
(7) Reinforce and reward positive coping strategies by patient and family
(8) Use preventive treatment mode with nonnarcotic and combination pharmacologic therapies
(9) Effectively manage other symptoms, e.g., insomnia, depression, etc.
(10) Involve patient and family in discharge planning for outpatient follow-up

3. Ineffective coping mechanisms related to drug dependence, premorbid ineffective coping ability, personality characteristics, chronic benign pain and disease state, and lack of control

a. Expected outcomes
(1) Patient participates in prescribed plan of care
(2) Patient discusses problems with appropriate family and resource persons
(3) Patient verbalizes appropriately and uses effective coping strategies

b. Nursing interventions
(1) Assess ineffective or maladaptive behaviors
(2) Treat pain and disease state adequately with nonnarcotic and physical analgesic modalities
(3) Establish mutually formulated goals
(4) Assign consistent caregivers who use the same approaches to patient's pain management
(5) Positively reinforce specific goal-oriented behaviors
(6) Encourage patient participation in all aspects of care
(7) Collaborate with resource persons to develop and implement a consistent treatment plan

References

1. Subcommittee on Taxonomy; International Association for the Study of Pain. (1979). Pain terms: A list with definitions and notes on usage. *Pain, 6*, 250.
2. McCaffery, M. (1980). Understanding your patient's pain. *Nursing, 10*(9), 26.
3. Halpern, L. M. (1984). Drugs in the management of pain: Pharmacology and appropriate strategies for clinical utilization. In C. Benedetti, R. Chapman & G. Morrico (Eds.), Recent advances in the management of pain. *Advances in pain research and therapy* (Vol. 7., pp. 147–172). New York: Raven Press.
4. McCaffery, M., & Beebe, A. (1989). *Pain: Clinical manual for nursing practice* (p. 16). St. Louis: C. V. Mosby Co.
5. American Pain Society. (1988). Relieving pain: An analgesic guide. *American Journal of Nursing, 88*(6), 825.
6. World Health Organization. (1986). *Cancer pain relief.* Geneva: Author.
7. Porter, J., & Jick, H. (1980). Addiction rare in patients treated with narcotics. *New England Journal of Medicine, 302*(2), 123.
8. Jasinski, D. R., Johnson, R. E., & Kocher, T. R. (1985). Clonidine in morphine withdrawal. *Archives of General Psychiatry, 42*(11), 1063–1071.

Suggested Readings

Christoff, S. B. (1988). Pain. In M. R. Kinney, D. R. Packa & S. B. Dunbar (Eds.), *AACN's clinical reference for critical care nursing* (2nd ed., pp. 372–398). New York: McGraw-Hill.

Cousins, M. J., & Phillips, G. D. (Eds.). (1986). *Clinics in critical care medicine: Acute pain management.* New York: Churchill Livingstone.

Jacox, A. (1979). Assessing pain. *American Journal of Nursing, 79*(5), 895–900.

Mlynczak, B. (1989). Assessment and management of the trauma patient in pain. *Critical Care Nursing Clinics of North America, 1*(1), 55–65.

Radwin, L. E. (1987). Autonomous nursing interventions for treating the patient in acute pain: A standard. *Heart and Lung, 16*(3), 258–266.

Raj, P. P. (Ed.). (1986). *Practical management of pain.* Chicago: Year Book Medical Publishers.

MODULE 15
PSYCHOSOCIAL RESPONSE TO TRAUMA

Joanne Michener, MSN, RN, CS
Nancy Vanore-Black, MSN, RN

Prerequisite

Basic knowledge of psychosocial nursing.

Objectives

1.0 List the effects of trauma and the normal stages of psychological coping.
2.0 Identify major components of crisis theory.
2.1 Describe stages of crisis response.
2.2 Identify pathological responses to crises.
2.3 Describe crisis intervention techniques.
3.0 Describe the psychopharmacologic agents sometimes indicated, including side effects and contraindications.
4.0 Describe the spectrum of emotional response that may occur during the recovery phase of traumatic injury.
5.0 Explain posttraumatic stress response.
6.0 Describe the method of psychosocial assessment for patients and families during acute phase of traumatic injury.
6.1 Identify components of psychosocial history preinjury.

6.2 Identify major components of mental status exam to be included in patient/family assessment.

7.0 List common nursing diagnoses related to psychosocial responses of patients and families to a traumatic injury.

8.0 Identify psychosocial nursing interventions with rationale for patients experiencing traumatic injury.

9.0 Evaluate patient and family responses to psychosocial nursing interventions, including coping skills, and patient's/family's level of adaptation.

A. PSYCHOSOCIAL EFFECTS OF TRAUMA

1. **Common effects of trauma (1)**
   a. Trauma is an unplanned, unpredictable event
   b. Victims confront their own vulnerability and mortality
   c. Victims faced with many unknowns—unknown extent of injury, number of procedures to be endured, length of hospitalization, and functional outcome
   d. Victims experience helplessness, humiliation, and changes in body image
   e. Victims are isolated from normal support systems
   f. Possible prolonged dependency
   g. Severe physical injuries often cause patients/families to relive other intense emotional experiences and reactivate disturbances, e.g., disturbed self-image
2. **Many psychological/behavioral factors actually increase the probability of trauma**
   a. Alcohol abuse
   b. Immature personalities
   c. Aggressiveness/hostility
   d. Nonconformity
   e. Disregard of authority
   f. Risk-taking tendency
3. **Factors affecting patient's response to injury (1,2)**
   a. Physical factors
      (1) Overall severity of injury
      (2) Loss of limb or sensory organ
      (3) Presence of brain damage
      (4) ICU psychosis related to sleep deprivation, sensory deprivation/overload, and/or medications
      (5) Complicating medical conditions, e.g., anoxia
      (6) Presence of drugs, alcohol, or abstinence syndromes
   b. Psychological factors
      (1) Patient's mental state at time of injury
      (2) Sense of responsibility for the injury
      (3) Reaction to injury, effects on others
      (4) Degree of memory for the event
      (5) Victim's developmental level
      (6) Usual coping skills under stress

c. Social factors
   (1) Availability of social support
   (2) Financial responsibility
   (3) Legal implications
   (4) Loss of significant other
   (5) Cultural determinants

B. RESPONSES TO TRAUMA

1. Patient/victim (3)

a. Acute stage
   (1) Patient uses defensive coping mechanisms, i.e., repression, denial, reaction formation, regression, projection, displacement, isolation
   (2) Affect may be absent, resigned, blunted, or constricted
   (3) Interventions
      (a) Ensure physiologic/safety needs are met
      (b) Do not confront denial
      (c) Communicate even if patient withdraws

b. Recovery phase—convalescent/rehabilitation phase
   (1) Changes assimilated and new behavior patterns developed
   (2) Stage often heralded by anger, hostility
   (3) Dysphoric moods seen

c. Abnormal reactions
   (1) Depressive reaction
   (2) Psychotic reaction
   (3) Indifference
   (4) Excessive anxiety—most common
   (5) Excessive dependency

2. Family responses (3)

a. Shock, protest, denial, numbness
   (1) Blunted, numb affect
   (2) Waves of somatic distress
   (3) Family needs comfort, support

b. Preoccupation with deceased
   (1) Anger, guilt, sadness
   (2) Somatic symptoms
   (3) Allow family members to relive situation

c. Factors affecting response
   (1) Nature of loss—unexpected
   (2) Social support network
   (3) Concurrent events

d. Adaptive responses—distancing, mistrust, anger, guilt, crying, detachment, helplessness

e. Abnormal response
   (1) Suspicion, hostility, rejection
   (2) Abnormal, delayed responses often seen in family spokesman or support person

(3) Distorted response
(a) Symptoms of deceased's final illness
(b) Medical illness
(c) Overactivity without sense of loss
(d) Social isolation
(e) Hostility to a specific person
(f) "Wooden" behavior
(g) Activities detrimental to social/economic existence
(h) Agitated depression

3. Stages of coping

a. Denial, disbelief, shock
b. Depression, immobility
c. Anger, acting out with inappropriate behavior
d. Coping, reintegrating

C. TRAUMA AS A CRISIS

1. Crisis

a. Defined an an upset to a steady state; can mean both danger and opportunity (4)
b. Affects cognitive, affective, and behavioral functioning
(1) Cognition—judgment impaired; confusion, disorganization, and "tunnel vision" may occur
(2) Affect—characterized by anxiety, panic, depression, agitation, helplessness, and hopelessness; interferes with problem solving
(3) Behavior—individual acts out or is unable to do ordinary tasks and self-care
c. Usually self-limited; lasts four to six weeks (4)
d. With its sudden disruption of normal life, few events are more likely to precipitate a crisis state for an individual or a family than traumatic injury
e. Changing situations may present problems not readily solved by coping mechanisms that have worked in the past

2. Pathological responses to crisis

a. Catastrophic reaction—immediately posttrauma
(1) Usually lasts four to five days
(2) Flat effect
(3) Answers questions in monosyllables
(4) Amnesic for entire experience
(5) Fearful—little interaction with caregiver
(6) Severe anxiety—inability to discuss fears
b. Euphoric response—usually within 24 hrs
(1) Usually ends in intermediate phase of hospitalization
(2) Exceptionally high activity level
(3) Very cheerful, even when discussing painful or upsetting events
(4) Speech is animated
(5) Memory is often intact
(6) Usually relates well with caregivers
(7) Extreme denial

c. Delirium—two to five days posttrauma
   (1) Often clears after first good sleep; may continue for weeks
   (2) Variable activity level—passive to combative
   (3) Variable affect—flat to depressed to angry
   (4) Speech level variable—may speak little or constantly; may be inappropriate
   (5) Gaps in memory—may reach total amnesia
   (6) Response to caregiver variable—may become paranoid and fearful of personnel
   (7) Contributing factors
      (a) Sleep deprivation
      (b) Sensory alterations
      (c) Microemboli
      (d) Drugs, medications
      (e) Head injury
      (f) Infection
      (g) Perfusion difficulties
      (h) Preincident psychological disturbance
d. Pathological mourning or agitated depression
   (1) Self-accusation
   (2) Tension
   (3) Agitation
   (4) Feelings of worthlessness
   (5) Insomnia
   (6) Need for "punishment"
   (7) Suicidal ideation

3. Crisis intervention

a. Inexpensive, short-term therapy that focuses on the immediate problem; offers help that a person needs to reestablish equilibrium (4)
b. Generic approach—useful for nonmental health professionals; emphasizes direct encouragement of adaptive behaviors, general support, environmental manipulation, and anticipatory guidance
c. Individual approach—uses professional assessment of the intrapsychic processes of the person in crisis; needed for those unresponsive to generic approach
d. Goals of crisis intervention
   (1) Identify the crisis and any precipitants
   (2) Minimize maladaptive behaviors
   (3) Mobilize internal and external support systems
   (4) Find positive methods of coping with current stressors
   (5) Return to "precrisis" level of functioning, or higher
e. Crisis intervention techniques
   (1) Assessment of individual—may require specialized assistance
   (2) Planning of therapeutic intervention
   (3) Intervention
      (a) Assist individual to gain an intellectual understanding of his/her crisis
      (b) Help the individual bring out feelings to which he/she may not have access
      (c) Explore coping mechanisms
      (d) Resolve the crisis

4. **Psychopharmacologic agents**
a. In early phase, pain and anxiety need to be managed
b. Pain management agents—narcotics, other analgesics administered by nurse or via patient-controlled devices
c. Antianxiety agents, i.e., lorazepam (Ativan) indicated for short-term relief of anxiety, drug withdrawal, and sleep disturbances, if no cognitive deficit (2)
d. Major tranquilizers, i.e., haloperidol (Haldol) indicated for management of concomitant psychotic features, e.g., ICU psychosis
e. Antidepressant agents may be indicated in rehabilitation phase
5. **Emotional responses during the recovery phase**
a. Grief reactions related to perceived losses
b. Injury to self-esteem
   (1) Body image dysfunction
   (2) Loss of independent functioning
   (3) Loss of position in family constellation
   (4) Reorganization of self-concept
c. Posttraumatic stress disorder
   (1) May develop at any time in response to a psychologically traumatic experience following bodily injury
      (a) Acute posttraumatic stress occurs in the first six months after event and lasts less than six months
      (b) Any symptoms that develop after six months are considered to be a chronic or delayed posttraumatic stress response
   (2) Specific acute clinical symptoms
      (a) Reexperiencing the event; rumination
      (b) Reexperiencing the emotions of the event
      (c) Nightmares and sleep disturbances
      (d) Hyperalertness and anxiety; exaggerated startle response
      (e) Loss of concentration; memory impairment
      (f) Irritability, agitation
      (g) Emotional anesthesia, withdrawal
   (3) Treatment
      (a) Obtain psychiatric support, consultation
      (b) Encourage brief discussions that focus on connecting feelings with events
      (c) Validate patient's concerns regarding posttraumatic stress response symptoms
      (d) Utilize short-term antianxiety or antidepressant medications as prescribed
      (e) Reassure patient about and reorient to current environment
      (f) During flashbacks, support the patient, reorient to environment, avoid confrontation, and help to decrease stimuli

D. PSYCHOSOCIAL ASSESSMENT OF PATIENT AND FAMILY

1. **Current level of functioning within the family constellation**
a. Patient's and family members' roles pre- and postinjury
b. Educational level
c. Occupation

2. Utilization of coping mechanisms

a. Use of alcohol and/or drugs
b. Methods of coping with prior events

3. Recent or precipitating life events

a. Recent losses
b. Contributing stressors

4. Mental status examination—an organized method for observing and analyzing data regarding a patient's affective and cognitive functioning (5)

a. Appearance—grooming, general appearance
b. Behavior—degree of activity, cooperativeness, eye contact, gestures, and general movements
c. Speech—ability to use right word, presence of pressured tone, rate of speech, degree of spontaneity
d. Thought processes
   (1) Thought content
      (a) Magical, bizarre, or unusual thoughts
      (b) Perceptions—presence of hallucinations, delusions, paranoid ideation
      (c) Suicidal or homicidal ideation
   (2) Thought process—clear, logical, organized
e. Mood/affect—depressed, euphoric, angry, anxious
f. Intellectual functioning
   (1) Orientation to time, place, and person
   (2) Registration and recall—e.g., can recall three unrelated objects
   (3) Attention and concentration, e.g., can count backwards from seven
   (4) Language—verbal discussion consistent with education and background
   (5) Memory—recent and remote
   (6) Thought patterns—proverbs
   (7) Insight—understanding of situation
   (8) Judgment—ability to compare and assess alternatives

E. NURSING DIAGNOSES, EXPECTED OUTCOMES, AND INTERVENTIONS

1. Initial crisis phase

a. Anxiety, patient and family, related to traumatic event and implications
   (1) Expected outcome—patient and family utilize coping skills effectively to keep anxiety at tolerable level
   (2) Nursing interventions
      (a) Assess patient/family for current level of anxiety and fear
      (b) Provide patient/family with explanations of all treatments and procedures
      (c) Support therapeutic use of defense and other coping mechanisms
      (d) Provide patient/family opportunities to discuss concerns and feelings through techniques of supportive listening
      (e) Administer antianxiety medication as prescribed
      (f) Teach relaxation techniques
      (g) Encourage visits from supportive family and significant others

b. Powerlessness related to restriction from normal activities and loss of function
   (1) Expected outcomes
      (a) Patient states increase in feelings of control
      (b) Patient demonstrates involvement in own care
      (c) Patient makes decisions regarding self
   (2) Nursing interventions
      (a) Provide patient/family with the explanations of all treatments, procedures, and progress
      (b) Give patient/family the opportunity to make all decisions appropriate to condition and knowledge levels
      (c) Support and encourage appropriate expressions of regaining control by the patient and family
      (d) Help patient identify personal strengths and realistic capabilities
      (e) Help patient identify and cope with dependency issues
c. Ineffective coping, individual and family, related to situational crises and role changes
   (1) Expected outcomes
      (a) Patient and family verbalize concerns and demonstate effective coping
      (b) Patient expresses needs, verbally or nonverbally, and participates in decisionmaking when possible
      (c) Patient and family return to precrisis adaptive level, or higher, or have plans for doing so
   (2) Nursing interventions
      (a) Assess individual and family system functioning/support system network
      (b) Recognize patient's and family's difficulty in reaching decisions; assist with problem-solving efforts as necessary
      (c) Provide family with referrals for assistance as appropriate
      (d) Support therapeutic use of defense and other coping mechanisms
      (e) Support patient and family during periods of inability to cope
      (f) Provide requested information; do not overwhelm with details
      (g) Identify and eliminate unnecessary stressors such as excess environmental noise and light, pain and discomfort, unnecessary sleep interruptions, inappropriate bedside conversations
      (h) Identify family spokesperson; utilize consistent people to care for patient
      (i) Help family identify and implement necessary role changes
d. Additional nursing diagnoses
   (1) Knowledge deficit related to lack of exposure and unfamiliarity with strategies and resources for coping with trauma sequelae
   (2) Sleep pattern disturbances related to unfamiliar environment, pain, and biochemical alteration
   (3) Altered thought processes related to psychological stress, unfamiliar environment, and organic dysfunction
   (4) Social isolation related to hospitalization
   (5) Impaired verbal communication related to altered mentation, aphasia, or artificial airway
   (6) Fear related to unknown outcome and unfamiliar environment
   (7) Potential for violence, self-directed or directed at others, related to head injury, panic, anger, and rage

2. Recovery phase

a. Body image disturbance related to injury and sequelae
   (1) Expected outcomes
      (a) Patient uses adaptive devices and techniques, e.g., prosthesis, cosmetics, clothing to enhance appearance
      (b) Patient expresses understanding of and adaptation to body changes
      (c) Patient incorporates changes into self-concept
      (d) Patient and family accept assistance with coping
   (2) Nursing interventions
      (a) Assess patient for current stage of perception of injuries and adaptation
      (b) Recognize denial as normal adaptive response during recovery phase
      (c) Offer patient and family opportunities to discuss concerns and feelings through techniques of supportive listening
      (d) Refer to appropriate resources, e.g., psychiatric clinical nurse specialist, neuropsychology, psychiatry, pastoral counseling, social services, plastic surgeons, or cosmetic consultants
      (e) Provide the patient/family with explanations of all treatments, procedures, and probable long-term results of injury and possible reconstructive/cosmetic therapy
      (f) Assist patient/family to cope with physical limitations resulting from injury
      (g) Use role-playing to help patient practice techniques for dealing with responses of others to changes in patient's body appearance
      (h) Promote independent activities, self-care
      (i) Give patient/family the opportunity to make all decisions appropriate to condition and knowledge level
      (j) Utilize and reinforce patient/family strengths and support network to enhance coping during recovery phase

b. Self-concept disturbance related to change in role performance
   (1) Expected outcomes
      (a) Patient and family verbalize a realistic view of required role changes
      (b) Patient/family return to precrisis adaptive level, or higher, or have plans for doing so
      (c) Family roles are fulfilled
   (2) Nursing interventions
      (a) Determine patient's role and role performance prior to injury
      (b) Assess nature and extent of role performance changes
      (c) Discuss and assist patient/family to develop strategies for dealing with role changes
      (d) Assist patient with reorganization of self-concept
         i) Grieving process for lost roles
         ii) Defining new role
         iii) Reeducation, retraining

c. Grieving, anticipatory and dysfunctional, related to loss of loved one, career, and/or body part
   (1) Expected outcomes
      (a) Patient and family progress through stages of grief at their own pace
      (b) Grief is expressed and resolved adequately

(c) Patient functions adequately in daily living
(2) Nursing interventions
(a) Assess patient and family losses
(b) Acknowledge grief; allow time for patient/family to express grief
(c) Offer therapeutic support; teach and reinforce effective coping techniques
(d) Refer to institutional and community resources, and mental health professionals
(e) Provide family opportunity for organ/tissue donation as appropriate

d. Additional nursing diagnoses
(1) Self-care deficit, various, related to functional loss
(2) Sexual dysfunction related to altered body structure or function, lack of knowledge, or emotional sequelae of trauma
(3) Social isolation related to hospitalization, restricted activity, altered mental status, and/or altered self-concept
(4) Altered health maintenance related to ineffective coping, dysfunctional grieving, or altered cognitive and physical function
(5) Posttrauma response related to extraordinary impact of traumatic event
(6) Rape trauma syndrome related to sexual assault

References

1. Lenehan, G. P. (1986). Emotional impact of trauma. *Nursing Clinics of North America, 21*(4), 729–740.
2. Peterson, L. G. (1986). Acute response to trauma. In L. G. Peterson & G. J. O'Shanick (Eds.), Psychiatric aspects of trauma. *Advances in Psychosomatic Medicine, 16,* 84–92.
3. Brown, J. T. (1986). Grief responses in trauma patients and their families. In L. G. Peterson & G. J. O'Shanick (Eds.), Psychiatric aspects of trauma. *Advances in Psychosomatic Medicine, 16,* 93–114.
4. Aguilera, D. C., & Messick, J. M. (1986). *Crisis intervention: Theory & methodology* (5th ed.). St. Louis: C. V. Mosby Co.
5. Lewis, S., Grainger, R. D. K., McDowell, W. A., Gregory, R. J., & Messner, R. L. (Eds.). (1989). *Manual of psychosocial nursing interventions: Promoting mental health in medical-surgical settings.* Philadelphia: W. B. Saunders Co.

Suggested Readings

Alspach, J. G. (Ed.). (1991). *Core curriculum for critical care nursing.* (4th ed.) Philadelphia: W. B. Saunders Co.

Braverman, M. (1980). Onset of psychotraumatic reactions. *Journal of Forensic Sciences, 25*(4), 821–825.

Craig, M., Copes, W., & Champion, H. (1988). Psychosocial considerations in trauma care. *Critical Care Quarterly, 11*(2), 51–58.

DiMaria, R. A. (1989). Posttrauma responses: Potential for nursing. *Journal of Advanced Medical Surgical Nursing,* 2(1), 41–48.

Folstein, M. F., Folstein, S. E., & McHugh, P. R. (1975). Mini-mental state: A practical method for grading the cognitive state of patients for the clinician. *Journal of Psychiatric Research, 12*(3), 189–198.

Fontaine, D. K. (1989). Physical, personal, and cognitive responses to trauma. *Critical Care Nursing Clinics of North America, 1*(1), 11–22.

Fought, S. G., & Throwe, A. N. (1984). *Psychosocial nursing care of the emergency patient.* New York: John Wiley & Sons.

Kleenan, K. M. (1989). Families in crisis due to multiple trauma. *Critical Care Nursing Clinics of North America, 1*(1), 23–31.

Kubler-Ross, E. (1982). *Living with death and dying.* New York: Macmillan.

Lilliston, B. A. (1985). Psychosocial responses to traumatic physical disability. *Social Work in Health Care, 10*(4), 1–13.

Mattsson, E. I. (1975). Psychological aspects of severe physical injury and its treatment. *The Journal of Trauma, 15*(3), 217–234.

McLean, A., Jr., Dikmen, S., Temkin, N., Wyler, A., & Gale, J. (1984). Psychosocial functioning at one month after head injury. *Neurosurgery, 14*(4), 393–399.

Modlin, H. (1983). Traumatic neurosis and other injuries. *Psychiatric Clinics of North America, 6*(4), 661–681.

Solursh, D. S. (1990). The family of the trauma victim. *Nursing Clinics of North America, 25*(1), 155–162.

Strange, J. (Ed.). (1987). *Shock trauma care plans.* Springhouse, PA: Springhouse Corp.

Whitsell, L. A., Patterson, C. M., Young, D. H., & Schiller, W. R. (1989). Preinjury psychopathology in trauma patients. *The Journal of Trauma, 29*(8), 1158–1162.

Section III
Comprehensive Topics in Trauma Nursing

MODULE 16
MEDICAL SEQUELAE OF TRAUMA

Nancy Bucher, MSN, RN, CCRN
Mary Jean Osborne, MSN, RN, CCRN

Prerequisite

Review anatomy and physiology of body systems and physical assessment techniques.

Objectives

1.0 **Identify and briefly discuss the pathophysiology and treatment goals for trauma patients who develop pressure sores, atelectasis, pneumonia, contractures, muscle atrophy, pulmonary or fat emboli, sepsis, adult respiratory distress syndrome (ARDS), acute renal failure (ARF), disseminated intravascular coagulation (DIC), and gastrointestinal, liver, or cardiac failure following injury.**

1.1 List specific trauma-related etiologic factors that precipitate these medical problems.

1.2 Identify significant elements in the past medical history, resuscitation phase, and physical assessment of a trauma patient which place the individual at risk for the development of medical sequelae of trauma.

1.3 List laboratory and radiologic studies required for a definitive medical diagnosis of major medical problems associated with trauma.

1.4 List specific medical interventions used to treat common sequelae of trauma.

2.0 Given specific patient data, identify pertinent medical and nursing activities that might prevent the medical problems that accompany trauma.

3.0 Using the nursing process, develop a plan of nursing care for patients who manifest medical sequelae of trauma.

3.1 Develop nursing diagnoses based on assessment data.

3.2 Anticipate and assist with medical interventions for the patient with various medical sequelae of trauma.

3.3 Identify expected patient outcomes and appropriate nursing interventions for patients with medical problems related to trauma.

4.0 Identify those injuries and their concomitant physiologic responses that predispose individuals to the hazards of immobilization.

4.1 List the major hazards of immobilization.

4.2 Briefly describe physiologic and pathologic responses to long-term immobility in the trauma patient.

5.0 Identify patients at risk for development of multiple systems organ failure (MSOF).

5.1 Describe events during resuscitation of the trauma patient which indicate potential for MSOF.

5.2 Identify injuries that, alone or in combination, predispose the patient to MSOF.

A. HAZARDS OF IMMOBILITY

1. Pressure sores (also see Module 26—Integumentary System—and Module 13—Wound Healing)

a. Defined as skin ulceration that occurs from sustained compression to soft tissues, and resultant obliteration of arteriolar and capillary blood flow

b. Precursors—medical or surgical conditions resulting in long periods of immobilization and/or direct skin tissue damage; those directly related to trauma include
   (1) Shock, inadequate tissue perfusion
   (2) Direct tissue trauma
   (3) Fractures of the long bones; compound, pelvic, hip, and vertebral fractures
   (4) Spinal cord injury
   (5) Vascular injury
   (6) Head trauma
   (7) Burns
   (8) Injuries requiring prolonged bed rest or other limitations of movement

c. Preventive interventions
   (1) Early aggressive treatment of shock
   (2) Prevention of tissue hypoxemia
   (3) Early immobilization of fractures to allow ambulation
      (a) Use of external fixation devices
      (b) Open reduction and internal fixation
      (c) Use of casts, cast braces, or other types of braces and assistive devices

(4) Early use of kinetic treatment table, e.g., rotating bed, for patients with spinal cord injuries, vertebral fractures, or unstable pelvic fractures
(5) Expedient surgical repair of vascular injuries
(6) Frequent turning, repositioning, ambulation
(7) When early mobilization is contraindicated, the use of special beds is advocated, e.g., air-fluidized or oscillating low air loss
(8) Early nutritional assessment and intervention

d. Assessment
 (1) Interview
  (a) Report of sore areas or areas where pressure is felt
  (b) Past medical history including allergies, particularly skin allergies, skin problems, peripheral vascular disease, diabetes mellitus, nutritional habits, and previous wound healing
 (2) Physical examination
  (a) Inspect sacrum, buttocks, hips, knees, heels, dorsal aspect of feet, ears, and occipital area of head; inspect for redness, edema, taut shiny skin, and signs of vascular compromise, including pain, pallor, poor capillary refill, diminished pulses
  (b) Note open wounds, lacerations, ecchymoses, shearing effects
  (c) Check for pressure secondary to tight casts, dressings, traction, braces
  (d) Overall appearance—cachexia, obesity, condition of nails and mucous membranes, texture of hair, presence of rashes, skin turgor

e. Classification—four-point scale (1)
 (1) Grade I—erythema, induration, and ulceration to the epidermis
 (2) Grade II—ischemic area extending to the fat layer
 (3) Grade III—ischemic area extending through the fat layer, including dermis, muscle, joint involvement
 (4) Grade IV—sore extends to bone and joint structures involving all tissue

f. Nursing diagnoses, expected outcomes, and interventions
 (1) Impaired skin integrity, actual or potential, related to direct tissue trauma, vascular trauma or compromise, and/or nutritional deficit
  (a) Expected outcomes—skin is intact; wounds heal adequately
  (b) Nursing interventions
   i) Obtain and document a complete baseline skin assessment; reassess every eight hours
   ii) Document size, location, and description of wounds
   iii) Examine all bony prominences at least every four hours
   iv) Perform peripheral neurovascular check every four hours
   v) Turn and reposition patient every two hours; when frequency of turning and repositioning is limited, obtain air-fluidized, Roto-Rest, or water bed, heel and elbow protectors, sheepskin
   vi) Keep skin clean and dry; use mild soap; bag draining wounds; lubricate prominences
   vii) Secure dressings with paper tape or use nonadhesive method; remove tape gently
   viii) Use smooth plastic transfer board to prevent shearing force when moving patient from bed to stretcher or chair
   ix) Monitor casts and dressings for tightness and pressure areas; notify physician if necessary; have cast cutter available

x) Cover and pad sharp edges on casts; reinsert cast windows, and wrap with Kling or elastic bandage to prevent edema and breakdown around window edge
xi) Place protective covers on external fixator pin ends
xii) Keep heels off bed, especially if casts or traction are present; inspect dorsum and heel of foot, if Buck's boot is used
xiii) Keep straps on abductor pillows loose and nonconstrictive
xiv) Instruct patient with hip and extremity fractures to relieve pressure on sacrum frequently
xv) Assist with early ambulation

(2) Potential for infection related to loss of skin integrity and wound contamination
(a) Expected outcomes
i) No signs or symptoms of local infection
ii) Afebrile
iii) Normal WBC
iv) Negative wound cultures
(b) Nursing interventions (see Module 12—Infection)

(3) Nutritional deficits, actual or potential, related to increased metabolic requirements secondary to loss of tissue proteins and wound healing
(a) Expected outcomes
i) Minimal weight loss
ii) Normal serum albumin
iii) Normal wound healing
(b) Nursing interventions (see Module 11—Nutrition)

(4) Alteration in comfort—pain related to presence of open wound, pressure sore, and/or wound care
(a) Expected outcomes—patient indicates absence of or minimal pain through verbal and nonverbal expressions
(b) Nursing interventions (see Module 14—Pain)

2. Atelectasis and pneumonia

a. Atelectasis is characterized by airless lung tissue secondary to occluded air passages
b. Pneumonia implies inflammation of the alveolar spaces due to infection
c. Precursors related to trauma are frequently related to pain and other factors that inhibit deep breathing, adequate coughing, and turning
(1) Cardiothoracic trauma—blunt, penetrating, fractured ribs, flail chest, pulmonary contusions
(2) Intrapulmonary hematomas
(3) Pneumothorax, hemothorax
(4) Abdominal trauma
(5) Head trauma
(6) Spinal cord trauma
(7) Musculoskeletal trauma
(8) Inhalation injury
(9) Aspiration of blood, gastric contents
d. Assessment
(1) Interview

(a) Subjective problems—dyspnea, pleuritic pain, anxiety
(b) Past medical history—allergies, smoking habits, pulmonary illness
(2) Physical examination
(a) Inspect chest for movement, symmetry, respiratory rate and rhythm, use of accessory muscles for breathing
(b) Note color of lips, conjunctivae, extremities
(c) Observe for restlessness
(d) Note color and consistency of sputum
(e) Palpate for respiratory excursion, areas of tenderness, tactile fremitus
(f) Percuss—dullness vs resonance and level of diaphragm; high level suggests possible atelectasis or pneumonia
(g) Auscultate for diminished breath and adventitious sounds, vocal fremitus, pleural friction rub, tachycardia

e. Diagnostic indicators
(1) High index of suspicion related to type of injury, long-term mechanical ventilation, and long periods of immobility
(2) Diminished breath sounds, crackles
(3) Deteriorating ABGs
(4) Elevated temperature
(5) Positive chest x-ray
(6) Elevated WBC
(7) Positive sputum culture
(8) Hypoxemia refractory to high levels of inspired oxygen
(9) Respiratory alkalosis secondary to hyperventilation
(10) Hypercapnia—late sign
(11) Increased peak inspiratory pressure
(12) Respiratory compliance less than 50 ml/cm H_2O
(13) Decreased functional residual capacity (FRC)
(14) Increased alveolar-arterial (A-a) gradient

f. Nursing diagnoses, expected outcomes, and interventions
(1) Potential for alteration in gas exchange secondary to reduced surface area for oxygen and carbon dioxide diffusion
(a) Expected outcomes
i) Clear breath sounds and chest x-ray
ii) Normal rate and quality of respirations
iii) Normal ABGs, compliance, FRC, A-a gradient, temperature, and WBC
(b) Nursing interventions
i) Assess respiratory status frequently
ii) Maintain patent airway; assist with intubation if needed
iii) Administer high flow humidified oxygen
iv) Mechanically ventilate if needed; deliver periodic volumes (sighs) greater than tidal volume
v) Monitor arterial oxygen saturation (SaO_2) with pulse oximeter; monitor ABGs
vi) Encourage coughing and deep breathing; suction as needed to remove secretions
vii) Elevate head of bed; turn or reposition every two hours
viii) Chest physiotherapy

ix) Keep well-hydrated
x) Administer bronchodilators as prescribed; provide nebulizer treatments

(2) Knowledge deficit regarding prevention of posttrauma atelectasis or pneumonia
(a) Expected outcomes—patient will demonstrate knowledge and self-care related to prevention of atelectasis and pneumonia
(b) Nursing interventions
i) Teach patient to cough and deep breathe, splinting chest and abdominal incisions
ii) Teach patient to change positions frequently, and assist patient to sit and ambulate
iii) Teach and encourage use of incentive spirometry

3. Muscle atrophy and contractures

a. Muscle atrophy is characterized by reduction in size and degeneration of a muscle or muscle group
b. Contractures are caused by shortening of muscle fibers and commonly decrease joint range of motion
c. Precursors—immobility secondary to any type of traumatic injury; the highest incidence occurs with
(1) Head injury
(2) Spinal cord trauma
(3) Musculoskeletal trauma
(4) Burns
(5) Amputations
d. Assessment
(1) Interview
(a) Subjective problems including muscle weakness and impaired body image
(b) Past medical history—related neurological or musculoskeletal illness
(2) Physical examination
(a) Look for obvious deformities
(b) Observe for limb shortening or decreased muscle mass
(c) Note muscle weakness and loss of function
(d) Compare range of joint motion (ROM) to normal range
(e) Note pressure areas, edema, discoloration
(f) Perform neurovascular assessment (see Module 24—Musculoskeletal Injury)
e. Nursing diagnoses, expected outcomes, and interventions
(1) Potential for impaired mobility secondary to muscle atrophy or contractures
(a) Expected outcomes—patient maintains muscle mass and optimal function of all joint areas
(b) Nursing interventions
i) Do ROM for all extremities every four hours; include hips and shoulders
ii) Teach patient and family to do ROM
iii) Apply splints to patients with spasticity and/or decreased level of consciousness
iv) Consult physical and occupational therapists

(2) Self-care deficit related to limited motion from joint contractures and/or weakness from muscle atrophy
  (a) Expected outcome—patient accomplishes activities of daily living
  (b) Nursing interventions
    i) Initially assist patient with activities of daily living; gradually increase patient involvement
    ii) Provide and teach use of self-help devices
    iii) Encourage independence and reinforce mastery of self-care
(3) Impaired self-concept related to physical and functional changes in body image
  (a) Expected outcome—patient verbalizes concerns regarding changes in body image and adapts to these changes
  (b) Nursing interventions
    i) Encourage patient to verbalize feelings regarding changes in body appearance and function
    ii) Bolster self-esteem and confidence by pointing out patient's strengths and abilities
    iii) Encourage active participation in physical therapy, nutrient consumption, and decisionmaking

B. PULMONARY EMBOLI

1. Defined as venous thrombi or clots that occlude the pulmonary vasculature
2. Precursors—predispose person to Virchow's triad (stasis of blood, coagulation abnormalities, and vessel wall damage); those directly related to trauma include
a. Shock, inadequate tissue perfusion
b. Fractures of pelvis or lower extremities
c. Multisystem trauma
d. Vascular, spinal cord, or head trauma
e. Prolonged immobilization
3. Preventive interventions
a. Restore normotensive state and adequate circulating volume as soon as possible
b. Mobilize as soon as possible
c. If unable to mobilize
  (1) Implement elastic stockings or pneumatic sequential compression device
  (2) Elevate extremities to promote venous return
  (3) Teach leg exercises
  (4) Anticoagulate, if not contraindicated
4. Assessment
a. Interview
  (1) Subjective problems including dyspnea, calf or leg tenderness, chest pain, anxiety
  (2) Past medical history—allergies, smoking habits, medications, e.g., birth control pills, related illness, e.g., phlebitis
b. Physical examination

(1) Inspect color of skin, lips, conjunctivae, and extremities; skin turgor; swelling or redness of extremity; chest movement; respiratory rate and rhythm; restlessness; level of consciousness
(2) Palpate for respiratory excursion, warmth of extremity, pain of extremity on dorsiflexion, and neck vein engorgement
(3) Percuss to evaluate aeration of all lung fields and level of diaphragm
(4) Auscultate breath sounds, adventitious sounds, vocal fremitus, apical heart rate and rhythm, and pleural friction rub

5. Diagnostic indicators

a. High index of suspicion related to precipitating factors
b. Acute onset of shortness of breath, pleuritic chest pain
c. Hypoxia, hypocarbia
d. Respiratory alkalosis secondary to hyperventilation
e. Increased A-a gradient
f. Increased temperature and WBC
g. Nonspecific changes on chest x-ray
h. Nonspecific changes on ECG; possible ischemia
i. Ventilation/perfusion (V_A/Q) scan may reveal normal ventilation and decreased or absent perfusion; not definitive
j. Pulmonary angiogram confirms diagnosis of PE; defines areas of decreased perfusion
k. Decreased blood pressure and increased pulmonary artery pressure

6. Nursing diagnoses, expected outcomes, and interventions

a. Anxiety related to sudden onset of dyspnea and chest pain
  (1) Expected outcomes—verbal and nonverbal indications of decreased anxiety
  (2) Nursing interventions
    (a) Assess level of anxiety
    (b) Stay with and reassure patient
    (c) Explain procedures
    (d) Encourage verbalization of fears
    (e) Sedate if needed
b. Alteration in tissue perfusion related to deep vein thrombosis and/or thromboembolism
  (1) Expected outcomes—improved perfusion of affected tissues without bleeding
  (2) Nursing interventions
    (a) Assess extremities frequently for edema, warmth, local erythema, measured circumference, Homans' sign (pain on dorsiflexion)
    (b) Monitor temperature and WBC
    (c) Prepare patient for venogram, ultrasound, or impedance plethysmography
    (d) Administer anticoagulants as prescribed
      i) Monitor partial thromboplastin time if heparin is used
      ii) Monitor prothrombin time if Coumadin is used
    (e) Continue elastic antiembolic stockings
    (f) Discontinue sequential compression device if thromboembolism occurs
    (g) Monitor for signs of bleeding
    (h) Keep protamine or vitamin K available
    (i) Avoid intramuscular injections
    (j) Maintain bed rest; avoid use of pillows or knee gatch

(k) Instruct patient not to cross or massage legs

c. Alteration in gas exchange related to pulmonary vessel occlusion
   (1) Expected outcomes—improved gas exchange as evidenced by absence of signs or symptoms of hypoxia; improved PaO_2 relative to FiO_2; decreased A-a gradient; normal serum pH
   (2) Nursing interventions
      (a) Prepare patient for vena cava umbrella or Greenfield filter insertion
      (b) Assess respiratory status every two to four hours
      (c) Administer oxygen as prescribed
      (d) Assist with intubation, if needed
      (e) Mechanically ventilate, if needed
      (f) Obtain and monitor ABGs; insert arterial line if monitoring ABGs frequently
      (g) Administer thrombolytic agents as prescribed; monitor coagulation profile and signs of bleeding
      (h) Elevate head of bed; reposition patient frequently
      (i) Encourage coughing and deep breathing
      (j) Provide adequate fluid intake
      (k) Monitor oxygen saturation with pulse oximeter
      (l) Monitor pulmonary artery pressures for signs of right ventricular failure
d. Alteration in comfort—pain related to pulmonary vascular occlusion
   (1) Expected outcome—patient will verbalize relief of pain
   (2) Nursing interventions
      (a) Assess cardiovascular status every one to two hours
      (b) Assess patient for pleuritic-type pain
      (c) Administer morphine or other prescribed analgesics
      (d) Position patient for comfort

C. FAT EMBOLUS

1. **Defined as an occlusion of the pulmonary vessels from a fat globule; usually occurs subsequent to long bone trauma, but may follow other injuries**
2. **Onset usually 24 to 48 hrs postinjury; earlier than pulmonary embolus**
3. **Precursors**

a. Long bone fractures
b. Multiple fractures
c. Multisystem trauma
d. Massive soft tissue injuries
e. Crush injury
f. Burns

4. **Preventive interventions**

a. Gentle handling and early immobilization of fractures and soft tissue injuries
b. Early open reduction and internal fixation of fractures

5. **Assessment**

a. Interview for symptoms including dyspnea, anxiety, and chest pain

b. Physical examination
  (1) Inspection
    (a) Color of skin, lips, conjunctivae, and extremities
    (b) Presence of petechiae on chest, axilla, oral mucosa, and flank
    (c) Urine for presence of fat globules
    (d) Chest movement, respiratory rate and rhythm
    (e) Cough, description of sputum
    (f) Mental status, confusion, restlessness, altered level of consciousness
  (2) Palpation for respiratory excursion and tactile fremitus
  (3) Percussion to evaluate aeration of lung fields and level of diaphragm
  (4) Auscultation of breath sounds, adventitious sounds, vocal fremitus, and apical heart rate and rhythm

6. Diagnostic indicators

a. High index of suspicion related to usual precursors
b. Acute onset of shortness of breath, diaphoresis, tachycardia
c. PaO_2 less than 60 mm Hg
d. Elevated WBC and temperature
e. Decreased platelet count
f. Elevated lipase, free fatty acids, and fibrin-split products
g. Urine or sputum analysis reveals fat globules
h. Chest x-ray demonstrates fluffy infiltrates
i. Nonspecific changes on ECG
j. Possible decreased hemoglobin and hematocrit

7. Nursing diagnoses, expected outcomes, and interventions

a. Anxiety related to sudden onset of dyspnea; family anxiety related to changes in patient's mentation or decreasing level of consciousness
  (1) Expected outcomes—patient and family will verbalize or display a decreased level of anxiety
  (2) Nursing interventions
    (a) Assess level of patient and family anxiety
    (b) Stay with and reassure patient
    (c) Explain all procedures and changes in patient condition to patient and family
    (d) Encourage verbalization of fears
    (e) Sedate as needed
b. Potential for alteration in gas exchange related to occlusion of pulmonary vessels
  (1) Expected outcomes—adequate gas exchange evidenced by PaO_2 greater than 80 mm Hg, normal respiratory rate and A-a gradient
  (2) Nursing interventions
    (a) Prevention and early detection are most important
      i) Handle all fractures and soft tissue injuries gently; maintain traction when repositioning
      ii) Identify patients at risk for fat emboli, and monitor neurological and respiratory status every one to two hours
    (b) Check temperature every four hours
    (c) Monitor urine and sputum for fat globules
    (d) Inspect skin for petechiae
    (e) Utilize pulse oximetry

c. Actual alteration in gas exchange related to occlusion of pulmonary vessels
   (1) Expected outcomes—adequate gas exchange as evidenced by
      (a) Arterial blood pH 7.35 to 7.45
      (b) PCO_2 less than 45 mm Hg; PO_2 greater than 80 mm Hg
      (c) Oxygen saturation more than 95%
   (2) Nursing interventions
      (a) Administer high flow humidified oxygen
      (b) Monitor ABGs and oxygen saturation via pulse oximetry
      (c) Anticipate need for intubation and mechanical ventilation; provide as needed
      (d) Administer medications as ordered, e.g., heparin, steroids, 5% alcohol, low molecular weight dextran

D. SEPSIS

1. **Defined as an acute systemic response to bacterial invasion which often results in septic shock (2)**
2. **Frequently a cause of late trauma deaths, several weeks after injury**
3. **Often related to adult respiratory distress syndrome, acute renal failure, and failure of other, often multiple, organs**
4. **Characterized by a syndrome of continuing phagocytosis in the presence of protein malnutrition (3), impaired lymphocyte function, regional tissue malperfusion and ischemia, and the generation of various endogenous mediators that cause proteolysis and increase hypermetabolism**
5. **Mechanisms implicated in the pathogenesis of sepsis (2)**
a. Mechanical obstruction of the microvasculature by cellular elements of blood
b. Regional vasoconstriction despite dilation of peripheral vessels
c. Activation of complex biochemical cascades, e.g., complement, clotting, resulting in release of mediators
d. Altered oxidative metabolism at the cellular level (4)
6. **Myocardial depression and pump failure contribute to mortality**
7. **For related medical and nursing interventions, see Module 10—Shock (septic)—and Module 12—Infection)**

E. ADULT RESPIRATORY DISTRESS SYNDROME (ARDS)

1. **Characterized by damage to the alveolar-capillary unit and increased pulmonary microvascular permeability, resulting in severe alteration in gas exchange and decreased lung compliance**
2. **Also known as shock lung, Da Nang lung, stiff lung, and traumatic wet lung**
3. **Pathophysiology**

a. Stage I—period of initial injury, characterized by initial lactic acidosis, spontaneous hyperventilation, leading to hypocarbia and mixed metabolic and respiratory alkalosis
b. Stage II—hemodynamic stability, continued persistent hyperventilation, and deteriorating arterial blood gases
c. Stage III—progressive pulmonary insufficiency, requiring ventilatory intervention and administration of 100% oxygen
d. Stage IV—terminal hypoxemia leading to coma, bradydysrhythmias, and death

4. Precursors—any medical or surgical condition resulting in lung injury may precipitate ARDS, often within 48 hrs of injury; those directly related to trauma include

a. Shock, inadequate tissue perfusion
b. Thoracic and nonthoracic trauma
c. Pulmonary contusions
d. Massive blood transfusions
e. Microemboli from tissue trauma or transfusion; disseminated intravascular coagulation
f. Fracture of long bones
g. Thromboembolism
h. Fat emboli
i. Smoke inhalation
j. Noxious gas inhalation
k. Oxygen toxicity
l. Aspiration of gastric contents
m. Near-drowning, fresh or salt water
n. Overhydration
o. Nosocomial infections, pneumonia, and sepsis are often associated with later (5 to 21 days postinjury) manifestations of ARDS

5. Preventive interventions

a. Treat shock early and aggressively
b. Prevent hypoxemia; administer 100% oxygen
c. If ventilatory effort inadequate, intubate and mechanically ventilate
d. Give fresh, warmed, filtered blood, when possible, to avoid the introduction of particulate matter procoagulants
e. Immobilize fractures early
f. Monitor carboxyhemoglobin levels in inhalation injury patients
g. Decompress stomach and prevent aspiration
h. Initiate thromboembolic prophylaxis

6. Assessment

a. Interview
   (1) Specifics of resuscitation
   (2) Subjective problems—dyspnea, anxiety
   (3) Past medical history—allergies, smoking habits, pulmonary illness
   (4) Occupation
b. Physical examination
   (1) Inspect for chest movement; respiratory rate and rhythm; color of lips, conjunctivae, and extremities; use of accessory muscles for breathing; restlessness

(2) Palpate for respiratory excursion, tenderness, tactile fremitus
(3) Percussion—dullness vs resonance; level of diaphragm
(4) Auscultate breath sounds, adventitious sounds, vocal fremitus, pleural friction rub, apical heart rate and rhythm

c. Physical findings
(1) Tachypnea and tachycardia
(2) Breath sounds—no characteristic findings, but may be tubular; rales unusual in absence of cardiac component

7. **Diagnostic indicators**

a. High index of suspicion related to precipitating factors
b. Hypoxemia refractory to high levels of inspired oxygen (PaO_2 less than 60 mm Hg on FiO_2 greater than or equal to 50%)
c. Respiratory alkalosis secondary to hyperventilation
d. Hypercapnia (late sign)
e. Diffuse interstitial and alveolar infiltrates on chest x-ray; extreme shows "white out"
f. Increased peak inspiratory pressures
g. Respiratory compliance less than 50 ml/cm H_2O
h. Decreased functional residual capacity (FRC)
i. Increased right to left shunt (Q_S/Q_T greater than 20% of cardiac output)
j. Increased deadspace ventilation (V_D/V_T)
k. Increased A-a gradient
l. Increased ventilation perfusion mismatch
m. Low to normal pulmonary capillary wedge pressure (PCWP)

8. **Medical interventions**

a. Insert endotracheal tube for
(1) Subjective respiratory distress
(2) Tachypnea
(3) Vital capacity less than 12 to 15 cc/Kg
(4) PaO_2/FiO_2 ratio—250 to 300
(5) A-a gradient greater than 300 to 350 mm Hg
(6) Q_S/Q_T greater than 15 to 20%

b. Correct hypoxemia
(1) Administer lowest possible oxygen concentration to achieve adequate oxygenation
(2) Continuous positive airway pressure (CPAP)
(3) Mechanically ventilate
(4) Positive end expiratory pressure (PEEP)

c. Insert arterial line to monitor blood pressure and obtain blood gases
d. Insert pulmonary artery catheter to monitor fluid status, obtain cardiac outputs and mixed venous oxygen saturation, and calculate shunt fraction
e. Prescribe antibiotics for documented infection

9. **Nursing diagnoses, expected outcomes, and interventions**

a. Anxiety related to dyspnea and fear of death
(1) Expected outcomes—patient verbalizes decreased anxiety and fear of death
(2) Nursing interventions
(a) Assess level of anxiety
(b) Stay with and reassure patient

(c) Explain all procedures
(d) Encourage verbalization of fear
(e) Minimize activity level and provide sedation as required
(f) Provide supplemental oxygen

b. Impaired gas exchange related to injury to the alveolar-capillary interface, and interstitial edema in lung parenchyma
(1) Expected outcomes
(a) Pulmonary function within normal limits
(b) Respiratory rate within normal limits
(c) Absence of subjective dyspnea
(d) Improved PaO_2 relative to FiO_2, e.g., PaO_2 greater than or equal to 80 mm Hg on FiO_2 less than 50%
(e) Increased FRC and compliance
(f) Decreased shunting, A-a gradient, and V_D/V_T
(g) Mixed venous oxygen saturation between 60 and 80%
(h) Arterial oxygen saturation greater than 95%
(i) Clear breath sounds and chest x-ray
(2) Nursing interventions
(a) Assess respiratory status frequently; auscultate breath sounds
(b) Maintain patent airway; suction p.r.n.
(c) Administer high flow humidified oxygen
(d) Assist with intubation, if needed
(e) Mechanically ventilate, if needed
(f) Administer paralyzing agents as prescribed
(g) Maintain PEEP as prescribed
(h) Suction p.r.n. using Ambu bag with PEEP valve
(i) Obtain ABGs per protocol; pay strict attention to oxygen saturation, which should be greater than 95%
(j) Monitor oxygen saturation with pulse oximeter or oximetry
(k) Monitor trends in mixed venous oxygen saturation
(l) Elevate head of bed; reposition patient frequently; evaluate response to turning to injured side
(m) Encourage deep breathing and coughing; provide chest physiotherapy
(n) Place in kinetic therapy bed to allow for continuous turning
(o) Monitor cardiac rhythm; observe for tachycardia and dysrhythmias
(p) Monitor pulmonary artery and capillary wedge pressure (PAP and PCWP); maintain arterial lines
(q) Administer steroids as prescribed
(r) Monitor and maintain fluid balance; avoid overload

c. Potential for decreased cardiac output secondary to increased pulmonary vascular resistance and high levels of PEEP
(1) Expected outcomes
(a) Cardiac output within normal limits
(b) Normal PCWP
(c) Normal sinus rhythm
(2) Nursing interventions
(a) Assess for signs and symptoms of pneumothorax and barotrauma related to increased levels of PEEP

(b) Measure cardiac output, cardiac index, and systemic vascular resistance every four hours
(c) Administer vasoactive medications as prescribed

F. ACUTE RENAL FAILURE

1. **Defined as an acute deterioration in renal function related to varying etiologies; classified as prerenal, intrarenal, or postrenal**
2. **Precursors**
a. Prerenal—diminished blood volume to renal structures causing hypoperfusion of the kidney and protracted renal ischemia
   (1) Hypovolemia due to hemorrhage or third spacing of fluids as in burns, spinal shock, sepsis
   (2) Cardiovascular dysfunction, e.g., myocardial infarction, tamponade
   (3) Vascular trauma involving interruption or transection of the aorta, renal artery, or other major blood vessel
   (4) Renal vascular thrombosis
   (5) Intracardiac trauma, with prolonged cross-clamping of the aorta during open thoracotomy or operative procedures for vascular trauma
   (6) Intraabdominal or retroperitoneal hemorrhage
   (7) Administration of potent vasopressors
b. Renal—intrarenal factors related to direct parenchymal injury or acute tubular necrosis (ATN)
   (1) Ischemia of the kidney from a low flow state
   (2) Direct renal trauma
   (3) Rhabdomyolysis, e.g., crush or deep burn injury producing myoglobinuria
   (4) Hemolytic transfusion reactions
   (5) Nephrotoxic antibiotics or radiographic contrast media
   (6) Disseminated intravascular coagulation
c. Postrenal—related to structural interruption of the urinary collecting system
   (1) Direct trauma to upper urinary tract
   (2) Bladder rupture
   (3) Obstruction of lower urinary tract, e.g., urethral transection, neurogenic bladder, prostatic hypertrophy, urinary catheter blockage
   (4) Ureteral compression from retroperitoneal hematoma
3. **Preventive interventions**
a. Restore normotensive state and adequate circulating volume as soon as possible after injury
b. Promptly restore vascular integrity
c. Minimize aortic cross-clamping time
d. Use vasopressors judiciously
e. Provide prompt surgical repair of visceral trauma and genitourinary structures
f. Promptly diagnose myoglobinuria and treat early; increase fluid intake and administer osmotic diuretics, if prescribed
g. Handle traumatized tissue gently; immobilize and fix fractures early
h. Check blood products carefully; type and cross-match when time permits; use type-specific and/or universal donor when necessary

i. Monitor peak and trough levels of nephrotoxic antibiotics
j. Hydrate adequately before and after radiographic dye studies
k. Prevent disseminated intravascular coagulation (see next section of this module)

4. **Assessment**

a. Interview
  (1) Specifics of resuscitation
    (a) Inadequate volume resuscitation
    (b) Use of I.V. contrast material
  (2) Presence of injuries that cause release of myoglobin, e.g., tissue trauma, massive muscle damage, crush injury, multiple fractures with associated soft tissue injury
  (3) Presence of bladder and genitourinary trauma
  (4) Subjective symptoms, including headache, anorexia, tachypnea, nausea, anxiety, weakness, drowsiness, insomnia, flank pain, pruritus, ammonia taste in mouth
  (5) Past medical history
    (a) Current medications, e.g., diuretics, antihypertensives, antibiotics, cardiac
    (b) History of related illness, e.g., chronic renal disease, urinary tract or kidney infections, enlarged prostate gland, hypertension, renal insufficiency, diabetes, lupus, previous nephrectomy, kidney or urologic surgery, cardiac or vascular disease
    (c) Current or past substance abuse
    (d) Recent exposure to radiographic dye
    (e) Recent radiation therapy

b. Physical examination
  (1) Inspection
    (a) Color of skin, lips, conjunctivae, and extremities
    (b) Skin turgor, condition of mucous membranes
    (c) Edema of hands, feet, legs, sacrum, and periorbita
    (d) Uremic frost
    (e) Changes in mentation, level of consciousness, restlessness
    (f) Muscle twitching, hyporeflexia, hiccups
    (g) Color and amount of urine; amounts less than or equal to 400 cc in 24 hrs may indicate renal failure
    (h) Dyspnea, Kussmaul's respirations
  (2) Palpation
    (a) Amount and location of edema
    (b) Pain, especially in flank area
    (c) Pulse, rhythm, rate, quality
  (3) Percussion—evaluate lung fields; note areas of tenderness
  (4) Auscultation
    (a) Presence of S_3, S_4
    (b) Presence of pericardial friction rub
    (c) Rhonchi, moist crackles
    (d) Blood pressure

5. **Diagnostic indicators**

a. High index of suspicion related to pre-, intra-, and postrenal precipitating factors
b. Acute onset of oliguria, less than 400 cc per 24 hrs

c. Central nervous system disturbances—lethargy, confusion, stupor, muscle twitching, weakness
d. Pulmonary symptomatology—Kussmaul's breathing, uremic breath odor
e. Cardiovascular disturbances—hypertension, tachycardia, dysrhythmias, pericarditis
f. Integumentary manifestations—dry skin, poor skin turgor, pruritis, uremic frost
g. Gastrointestinal changes—anorexia, nausea, vomiting, diarrhea
h. Hematological findings—ecchymosis, anemia, coagulopathies
i. Increased susceptibility to local and systemic infection; elevated WBC
j. Inadequate response to diuretics and fluids
k. Pulmonary artery pressures confirm absence of hypovolemia or cardiac etiology
l. Laboratory data
   (1) Elevated blood urea nitrogen (BUN) and serum creatinine
   (2) Elevated serum potassium, magnesium, and phosphate; decreased serum sodium and calcium
   (3) Decreased hemoglobin, hematocrit, and platelets
   (4) Increased serum renin levels
   (5) Urine specific gravity greater than 1.020, prerenal; varies with intra- and postrenal
   (6) Elevated urine osmolality, prerenal
   (7) Elevated urine sodium, renal; decreased urine sodium, prerenal
   (8) Urine positive for protein, tubular casts, epithelial cells, RBCs, WBCs, myoglobin
   (9) ABGs indicative of metabolic acidosis
m. Diagnostic studies
   (1) Intravenous pyelogram to rule out obstruction
   (2) Cystogram to rule out obstruction
   (3) X-ray of kidney, ureter, bladder (KUB)
   (4) Renal tomogram
   (5) CAT of abdomen
   (6) Renal ultrasound
   (7) Arteriogram
   (8) Renal scan
   (9) Renal biopsy

6. **Medical interventions**

a. Prescribe diuretics—may convert oliguric renal failure to nonoliguric type; can cause ototoxicity
   (1) Mannitol—osmotic diuretic
      (a) Decreases proximal tubular sodium reabsorption
      (b) Increases glomerular filtration rate, renin secretion, and washout of tubular casts
      (c) Dilates renal arterioles
      (d) Shrinks swollen glomerular capillary endothelial cells
   (2) Furosemide—inhibits active sodium and chloride transport in the ascending loop of Henle
   (3) Dopamine—to maximize renal blood flow
      (a) Use low dose, 3 to 5 mcg/kg/min
      (b) Increases renal vasodilation without systemic vascular effects; shifts flow from medulla to renal cortex

(4) Calculate fluid requirements and prescribe accordingly
(5) Limit sodium intake in diet and medications
(6) Monitor and treat hyperkalemia
(a) Kayexalate, per nasogastric tube or rectally, binds potassium
(b) Intravenous administration of glucose and insulin forces potassium into the cells, decreasing serum levels
(7) Prescribe aluminum-based antacids
(8) Initiate dialysis—continuous arteriovenous hemofiltration, peritoneal, or hemodialysis
(1) Decreases uremia
(2) Removes excess fluids
(3) Corrects acidosis, hyponatremia, and hyperkalemia
(4) Liberalizes fluid and electrolyte restrictions
(9) Calculate nutritional requirements to provide adequate carbohydrate and calories and promote positive nitrogen balance

7. **Nursing diagnoses, expected outcomes, and interventions**

a. Fluid volume excess, actual or potential, related to inadequate renal function
(1) Expected outcomes—normovolemia as evidenced by
(a) Normal vital signs and CVP
(b) Stable weight
(c) PCWP within normal limits
(d) Absence of peripheral edema
(2) Nursing interventions
(a) Weigh daily; observe for acute weight gain
(b) Monitor fluid intake and output hourly; measure urine specific gravity
(c) Administer fluids as prescribed
i) Administer large amounts of fluid in presence of myoglobinuria to prevent further tubular damage
ii) With loss of renal function, restrict fluids; replace insensible and measured fluid losses
(d) Administer diuretics, antihypertensive and cardiac medications as prescribed
(e) Monitor hemodynamic status, including blood pressure, central venous pressure, PAP, and PCWP
(f) Assess for tachycardia, presence of S_3 and S_4, and pericardial friction rub
(g) Restrict sodium intake in diet and medication
(h) Assess skin turgor, condition of mucous membranes, distended neck veins, peripheral, sacral, and periorbital edema
(i) Monitor results of urine and serum osmolality
(j) Assess breath sounds frequently; note moist crackles, dyspnea, frothy pink sputum
(k) Perform or assist with dialysis

b. Alteration in electrolyte balance related to impaired renal function
(1) Expected outcomes—serum and urine electrolytes within normal limits; absence of systemic signs of electrolyte imbalance
(2) Nursing interventions
(a) Observe for signs and symptoms of imbalances of major electrolytes, including potassium, calcium, phosphorus, sodium, and chloride

(b) Perform frequent neurological assessments
(c) Monitor results of serum electrolytes, blood urea nitrogen, and creatinine
(d) Follow dialysis protocols as prescribed

c. Alteration in cardiac output secondary to dysrhythmias produced by acid-base or electrolyte imbalance
  (1) Expected outcomes—normal cardiac rhythm and cardiac output
  (2) Nursing interventions
    (a) Review baseline ECG; obtain and review rhythm strip at least every eight hours, and more often if dysrhythmias noted; report to physician
    (b) Monitor cardiac rhythm continuously
    (c) Administer supplemental oxygen
    (d) Monitor for metabolic acidosis; ABGs every four hours
    (e) Administer sodium bicarbonate, if indicated
    (f) Monitor oxygen saturation with pulse oximeter
    (g) Monitor for signs and symptoms of electrolyte imbalance, especially potassium, sodium, calcium, phosphorus, and magnesium
    (h) Administer prescribed treatment for hyperkalemia—cation exchange resins (e.g., Kayexalate), calcium, sodium bicarbonate, or I.V. glucose and insulin
      i) Restrict all potassium intake from I.V.s and drugs
      ii) Avoid administration of banked blood, high in potassium, in favor of fresh blood
    (i) Restrict sodium intake with hypernatremia
    (j) Replace calcium as needed; administer vitamin D to enhance absorption
    (k) Administer antacid-phosphate binders to decrease hyperphosphatemia; avoid magnesium-based antacids

d. Impaired gas exchange related to volume overload and pulmonary edema
  (1) Expected outcomes—normal gas exchange as evidenced by
    (a) PaO_2 greater than 80 mm Hg and $PaCO_2$ 40 mm Hg or less
    (b) Oxygen saturation greater than 95%
  (2) Nursing interventions
    (a) Monitor respiratory status frequently; be alert for moist crackles, tachypnea, or dyspnea
    (b) Obtain ABGs as needed
    (c) Administer high flow humidified oxygen
    (d) Elevate head of bed
    (e) Monitor oxygen saturation with pulse oximetry
    (f) Monitor cardiac rhythm and status continuously
    (g) Observe for neck vein distension
    (h) Assess for elevated CVP, PAP, PCWP
    (i) Administer diuretics, cardiac glycosides, and morphine sulfate as prescribed
    (j) Maintain patent airway; assist with intubation and mechanical ventilation as needed
    (k) Follow protocols to reduce fluid load, including fluid restriction and dialysis

e. Alteration in nutrition related to uremic syndrome, abnormal gastrointestinal function, and hypermetabolism

(1) Expected outcomes—nutritional requirements will be met and positive nitrogen balance maintained
(2) Nursing interventions
(a) Administer prescribed nutritional regime to meet calorie and protein needs in uremic syndrome
(b) Administer antiemetic and antidiarrheal medications as needed (see Module 11—Nutrition—for detailed information)

f. Potential alteration in skin integrity due to pruritus, uremia, and negative nitrogen balance
(1) Expected outcomes—patient states relief of pruritus; skin remains intact
(2) Nursing interventions
(a) Assess skin frequently
(b) Turn and reposition every two hours; out of bed (OOB) if possible
(c) Massage bony prominences; relieve pressure
(d) Give frequent tepid baths to remove uremic frost
(e) Administer antipruritic medications as needed
(f) Encourage patient not to scratch skin, to keep fingernails short, and use hand mitts
(g) Utilize sheepskin, egg crate mattress, or air-fluidized bed when repositioning of patient is limited by specific injuries

g. Additional nursing diagnoses
(1) Potential for renal injury related to altered metabolism of medications, myoglobinuria, or use of contrast media
(2) Potential for injury related to uremic encephalopathy
(3) Altered thought processes related to uremic encephalopathy

G. DISSEMINATED INTRAVASCULAR COAGULATION (DIC)

1. **Defined as an acquired clotting factor deficiency that occurs secondary to another pathological process that releases tissue thromboplastin; this event accelerates normal clotting and subsequently decreases available clotting factors and platelets**
2. **Precursors—medical or surgical conditions that activate the clotting cascade by causing damage to the vascular endothelium or general destruction of tissue; those directly related to trauma include**

a. Shock, inadequate tissue perfusion
b. Multisystem trauma
c. Massive blood transfusion; mismatched transfusion
d. Liver or spleen trauma
e. Acute hemolysis due to infection and septicemia
f. Near-drowning
g. Open and closed chest trauma
h. Severe head injury
i. Burns
j. Massive soft tissue trauma
k. Septic abortion and other obstetric complications

l. Snake bites

3. **Preventive interventions**

a. Early aggressive treatment of shock
b. Give fresh, warmed, filtered blood for transfusion whenever possible

4. **Assessment**

a. Interview
   (1) Subjective complaints of nausea; pain in abdomen, back, muscles, joints; anxiety, headache, visual changes, numbness in lower extremities, orthopnea
   (2) Past medical history, including allergies, current medications, e.g., aspirin, Coumadin; presence of related illness, e.g., anemia, bleeding
b. Physical examination
   (1) Inspection
      (a) Overt bleeding at I.V. sites, orifices, incisional sites
      (b) Examine skin for ecchymosis, hematomas, petechiae, purpura, acrocyanosis
      (c) Note color, temperature, and turgor of skin
      (d) Check for hematuria, hemoptysis, gingivitis, epistaxis, hematemesis, hematochezia
      (e) Expanding abdominal girth from intraabdominal bleeding
      (f) Changes in mentation; restlessness
   (2) Palpation
      (a) Check for joint tenderness, edema
      (b) Check for liver, spleen, abdominal, or flank tenderness
      (c) Check for deep vein thrombosis (DVT) symptomatology
   (3) Percussion—do not percuss if DIC suspected
   (4) Auscultation—breath sounds and adventitious sounds; hypotension and tachycardia

5. **Diagnostic indicators**

a. High index of suspicion related to traumatic precipitating factors
b. Bleeding from single or multiple sites
c. Cool, mottled, cyanotic distal extremities
d. Decreased hemoglobin and hematocrit
e. Decreased platelet count and fibrinogen levels
f. Increased prothrombin, activated partial thromboplastin, plasma thrombin, and Lee-White (whole blood) clotting times
g. Increased fibrin-split products
h. Protamine sulfate test strongly positive
i. Clotting factor analysis to determine which factors are being consumed

6. **Medical interventions**

a. Treat underlying cause
b. Control bleeding
c. Normalize clotting factor levels through administration of blood products, including fresh frozen plasma, cryoprecipitate, and platelets
d. Cautiously administer intravenous heparin to slow intravascular coagulation
e. Treat underlying acidosis
f. Provide supplemental oxygen

7. **Nursing diagnoses, expected outcomes, and interventions**
a. Anxiety of patient and family, related to recurrent bleeding and inadequate knowledge of DIC
   (1) Expected outcomes—patient and family will manifest decreased levels of anxiety
   (2) Nursing interventions
      (a) Assess level of patient and family knowledge
      (b) Provide explanation of disease process and treatment
      (c) Encourage patient and family to verbalize fears and questions
b. Potential for hemorrhage related to inability to form a stable clot
   (1) Expected outcomes
      (a) Hemoglobin and hematocrit within normal range
      (b) Absence of bleeding
      (c) Normal coagulation profile
      (d) Normal vital signs
   (2) Nursing interventions
      (a) Protect patient from injury; minimize invasive procedures, including injections, to avoid injury and bleeding
      (b) Monitor for presence and amount of bleeding; test body secretions for occult bleeding
      (c) Apply cold packs and pressure to bleeding sites
      (d) Administer fluids, blood, and blood components as prescribed
      (e) Closely monitor hemoglobin, coagulation profiles, and vital signs
      (f) Administer anticoagulants or antifibrinolytics as prescribed
c. Alteration in tissue perfusion related to microcirculatory thrombosis
   (1) Expected outcomes—tissue perfusion adequate as evidenced by normal organ function
   (2) Nursing interventions
      (a) Assess function of body systems at least every four hours
         i) Monitor ABGs, central and peripheral oxygen saturation, PA pressure
         ii) Monitor urine character and volume
         iii) Monitor BUN and serum creatinine levels
      (b) Administer fluids to maintain normovolemia
      (c) Handle affected extremities gently
      (d) Provide high flow humidified oxygen and mechanical ventilation as needed
d. Additional nursing diagnoses
   (1) Fluid volume deficit related to hemorrhage
   (2) Alteration in comfort related to inadequate tissue perfusion and ischemia
   (3) Potential alteration in gas exchange related to anemia

H. GASTROINTESTINAL FAILURE

1. **Characterized by bacterial translocation of enteric organisms to systemic circulation, causing persistent macrophage activation and organ injury**
2. **Precursors include ileus, mucosal atrophy in absence of enteral feeding, and gastric or duodenal ischemia in shock**
3. **Assessment findings**
a. Gastrointestinal bleeding

b. Heme in nasogastric drainage or stool
c. Decreased or absent bowel sounds
d. Increased abdominal girth

4. Diagostic studies are used to find a septic focus

a. Ultrasound
b. Computerized axial tomography (CAT)
c. X-rays
d. Blood cultures

5. Medical interventions

a. Decompress stomach; nasogastric tube to suction
b. Prescribe pharmacologic therapy
   (1) Antacids to keep gastric pH above 5
   (2) Histamine blockers to reduce hydrochloric acid production
   (3) Carafate to coat gastric mucosa and promote healing
c. Initiate early enteral nutrition; duodenal feedings may begin intraoperatively
d. Provide adequate fluids

6. Nursing diagnoses, expected outcomes, and interventions

a. Inadequate gastrointestinal function related to surgical manipulation of the bowel, absence of enteral feeding, or shock state
   (1) Expected outcomes
      (a) Active bowel sounds on auscultation
      (b) Tolerates enteral feeding without diarrhea or large residual
      (c) Normal body temperature and WBC
      (d) Gastric pH greater than 5, if histamine blockers or antacids are used
   (2) Nursing interventions
      (a) Auscultate bowel sounds every four hours
      (b) Monitor volume of NG aspirate at least every eight hours
      (c) Administer enteral feedings; monitor tolerance by checking residual every four hours
      (d) Observe for abdominal distension and diarrhea; note subjective complaints of discomfort
      (e) Monitor temperature and WBC for early signs of infection
b. Potential for hemorrhage related to gastro/duodenal ischemia and ulceration
   (1) Expected outcomes—absence of gastrointestinal bleeding, as evidenced by heme-negative results when gastric drainage or stools are tested
   (2) Nursing interventions
      (a) Monitor gastric pH every four hours
      (b) Administer histamine blockers, antacids, and Carafate as prescribed; monitor response
      (c) Monitor nasogastric drainage and stools for blood

I. LIVER FAILURE

1. Characterized by toxic accumulation of amino acids, impaired glucose and protein production, deposition of fat, and cholestasis

2. May be caused by direct hepatic injury or biliary stasis

3. Associated with pneumonia and intraabdominal sepsis

4. **Assessment findings**
a. Elevated bilirubin with no demonstrable cause such as obstruction, or resolving hematoma
b. Jaundice from failure to metabolize bilirubin
c. Elevated SGPT, SGOT, alkaline phosphatase
d. Decreased serum albumin due to decreased liver synthesis
e. Ascites due to decreased albumin levels
f. Elevated serum ammonia level
g. Decreased level of consciousness due to accumulation of waste products in brain tissue
h. Occult or frank bleeding due to inadequate coagulation factors, and prolonged coagulation time
i. Petechiae
j. Blood in nasogastric drainage and/or stools
5. **Diagnostic indicators**
a. Hemoglobin, hematocrit, WBC
b. SGOT and gamma GT may indicate hepatocellular inflammation
c. Bilirubin (total and direct) and alkaline phosphatase (increases indicate hepatic obstruction)
d. Serum albumin, PT, PTT to assess the liver's synthesis ability
e. Abdominal ultrasound to rule out biliary obstruction
f. Electroencephalogram—hepatic encephalopathy may cause diffuse, generalized slowing of frequency
g. Abdominal CAT scan to identify intraabdominal abscess formation
6. **Medical and surgical interventions**
a. Prescribe antibiotic therapy
b. Drain and irrigate abdominal cavity, e.g., with abscesses or peritonitis
c. Prescribe lactulose and neomycin to decrease ammonia level
d. Initiate total parenteral nutrition with branch-chain amino acids
e. Initiate enteral feeding with special hepatic formulas, e.g., Hepataid
f. Prescribe albumin I.V. to keep serum albumin above 2.5 gms/dl
g. Prescribe blood component therapy to treat clotting deficiencies and blood loss
7. **Nursing diagnoses, expected outcomes, and interventions**
a. Alteration in nutrition, less than body requirements, related to inadequate hepatic function
   (1) Expected outcomes—nutritional indicators within normal limits; minimal weight loss; nutrient intake meets energy demands
   (2) Nursing interventions
      (a) Weigh daily
      (b) Monitor results of liver function studies, e.g., bilirubin, SGOT, SGPT, alkaline phosphatase
      (c) Monitor nutritional parameters, e.g., albumin, prealbumin, transferrin, nitrogen balance
      (d) Provide enteral or parenteral feedings as prescribed (see Module 11—Nutrition—for additional information)
b. Inadequate liver function related to sepsis and/or direct injury
   (1) Expected outcome—liver function studies within normal parameters
   (2) Nursing interventions
      (a) Monitor results of liver function studies (bilirubin, SGOT, SGPT, alkaline phosphatase)

(b) Monitor results of coagulation studies
(c) Monitor for therapeutic and toxic effects of medications that require hepatic breakdown or storage
(d) Observe for development of jaundice

c. Potential alteration in neurologic status related to the accumulation of ammonia in brain tissue
(1) Expected outcomes—level of consciousness remains unchanged; patient alert and oriented
(2) Nursing interventions
(a) Monitor neurologic status at least every four hours
(b) Monitor results of ammonia levels
(c) Consider cumulative effects of sedation if liver function is inadequate
(d) Administer neomycin via nasogastric tube to decrease gastrointestinal ammonia formation
(e) Administer lactulose via nasogastric tube to induce diarrhea and facilitate ammonia excretion

d. Potential hemorrhage related to inadequate synthesis of clotting factors
(1) Expected outcomes—no evidence of bleeding; hemoglobin and hematocrit within normal range
(2) Nursing interventions
(a) Monitor results of coagulation studies
(b) Monitor results of hemoglobin and hematocrit
(c) Hematest all stools and nasogastric drainage
(d) Administer blood component therapy as prescribed
(e) Protect patient from injury; minimize invasive procedures

e. Potential loss of skin integrity related to immobility, ascites, and peripheral edema
(1) Expected outcome—skin intact
(2) Nursing interventions (see section on pressure sores, pp. 185–187)

J. MYOCARDIAL FAILURE

1. **Myocardial depression may result from sepsis and the production of myocardial depressive factor from the ischemic gut during shock**
2. **Precursors also may include myocardial infarction, myocardial contusion, reduction of preload by high levels of PEEP, and hypovolemic shock**
3. **Assessment findings**

a. Arrhythmias associated with hypoxemia, hyperkalemia, acid-base imbalance, drugs, e.g., anesthetics, aminophylline, cocaine
b. Elevated pulmonary artery pressures
c. Decreased cardiac output

4. **Diagnostic studies**

a. Two-dimensional echocardiography to evaluate ventricular wall motion
b. CPK isoenzymes—specifically myocardial band (MB) fraction
c. Swan-Ganz catheter placement to determine left ventricular filling pressures

d. 12-lead ECG
5. **Medical interventions**
a. Insert pulmonary artery line for hemodynamic monitoring
b. Prescribe inotropic and antiarrhythmic drugs
c. Prescribe fluid replacement
d. Treat underlying sepsis
6. **Nursing diagnoses, expected outcomes, and interventions**
a. Decreased cardiac output related to inadequate circulating fluid volume (see Module 10—Shock)
b. Decreased cardiac output related to myocardial injury (see Module 22—Cardiothoracic Trauma)
c. Decreased cardiac output related to arrhythmias
 (1) Expected outcomes—cardiac function within normal limits as evidenced by
  (a) Apical pulse 60 to 100 beats/min
  (b) Normal sinus rhythm
  (c) Cardiac output 3 to 6 liters/min
 (2) Nursing interventions
  (a) Monitor ECG continuously; observe for arrhythmias, particularly after administration of medications, e.g., Pavulon, aminophylline
  (b) Monitor cardiac output
  (c) Monitor oxygen saturation via pulse oximeter
  (d) Monitor serum electrolytes
  (e) Titrate inotropic and antiarrhythmic medications as indicated

K. MULTIPLE SYSTEM ORGAN FAILURE (MSOF)

1. **Characterized by progressive deterioration of organ systems usually beginning with the lungs, and followed by the liver, kidneys, gastrointestinal tract, heart, and central nervous system (4)**
2. **Factors that increase risk of MSOF include hemorrhagic shock, pelvic or retroperitoneal hematoma, multiple transfusions, thoracic trauma, inadequate fluid resuscitation, sepsis, and presence of necrotic tissue**
3. **Patterns of organ failure may be sequential or simultaneous; mortality increases with greater number of organs involved**
4. **Pathophysiology**
a. Alteration in host defense
 (1) Generalized inflammatory response
 (2) Activation of complement cascade, which produces cell-damaging end products
 (3) End products of cascade activation cause cellular infiltration, interstitial edema, malperfusion, and defective tissue oxygen supply
b. Hypermetabolism
 (1) Increased oxygen demands in all tissues with decreased supply
 (2) Increased protein catabolism
 (3) Increased hepatic glucose production

(4) Cells resist carbohydrate utilization
(5) Increased lactate production resulting in lactic acidosis

5. Prevention strategies

a. Assessment of risk
   (1) Determine preinjury medical history
   (2) Review initial medical interventions and patient response
   (3) Monitor early signs of inadequate oxygen transport and elevated filling pressures
b. Vigorously restore intravascular volume
   (1) Control bleeding
   (2) Provide fluid and blood resuscitation
c. Maximize oxygen transport
d. Support ventilation if indicated by pulmonary function test, ABGs, physical examination
e. Fix fractures early to decrease probability of ARDS, reduce inflammatory response, and permit early mobilization
f. Clean wounds and debride devitalized tissue early
g. Avoid immobilization by aggressive efforts to reposition, turn, get patient out of bed, and ambulate
h. Provide early and vigorous nutritional support, preferably by enteral route

References

1. Shea, J. D. (1975). Pressure sore classification and management. *Clinical Orthopedics, 112*, 89–100.
2. Littleton, M. T. (1989). Complications of multiple trauma. *Critical Care Nursing Clinics of North America, 1*(1), 75–84.
3. Wilkerson, E. (1988). Inflammation, infection, and wound healing. In E. Howell, L. Widra & M. G. Hill (Eds.), *Comprehensive trauma nursing: Theory and practice* (pp. 326–362). Glenview, IL: Scott, Foresman & Co.
4. DeCamp, & Demling, R. (1988). Posttraumatic multisystem organ failure. *Journal of the American Medical Association, 260*(4), 530–534.

Suggested Readings

Alspach, J. G. (Ed.). (1991). *Core curriculum for critical care nursing* (4th ed.). Philadelphia: W. B. Saunders Co.

Barke, R., & Cerra, F. B. (1988). Multiple system organ failure. *Topics in Emergency Medicine, 9*(4), 1–12.

Bates, B. (1987). *A guide to physical examination and history taking* (4th ed.). Philadelphia: J. B. Lippincott Co.

Cerra, F. B. (1987). The hypermetabolic organ failure complex. *World Journal of Surgery, 11*(2), 173–181.

Faist, E., Baue, A. E., Dittmer, H., & Heberer, G. (1983). Multiple organ failure in polytrauma patients. *The Journal of Trauma, 23*(9), 775–785.

Fry, D. E. (1988). Multiple system organ failure. *Surgical Clinics of North America, 68*(1), 107–122.

Johanson, B. C., Wells, S. J., Dungca, C. U., & Hoffmeister, D. (Eds.). (1988). *Standards for critical care* (3rd ed.). St. Louis: C. V. Mosby Co.

Kenner, C. V., Guzzetta, C. E., & Dossey, B. M. (Eds.). (1985). *Critical care nursing: Body, mind, spirit.* Boston: Little, Brown, & Co.

Knezevich, B. A. (Ed.). (1986). *Trauma nursing: Principles and practice.* Norwalk, CT: Appleton-Century-Crofts.

Shires, G. T. (Ed.). (1979). *Care of the trauma patient* (2nd ed.). New York: McGraw-Hill.

Strange, J. M. (Ed.). (1987). *Shock trauma care plans.* Springhouse, PA: Springhouse Corp.

MODULE 17
REHABILITATION

Mary Pat Erdner, MSN, RN, CRRN
Cyndy Kraft-Fine, MSN, RN, CRRN

Objectives

1.0 Describe the rehabilitation process.
1.1 Define rehabilitation and list five major goals.
1.2 Identify, briefly, the hierarchy of the rehabilitation process.
2.0 Describe components of the interdisciplinary plan of care.
3.0 Identify functions of the interdisciplinary rehabilitation team.
3.1 Identify the role of the rehabilitation nurse in the rehabilitation process.
3.2 List several members of the specialty rehabilitation teams.
4.0 List relevant theories that direct nursing practice for the trauma/ rehabilitation patient.
5.0 Describe components of assessment in rehabilitation nursing practice.
5.1 Define immediate, short- and long-term memory.
5.2 List memory assessment questions for each type of memory.
5.3 List assessment questions for orientation, judgment, problem solving, proverbs, similarities, and simple math.
5.4 Describe the difference between speech and language.
5.5 List and define the disorders of speech.
5.6 List and define the disorders of language.
5.7 Identify the components of a speech and language assessment.
5.8 Describe the evaluation of the cerebellum.
5.9 Identify several major rehabilitation outcome measures.

5.10 Identify types of information elicited during the psychosocial evaluation.

6.0 Describe common nursing diagnoses during acute and convalescent phases of rehabilitation.

7.0 List nursing interventions related to specific nursing diagnoses during acute and convalescent phases of rehabilitation.

8.0 Define measurable criteria for expected outcomes in the evaluation of patient and family responses to acute and convalescent rehabilitation.

9.0 Describe the discharge planning process for the patient returning to the community.

9.1 Identify the goals of discharge planning.

9.2 List factors influencing the discharge plan.

9.3 Identify the major steps of the discharge process.

9.4 List several community care options.

9.5 Identify problems related to evaluating a medical equipment supplier.

9.6 Identify transportation considerations for the disabled within the community.

9.7 Identify several vocational problems for the disabled.

10.0 Anticipate client needs and assist with appropriate interventions in the transition from hospital to community.

10.1 Describe several potential postdischarge feelings and issues of adjustment.

10.2 List the steps in early home adjustment.

10.3 Identify the components of a lifetime follow-up care program.

A. GENERAL REHABILITATION CONCEPTS

1. Definitions of rehabilitation

a. Rehabilitation is a creative process that begins with immediate preventive care in the first stage of an accident or illness; it is continued through the restorative phase of care and involves adaptions of a whole being to a new life; the individual is restored to the fullest physical, mental, social, vocational, and economic capacity of which he/she is capable (1)

b. A dynamic process that restores an individual to the highest level of possible function; the emphasis is placed on the individual's remaining abilities rather than disabilities (2)

2. Goals of rehabilitation

a. Prevent disability and its complications

b. Treat disability

c. Promote high quality of life with disability (3)

d. Achieve maximum potential function and independence

e. Identify and develop goals of the patient for an acceptable quality of life with a disability

f. Promote health and wellness

g. Reintegrate patient into community successfully

3. Rehabilitation hierarchy (4)

a. Trauma and early posttrauma phase—stabilization of body systems and early psychological intervention

b. Early rehabilitation intervention—physical and occupational therapy; bowel and bladder programs for continence; social service financial planning and support
c. Independent self-care activities—wheelchair or mobility activities; learning about disability and self-care
d. Successful adjustment to living at home
e. Integration into the community
f. Gainful employment

B. THE INTERDISCIPLINARY PLAN

1. **Components of plan**
a. Assessment and identification of patient's current functional level, strengths, and weaknesses
b. Development of goals with measurable behavioral outcomes related to functional capabilities and needs of patient
c. Treatment plan updated at least weekly or biweekly, reflecting reevaluation of goals
d. Discharge plan reviewed with patient and family on the day of admission and reevaluated periodically
2. **Roles and functions of core team members**
a. The patient/family
   (1) Members of the team as defined by hospital accreditation and regulatory standards (5)
   (2) Active participants in the development of goals, treatment, and discharge plan
   (3) Understand the scope of illness and disability
   (4) Make decisions related to maintaining health and wellness, and perform or direct all aspects of care
   (5) Commit to goal achievement and successful completion of the rehabilitation program
b. Rehabilitation nurse
   (1) Provides nursing care directed at prevention, maintenance, and/or restoration of function with the goal of patient's adoption of a different lifestyle
   (2) Coordinates and implements activities of various therapies, including daily living skills, ambulation, wheelchair mobility, and cognitive strategies
   (3) Actively participates in the discharge plan; identifies impact of daily care and potential hardships for the care provider
c. Additional roles include physical therapist, occupational therapist, speech pathologist, recreational therapist, psychologist, social worker, physiatrist, and vocational counselor (see Module 8—The Trauma Team—for detailed role functions)
3. **Specialty team members**
a. Within a rehabilitation setting, additional members are added to specific disability teams to provide specialized care
b. Brain injury team members and consultants include neuropsychologist,

neurologist, neurosurgeon, job coach, neurophthalmologist, dentist/orthodontist, psychiatrist, and educational specialist

c. Spinal cord injury team members and consultants include urologist, plastic surgeon, orthopaedic surgeon, educational specialist

C. REHABILITATION CONCEPTS THROUGHOUT THE TRAUMA CONTINUUM

1. **Adjustment and adaptation**
2. **Change**
3. **Health and wellness**
4. **Learning**
5. **Self-care theory**

D. ASSESSMENT WITH A REHABILITATION FOCUS

1. **Physiologic assessment**

a. Neurocognitive assessment done as screening tool for individuals with suspected head injury
- (1) Assess cranial nerves as outlined in Module 20 (Head Injury)
- (2) Cognitive evaluation
  - (a) General appearance—grooming, hygiene, dress
  - (b) Memory—the ability to learn and remember new information; attention, concentration, categorization, and language influence memory
    - i) Immediate memory—immediate recall; reflects attention and concentration; ask patient to
      - a) Repeat a series of numbers after you, starting with three and progressing to six numbers
      - b) Repeat the alphabet stating every other letter
      - c) Subtract 7 from 100 and continue from each calculation
    - ii) Short-term memory—recently learned visual or verbal information
      - a) Ask patient to remember three common, unrelated objects, e.g., a typewriter, rose, and number eight
      - b) Test recall, with or without clues, immediately, at three minutes and at five minutes
      - c) Present three geometric pictures with three abstract words underneath each picture
      - d) Ask patient to copy the items
      - e) Ask patient to study the pictures and words as long as necessary; remove items and ask patient to replicate them
      - f) Repeat test in 5 and 10 minutes

iii) Past memory—ask patient to name several past presidents and identify important family dates

(c) Orientation

i) Determine orientation to person, place, time, and situation

ii) Assess ability to relate to environmental clues, e.g., snow on the ground means winter

(d) Judgment/abstract thought—ask patient to

i) Interpret common situations and proverbs

ii) Identify common aspects of two objects—how are a table and a chair alike? How is a tree and alcohol alike?

(e) Following directions—note how many steps of information an individual can follow

(f) Topographical orientation—patient's ability to find his/her way around the room, go to the nurses' station and back to the room, or negotiate neighborhood using appropriate landmarks and clues

(g) Math concepts—assess simple math by using paper and calculating figures in his/her head

b. Communication

(1) Speech: "Mechanical process of an individual's ability to communicate with oral language, utilizing the combination of appropriate neuromuscular actions necessary for phonation and articulation" (6, p. 125)

(2) Dysarthria—disorder of speech resulting from lack of neuromuscular control; affects elements of basic speech processes, e.g., respiration, phonation, resonance, articulation, and prosody

(a) Flaccid dysarthria—breathy voice quality; hypernasality; consonant imprecision secondary to flaccid paralysis and muscle atrophy (6)

(b) Spastic dysarthria—strained, harsh voice; hypernasality; slow rate of speech; consonant imprecision and limited range secondary to upper motor neuron lesion from trauma or cerebrovascular accident (CVA) (6)

(c) Ataxic dysarthria—imprecise consonants; irregular articulation; slow mouth movement; difficulty handling secretions secondary to cerebellar lesion from trauma or CVA (6)

(3) Apraxia—articulation disorder affecting the ability to position speech muscles and sequence muscle movements to produce speech; no muscle weakness, slowness, or incoordination present (6)

(a) Prosody alterations—changes in loudness, pitch, articulation time, and pauses during speech (6)

(b) Difficulty with phonation, repetition, word substitution, and prolongation of syllables or words (6)

(c) Slow speech with words and syllables evenly stressed and spaced (6)

c. Communication assessment

(1) Cranial nerves (see Module 20—Head Injury)—assess muscle strength, sensation, and coordination of mouth and tongue

(2) Assess respiratory system; note breathing patterns while speaking; breathiness, duration, and loudness

d. Language—"Ability to communicate through use of symbols, comprehension, decoding, and encoding" (6, p. 126)

(1) Aphasia—language disorder characterized by an inability to interpret and formulate language symbols or words (6)

(a) Nonfluent aphasia—verbal expression characterized by decreased output, less than 50 words per minute; speech with decreased phrase lengths, facial grimaces, and dysrhythmic phrases
(b) Fluent aphasia—verbal expression characterized by quantity of verbal output ranging from low-normal to approximately 200 words per minute; speech without effort; normal articulation but with substitute word or words that convey no information
(c) Anomia—difficulty finding correct word to convey information; characterized by descriptive phrases about the word without saying the word, or hesitation before speaking the correct word

(2) Assessment of language
(a) Evaluate word fluency, vocabulary, complexity, and ease of language and conversation
(b) Evaluate initiation of conversation, organization of thoughts and sentences
(c) Observe characteristics—preservation, quantity of jargon, rhythm and rate, paraphasias (substitution within a word or syllable such as "cat" instead of "hat")
(d) Assess verbal comprehension; note answers to yes-no questions; note number of commands patient can follow; ask patient to point to pictures and words and identify them
(e) Ask patient to name common and uncommon items
(f) Evaluate patient's reading and writing abilities

e. Cerebellar evaluation
(1) Assess gait for high level balance and righting reaction deficits related to cerebellum and vestibular system; ask patient to
(a) Walk heel-to-toe in a straight line forward and backward
(b) Walk on his/her toes and heels
(c) Cross one foot in front of the other and walk in a line
(2) Perform a Romberg test
(a) Ask patient to stand with feet together, eyes shut, and hands out in front
(b) The patient with Romberg's sign will have difficulty maintaining balance
(3) Perform rapid alternating movements; ask patient to
(a) Pat each leg as fast as he/she can with each hand
(b) Turn each hand over and back as rapidly as possible
(c) Touch each of his/her fingers with the thumb, in rapid sequence
(d) Tap the floor with the ball of his/her foot, one at a time
(4) Point-to-point testing; ask patient to
(a) Touch examiner's index finger and then his/her nose repeatedly; examiner should move finger about so patient has to alter directions and extend arm fully
(b) Place his/her heel on the opposite knee, then run it down the shin to the big toe (7)

f. Sensory testing
(1) Assess for pain, light touch, and temperature in each dermatome and along major peripheral nerves, bilaterally
(2) Assess proprioception by grasping patient's toe and moving it up and down; ask patient to close his/her eyes and to identify toe's position as you move it; repeat process with fingers

(3) Stereognosis—place small familiar objects in patient's hand and ask to identify object with his/her eyes closed

g. Integumentary system
   (1) Assess skin several times a day; measure width, length, and depth of lesions; serial photographs are helpful
   (2) Describe exudate, level of induration, temperature, and characteristics of surrounding areas
   (3) Pressure sores are graded on a four-point scale, I to IV (see Module 16—Medical Sequelae)

h. Outcome scales measuring physiologic or functional rehabilitation outcomes
   (1) Functional assessment—PULSES profile developed in 1957 by Moskowitz (8)
      (a) P = physical condition
      (b) U = upper extremity function
      (c) L = lower extremity function
      (d) S = sensory component
      (e) E = excretory function
      (f) S = mental and emotional status
   (2) Cognitive tools
      (a) Glasgow Coma Scale—developed to quantitatively describe severity of head injury; relates consciousness to motor response, verbal response, and eye opening on a scale of 3 to 15 (9) (see Table 19.1, p. 261)
      (b) Rancho Los Amigos Scale of Cognitive Levels and Expected Behavior describes levels of cognitive and behavioral recovery after traumatic brain injury (10)
         i) Level I—no response
         ii) Level II—generalized response
         iii) Level III—localized response
         iv) Level IV—confused-agitated
         v) Level V—confused, inappropriate, nonagitated
         vi) Level VI—confused-appropriate
         vii) Level VII—automatic-appropriate
         viii) Level VIII—purposeful and appropriate
      (c) Disability Rating Scale—0-to-30-point scale that measures arousal, awareness, responsiveness, cognitive ability for self-care activities, dependence on others, and psychosocial adaptabilty (11)
   (3) Program evaluation tools
      (a) PECS—patient evaluation conference system
         i) Interdisciplinary method of functional performance; assesses 15 categories, which represent potential outcomes
         ii) Each item scored on scale from 1 to 7; 1 to 4 represents dependence, and 5 to 7 represents independence
      (b) FIM-functional independence measure (12)
         i) Tool comprises six items—self-care, sphincter management, mobility, locomotion, communication, and social cognition
         ii) Scores within each category are on a four- or seven-point scale; the seven-point scale demonstrates more accurate outcomes

2. Psychologic assessment

a. Premorbid personality, previous coping patterns, and defenses

b. Developmental stage of patient
c. Availability of support systems including financial resources for ongoing therapy
d. Current behaviors, including grief and mourning, depression, anxiety, and defense mechanisms

3. **Social assessment**
a. Identification and assessment of primary care provider
   (1) Includes realistic commitment and desire for care/supervision of disabled individual
   (2) Health of primary caregiver—endurance and strength to provide physical care of patient, including transfers and positioning, and ability to withstand sleep interruptions
   (3) Attitudes toward disability and assumption of conflicting or new roles
   (4) Impact of disability on long-term life goals for family
   (5) Financial resources available to provide care
b. Family assessment
   (1) Previous coping strategies
   (2) Family composition—number of family members living in area, their roles, and current living situation
   (3) Patterns of communication, decisionmaking, and power within family
   (4) Educational level
   (5) Resources available to family
   (6) Ethnic and religious customs and beliefs
   (7) Beliefs and values about illness and disability
c. Assessment of other support systems
   (1) Identify friends and type of help they are able to provide; evaluate their time commitments and availability
   (2) Perceptions and values regarding disability
d. Economic status
   (1) Family financial status, monthly income, and expenses
   (2) Type of insurance for hospitalization, rehabilitation, and aftercare
   (3) Eligibility for benefits, e.g., social security, disability programs, and government grants
e. Occupational history
   (1) Current job, employer, and duration of employment; obtain job description from patient and employer
   (2) Past job experiences, including type of work
   (3) Degree of support from employer, availability of patient's current job, and functional ability to perform job
   (4) Potential for return to work
   (5) Attitude of employer toward disability
f. Home and community assessment
   (1) Home accessibility—number of steps into house and to bathroom; size of living area, including kitchen and bedroom; description of furniture placement; dimensions of doorways
   (2) Transportation
      (a) Community transportation, e.g., city bus service for the disabled
      (b) Ability to drive, current license, potential for returning to driving
   (3) Leisure activities and hobbies
   (4) Daily living routine

E. NURSING DIAGNOSES, EXPECTED OUTCOMES, AND INTERVENTIONS IN ACUTE ILLNESS

1. **Potential impaired skin integrity related to immobility or stabilization devices**

a. Expected patient/family outcomes
   (1) Skin intact—no signs of pressure sores
   (2) Identify strategies for pressure relief and perform skin care and pressure relief activities
   (3) Manage orthotic devices as directed
   (4) Skin remains intact during use of orthotic devices

b. Nursing interventions
   (1) Turn and position patient at least every two hours to keep skin adequately perfused; inspect bony prominences with each position change
   (2) Use an appropriate bed and mattress
   (3) Assist patient to sit properly in wheelchair with weight evenly distributed on both ischia; edge of chair approximately two to three fingers' width from the popliteal space; feet flat on footplates; knees and hips at 90° angle
   (4) Consult dietitian to plan for excellent nutrition and hydration
   (5) Keep skin clean and dry; avoid shearing and friction
   (6) Assist patient/family to identify appropriate seating and positioning techniques
   (7) Check skin under braces at least daily; request the orthotist to evaluate p.r.n.
   (8) If a stabilization device creates skin problems, or appears unsafe, keep patient on bed rest until adjusted

2. **Altered bowel elimination related to cognitive and perceptual impairments regarding knowledge of need to defecate and/or diminished or lost sphincter control**

a. Expected patient/family outcomes
   (1) Achieve predictable, regular, convenient bowel elimination schedule that reduces accidents or constipation
   (2) Identify interventions that may be necessary for constipation, impaction, diarrhea, and hemorrhoids
   (3) Demonstrate good health practices, including diet choices, mobilization, and adequate fluid intake, which may influence effective bowel program
   (4) Demonstrate psychomotor skills necessary for bowel elimination

b. Nursing interventions
   (1) Assess premorbid and present activity level, diet changes, medications, including enemas or use of laxatives, and neurologic sequelae of illness; assess previous bowel elimination routine and patterns
   (2) Determine caretaker and family schedule upon patient's discharge to coordinate patient's bowel elimination routine
   (3) Initiate a toileting schedule; consider any consistent premorbid or current toileting pattern
   (4) Note color, consistency, frequency, and amount of stool; document for ongoing evaluation
   (5) Position patient in upright position on commode, if possible, to facilitate evacuation utilizing gravity

(6) Consult dietitian to assist patient with food and fluid intake; use bulk and fruits when possible
(7) Provide privacy
(8) Upon initiation of toileting program
(a) Assess bowel sounds and cleanse lower rectum using laxatives or suppositories, if impacted
(b) Use stool softeners to increase fluid to stool; eliminate use if stool becomes too soft
(9) Administer bulk formers (methylcellulose products) to stimulate peristalsis and form stool; bulk formers may cause impaction if fluids are restricted
(10) Toilet individual at same time daily to establish pattern; timing can be determined by effectiveness of routine, past patterns, or postprandial gastrocolic reflex
(11) Temporarily initiate use of suppositories (glycerin or Fleet Bisacodyl) to establish routine; administer medication and wait approximately 20 min for effectiveness
(12) Assist patient/family to identify potential problems, including constipation, diarrhea, impaction, limited exercise, diet, and fluid restrictions

3. Altered bowel elimination related to upper neuron or reflexic neurogenic bowel

a. Expected patient/family outcomes (see E.2.a.)
b. Nursing interventions
(1) Administer bowel medication at timed intervals; give laxatives six hours before suppository
(2) Digitally stimulate S2 to 4 by placing a gloved, lubricated finger in the rectum and making a gentle circular motion, which relaxes sphincter, stimulates peristalsis, and results in effective evacuation
(3) Maintain bowel program even if patient is incontinent
(4) Prevent fecal impaction, which may stimulate autonomic dysreflexia
(5) Additional interventions (see E.2.b.)

4. Altered bowel elimination related to lower motor neuron or areflexic bowel secondary to lumbosacral nerve root and cord injury; manifested by flaccid rectum, diminished sensation to defecate, and incontinence with physical activity

a. Expected patient/family outcomes (see E.2.a.)
b. Nursing interventions
(1) Utilize daily bisacodyl suppository to keep rectum empty
(2) Instruct patient to get up on the commode, when possible, and use Valsalva's maneuver to increase the intraabdominal pressure and empty bowel
(3) Identify foods and medications that increase episodes of incontinence
(4) Additional interventions (see E.2.b.)

5. Altered pattern of urinary elimination related to neural dysfunction

a. Expected patient/family outcomes
(1) Achieves continence and independence with safe, simple, inexpensive, long-term urinary elimination routine that is integrated into lifestyle
(2) Identify potential complications related to bladder management, indwelling catheters, and intermittent catheterization
(3) Urine free of infection

b. Nursing interventions
  (1) Assess type of bladder dysfunction
    (a) Uninhibited bladder—failure of inhibitory fibers of corticoregulatory tract to suppress involuntary detrusor contractions; characterized by urgency, frequency, and incontinence (13)
    (b) Reflex neurogenic bladder—disruption in both sensory and motor nerve tracts above the spinal reflex arc, S2 to 4; characterized by decreased bladder capacity and incomplete voiding
    (c) Areflexic neurogenic bladder—disruption of lower motor neurons caused by injury to the micturition center in the spinal cord (S2 to 4), cauda equina, or sacral roots and nerves
  (2) Review diagnostic and laboratory data for BUN, serum creatinine, urinalysis, urine culture and sensitivity
  (3) Assess activity level, i.e., hours in bed, in chair, in PT gym
  (4) Assess hydration, fluid intake, and output
  (5) Initiate bladder management program
    (a) Uninhibited bladder
      i) Time voiding and medication—place the individual on a routine toileting program, e.g., every two hours
        a) As individual's ability to retain urine increases, increase time between toileting, e.g., increase to every $2\frac{1}{2}$ hrs, then 3 hrs
        b) Medication may be necessary to decrease bladder irritability, increase contractility, or treat urinary tract infections
        c) Facilitate reflex voiding by tapping the bladder or by Credé's method (suprapubic manual pressure) every 2 to 4 hrs
      ii) Maintain 2000 ml fluid intake
      iii) Check skin for breakdown, rash, and excoriation
      iv) Consider urinary catheter or diapering, if program unsuccessful
    (b) Neurogenic bladder
      i) Initiate clean or sterile, intermittent catheterization schedule
      ii) Establish routine, approximately every 4 hrs, and increase intervals as postvoid residuals remain low and voiding occurs in between
      iii) Restrict fluids to about 1800 ml/day to prevent overdistension
      iv) Utilize an external collecting device between catheterizations
      v) Consider urinary catheter only for urinary tract infections or reflux
      vi) Medications may include Dibenzyline, for tight or spastic internal sphincter, and/or Urecholine, for nonobstructive urinary retention in individuals with high urine residuals

6. **Impaired physical mobility related to heterotopic ossification, increased tone, spasticity, and contractures**

a. Definitions
  (1) Heterotopic ossification—osteogenesis in soft tissue below the level of injury in spinal cord or head injury
    (a) Always extraarticular and extracapsular; typically near large joints, i.e., knees, hips, shoulders, elbows, and spine
    (b) Early signs and symptoms—swelling, warmth, decreased range of motion, erythema, and increased alkaline phosphatase
  (2) Increased tone—levels describing postural muscle tone

(a) Rigidity—resistance to all motion; makes body parts stiff and immobile; type of rigidity depends on location of lesion, i.e., decerebrate, decorticate, and Parkinson's
(b) Spasms—spontaneous, involuntary, convulsive contractions of specific muscle groups; can occur anywhere in the body (14)
(c) Spasticity—result of intact reflex arcs below level of injury in spinal cord or head injury; characterized by hypertonicity, hyperactive stretch reflexes, and clonus
(d) Contractures—develop with prolonged shortening of structures across and around a joint; result in decreased ROM; initially involve changes in muscle tissue but progress to involve capsular and pericapsular changes

b. Expected patient/family outcomes
(1) Identify signs and symptoms of heterotopic ossification, spasticity, increased tone, and contractures, and follow prescribed regimen
(2) Tone and spasticity do not interfere with patient's daily living routine or safety
(3) Maintain patient's mobility and range of motion within normal limits

c. Nursing interventions
(1) Assess range of motion of joints daily
(2) Assess patient's functional level and area of lesion—depending on area of lesion, tonal patterns will differ and may interfere with functional abilities of the individual
(3) Assess discomfort and pain; administer pain medications p.r.n. and prior to ROM exercises
(4) Assess degree and pattern of spasticity, increased tone, and posturing; identify precipitating factors
(5) Assess for decreased ROM, redness, swelling, or heat around joints; compare to baseline and joints on other side
(6) Monitor serum calcium, phosphorus, alkaline phosphatase, and liver function tests if using antispasticity medications
(7) Provide adequate periods of rest between activities
(8) Describe and instruct patient and family about spasticity and increased tone; describe positive aspects of spasticity to patient, including ease of transfers and positioning
(9) Assist patient to identify triggers for spasticity and possible appropriate use of triggers
(10) If tone or spasticity suddenly increases, investigate acute causes such as fractures, thrombophlebitis, urinary tract infection, or other noxious stimuli
(11) Perform or encourage ROM exercises, at least b.i.d., to point of pain, unless contraindicated
(12) Utilize seating/positioning techniques and splints to maintain ROM and minimize "abnormal tone," i.e., spasticity, rigidity, spasms
(13) Pad side rails, if necessary, for safety

7. Potential for injury related to orthostatic hypotension

a. Expected patient/family outcomes
(1) Identify signs and symptoms of hypotension
(2) Maintain safety during episodes of hypotension
(3) Use coping techniques to decrease hypotensive episodes

b. Nursing interventions

(1) Assess and document baseline blood pressure
(2) Apply elastic hose and abdominal binder before getting patient out of bed
(3) Raise head of the bed gradually, to approximately 70°, before transfer; monitor blood pressure
(4) If patient is unable to tolerate upright wheelchair, use reclining wheelchair with elevated leg rests; monitor blood pressure with each position change
(5) Stay with patient after transfer to ensure safety; if patient complains of light-headedness or dizziness, tilt wheelchair back or lower head of bed; check blood pressure and elevate legs
(6) Assess for dehydration and replace fluids if necessary
(7) Review patient medications for hypotensive effects

8. **Altered thought process: attention and concentration deficit related to head injury**

a. Definition of terms (15)
(1) Arousal—organism's general state of readiness to respond to environment
(2) Attention—process by which one selectively responds to a specific event and inhibits responses to simultaneous events
(3) Focused attention—ability to respond discretely to specific auditory, visual, or tactile stimuli, often disrupted in early stages of emergence from coma when patient responds primarily to internal stimuli
(4) Sustained attention—ability to maintain consistent behavioral response during continuous and repetitive activity, i.e., patient can only focus on task for seconds to minutes
(5) Selective attention—ability to focus on task/event at hand, including external stimuli (sights and sounds) and internal stimuli (worries and important thoughts)
(6) Alternating attention—ability to shift focus of attention between tasks, e.g., secretary who must type, answer phone, and respond to inquiries
(7) Divided attention—ability to perform two tasks simultaneously, e.g., drive car and change radio station

b. Expected patient/family outcomes
(1) Maintain arousal in environment with increasing consistency
(2) Demonstrate attention to self and environment
(3) Attend to tasks even when distracted
(4) Complete tasks with increasing accuracy
(5) Follow increasingly complex directions

c. Nursing interventions
(1) Minimize external distractions such as movement, noise, and visual input, e.g., assess housekeeping schedules
(2) Maintain consistent staff, caregivers, and schedule
(3) Limit presentation of competing stimuli
(4) Keep verbal information simple and allow time for delayed response
(5) To minimize confusion, structure daily schedule to allow time for rest and activity
(6) Utilize and encourage familiar and overlearned behaviors
(7) Provide sensory stimulation program
(a) Principles of stimulation techniques not established by scientific investigation

(b) Control environment with least amount of distraction
(c) Apply stimuli, one at a time, and observe response; if response is seen, try to elicit same response with different modality
(d) Ask for and demonstrate desired response, e.g., stick out your tongue
(e) Sessions should be brief
(f) With family, identify stimuli that have emotional significance for patient, and encourage family members to use stimuli to elicit patient's response, e.g., tape recorded messages, cologne, or music
(g) Attempt to stimulate all five senses
(h) Once consistent responses appear, direct program toward establishing a communication system

(8) Assess medications for potential sedative effects; collaborate with physician to eliminate or replace those medications, if possible
(9) Provide adequate sleep/wake schedules; individualize schedules to consider patient's unique pattern and need for rest
(10) Introduce background stimuli gradually during task performance
(11) When distractions occur, redirect patient's attention back to task by visually and verbally refocusing patient's attention on nurse and task

9. Altered thought process: agitation/irritability related to head injury

a. Characteristics include outbursts from overstimulation, fear, or confusion; patient can become verbally or physically combative or assaultive
b. Expected patient/family outcomes
(1) Maintain safety in environment
(2) Outbursts decrease in frequency; patient remains calm
c. Nursing interventions
(1) Maintain quiet, calm environment
(2) Utilize orientation interventions
(3) Give calm, controlled, and firm redirection
(4) Utilize one-to-one staffing
(5) Identify activities that precipitate outbursts, fear, or confusion
(6) Redirect patient to familiar tasks that are nonthreatening
(7) Immediately reward patient with praise as outbursts diminish
(8) Use nonthreatening verbal and body language
(9) Use minimum of physical restraints
(10) Encourage patient to move as much as possible within controlled boundaries, e.g., Craig bed, floor mats, a quiet room
(11) Limit use of chemical restraints and medications that alter cognition
(12) Move patient around facility as little as possible
(13) Progress therapy from patient's room, to quiet room, to treatment area
(14) Model quiet, controlled behavior

10. Altered thought process: memory deficit related to head trauma

a. Types of memory deficits (15)
(1) Impaired memory related to attention deficit—difficulty with focused, sustained, selective, alternating, and divided attention; related to brain stem dysfunction, diffuse bilateral depression of subcortical mechanisms, thalamic or frontal areas
(2) Impaired memory secondary to encoding—difficulty integrating language processing and visual processing; confused about words, difficulty with organization, and categorization

(3) Impaired memory related to storage—immediate and short-term memory present; long-term memory impaired as a result of hippocampal injury, anoxia, or herpes encephalitis
(4) Impaired memory related to retrieval—difficulty with retrieving stored information; can remember better with cues

b. Expected patient/family outcomes
(1) Demonstrate improved memory using less cues
(2) Use strategies recommended by the therapy team

c. Nursing interventions
(1) Use lists and strategies recommended by therapy team and assist patient to practice activities
(2) Implement role-play activities with patient and use listed steps for daily living tasks
(3) Use internal memory guides such as mnemonic strategies, visual imagery, anchor words, and other verbal associations; not necessarily effective for memory disorders related to head injury (16)
(4) Use simple memory devices—alarms, calendars, buzzers, and watches
(5) Use environmental modifications—posted reminders on mirrors, labeled shelves, alphabetized cupboards
(6) Use storage devices—diaries, lists, notebooks, and computers
(7) Additional interventions (see E.8.c. and E.9.c.)

11. **Impaired verbal communication related to speech or language deficit, resulting from head trauma or artificial airway**

a. Expected patient/family outcomes
(1) Use words and sentence structures to convey ideas
(2) Follow simple commands
(3) Demonstrate increasing comprehension of ideas and words
(4) Convey needs to staff and family
(5) Use communication strategies effectively

b. Nursing interventions
(1) Anticipate patient's needs and develop a predictable, daily routine with patient
(2) Encourage patient to verbalize thoughts; establish simple means of communication with yes/no responses
(3) Use mouth-controlled device for cervical injury patients who have poor to absent arm function
(4) Use call system on which the patient can tap with intact muscles; use for patients with triceps function
(5) Keep verbalizations to patient simple and repeat words in a normal tone; simultaneously use gestures and verbalizations while communicating with patient
(6) Limit communication to one person speaking at a time
(7) Allow for processing time and delayed responses
(8) Verify accuracy of responses with family
(9) Provide alternative methods of communication—pad and paper, alphabet board, common pictures representing daily needs, and commercial communicators
(10) Collaborate with speech therapist to develop additional interventions

12. **Visual perceptual deficit related to head trauma**
   a. Characteristics
      (1) Visual changes, including double vision, blurry vision, light sensitivity, and difficulty judging distances; visual-spatial confusion, slow visual-motor integration, and unilateral neglect
      (2) May see patient squinting, misjudging objects, making errors in reaching for items, running into walls, or falling
   b. Expected patient/family outcomes
      (1) Familiar and safe environment is provided
      (2) Use compensatory strategies effectively
   c. Nursing interventions
      (1) Assess visual acuity, visual field cuts, and extraocular movements
      (2) Encourage optometry/neuroophthalmology consultations to evaluate and prescribe glasses, patches, prism lenses, and/or fusion training
      (3) Encourage scanning activities, e.g., reading
      (4) Encourage optic activities that concentrate on tracking, focusing, and eye-hand coordination
      (5) Encourage use of affected side in activities
      (6) Emphasize input to affected side through visual and tactile cuing
      (7) Encourage practice of bimanual activities
      (8) Stress and teach the family safety techniques related to deficits in patient's visual perception
      (9) Encourage and recommend leisure activities that utilize compensatory strategies
13. **Impaired swallowing related to dysphagia, resulting from impaired level of consciousness, oromotor deficits, or bronchotracheal impairment**
   a. Expected patient/family outcomes
      (1) Maintain adequate nutritional intake
      (2) Demonstrate recommendations of therapy team, including use of positioning, seating, food choices, and eating sequences
      (3) Use most appropriate and safe route of nutrition
      (4) Experience no aspiration or choking
   b. Nursing interventions
      (1) Assess cranial nerves V, VII, IX, X, and XII
      (2) Assess cognitive status and level of alertness
      (3) Assess premorbid height, weight, and weight loss secondary to trauma
      (4) Assess seating and positioning for effective eating and swallowing
      (5) Assess dietary habits and regular 24-hour diet pattern
      (6) Assess ability to self-feed, swallow, and time needed for oral intake to satisfy caloric and fluid needs
      (7) Assess insurance and financial limitations, and patient's daily caloric needs for enteral or parenteral feeding program
      (8) Assess bowel and bladder alterations
      (9) Assess hyperglycemia, hypoglycemia, diarrhea, nausea, vomiting, and cramping
      (10) Assess rate and type of enteral feeding related to above side effects
      (11) Make referrals to dietitian and occupational and speech therapists
      (12) Assist in choosing alternate methods of feeding patient, including venous access, enteral, or nasogastric tube

(13) Review lab values—creatine excretion, serum albumin, total lymphocyte count, serum transferrin, and total protein
(14) Weigh patient weekly and document; if in wheelchair, make sure chair weight is constant week to week
(15) Assess patient's level of activity and disability, and inform dietitian to assess caloric needs accurately
(16) Maintain good oral hygiene
(17) Utilize techniques for positioning, seating, swallowing strategies, and feeding devices prescribed by the team
(18) Maintain intake/output and caloric records as needed
(19) Allow adequate time for eating and provide appropriate environment

14. **Additional nursing diagnoses in acute phase**
a. Potential impairment in circulation—deep vein thrombosis (see Module 16—Medical Sequelae)
b. Dysreflexia related to impaired regulation of the autonomic nervous system, after injury to the spinal cord above T7, or head injury (see Module 21—Spinal Cord Injury)
c. Altered thought process—orientation deficit related to head injury (see Module 20—Head Injury)

F. NURSING DIAGNOSES, EXPECTED OUTCOMES, AND INTERVENTIONS DURING CONVALESCENCE

1. **Potential for activity of daily living deficit related to functional losses**
a. Expected patient/family outcomes
(1) Participate in daily living activities as functionally and cognitively able
(2) Assume roles and functions within home and community at functional capacity
(3) Perform daily living tasks safely
(4) Demonstrate energy conservation and work simplification
(5) Incorporate physical routines into daily schedule
b. Nursing interventions
(1) Collaborate with therapists to carry over activity program
(2) Allow time for, and encourage use of, daily living skills
(3) Work with patient to provide rest periods and conserve energy during daily tasks; teach pacing of activities
(4) Encourage use of adaptive equipment
(5) Provide verbal cues and modeling, as needed
(6) Provide written instructions and sequences, as necessary

2. **Alteration in physical mobility related to functional changes and losses**
a. Expected patient/family outcomes
(1) Mobilize as functionally and cognitively able
(2) Safely perform mobility tasks
(3) Conserve energy while mobile

b. Nursing interventions
   (1) Explain the importance of using muscles and mobilizing extremities
   (2) Incorporate ROM, active or passive, into patient's daily routine
   (3) Work with therapists to incorporate exercise routine into functional activities
   (4) Medicate p.r.n. for pain before mobilization activities
   (5) Encourage pacing of activities
   (6) Assist patient with activities recommended by therapists, including wheelchair mobility, transfers, ambulation, and bimanual activities

3. Potential sexual dysfunction related to sensory and motor deficits, autonomic dysfunctions, hormonal dysfunction, disfigurement, cognitive, and psychosocial sequelae of traumatic injury

a. Expected patient/family outcomes
   (1) Describe changes in sexual functioning and sexuality resulting from disability, and identify methods to remain sexually active
   (2) Describe medication side effects that may interfere with sexual function or sexuality

b. Nursing interventions
   (1) Assess preinjury knowledge and attitudes of patient regarding sexuality and sexual function
   (2) Discuss available resources that address issues and concerns regarding sexual function
   (3) Assist the patient/significant other in problem solving, including management of bowel and bladder, spasticity, positioning, conception, and birth control
   (4) Provide information regarding normal structure and function of sexual organs
   (5) Describe alterations in patient's sexual response following a disability
   (6) Assist in identifying alternate types of sexual expression and options that may provide sexual satisfaction
   (7) Discuss alterations in roles related to sexuality, including the lover/caretaker and spouse

4. Potential ineffective individual and/or family coping related to catastrophic disability and/or previous dysfunctional coping patterns

a. Expected patient/family outcomes
   (1) Demonstrate effective coping strategies during and after the crisis
   (2) Make decisions and solve problems related to self and premorbid roles
   (3) Increase socialization

b. Nursing interventions
   (1) Assess previous styles of coping with crises
   (2) Assess coping options available to patient and methods he/she is currently using
   (3) Assess and communicate, with family and therapy team, patient's perception of coping behaviors
   (4) Monitor effectiveness of coping behavior when assisting patient to deal with stress; if coping behaviors interfere or are ineffective, plan alternative approaches with the team
   (5) Identify community health services and outpatient resources available to patient and family
   (6) Discuss anticipated changes in home and family life with family and patient

(7) Role play and rehearse potential coping strategies with the patient
(8) Provide private time for patient and family

5. **Potential/actual disturbance in self-concept related to dependency, disability, helplessness, and changes in body image, self-esteem, role performance, and personal identity**

a. Expected patient/family outcomes
(1) Verbalize concerns regarding changed body image and functions
(2) Look at and touch body and discuss the changes
(3) Identify strengths and weaknesses about herself/himself
(4) Begin to participate in daily living skills and plan for future community reintegration

b. Nursing interventions
(1) Initiate early assessment of patient's self-concept and coping mechanisms; institute appropriate referrals for psychosocial counseling
(2) Encourage patient to view self in full-length mirror
(3) Encourage good hygiene, dressing, grooming, and care about appearance
(4) Encourage patient to touch affected limbs and participate in positioning, dressing, and bathing, if possible
(5) Encourage and allow choices in patient's daily schedule and care, as much as possible, setting limits as needed
(6) Provide positive feedback when patient attends to appearance, posture, dress, and grooming
(7) Discuss feelings of dependency and their effects on patient; help patient maintain control whenever possible
(8) Utilize peer counselors, when appropriate, to provide role models and give credibility to patient teaching
(9) Discuss changes in body appearance and patient's perception of body with patient, family, and friends
(10) Involve patient in decisionmaking and goal setting, e.g., negotiate aspects of personal care patient considers most important to maintain
(11) Encourage family to include patient in family decisions while he/she is hospitalized
(12) Encourage identification of strengths and weaknesses
(13) Encourage socialization and new recreational endeavors

6. **Additional nursing diagnoses in recovery phase**

a. Activity intolerance
b. Fatigue
c. Sleep pattern disturbance
d. Diversional activity deficit
e. Impaired home maintenance management
f. Altered health maintenance
g. Feeding self-care deficit
h. Bathing/hygiene self-care deficit
i. Dressing/grooming self-care deficit
j. Toileting self-care deficit
k. Impaired social interaction
l. Social isolation
m. Altered role performance

G. REINTEGRATION WITH SOCIETY

1. Discharge planning goals
a. Maximize functional capabilities and maintain health and wellness
b. Promote self-care or directed care through patient/family education
c. Promote and facilitate community reintegration at home, work, school, and during leisure activities

2. Discharge plan
a. Determined by goals and outcomes related to the disability
b. Trauma/rehabilitation team devises plan with patient and family
c. Depends on the resources available

3. Discharge planning process
a. Begins upon admission of patient with assessments by all team members
b. Identify patient's disposition, primary care provider, and resources for discharge upon admission, and continue to assess these areas throughout stay
c. Interdisciplinary team identifies individual goals with patient
d. Considerations for patient's disposition include current and projected financial resources and long-term financial needs
e. Predischarge family meeting includes patient, interdisciplinary team, responsible payer, vocational counselor, insurance case manager, workmen's compensation representative
  (1) Confirm primary caregivers
  (2) Ensure feasibility of disposition
  (3) Assess knowledge base of health care providers and managers
  (4) Identify accessible family physician
  (5) Identify medical equipment supplier and drugstore
  (6) Identify amount of professional and attendant care, and ongoing therapy needs
  (7) Discuss support issues for the family/patient
f. Review individual's access to community resources, including social and recreational outlets, and transportation
g. Identify and justify needs for home modifications, special or modified equipment, software, continuous home health care services, skilled or attendant care, and follow-up/therapy plan
h. Consider a therapeutic pass—medically approved leave, several hours to one weekend, to evaluate patient's and caregiver's skills, patient's functional capabilities at home, and assess family's ability to cope with lifestyle changes

4. Community care options
a. Home health care programs
b. Hired attendant care
c. Extended care facilities
d. Day hospital and respite programs
e. Transitional living programs
f. Sheltered employment centers

5. Durable medical equipment
a. Long lead time needed for most items to be delivered

b. Confirm and comply with insurance guidelines before order is placed to ensure payment
c. Consider need for service when identifying vendor
d. Consider durability when selecting item
e. Equipment and features
   (1) Wheelchair and seating equipment
   (2) Beds—all electric, side rails, hi-low, Trendelenburg, double or king, specialty types
   (3) Mattresses—water, gel, air, egg crate
   (4) Bath equipment—shower commode chair, commode chair, hand-held shower hose
   (5) Transfer devices—Hoyer lift, transfer board
   (6) Respiratory equipment—portable suction, portable ventilator
   (7) Medical equipment—glucometer, dialysis equipment

6. **Medical nondurable/disposable supplies**

a. Choose supplier/vendor with patient; consider service and reliability, delivery to client's home, financial payment plans, and cost of products
b. Plan delivery two to three days before discharge and at routine intervals; consider space needed to store supplies
c. Consider durable products vs disposable products for convenience and cost to patient

7. **Transportation**

a. Accessible transportation facilitates patient's reintegration into the community
b. Consider functional abilities of patient, destination and frequency of travel, ease of access, and cost
c. Before evaluating patient's ability to drive, consider
   (1) Access to automobile and current driver's license
   (2) Health status, including seizure disorders, functional abilities, cognitive abilities, reaction time, vision, and knowledge of the driving laws
   (3) Driver's evaluation may require written test of laws, assessment of reaction time, and adaptions for functional disabilities; may require road test to evaluate individual's ability
   (4) Evaluation may indicate need for driving lessons in adapted automobile
   (5) Customized van evaluation and prescription may be completed to recommend accessible features for use by disabled
   (6) Community transportation availability must be evaluated by rehabilitation team and application made to appropriate agency
   (7) Patient education may include community advanced wheelchair skills, outside ambulation, and car transfers
      (a) Curbs
      (b) Wheelies
      (c) Crossing streets
      (d) Uneven surfaces
      (e) Getting up after falling out of wheelchair
      (f) Car transfers; putting wheelchair in/out of car
      (g) Cognitively impaired patients may require topographical orientation, short- or long-term supervised transportation use, map reading, evaluation and instruction in crossing streets safely

8. **Vocational evaluation**
a. Evaluation completed by interdisciplinary team to develop realistic goals and plan
b. Considerations for reemployment
  (1) Availability of job
  (2) Appropriateness of job for patient
  (3) Financial considerations
  (4) Transportation availability to place of work
  (5) Functional, cognitive, and social skills required for job
  (6) Funding for vocational program
c. Vocational programs may include
  (1) Vocational evaluation
  (2) Work hardening
  (3) Work adjustment and skills training
  (4) Supported employment and job coaching
9. **Leisure time evaluation**
a. Consider community, patient desires and hobbies, previous values of leisure time, functional and cognitive abilities
b. Counseling and adaptive devices may facilitate the leisure choices
c. Adapted activities may include sports/wheelchair sports, games, recreational activities, volunteer work, travel, reading, and the arts

H. POSTINJURY ADJUSTMENT AND FOLLOW-UP

1. **Common feelings of patient postdischarge**
a. Discomfort with lack of structured routine at home vs hospital
b. Accentuated helplessness and dependency without hospital personnel
c. Activities at home and in community seem difficult and time-consuming due to less accessible environment
d. Socialization outside of the home seems overwhelmingly inaccessible, as it takes a long time to get ready
e. Planning for problems, accessible environments, and accessible, available transportation can be frustrating
f. Misses supportive atmosphere and relationships with hospital or rehabilitation center staff and peers
2. **Early home adjustments**
a. Modify home and rearrange furniture
b. Ensure correct equipment and software
c. Ensure proper schedule and proficiency of caretaker
d. Begin to relearn new roles and responsibilities
e. Establish realistic schedule, for all care and daily routines, that considers entire family
f. Begin planning community reintegration for patient or spouse/caregiver, if possible
g. Assess financial plans

3. **Ongoing issues of adjustment**
a. Role changes
b. Changes in financial status
c. Unrealistic expectations for the disabled individual
d. Overwhelming fatigue of all individuals in household
e. Sexuality—changes in expression and sexual function
   (1) Male may have alterations in erection, sensation, ejaculation, libido, fertility, and orgasmic response
   (2) Females may have alterations in libido, sensation, orgasmic response, and reproduction
f. Drug and alcohol abuse may occur after discharge because of lack of alternatives for leisure time, and for release of tension and frustration
g. Long-term characteristics of the brain-injured population
   (1) Diminished social perceptiveness without self-criticism
   (2) Diminished self-control and self-regulation
   (3) Emotional alterations, including apathy, silliness, lability, irritability, and altered sex drive
   (4) Inability to learn from social situations

4. **Follow-up care**
a. Lifetime system of care recommended for optimal functional outcomes with less complications and recurrent hospitalizations (17)
b. Appointment to evaluate interdisciplinary plan for patient/family problems
c. Patient evaluated at 1, 3, 6, and 12 months postdischarge, then annually, and more often, if necessary; evaluation done by physiatrist, nurse, and social worker; other team members are consulted, if necessary
d. Repeated neurologic, cognitive, and functional evaluations completed with outcomes and recommendations for the patient
e. Laboratory and diagnostic studies completed; include genitourinary workup for spinal cord patients and seizure medication prophylaxis for head injury patients
f. Interim visits provide ongoing triage of medical, psychosocial, vocational problems, patient teaching, and emergency recommendations

I. RESOURCE AGENCIES

1. **Funding agencies**
a. Veterans Administration
b. Office of Vocational Rehabilitation—state agency
c. Social Security office—local district office
d. Local church and community services—Jaycees, Jewish Federation, Catholic Services
e. City specialty program—attendant care
f. State insurance commission—used to advise and facilitate insurance payment process
g. Crime victims programs

2. Specialty organizations

a. Paralyzed Veterans of America, 7315 Wisconsin Ave., Suite 301-W, Washington, DC 20014
b. National Spinal Cord Injury Association, 149 California St., Newton, MA 02158
c. National Easter Seal Society, 2023 W. Ogden Ave., Chicago, IL 60612
d. American Foundation for the Blind, 15 W. 16th St., New York, NY 10011
e. National Head Injury Foundation, P.O. Box 567, Framingham, MA 01701

3. Recreational and vocational resources

a. President's Committee on Employment of Handicapped, 1111 20th St., Washington, DC 20210
b. State vocational office
c. Sheltered employment service
d. *Resource Guide to Literature on Barrier Free Environments* (2nd ed., 1980), Architectural and Transportation Barriers Compliance Board, U.S. Government Printing Office, Washington, DC 20402
e. Association of Handicapped Artists, 1134 Rand Building, Buffalo, NY 14203
f. National Wheelchair Athletic Association, 40–24 62nd St., Woodside, NY 11377
g. National Park Guide for Handicapped (#2405-0286), Superintendent of Documents, U.S. Government Printing Office, Washington, DC 20402

References

1. Stryker, R. (1977). *Rehabilitative aspects of acute and chronic nursing care* (2nd ed.). Philadelphia: W. B. Saunders Co.
2. King, R. B., & Dodas, S. (1980). Rehabilitation of the patient with a spinal cord injury. *Nursing Clinics of North America, 15*(2), 225–243.
3. Walsh, A. (Ed.). (1980). *The expanded role of the rehabilitation nurse.* Thorofare, NJ: Charles B. Slack, Inc.
4. Hickey, J. (1986). *The clinical practice of neurological and neurosurgical nursing* (2nd ed.). Philadelphia: W. B. Saunders Co.
5. Commission on Accreditation of Rehabilitation Facilities. (1987). *Standards manual for facilities serving people with disabilities.* Tucson, AZ: Author.
6. Mumma, C. M. (Ed.). (1987). *Rehabilitation nursing: Concepts and practice: A core curriculum* (2nd ed., pp. 125–126). Evanston, IL: Rehabilitation Nursing Foundation.
7. Bates, B. (1987). A *guide to physical examination and history taking* (4th ed.). Philadelphia: J. B. Lippincott Co.
8. Moskowitz, E., & McCann, C. (1987). Classification of disability in the chronically ill and aging. *Journal of Chronic Diseases, 5*(2), 342–346.
9. Jennett, B., & Teasdale, G. (1981). *Management of head injuries.* Philadelphia: F. A. Davis Co.
10. Professional Staff Association of Rancho Los Amigos. (1980). *Rehabilitation of the head injured adult: Comprehensive management.* Rancho Los Amigos, CA: Los Amigos Hospital, Inc.
11. Rappaport, M., Hall, K. M., Hopkins, K., Belleza, T., & Cope, D. N. (1982). Disability rating scale for severe head trauma: Coma to community. *Archives of Physical Medicine & Rehabilitation,* 63(3), 118–123.

12. Granger, C., Hamilton, B. B., & Sherwin, F. S. (1986). *Guide for the use of the uniform data system for medical rehabilitation.* Buffalo, NY: State University of Buffalo.
13. Sayles, S. M. (1981). *Rehabilitation nursing: Concepts and practice.* Evanston, IL: Rehabilitation Nursing Institute.
14. O'Sullivan, S., & Schmitz, T. (1988). *Physical rehabilitation: Assessment and treatment.* Philadelphia: F. A. Davis Co.
15. Mateer, K., & Scheberg, I. (1989). *Introduction to cognitive rehabilitation: Theory & practice.* New York: Guilford Press.
16. Glisky, E. L., & Schacter, D. L. (1986). Remediation of organic memory disorders: Current status and future prospects. *Journal of Head Trauma Rehabilitation, 1*(3), 54–63.
17. Cioschi, H., & Staas, W. E. (1987). Follow-up care. In L. E. Buchanan & D. A. Nawaczenski (Eds.), *Spinal cord injury: Concepts and management* (pp. 219–234). Baltimore: Williams & Wilkins.

Suggested Readings

Buchanan, L. E., & Nawaczenski, D. A. (Eds.). (1987). *Spinal cord injury: Concepts and management.* Baltimore: Williams & Wilkins.

Church, C. S. (1981). Social work involvement with families at the acute stage of spinal cord injury. *SCI Digest,* 3(4), 49–53.

Cioschi, H. M., & LaMantia, J. G. (1983, December). Selecting a wheelchair cushion. *RX Home Care,* pp. 33–38.

Fuhrer, M. (1987). *Rehabilitation outcomes and measures.* Baltimore: Brookes Publishing Co.

Goldimond, I. (1973). A diary of self-modification. *Psychology Today,* 7(6), 95–102.

Granger, C., & Gresham, G. (1984). *Functional assessment in rehabilitation medicine.* Baltimore: Williams & Wilkins.

Harvey, R. F., & Jellinek, H. M. (1983). Patient profiles: Utilization in functional performance assessment. *Archives of Physical Medicine and Rehabilitation,* 64(6), 268–271.

Jacobs, B. W., & LaMantia, J. G. (1982). Lifetime follow-up care. *SCI Digest,* 2(4), 51–55.

Lezak, M. D. (1978). Living with the characterologically altered brain injured patient. *Journal of Clinical Psychiatry,* 39(6), 592–597.

Lindeman, J. E. (1981). Spinal cord injury. *Psychological and behavioral aspects of physical disability.* New York: Plenum Press.

Martin, N., Holt, N., & Hicks, D. (1981). *Comprehensive rehabilitation.* New York: McGraw-Hill Book Co.

Matthews, P. J., Carlson, C. E. (1987). *SCI: A guide to rehabilitation nursing.* Rockville, MD: Aspen Publishers, Inc.

Pallett, P. J., & O'Brien, M. T. (1985). *Textbook of neurological nursing.* Boston: Little, Brown, & Co.

Peterson, C. R., Carnes, G. D., & Frank, R. G. (1980). Who's in charge here? The rehabilitation team: Anatomy, physiology and pathology. *SCI Digest,* 3(3), 3–8.

Rosenthal, M., Griffith, E. R., Bond, M. R., & Miller, J. D. (1983). *Rehabilitation of the head injured adult.* Philadelphia: F. A. Davis Co.

Schneider, F. J. (1986). *Stroke/head injury: A guide to functional outcomes in physical therapy management.* Rockville, MD: Aspen Publishers, Inc.

Shontz, F. C. (1970). Physical disability and personality: Theory and recent research. *Psychological Aspects of Disability, 17,* 51–69.

Siev, E., Frieshtat, B., & Zolta, B. (1986). *Perceptual and cognitive dysfunction in the adult stroke patient.* Norwalk, CT: Appleton-Century-Crofts.

Treischmann, R. B. (1980). *Spinal cord injuries: Psychological, social and vocational adjustment.* Elmsford, NY: Pergamon Press.

Whiteneck, K. G., Adler, C., & Carter, R. E. (1989). *The management of high quadriplegia.* New York: Demos Publications.

Whyte, J., & Glenn, M. B. (1986). The care and rehabilitation of the patient in a persistent vegetative state. *Head Trauma Rehabilitation, 1*(1), 39–53.

MODULE 18
ORGAN AND TISSUE DONATION

Laura Coates Hammond, MSN, RN, CCRN

Objectives

1.0 Identify the scope of organ and tissue donation.
1.1 Identify the current need for organ donation.
1.2 Describe why potential donors are not recognized.
1.3 List the organs and tissues that can be donated.
2.0 Define the process of evaluation of the organ/tissue donor.
2.1 Describe the role of the nurse in the evaluation process.
2.2 Describe the role of the transplant coordinator in the evaluation process.
2.3 Define the specific criteria for each organ/tissue donated.
2.4 List the laboratory/diagnostic tests that are performed.
3.0 Identify the impact of required request legislation.
3.1 Define the difference between required request and routine inquiry.
3.2 Describe the goal of this legislation.
4.0 Describe the physiological changes associated with brain death.
4.1 List causes associated with the development of brain death.
4.2 Define the Monro-Kellie doctrine and its significance to brain death.
4.3 Describe the brain's response to increased intracranial pressure.
5.0 Identify the current standard criteria used for defining brain death in adults and children.
5.1 Describe the significance of the Uniform Determination of Death Act.
5.2 Identify potential complicating conditions that may arise in the diagnosis of brain death.

5.3 Identify corroborative tests that may be utilized.
5.4 Describe the differences in the determination of brain death in adults and children.
6.0 Define the role of the nurse in recognizing and assessing brain death.
7.0 Develop nursing diagnoses based on assessment data.
7.1 List the common nursing diagnoses related to brain death.
7.2 Identify signs and symptoms that validate the specific nursing diagnoses.
8.0 Identify nursing interventions required for the patient with brain death.
8.1 Relate interventions to specific nursing diagnoses.
8.2 Identify rationale for nursing interventions.
8.3 Given a patient scenario, prioritize the nursing interventions.
9.0 Identify nursing interventions required for the family of a patient diagnosed as brain dead.
9.1 Relate interventions to specific nursing diagnoses.
9.2 Identify rationale for nursing interventions.
10.0 Evaluate patient and family responses to medical and nursing interventions.
10.1 Define desirable outcomes for the patient diagnosed as brain dead.
10.2 Define desirable outcomes for the family of the patient diagnosed as brain dead.
10.3 List types of data to be included in nursing documentation.
11.0 Develop nursing diagnoses for the management of the organ donor.
11.1 List common nursing diagnoses related to maintaining organ function.
11.2 Identify specific etiological factors related to each diagnosis.
11.3 Identify signs and symptoms that validate the nursing diagnoses.
12.0 Identify the nursing interventions required for the organ donor.
12.1 Related interventions to specific nursing diagnoses.
12.2 Identify the rationale for nursing interventions.
13.0 Evaluate the organ donor's response to medical and nursing interventions.
13.1 Define the outcomes for the organ donor.
13.2 List the measurable criteria for each outcome.
13.3 List types of data to be included in nursing documentation.
14.0 Identify nursing interventions required for the family of the organ donor.
14.1 Relate interventions to specific nursing diagnoses.
14.2 Identify rationale for nursing interventions.
15.0 Evaluate the family's response to medical and nursing interventions.
15.1 List the desired outcomes for the family.
15.2 List the measurable criteria for each outcome.

A. ORGAN/TISSUE DONATION

1. **Defined as transplantation of organs or tissues from one person to another**

a. Initially considered experimental, but acceptance gained with the improved success rate associated with the use of antirejection drugs

b. Technology for transplantation has improved greatly and has gained credibility because a better quality of life, or life itself, has been provided for many

2. **Need**
a. The greatest need is for kidneys, with approximately 8000 people a year waiting for kidney transplant; waiting list also exists for all other organs
b. Approximately 20,000 people per year become potential organ donors; only 15% actually donate
3. **Why potential donors are not recognized**
a. Medical and nursing staff are uninformed about medical criteria necessary for donation
b. Staff dislike discussing matter with family at a time of intense grief; many feel it creates an added grief
c. Lack of knowledge about procedures for contacting an organ procurement agency
d. Difficulty in perceiving patient as an "organ donor"
e. Lack of time due to critical condition of the patient
f. Concerns about legal aspects
4. **Organs and tissues that can be donated are limited only by the technology, transplant techniques, and survival rates**
a. Tissues—corneas, bone, skin, and heart valves (see Table 18.1)
b. Organs—heart, heart and lung, lung, kidney, liver and pancreas (see Table 18.2)
5. **Required request legislation**
a. Initiated as federal legislation in 1986 to increase public awareness about the benefits and options of organ and tissue donation
b. A result of the rapid growth in organ transplantation and the scarcity of donors
c. A part of state legislation in 47 out of 50 states
d. Law incorporates "routine inquiry" or "required request" language

Table 18.1

Tissue donation for transplant purposes. Reprinted with permission of John R. Kately, Michigan Tissue Bank; revised with assistance of Delaware Valley Transplant Program.

Tissue	*Age Limit**	*Removal Time Limit*	*Exclusion for Transplant*	*Benefit*
Bone	5–65	24 hrs	Cancer and infection at time of death	Used for spinal fusion and neurosurgical repair
Eye	none	6 hrs	Infection at time of death	Used for corneal transplant
Skin	15–65	24 hrs	Cancer and infection at time of death	Used as dressing for patients with extensive full-thickness burns
Heart valves	0–55	12 hrs	Cancer and infection at time of death; existing severe cardiac disease	Aortic and pulmonary valves used for cardiac replacement surgery

*Note: Age limits are approximate; medical suitability will be determined by the procurement organization. Full-term newborn = 0 years.

Table 18.2

Organ donation for transplant purposes. Reprinted with permission of John R. Kately, Michigan Tissue Bank; revised with assistance of Delaware Valley Transplant Program.

Organ	*Age Limit**	*Exclusion for Transplant*	*Benefit*	*Miscellaneous*
Kidney	0–65	Metastatic cancer and infection at time of death; prolonged untreated hypertension; existing renal disease	For treatment of patients with end-stage renal disease (patients on dialysis)	Donor and recipient must have compatible blood and tissue type
Liver	0–60	Cancer and infection at time of death	For treatment of patients with end-stage liver disease with a life expectancy of less than one year	Donor and recipient must match for weight and size and must have compatible blood type
Heart	0–60	Cancer and infection at time of death	For treatment of patients with end-stage heart disease, usually with survival potential of a few months to one year	Donor and recipient must match for weight and size and have compatible blood and tissue type
Heart-lung	0–60	Cancer and infection at time of death	For treatment of patients with end-stage heart disease with pulmonary complications	Donor and recipient must match for weight and size and have compatible blood and tissue type
Pancreas	5–60	Cancer and infection at time of death	For treatment of patients with long-term, insulin-dependent diabetes who are suffering from complications of diabetes	
Lung	0–60	Cancer and infection at time of death	For treatment of patients with end-stage pulmonary disease	

*Note: Age limits are approximate; medical suitability will be determined by procurement organization. Full-term newborn = 0 years.

(1) Routine inquiry requires hospitals to develop protocols to ensure that families of patients who die under conditions that would make them suitable candidates for organ donation are "offered the opportunity," or "informed of the option" of donation

(2) Required request uses stronger language; requires that the family of a potential donor actually be asked to donate organs

e. Goal of either is to provide families of all donor candidates the opportunity to make their own decisions about donation, rather than have the decision made for them because of lack of information

B. EVALUATION OF THE ORGAN DONOR

1. **All patients should be considered potential donors**
2. **Organs can be donated only in situations of brain death, since organs require maintenance of tissue perfusion through an intact cardiac and pulmonary status**
3. **Tissues can be donated in all instances of death**
4. **General considerations for organ donor**

a. Age of donor
b. Absence of infection and/or communicable disease
c. Absence of cancer, except primary brain tumor
d. Known past medical history, including history of diabetes mellitus and hypertension, or specific organ dysfunction, e.g., prior MI, renal insufficiency, etc.
e. Acceptable hemodynamic status and organ function

5. **Organ-specific criteria (refer to Table 18.2)**

a. Depending upon which organs will be transplanted, additional specific criteria will be evaluated
b. Specific age limits for various organs donated
c. Size and weight comparisons necessary for extrarenal organs

6. **Laboratory/diagnostic evaluation**

a. Serum BUN, creatinine, and urinalysis
b. Blood type
c. Urine culture and sensitivity
d. Blood cultures
e. Chest x-ray
f. Hepatitis studies
g. HIV and VDRL
h. Liver enzymes
i. Cardiac enzymes
j. Echocardiogram and ECG

7. **Time limitations**

a. Organs must be transplanted within a specific time period from the time of removal from the donor
b. Distance between donor and recipient hospital sites may preclude specific organ donation

C. BRAIN DEATH

1. **Definition: Irreversible condition in which there is cessation of function of the entire brain and brain stem**
2. **Causes**
 a. Trauma
 b. Anoxia, suffocation
 c. Near-drowning
 d. Intracerebral hemorrhage
 e. Cerebral tissue swelling
 f. Metabolic disturbances
 g. Drug overdose
3. **Pathophysiology**
 a. Anatomy
  (1) Skull is a fixed, rigid container housing the brain tissue
   (a) Skull cannot expand or contract with changes in cranial volume
   (b) Increased volume within in the skull causes a concomitant rise in intracranial pressure
  (2) Foramen magnum is the only opening in the skull
  (3) All blood supply to the brain is via carotid and vertebral arteries, which enter the skull through the foramen magnum along the brain stem
  (4) Components of the cranial vault
   (a) Brain tissue, approximately 87% of volume
   (b) Blood, approximately 3 to 4% of volume
   (c) Cerebrospinal fluid (CSF), 9 to 10% of volume
   (d) These three components normally account for 100% of the volume within the cranial vault
  (5) Monro-Kellie doctrine
   (a) If the volume of one component increases, there must be a reciprocal decrease in one or both of the other two components, or pressure rises in the skull
   (b) Increased volume within the skull causes a reciprocal increase in pressure
 b. Physiology
  (1) Causes of changes in cranial volume
   (a) Space-occupying lesion, e.g., blood clot or hemorrhage, tumor, abscess/empyema, or foreign body (bullet, skull fragments)
   (b) Hydrocephalus—increased cerebrospinal fluid
    i) Overproduction of CSF
    ii) Blockage of sinuses that drain CSF from the cranium
   (c) Tissue edema—retention of sodium and water in brain cells secondary to inflammation or injury
  (2) Increased intracranial pressure
   (a) As volume in the skull increases, pressure increases causing compression of all structures within the skull
   (b) Brain tissue shifts toward area of lesser pressure
   (c) An early sign of increased pressure is a shift of structures away from the site of lesion or injury; visualized on CAT scan

(d) As pressure builds, it is exerted through the opening in the skull, the foramen magnum, and the brain stem is compressed

(e) When pressure in the skull exceeds systemic pressure, blood cannot flow into the skull against the pressure gradient, causing cessation of cerebral blood flow

(f) Measured by a calculation of the cerebral perfusion pressure (CPP)

i) CPP = MAP − ICP

a) MAP is the mean arterial pressure calculated as

$$\text{MAP} = \text{diastolic pressure} + \frac{\text{systolic pressure} - \text{diastolic pressure}}{3}$$

b) ICP is the intracranial pressure as measured from a pressure monitoring device

ii) CPP reflects the difference between MAP and ICP; changes in either parameter will affect the CPP

iii) Normal CPP is greater than 60 mm Hg; less than 60 indicates inadequate blood flow to the brain, and, if sustained over a short period of time, causes cerebral cell death

(3) Herniation

(a) Shifting of cerebral structures as a result of increased pressure

(b) Initially, structures shift across the midline; called central herniation

(c) Subsequently, shifting occurs downward across the tentorium and onto the brain stem; called transtentorial herniation

4. Criteria for determining brain death

a. Harvard criteria (1)

(1) Established in 1968

(2) First standard for diagnosis of brain death

(3) Defined brain death when there was

(a) 24-hour persistence of deep coma

(b) Total areflexia

(c) Apnea

(d) Exclusion of sedative drug overdose

b. Guidelines for Determination of Death (2)

(1) Accepted as the current clinical standard

(2) Set forth by the President's Commission for the Study of Ethical Problems in Medicine and Biomedical and Behavioral Research, 1981

(3) An individual with irreversible cessation of all functions of the entire brain, including the brain stem, is dead

(a) Cessation is recognized when

i) Cerebral functions are absent

ii) Brain stem functions are absent, including pupillary, corneal, oculovestibular (calorics), oculocephalic (doll's eyes), and respiratory reflexes

iii) Peripheral nervous system activity and spinal cord reflexes may persist after death

(b) Irreversibility is recognized when

i) The cause of coma is established and accounts for the loss of brain function
ii) The possibility of recovery is excluded
iii) The cessation of all brain functions persists for an appropriate period of observation and/or trial of therapy (usually 6 to 24 hrs)

(c) Complicating conditions may invalidate the usual criteria and require special examinations to establish brain death
i) Shock
ii) Hypothermia
iii) Drug and metabolic intoxication
iv) Immaturity, especially children under five years of age

(d) Corroborative tests are used to support clinical diagnosis but are not diagnostic alone
i) EEG
a) An absence of recordable brain waves supports the diagnosis of brain death; called "electrocerebral silence," "isoelectric," or "flat line"
b) Focus of concern is the inability to obtain artifact-free tracing in a busy intensive care unit
c) Use caution when determining brain death in children, since there are studies demonstrating survival of the immature nervous system after significant periods of electrocerebral silence
d) Advantages are that the test is portable, available, and relatively reliable

ii) Cerebral blood flow studies
a) Demonstrate absence of cerebral blood flow above the cervical portion of the internal carotid artery
b) Used only for exceptional cases, i.e., children under five years and when etiology of brain death is unknown
c) Disadvantages include invasiveness of study and need to transport patient to radiology suite

iii) Radionuclide isotope perfusion scan demonstrates the same information as cerebral blood flow study, but is noninvasive and can be done at bedside

c. Criteria for determining brain death in children
(1) Use caution when applying brain death criteria to children, since their neurologic responses to stimuli are altered
(2) Absence of spontaneous movement and reflexes
(a) Brains of infants and children seem to have an increased resistance to hypoxemia, so apnea testing may be inconsistent or inconclusive
(b) Cases have been reported of children who have substantially recovered, even after they have exhibited unresponsiveness to neurologic examination for longer periods than expected
(3) Absence of cerebral function; cerebral blood flow studies are the most reliable indicator
(4) Time interval—period of observation for cessation of all brain function may be longer for children than adults; 24 to 72 hrs suggested
(5) Complicating conditions

(a) Shock
(b) Hypothermia—may be related to immature nervous system or externally caused hypothermia, e.g., cold-water near-drowning; must be corrected before brain death criteria can be fulfilled
(c) Drug and metabolic intoxication—the child's immature renal and hepatic system may prolong excretion of drugs and metabolites; serum levels should be measured prior to determination of brain death in the child, as well as the adult

5. **Uniform Determination of Death Act**
a. Prior to adoption of this statute, a state's common law defined death as the cessation of cardiac and respiratory function; it did not recognize brain death
b. Act established single standard for use by all physicians in determining death
c. Has not yet been adopted in all states
d. The act's expanded definition states: "An individual, who has sustained either 1) irreversible cessation of circulatory and respiratory function, or 2) irreversible cessation of all functions of the entire brain, is dead. A determination of death must be made in accordance with accepted medical standards." (3)

6. **Removal of ventilatory support**
a. Once the criteria for brain death have been met, the patient is pronounced dead and ventilatory support is discontinued, if the patient is not to be an organ donor
b. Family permission for removal of ventilatory support should not be solicited—the patient is dead
c. If organ donation is being pursued, all support systems, assessments, and documentation are maintained

7. **Nurse's role in determining brain death**
a. Assessment
(1) Recognition of causative factors and identification of those patients whose conditions may progress to brain death
(2) Loss of brain functioning may progress slowly over time and may not be consistent from one assessment to the next
(3) Careful documentation of assessment findings and/or trends is crucial
(4) Cerebral and brain stem function
(a) Determination of level of consciousness and highest level of response to stimuli
(b) Cephalic reflexes
i) Absence of cough, gag, swallowing reflexes
ii) Abscence of pupillary and corneal reflexes
iii) Absence of "doll's eyes" phenomenon
(c) Absence of spontaneous respirations
i) Initial assessment performed during suctioning of the endotracheal tube
ii) Confirmation with apnea test performed by physician—patient is ventilated with pure oxygen for 10 min, then the ventilator is disconnected, and the patient receives a passive flow of oxygen for an additional 10 min
iii) Close observation for any spontaneous respiratory activity
(d) Spinal reflexes may be present even with confirmed diagnosis of brain death

(5) Body temperature must be at least 97°F (37°C) to eliminate hypothermia as a complicating condition during brain death evaluation
(6) Family dynamics
  (a) Level of understanding of the concept of brain death
  (b) Role relationships among family members and to patient
  (c) Presence of effective or ineffective coping behaviors
  (d) Support systems available and utilized by family members
  (e) Ongoing assessment of family's needs to promote supportive environment

D. COORDINATION OF DONATION EFFORT

1. **Coordination of the donation and transplantation of organs is the responsibility of an organ procurement agency; the transplant coordinator is responsible for**
a. Evaluating the patient's suitability for donation
b. Establishing the need for specific organs through a national computer bank
c. Coordinating activities of single or multiple transplant teams
d. Consulting with family and staff to answer questions and obtain consent
e. Contacting local agencies if the case is under the jurisdiction of the medical examiner
f. Assisting medical and nursing staff with donor management
g. Providing resources for education of health care personnel about organ donation
2. **The organ procurement agency personnel are available 24 hrs a day; a national referral telephone number identifies the coordination agency for a specific area, 1-800-24-DONOR**

E. CARE OF THE ORGAN DONOR

1. **The goal is maintenance of optimal conditions for all body systems to promote as normal an environment as possible for organ retrieval**
2. **In general, maintenance of a donor for optimal kidney function will protect other organs as well**
3. **Nursing diagnoses, expected outcomes, and interventions**
a. Fluid volume deficit related to inadequate fluid resuscitation; therapeutic dehydration; large volume urinary losses from diabetes insipidus; third spacing of fluids
  (1) Expected outcomes
    (a) Urine output of 1.5 to 2.0 ml/kg/hr
    (b) Central venous pressure reading of 10 to 12 cm H_2O (adult)
    (c) Ability to decrease or discontinue vasopressor support
    (d) Maintenance of systolic BP at 100 mm Hg or higher

(2) Nursing interventions
   (a) Assess for source of hypovolemia
   (b) Monitor hemodynamic parameters hourly and note trends or deviations
      i) Cardiac rate and rhythm (continuously)
      ii) Arterial blood pressure
      iii) Central venous or pulmonary artery pressures if catheters in place
      iv) Fluid intake
      v) Urine output
   (c) Administer crystalloid and/or plasma volume expanders through large bore intravenous lines to restore normovolemia
   (d) Administer blood products when obvious bleeding is noted or hematocrit is low
   (e) Administer aqueous Pitressin by intravenous bolus, or by drip if diabetes insipidus (DI) develops
   (f) Replace large urine outputs from DI, milliliter for milliliter, on an hourly basis
   (g) Monitor electrolytes for development of hypokalemia or hypernatremia, and alter fluid administration to correct imbalances
   (h) Monitor urine-specific gravity hourly

b. Altered tissue perfusion related to fluid volume deficit, and/or failure of the vasomotor center of the brain to regulate sympathetic motor tone and effective vascular resistance
   (1) Expected outcomes
      (a) Maintenance of systolic BP at 100 mm Hg or higher
      (b) Normal arterial blood gas pH
      (c) Absence of cyanosis
      (d) Urine output of 1.5 to 2.0 ml/kg/hr
   (2) Nursing interventions
      (a) Monitor hemodynamic parameters hourly; note trends and deviations
      (b) Correct hypovolemia
      (c) Administer vasopressors if vasomotor tone is altered; dopamine is the agent of choice
      (d) Monitor ECG; correct cardiac dysrhythmias

c. Impaired gas exchange related to loss of cerebral control of respiratory mechanics; inadequate ventilatory settings; associated chest or lung trama; development of pneumonia, atelectasis, or pulmonary edema, which cause decreased compliance and/or increased airway pressures
   (1) Expected outcomes
      (a) Arterial blood gases remain stable
      (b) Arterial pH within normal limits
      (c) Prevention of atelectasis or pneumonia
   (2) Nursing interventions
      (a) Assess pulmonary parameters and status
         i) Auscultate lung fields
         ii) Monitor mechanical ventilator setting and alarm parameters
         iii) Monitor presence, color, and consistency of sputum
         iv) Arterial blood gas determinations
      (b) Identify mechanism of injury; maintain high index of suspicion for associated traumatic injuries

(c) Maintain airway patency utilizing sterile suctioning technique to remove secretions
(d) Reposition patient every two hours
(e) Obtain chest x-ray to determine proper endotracheal tube placement and change in pulmonary parenchymal status

d. Potential for infection related to invasive lines and/or mechanical ventilation
(1) Expected outcomes
(a) Temperature within normal limits
(b) Negative culture reports
(2) Nursing interventions
(a) Utilize aseptic technique for all dressing changes and pulmonary toilet
(b) Monitor temperature, WBC
(c) Obtain wound, urine, or sputum cultures for changes in drainage, presence of odor, symptomatology
(d) Obtain blood cultures when temperature spikes

e. Potential alteration in organ function related to inadequate tissue perfusion and oxygenation; alteration in electrolytes; presence of infection; cardiac dysrhythmias and arrest
(1) Expected outcome—early recognition of potentially dysfunctional organs
(2) Interventions
(a) Monitor specific laboratory/diagnostic tests to determine adequacy of organ function, i.e., liver function studies, ECG, echocardiogram, etc.
(b) Inform physician/transplant surgeon of indications of organ failure

F. CARE OF THE DONOR FAMILY

1. **Families often look for meaning in tragedy and death; organ donation may provide a feeling that the death will help someone else**
2. **Research**

a. One study shows that 80% of families who are approached are agreeable to organ donation (4)
b. 69% of families who donated felt donation was a source of comfort; 87% said they would donate again (5)

3. **Many families do not consider organ donation on their own and appreciate being offered the option by medical and nursing personnel**
4. **Nurse's role**

a. The nurse is the person with whom the family has the most contact and communication
b. The family views the nurse as a resource for information and interpretation of information
c. The nurse needs to evaluate his/her own feelings and attitudes toward organ donation to be a positive support to the family
(1) The nurse must understand and accept the concept of brain death
(2) The situation forces the nurse to cope with thoughts of his/her own mortality

(3) The nurse may feel frustrated at not being able to save the donor

d. Regardless of the other personnel involved, i.e., transplant coordinator, clergy, social worker, or physician, the nurse has the crucial role in supporting the family

e. The nurse can make the difference in the way the public perceives the concept of organ donation

5. Approaching the family

a. Determine who should take responsibility to approach the family

b. The requester should be comfortable with the task, clear about own feelings, and view donation as a positive option for the family

c. Investigate family dynamics
   (1) Identify the role of the patient in the family structure
   (2) Identify one family member who has emerged as spokesperson
   (3) Define who is legal next of kin
   (4) Identify relationships between family and friends

d. The discussion should take place in a private room with all family members and/or significant others present

e. Contact family's clergy, or other support systems, if family wishes

f. Assess family's understanding of patient status; what has been explained thus far

g. Clarify family's understanding of brain death

h. Allow time for family to process and accept the terminal diagnosis prior to discussion of organ donation

i. Elicit from family if patient expressed a wish to be an organ donor, i.e., signed an organ donor card

j. Ask if family is interested in more information on organ donation

k. Answer all of the family's questions honestly; questions frequently concern religious beliefs, confidentiality, time frame, effects on funeral arrangements, financial obligations, and information about the organ recipients

6. Nursing diagnoses, expected outcomes, and interventions

a. Anticipatory grieving of family related to pending loss of loved one
   (1) Expected outcomes
      (a) Family is aware of the grieving process
      (b) Family participates in decisionmaking
      (c) Family members express grief
      (d) Family members demonstrate positive coping behaviors
   (2) Nursing interventions
      (a) Allow frequent visitation
      (b) Explain brain death and organ donation procedures
      (c) Allow expression of grief emotions, e.g., anger, fear, guilt, etc.
      (d) Consult social worker, pastoral care counselor, transplant coordinator, etc.

b. Altered family process related to pending death
   (1) Expected outcome—family vocalizes what loss will mean
   (2) Nursing interventions (see interventions F. 6. a. (2))
      (a) Identify the role relationships of patient to family and how loss will affect members
      (b) Assist the family to identify its strengths

c. Family knowledge deficit related to brain death and organ donation
   (1) Expected outcomes
      (a) Family states understanding of brain death and organ donation process

(b) Family makes final decision about organ donation
(c) Family is comfortable with decision

(2) Nursing interventions
(a) Provide information at family's level of understanding
(b) Provide concise, consistent information
(c) Recognize family's inability to process all information, and repeat explanations frequently
(d) Keep family informed about testing procedures for brain death and implications of organ donation
(e) Allow family to ask questions
(f) Provide time for family to consult with transplant coordinator
(g) Allow time for private discussion among family members without the presence of health care providers
(h) Discuss all options available to family

References

1. Ad Hoc Committee of the Harvard Medical School. (1968). A definition of irreversible coma: Report of the Ad Hoc Committee of the Harvard Medical School to examine the definition of brain death. *Journal of the American Medical Association, 205*(6), 337–340.
2. Guidelines for the determination of death. (1981). Report of the medical consultants on the diagnosis of death to the President's Commission for the Study of Ethical Problems in Medicine and Biomedical and Behavioral Research. *Journal of the American Medical Association, 246*(19), 2184–2186.
3. McCabe, J. M. (1981). The new determination of death act. *American Bar Association Journal, 67*(11), 1476–1478.
4. Cox, J. (1986). Organ donation: The challenge for emergency nursing. *Journal of Emergency Nursing, 12*(4), 199–204.
5. Skelley, L. (1985). Practical issues in obtaining organs for transplant. *Law, Medicine & Health Care, 13*(1), 35–37.

Suggested Readings

American Hospital Association, American Medical Association, and United Network for Organ Sharing. (1988, September). *Required request legislation: A guide for hospitals on organ and tissue donation.* (Available from American Hospital Association, Chicago.)

Brent, N. J. (1983). Uniform determination of death act: Implications for nursing practice. *Journal of Neuroscience Nursing, 15*(5), 265–267.

Davis, K. M., & Lemke, D. (1987). Brain death: Nursing roles and responsibilities. *Journal of Neuroscience Nursing, 19*(1), 36–39.

Delaware Valley Transplant Program. *Organ procurement manual.* Philadelphia: Author.

Diggs, C. L. (1986). Recognition and nursing care of organ donors. *Journal of Emergency Nursing, 12*(4), 199–204.

Goldsmith, J., & Montefusco, C. (1986). Nursing care of the potential organ donor. *Critical Care Nurse, 5*(6), 22–29.

Hannegan, L. (1987). Brain death: Diagnosis and dilemma. *Critical Care Nurse Quarterly, 10*(3), 83–91.

Hart, D. (1986). Helping the family of the potential organ donor: Crisis intervention and decision making. *Journal of Emergency Nursing, 12*(4), 210–212.

Hazinski, M. F. (1987). Organ donation: What the new "required request" law means to you. *Pediatric Nursing, 13*(6), 415, 439.

Kozlowsi, L. (1988). Case study in identification and maintenance of an organ donor. *Heart and Lung, 17*(4), 366–371.

Malecki, M. (1987). A personal perspective: Working with families who donate organs and tissues. *AD Nurse, 2*(4), 12–14.

Skelley, L. (Ed.). (1989). Organ and tissue transplantation. *Nursing Clinics of North America, 24*(4).

Slemenda, M. B. (1983). Brain death determination and management in children. *Critical Care Nurse.* 3(3), 63–66.

Stark, J., Reilly, P., Osiecki, A., & Cook, L. (1984). Attitudes affecting organ donation in the intensive care unit. *Heart and Lung, 13*(4), 400–404.

Stephenson, C. (1987). Brain death in children: Is there a difference? *Focus on Critical Care, 14*(1), 49–56.

Strange, J M., (Ed.). (1987). *Shock trauma care plans.* Springhouse, PA: Springhouse Corp.

Weber, P. (1985). The human connection: The role of the nurse in organ donation. *Journal of Neuroscience Nursing, 17*(2), 119–122.

Section IV
Systematic Approach to Trauma Nursing

MODULE 19
NURSING ASSESSMENT

Barbara Wakefield Esposito, RN, CEN

Objectives

1.0 Describe types of information obtained in the interview process.
1.1 List sources commonly used to provide patient history and an account of the traumatic event.
1.2 Identify information required for the patient data base, including injury scenario, presenting problem, and past health history.
1.3 Describe important subjective information that may be helpful in assessment of the patient.
1.4 Identify aspects of the family history that should be included in the data base.
2.0 Describe the sequence of physical assessment.
2.1 Identify steps and purposes of the primary survey to diagnose and manage life-threating injuries.
2.2 List important items in the initial examination which differentiate between normal/acceptable and life-threatening conditions.
2.3 Briefly list major types of life-threatening injuries that require immediate intervention.
2.4 List common nursing diagnoses related to life-threatening injuries.
2.5 Anticipate, prioritize, and assist with appropriate medical-surgical interventions.
2.6 Identify data obtained to complete the secondary survey.
3.0 Describe diagnostic studies obtained during the initial phase of treatment.
3.1 List laboratory studies commonly ordered.
3.2 List radiologic studies obtained for definitive diagnosis.

3.3 Identify special procedures utilized for definitive diagnosis.
4.0 Describe important elements in monitoring the response to resuscitation.
4.1 Identify medical and nursing interventions based on actual/potential injuries.
4.2 Evaluate patient response to medical and nursing interventions.
4.3 Define desirable outcomes for the resuscitation.
4.4 List measurable criteria for each outcome.
4.5 List types of data to be included in nursing documentation.
5.0 Describe preparation for transfer to definitive care.
5.1 List additional medical and nursing interventions that may be required to complete the initial phase of treatment.
5.2 Identify types of information that must be provided to the receiving inpatient unit.
5.3 Identify types of information that must be provided to the receiving hospital for intrahospital transfer.

A. INTERVIEW PROCESS

1. Patient history

a. Source
  (1) Patient
  (2) Family, significant others
  (3) Prehospital personnel
  (4) Bystander(s)
  (5) Personal belongings—wallet, medic alert cards, jewelry

b. Injury scenario and mechanism of injury
  (1) Motor vehicle accident
    (a) Type of vehicle
    (b) Collision speed
    (c) Type of collision; direction of force
    (d) Use of safety restraint, helmet, air bag
    (e) Ejection from vehicle
    (f) Position in vehicle before and after collision
  (2) Fall
    (a) Precipitating event
    (b) Distance of fall
    (c) Position of landing
    (d) Type of surface
  (3) Struck by blunt object
    (a) Precipitating agent
    (b) Impact force
    (c) Body area involved
  (4) Penetrating wound
    (a) Precipitating agent
    (b) Velocity
    (c) Estimated depth of penetration

(d) Entry site, angle
(e) Position of assailant
(5) Thermal wound
(a) Precipitating agent
i) Heat
ii) Chemical
iii) Electrical—power source
iv) Radiation
v) Cold—frostbite, hypothermia
(b) Length of exposure
(6) Other
(a) Abuse—child, adult, elder, sexual; injury pattern inconsistent with stated mechanism
(b) Alleged perpetrator

c. Presenting problem as stated by patient, prehospital personnel, or significant other
d. Past health history—A M P L E
(1) A—allergy(ies)
(2) M—current medication(s)
(3) P—past illnesses, medical history
(a) Comorbid conditions
i) Respiratory disease, smoking history
ii) Cardiovascular disease
iii) Endocrine disease
iv) Neurological disease
v) Splenectomy
vi) Other
(b) Tetanus immunization
(c) Previous/current infectious disease or I.V. substance abuse
(d) Female—date of last menstrual period; whether sexually active
(4) L—time of last meal; liquid ingested
(5) E—events preceding injury; time of injury
(6) Weight, height
(7) Place of occurrence

e. Routine demographic and financial data for institutional admission

2. Other subjective data

a. Pain
(1) Location
(2) Intensity, using a 1-to-10 scale
(3) Quality
(4) Radiation
(5) Precipitating factor(s)
(6) Relieved by

b. Nausea, vomiting
c. Dyspnea, dysphagia

3. Family/social history

a. Occupation
b. Marital status; number of children

c. Religion
d. Extended family; other support persons
e. Role in family structure
f. Financial concerns

B. PHYSICAL ASSESSMENT

1. Primary: rapid assessment to simultaneously identify and intervene in life-threatening injuries—A, B, C, D, E

a. Airway maintenance and cervical spine control
  (1) Airway assessment
    (a) Patent airway
      i) Patient speaks or makes sounds appropriate for age
      ii) Chest rises and falls easily with respirations/positive pressure ventilation
      iii) Foreign material not visible in upper airway
    (b) Compromised/obstructed airway
      i) Unable to speak or make sounds appropriate for age
      ii) Substernal/intercostal retractions
      iii) Inspiratory/expiratory stridor
      iv) Delayed capillary refill; cyanosis, especially in mucous membranes
      v) Nasal flaring in infants
      vi) Altered level of consciousness
      vii) Apnea, agonal respirations
  (2) Etiology of airway obstruction
    (a) Tongue
    (b) Secretions
    (c) Vomitus
    (d) Blood
    (e) Teeth, dental plate
    (f) Foreign debris
    (g) Edema
    (h) Airway injury
    (i) Facial injury
    (j) Inhalation injury
  (3) Cervical spine **must** be stabilized during airway intervention(s) by most effective means—manual in-line stabilization, cervical collar, sandbags, taping, other specialized immobilization devices
  (4) Potential nursing diagnosis and interventions in priority order—ineffective airway clearance
    (a) Chin lift/jaw thrust
    (b) Suction—rigid suction device, tonsil tip suction
    (c) Insert airway—oropharyngeal or nasopharyngeal
    (d) Prepare for and assist with orotracheal or nasotracheal intubation

(e) Prepare for and assist with surgical airway; inability to intubate is the only indication for this
i) Surgical cricothyroidotomy
ii) Tracheotomy
iii) Needle cricothyroidotomy; preferable for children under 12 years

b. Breathing and ventilation
(1) Assessment
(a) Normal/acceptable
i) Spontaneous, unlabored respirations
ii) Chest expansion equal bilaterally
iii) Breath sounds bilaterally
(b) Compromised
i) Apnea
ii) Respiratory rate less than 10/min; weak, shallow respirations
iii) Adult respiratory rate greater than 24/min; labored, retractions
iv) Pediatric—respiratory rate greater than parameters appropriate for age; labored, retractions, nasal flaring
v) Diminished or absent breath sounds
vi) Paradoxical respirations
vii) Unequal pulmonary excursion
viii) Cyanosis, especially mucous membranes
ix) Tracheal deviation
x) Distended neck veins
xi) Anxious, restless, confused, stuporous, or comatose
xii) External signs of trauma to chest, contusions, abrasions
xiii) Open chest wound
xiv) Subcutaneous emphysema
(2) Life-threatening conditions that impair adequate ventilation must be treated at time of diagnosis
(a) Tension pneumothorax
(b) Large flail segment with pulmonary contusion
(c) Open pneumothorax
(d) Occasionally, massive hemothorax
(3) Potential nursing diagnoses and interventions
(a) Ineffective breathing pattern
i) Provide supplementary oxygen to ensure adequate volume and FiO_2 greater than 85%; use bag-valve mask device, nonrebreather face mask, or nasal prongs
ii) Prepare for and assist with needle thoracostomy or tube thoracostomy
iii) Cover open chest wound with three-sided occlusive dressing; one side left open to act as flutter valve
iv) Intubate patient and provide mechanical ventilation as needed
(b) Ineffective gas exchange
i) Provide supplementary oxygen to ensure adequate volume and FiO_2 greater than 85%; use bag-valve mask device, nonrebreather face mask, or nasal prongs
ii) Reassess for tension pneumothorax
iii) Intubate patient and provide mechanical ventilation as needed

c. Circulation with hemorrhage control—blood volume, cardiac output
  (1) Assessment
    (a) Normal/acceptable
      i) Patient conscious; answers questions appropriately
      ii) Skin pink, warm, dry; capillary refill within two seconds
      iii) Full, slow, regular peripheral pulses
      iv) Pulse rate—adult rate above 50 and below 120 beats per minute (bpm); pediatric rate within parameters appropriate for age
      v) No obvious uncontrolled external bleeding
    (b) Compromised/potentially compromised
      i) Altered level of mentation/consciousness
      ii) Skin pale, cool, diaphoretic
      iii) Capillary refill greater than two seconds
      iv) Pulse
        a) Adult rate less than 50 and greater than 120 bpm; pediatric rate above or below parameters appropriate for age
        b) Thready, irregular central pulse unobtainable at more than one site
      v) Systolic blood pressure less than 90 mm Hg
      vi) External exsanguinating hemorrhage
  (2) Life-threatening conditions that impair circulation
    (a) Hypovolemia is the assumed etiology until proven otherwise
    (b) Pericardial tamponade
      i) Beck's triad—distended neck veins, systemic hypotension, muffled heart sounds
      ii) Narrowed pulse pressure
      iii) Elevated CVP
  (3) Potential nursing diagnoses and interventions
    (a) Fluid volume deficit secondary to hemorrhage
      i) Supplemental oxygen therapy as discussed in 1.b.—breathing
      ii) As appropriate for patient condition, establish large caliber I.V. catheters
        a) Minimum of two is recommended
        b) Draw blood for baseline laboratory studies
        c) Replace volume with warmed, balanced salt solution and, as necessary, blood or blood products
      iii) Control exsanguinating external hemorrhage
        a) Direct pressure
        b) Pneumatic splints are controversial
        c) Application and inflation of pneumatic antishock garment may control, or significantly reduce, abdominal or lower extremity hemorrhage; may use to splint lower extremity fractures
      iv) Apply ECG leads
      v) Monitor pulse
      vi) Prepare for autotransfusion
    (b) Decreased cardiac output secondary to compression of myocardium by blood accumulation in pericardial sac
      i) Consistent with injury, prepare for and assist with pericardiocentesis
      ii) Monitor for reaccumulation of tamponade

d. Disability—brief neurologic survey of level of consciousness and pupil response; more detailed assessment performed as part of secondary survey
   (1) AVPU—mnemonic designating level of consciousness in response to a stimulus
      (a) A = alert
      (b) V = verbal
      (c) P = pain
      (d) U = unconscious
   (2) Assessment
      (a) Normal/acceptable
         i) Alert; answers questions appropriately
         ii) Pupils equal; react to light
         iii) Appropriate motor and sensory response
      (b) Compromised/potentially compromised
         i) Unconscious; altered level of consciousness
         ii) Ipsilateral pupillary dilation; fixed pupils
         iii) Loss of, or decrease in, motor or sensory response
   (3) Potential nursing diagnosis and interventions—ineffective airway clearance related to loss of self-protective mechanisms
      (a) Open and maintain airway
      (b) Suction airway for secretions and debris
e. Exposure—patient must be completely undressed to facilitate thorough evaluation
f. Lifesaving interventions **must** be initiated when the problem is identified rather than at the end of the primary survey

2. **Secondary survey—complete head-to-toe examination; begun after completing primary survey and ensuring that resuscitation is in progress (resuscitation is addressed in part 3., below)**

a. Head
   (1) Check scalp for lacerations, contusions, swelling, other signs of trauma
   (2) Examine skull for depressions, deformities, penetrating wounds
      (a) Signs of basilar skull fracture
         i) Battle's sign—mastoid ecchymosis
            a) Delayed appearance of bruise behind ear at 24 to 72 hrs postinjury
            b) Etiology—fracture of basal portion of temporal bone
         ii) Raccoon's eyes—periorbital ecchymosis seen with fracture of orbital roof or anterior portion of cranial vault
   (3) Check for otorrhea, rhinorrhea, or blood draining from the nose and ears
   (4) Check pupils for size, reactivity, equality; inspect eyes and eyelids; note color of inner surfaces of eyelids
   (5) Palpate bony prominences of face for deformity; note contusions, lacerations, abrasions, areas of ecchymosis, entrance or exit wounds
   (6) Check mouth for blood, vomitus, loose teeth, dentures
b. Neck
   (1) Palpate carefully for tenderness over the cervical spine area
   (2) Maintain neck stabilization through methods previously mentioned, until adequate radiologic evaluation is completed
   (3) Evaluate for distended or flat neck veins and tracheal deviation

(4) Examine for contusions, abrasions, lacerations, swelling, ecchymosis, entrance or exit wounds, subcutaneous emphysema
(5) Note hoarseness

c. Chest
(1) Inspect for contusions, abrasions, lacerations, ecchymosis, penetrating wounds, impaled objects, sucking wounds
(2) Look for equal expansion; note paradoxical breathing
(3) Auscultate breath sounds and heart sounds
(4) Palpate clavicles, rib cage, sternum; note subcutaneous emphysema
(5) Evaluate cardiac rhythm

d. Abdomen
(1) Inspect for contusions, abrasions, lacerations, ecchymosis, penetrating wounds, impaled objects
(2) Auscultate for bowel sounds
(3) Perform light and deep palpation; note guarding, tenderness, rigidity

e. Pelvis—assess for fracture(s) by compressing iliac crests toward midline and rocking the pelvis

f. Genital area
(1) Inspect for obvious injuries
(2) Note external bleeding at meatus
(3) Inspect for scrotal hematoma
(4) Assist with rectal examination; a high-riding prostate is a contraindication to urinary catheter placement

g. Extremities
(1) Lower
(a) Inspect for swelling, deformity, dislocation, protruding bone, bleeding, obvious fracture
(b) Palpate for point tenderness
(c) Evaluate for neurovascular compromise
(d) Check pedal pulses bilaterally
(2) Upper
(a) Assess as in (a), (b), (c), above
(b) Check radial pulses bilaterally

h. Back—carefully logroll patient onto side, maintaining spinal alignment
(1) Inspect for contusions, abrasions, lacerations, ecchymosis, penetrating wounds, impaled objects
(2) Palpate for deformities and point tenderness over thoracic and lumbar spine

i. Neurologic
(1) Reevaluate level of consciousness using the Glasgow Coma Scale (1) (Table 19.1)
(2) A decreased level of consciousness since primary survey may indicate decreased cerebral oxygenation and/or perfusion; oxygenation, ventilation, and perfusion must be immediately reassessed
(3) Sensory loss
(4) Motor impairment
(5) Pupil reaction
(6) Potential for neurologic deterioration related to increased intracranial pressure, secondary to expanding, space-occupying lesions and cerebral edema

Table 19.1

Glasgow Coma Scale

Subscale	*Stimulus/Response*	*Points*
Eye Opening	Spontaneous	4
	To voice	3
	To pain	2
	No eye opening	1
Verbal	Converses—oriented	5
	Converses—disoriented	4
	Verbalizes	3
	Vocalizes	2
	No sound	1
Motor	Follows commands	6
	Localizes	5
	Withdraws from pain	4
	Flexion to pain—decorticate	3
	Extension to pain—decerebrate	2
	No movement	1
		Total Score 3 to 15

j. A more focused secondary survey may be done if patient presentation or exposure reveals localized injury

3. Resuscitation and monitoring for trends and changes—implemented with primary survey and ongoing throughout emergency department phase of treatment

a. Resuscitation
  (1) Continue initial interventions from the primary survey, i.e., maintain airway and breathing, and provide humidified oxygen
  (2) I.V. therapy and volume replacement
    (a) Urgency, number, and sizes of I.V. catheters depend on degree of shock and apparent rate of bleeding; suggested guidelines
      i) Hemodynamically stable with minimal injury—use one 16- or 18-gauge percutaneous catheter
      ii) Shock and significant injury—use a minimum of two 14- to 16-gauge percutaneous catheters
      iii) Profound shock and massive injuries—assist with placement of venous cutdowns at multiple sites
      iv) Subclavian or jugular lines not advised initially due to difficult access and potential complications
    (b) Fluid selection (see Module 10—Shock)
      i) Two to three liters warmed, balanced salt solution, e.g., lactated Ringer's solution
      ii) If no improvement in vital functions, blood therapy is initiated in the following order of preference
        a) Whole blood is best but generally not available

b) Use low titer, type O-negative red blood cells for women; either type O-negative or type O-positive for men, if unable to wait for type-specific blood
c) Type-specific red blood cells
d) Typed and cross-matched blood, if time permits

(3) Pneumatic antishock garment (PASG) applied and removed by physician order and protocol
  (a) Indications for use
    i) Inadequate response to fluid replacement
    ii) Hemostasis
    iii) Stabilization of pelvis and/or lower extremity fracture(s)
  (b) Generally contraindicated for patients with
    i) Bleeding thoracic wound
    ii) Impaled object in abdomen
    iii) Abdominal evisceration
    iv) Tension pneumothorax
    v) Pericardial tamponade
    vi) Controversial in head injury

(4) Insert urinary bladder catheter
  (a) For male patient, only after rectal examination by physician
  (b) Contraindicated if
    i) Blood at urethral meatus
    ii) Blood in scrotum
    iii) Prostate is high-riding or cannot be palpated

(5) Insert nasogastric tube—use orogastric tube for patient with potential cribriform plate fracture

(6) Prevent hypothermia
  (a) Warm I.V. solutions, blood products, and lavage solutions
  (b) Cover patient with warm blankets
  (c) Overhead warming lamps
  (d) Warm humidified oxygen

(7) Prepare for and assist with peritoneal lavage—quick diagnostic procedure to determine intraabdominal bleeding
  (a) Indicated when results of physical examination are equivocal or patient is unable to participate in abdominal evaluation
  (b) Nasogastric tube and urethral catheter must be placed prior to procedure
  (c) Warmed, balanced salt solution is used for irrigation fluid
  (d) Some physicians may prefer abdominal computerized axial tomography (CAT) scan for diagnosis rather than peritoneal lavage

b. Continuous monitoring for trends and changes or positive response to resuscitation
  (1) Normal/acceptable evaluation
    (a) Vital signs
      i) Heart rate greater than 60 bpm and less than 100 bpm
      ii) Systolic blood pressure greater than 90 mm Hg
      iii) Respiratory rate above 12 and below 24/min
    (b) Abscence of cardiac dysrhythmias
    (c) Neurologic status

i) Level of consciousness—no decrease in mentation
ii) Improvement or maintenance of Glasgow Coma Score, motor, or sensory level
iii) Pupils equal and reactive

(d) Temperature—normothermia
(e) Warm, dry skin; capillary refill less than or equal to two seconds
(f) Urine output greater than 0.5 to 1 ml/kg/hr
(g) Arterial pH above 7.30

(2) If positive responses are not demonstrated, notify physician and reevaluate plan of care
(3) Documentation on data flowsheet

i) Physiologic parameters
ii) Timed entries of treatment and responses to interventions
iii) Laboratory values

4. Diagnostic studies

a. Blood for trauma profile should be drawn when first I.V. catheter is placed

(1) Type and cross-match
(2) Complete blood count (CBC) with differential
(3) Glucose
(4) Blood urea nitrogen (BUN)
(5) Electrolytes
(6) Creatinine
(7) Amylase
(8) Toxicology, alcohol and drug levels, as indicated
(9) Coagulation studies

b. Other blood studies

(1) Human immunodeficiency virus (HIV) with patient consent
(2) Hepatitis profile
(3) Arterial blood gases

c. Urine for trauma profile—complete urinalysis, dipstick for blood, and toxicology, as indicated

d. Other specimens

(1) Peritoneal lavage fluid
(2) Other fluids, e.g., gastric

e. Radiologic studies

(1) Routine

(a) Cervical spine
(b) Chest
(c) Pelvis
(d) Others as appropriate for injury

(2) Special studies as indicated

(a) "One shot"—in resuscitation area or operating room, patient is injected with dye; one or two radiographs assist in diagnosis or determine function of renal system

i) Intravenous pyelogram (IVP) for possible kidney injury or kidney absence
ii) Cystogram for possible bladder injury
iii) Urethrogram for possible urethral injury

(b) Computerized axial tomography (CAT)
(c) Angiography
(d) Ultrasound
(e) Magnetic resonance imaging (MRI)

5. Prepare patient for transfer to definitive care

a. Assist with immobilization of fractures
b. Perform wound care consistent with protocol
c. Secure I.V. lines and all tubes
d. Provide continued oxygenation and ventilation
e. Administer medications as prescribed
  (1) Tetanus immunization
  (2) Antibiotics
  (3) Analgesics
  (4) Other
f. Ensure documentation is complete
  (1) All reports/results included
  (2) Intake/output totaled
g. In-house transfer
  (1) Provide operating room/inpatient receiving nurse with report of mechanism of injury, past health history, assessment, interventions, and response to interventions
  (2) Transfer patient to operating room/receiving inpatient unit with appropriate personnel and monitoring devices
h. External transfer
  (1) Provide flight nurse, mobile intensive care nurse (MICN), paramedic, or physician with report of mechanism of injury, past health history, assessment, interventions, and response to interventions
  (2) Copy and send all records and reports to receiving facility
  (3) Notify family of transfer
  (4) Assist with transfer of patient to transport vehicle with appropriate personnel and monitoring devices

Reference

1. Teasdale, G., & Jennett, B. (1974). Assessment of coma and impaired consciousness. *Lancet,* 2(13 July), 81–84.

Suggested Readings

American College of Surgeons Committee on Trauma. (1989). *Advanced trauma life support, student manual* Chicago: American College of Surgeons.

Beaver, B. M. (1990). Care of the multiple trauma victim: The first hour. *Nursing Clinics of North America,* 25(1), 11–22.

Cardona, V., Hurn, P., Mason, P., Scanlon/Schilpp, A., & Veise-Berry, S. (Eds.).

(1988). *Trauma nursing: From resuscitation through rehabilitation.* Philadelphia: W. B. Saunders Co.
Carpenito, L. (1987). *Nursing diagnosis: Application to clinical practice.* Philadelphia: J. B. Lippincott Co.
Hickey, J. V. (1986). *The clinical practice of neurological and neurosurgical nursing.* 2nd ed. Philadelphia: J. B. Lippincott Co.
Hoyt, K. S. (1986). Chest trauma assessment. *Trauma Quarterly,* 2(2), 1–8.
Joy, C. (Ed.). (1989). *Pediatric trauma nursing.* Rockville, MD: Aspen Publishers, Inc.
Kite, J. (1987). Cardiac and great vessel trauma: Assessment, pathophysiology, and intervention. *Journal of Emergency Nursing, 13*(6), 346–351.
McSwain, N., & Kerstein, M. (Eds.). (1987). *Evaluation and management of trauma.* Norwalk, CT: Appleton-Century-Crofts.
Maddox, K. L., Moore, E. E., & Feliciano, D. V. (Eds.). (1988). *Trauma.* East Norwalk, CT: Appleton & Lange.
Manley, L. K. (1987). Pediatric trauma: Initial assessment and management. *Journal of Emergency Nursing, 13*(2), 77–87.
Moorhouse, M., Geissler, A., & Doenges, M. (1987). *Critical care plans: Guidelines for patient care.* Philadelphia: F. A. Davis Co.
Pauley, S. Y. (1987). Massive hemorrhage in trauma. *Journal of the National Intravenous Therapy Association, 10*(6), 410–420.
Rea, R., Bourg, P., Parker, J., & Rushing, D. (1987). *Emergency nursing core curriculum.* Philadelphia: W. B. Saunders Co.
Sheehy, S., & Barber, J. (Eds.). (1985). *Emergency nursing: Principles and practice.* St. Louis: C. V. Mosby Co.
Strange, J. M. (Ed.). (1987). *Shock trauma care plans.* Springhouse, PA: Springhouse Corp.
Tyson, G. (1987). *Head injury management for providers of emergency care.* Baltimore: Williams & Wilkins.

MODULE 20
HEAD INJURY

Rae L. Conley, MSN, RN, CCRN

Prerequisite

Review neuroanatomy, neurophysiology, and the Monro-Kellie hypothesis.

Objectives

1.0 Describe common head injuries.
1.1 List major types of head injuries.
1.2 Briefly describe pathophysiology and major defining characteristics of each type of injury.
1.3 State frequent mechanisms of injury for each.
1.4 List diagnostic indicators helpful in discovering each injury.
2.0 Develop nursing diagnoses based on assessment data.
2.1 List common nursing diagnoses related to head trauma.
2.2 Identify specific etiologic factors related to each diagnosis.
2.3 Identify signs and symptoms that validate the specific nursing diagnoses.
3.0 Anticipate and assist with appropriate medical-surgical interventions for head injury.
3.1 Given specific patient data, recognize which medical-surgical interventions might be required.

3.2 Given specific patient data, state the equipment needed to assist with medical interventions.
3.3 Describe the pharmacologic agents most likely to be required for the patient with head injury and the rationale for each.
4.0 Identify nursing interventions required for the patient with head injury.
4.1 List common nursing interventions required in patients with head trauma.
4.2 Given a patient scenario, prioritize nursing interventions.
4.3 Relate interventions to specific nursing diagnoses.
4.4 Identify the rationale for nursing interventions.
5.0 Evaluate patient response to medical and nursing interventions.
5.1 Define desirable outcomes with specific, measurable criteria for the patient with head trauma.
5.2 List nursing activities required for continuous monitoring and evaluation of patient status.
5.3 List types of data to be included in nursing documentation.

A. PATTERNS OF INJURY IN HEAD TRAUMA: PATHOPHYSIOLOGY

1. Extracranial

a. Scalp injuries—may include abrasions, avulsions, burns, and lacerations (see Module 26—Integumentary and Soft Tissue Injury)
b. Skull fractures
   (1) Linear—an inbending of the skull at the point of injury with simultaneous outbending around the region of impact; most common type
      (a) Etiology—low-velocity blunt or compression trauma
      (b) Diagnostic indicators
         i) Standard skull film (SSF)
         ii) With linear fracture of the temporal bone, observe for signs and symptoms of epidural hematoma secondary to rupture and hemorrhage of the middle meningeal artery
   (2) Comminuted—a breakage of skull bone into multiple fragments
      (a) Etiology—moderate-velocity blunt or compression trauma
      (b) Diagnostic indicators include history of head trauma (HHT), SSF, and palpation of skull
   (3) Depressed—a fracture with an inward displacement of part of the skull
      (a) Etiology—usually associated with high-velocity blunt or compression trauma
      (b) Diagnostic indicators include HHT, SSF, and inspection and palpation of the skull
   (4) Compound or open—a combination of a depressed skull fracture and a scalp laceration; the dura may be torn
      (a) Etiology—blunt and/or penetrating trauma
      (b) Diagnostic indicators include SSF and inspection and palpation of the skull

(5) Basal—a fracture that involves the base of the skull, particularly the anterior and middle fossae; the dura is frequently torn
  (a) Etiology—blunt trauma to head, especially to the mandible, or when the vertebral column is driven against the occipital condyles, e.g., fall on the buttocks
  (b) Diagnostic indicators
    i) History of head trauma or fall on buttocks
    ii) SSF—not as reliable as with other skull fractures
    iii) Physical findings for anterior fossa fracture—e.g., fracture of the paranasal sinuses
      a) Rhinorrhea
      b) Epistaxis
      c) Visual defect—cranial nerve II
      d) Subconjunctival hemorrhage
      e) Anosmia—cranial nerve I
      f) Periorbital ecchymosis—raccoon's eyes
    iv) Middle and posterior fossae fractures associated with fracture of the temporal petrous bone; involves the middle ear
      a) Otorrhea
      b) Hemotympanum
      c) Conductive hearing loss—cranial nerve VIII
      d) Facial nerve palsy (Bell's palsy)—cranial nerve VII
      e) Ecchymosis over mastoid bone (Battle's sign)—24 to 36 hrs after injury

2. **Intracranial (for review of brain lobes, functions, and findings when injured, see Table 20.1)**

a. Parenchymal
  (1) Concussion
    (a) Mild concussion is defined as a temporary physiologic disturbance of neurologic function without loss of consciousness
    (b) Classical cerebral concussion is defined as a traumatic, reversible neurologic deficiency that results when there is temporary loss of consciousness, usually less than six hours, and some degree of retrograde and posttraumatic amnesia; often accompanied by subtle, residual neurologic impairments
    (c) Etiology—a strong, rapid acceleration-deceleration stimulus or a sudden sharp blow to the skull
    (d) Diagnostic indicators
      i) Nonspecific findings on neurologic examination
      ii) Postconcussion syndrome
        a) May be experienced for several weeks to one year after head injury
        b) Symptoms include headache, dizziness, nervousness and irritability, emotional lability, fatigability, insomnia, poor concentration and memory, difficulty with abstract thinking, difficulty with judgment, loss of inhibition, loss of libido, and avoidance of crowds
  (2) Contusion and laceration
    (a) A contusion is an actual bruising of brain tissue without puncture of the pial covering; found at the site of impact (coup), or in a line directly opposite the point of impact (contrecoup)

Table 20.1

Brain lobes and functions

Lobe	*Function*	*Finding When Injured*
Frontal	Primary motor cortex	Loss of movement on opposite side of the body
	Broca's speech center	Expressive aphasia
	Emotional expression and behavior	Quick mood changes; lack of inhibition regarding excretory, sexual, and social activities; easily distracted from intellectual pursuits
Parietal	Processing of sensory input	Loss of ability to localize a painful stimulus or measure the intensity of pain
	Stereognosis	Loss of ability to recognize the size, shape, texture, and consistency of common objects if touched
	Comprehension of the written word	Inability to understand what is read
	Two-point discrimination	Inability to distinguish between two simultaneous skin contacts
	Proprioception and position sense	Loss of awareness of body parts and their orientation in space
Temporal	Sound perception; determination of the source of sound and interpretation	Deafness; inability to recognize sounds
	Integration of the impulses from auditory, visual, and somatesthetic sources	Inability to understand the written and spoken word, and the use of language, in general
	Psychical cortex	Déjà vu experiences
Occipital	Visual cortex	Flash of light at the time of impact
	Visual associative areas	Inability to recognize or identify familiar objects

(b) Cerebral laceration is a traumatic tearing of the cortical surface of the brain

(c) Etiology—commonly found together beneath a depressed skull fracture and around penetrating injuries; can also occur with blunt head injuries

(d) Diagnostic indicators

i) Swelling and obvious laceration noted upon inspection and palpation

ii) Neurological examination may reveal a wide spectrum of neurologic deficits

iii) CAT scan; MRI

(3) Diffuse axonal injury (DAI)—a widespread disruption of neurologic function without any focal lesions noted; characterized by diffuse white matter degeneration, global neurologic dysfunction, and diffuse cerebral swelling

(a) Mild DAI (Grade 1)—abnormalities mainly restricted to the parasagittal white matter of the cerebral hemispheres; coma for 6 to 24 hrs

(b) Moderate DAI (Grade 2)—Grade 1 plus a focal lesion in the corpus callosum; coma for more than 24 hrs with little or no evidence of brain stem dysfunction
(c) Severe DAI (Grade 3)—abnormalities of the white matter of the cerebellum and the upper brain stem, and a greater degree of axonal hemispheric abnormalities than shown in Grades 1 or 2; coma for more than 24 hrs with consistent signs of brain stem dysfunction (1)
(d) Etiology—acceleration-deceleration movement to the brain, which causes a shearing injury to the axons
(e) Diagnostic indicators
  i) Depends on the severity of the DAI
  ii) Immediate, deep, prolonged coma lasting weeks to months, increased intracranial pressure, persistent brain stem reflexive decorticate or decerebrate posturing, hypertension, elevated temperature, hyperhidrosis
  iii) CAT scan shows characteristic small hemorrhagic lesions in the corpus callosum, superior cerebellar peduncles, or periventricular region
  iv) MRI

b. Hemorrhage
  (1) Epidural hematoma (EDH)
    (a) A collection of blood between the skull and dura; usually due to laceration of the middle meningeal artery associated with temporal bone fracture
    (b) Etiology—falls, direct blows to the head, MVC, sports injuries
    (c) Diagnostic indicators
      i) Progression of altered consciousness, e.g., momentary unconsciousness followed by a lucid period and return to unconsciousness; may rapidly progress from initial lucidity to drowsiness, confusion, and coma
      ii) Headache of increasing severity, possible seizures (Jacksonian or generalized) vomiting, ipsilateral or contralateral hemiparesis, dilated ipsilateral pupil that becomes fixed
      iii) SSF
      iv) CAT scan; MRI
  (2) Subdural hematoma (SDH)
    (a) A collection of blood between the dura mater and arachnoid layer of the meninges
      i) Classified as acute (within 48 hrs), subacute (2 to 14 days), and chronic (more than 14 days), depending on the time at which symptoms develop after injury
      ii) Hemorrhages of this type are usually venous, slower to develop than in EDH, and mostly unilateral
    (b) Etiology—MVC, industrial accidents, falls, assaults, and sports injuries; occur from frontal or occipital impact more often than from lateral impact
    (c) Diagnostic indicators
      i) Signs and symptoms
        a) Acute—headache, drowsiness, agitation, slow cerebration, confusion, ipsilateral dilated and fixed pupils, contralateral hemiparesis
        b) Subacute—similar to acute with failure to regain consciousness
        c) Chronic—headache that progresses in severity, slow cerebration, confusion, drowsiness, giddiness, possible seizure, papilledema, dilated ipsilateral pupil that is sluggish to light, ipsilateral or contralateral hemiparesis; hematoma may reaccumulate

ii) CAT scan; MRI
iii) Cerebral angiography
(3) Subarachnoid hemorrhage (SAH)
(a) A collection of blood located between the arachnoid mater and the pia mater
(b) Etiology—traumatic SAH is usually diffuse and does not form a definite hematoma; bleeding occurs from superficial cortical vessels and is associated with subdural hematoma
(c) Severe headache, deteriorating level of consciousness, nuchal rigidity, hemiparesis, ipsilateral dilated pupil
(d) NOTE: lumbar puncture should be avoided in patients with increased intracranial pressure because of risk of brain stem herniation; diagnosis is confused by blood in cerebral spinal fluid (CSF)
(4) Intracerebral hematoma—a deep contusion or tear in blood vessels that results in hemorrhage within the brain
(a) Etiology—single or multiple hematomas may occur from blows to the skull, rotational acceleration, missile-type injuries, and coup-contrecoup injuries; assocated with skull fractures, especially depressed fractures
(b) Diagnostic indicators
i) Headache, deteriorating consciousness to deep coma, hemiplegia on contralateral side, dilated pupil on the side with clot
ii) CAT scan; MRI
iii) Cerebral arteriogram
(5) Brain stem hemorrhage—bleeding into the midbrain, pons, or medulla
(a) Etiology
i) Primary—direct impact or torsion injuries of the brain stem
ii) Secondary—compression from increased intracranial pressure, cerebral edema, or laceration of temporal lobes
(b) Diagnostic indicators
i) Midbrain injury—deep coma, fixed pupils at midpoint or slightly wider, ophthalmoplegia, decerebration
ii) Pons injury—coma, small nonreactive pupils, ophthalmoplegia, decerebration
iii) CAT scan; MRI
c. Cranial nerve injury—injury to one or more of the 12 pairs of nerves that originate in the brain (see Figure 20.1)
(1) Etiology—direct trauma or alteration in blood flow
(2) Diagnostic indicators—neurological deficits (see Table 20.2—Cranial Nerve Assessment)
d. Vascular injury
(1) Traumatic aneurysm—occurs when the arterial wall is completely lacerated and local hemorrhage ensues
(a) Etiology—commonly blunt or penetrating injuries to the head; sometimes a congenital aneurysm will rupture and precede or cause the traumatic event
(b) Diagnostic indicators
i) Patient may be asymptomatic if aneurysm not ruptured
ii) If ruptured, signs and symptoms of increased intracranial pressure occur
iii) If blood has contacted the meninges, symptoms of meningeal irritation occur, e.g., stiff neck, Kernig's and Brudzinski's signs, photophobia (1)

Figure 20.1

The cranial nerves. (*A*) Inferior view of the brain showing the cranial nerves. (*B*) Lateral view of the brain showing a schematized version of the cranial nerves.
From L. S. Brunner & D. S. Suddarth (Eds.), *Textbook of medical surgical nursing* (6th ed.). Philadelphia: J. B. Lippincott Company, 1988, p. 1521. Reprinted with permission.

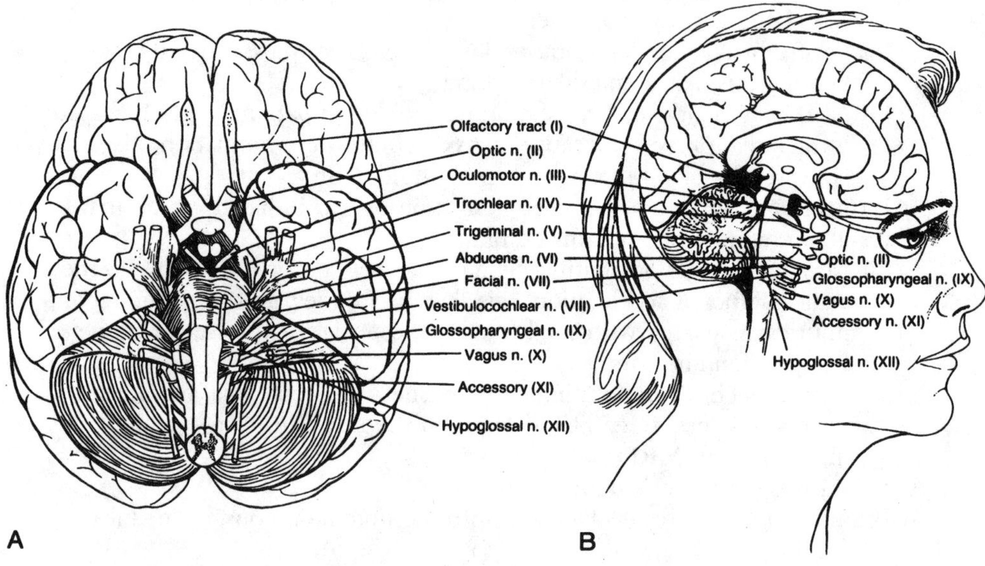

(2) Carotid cavernous fistula—a direct communication between the high pressure arterial blood of the internal carotid artery and the low venous pressure of the cavernous sinus
   (a) Etiology—head trauma, especially a basal skull fracture
   (b) Diagnostic indicators—bruit over the orbit of the eye, pulsating proptosis, conjunctival edema, orbital pain and chemosis, limitation of ocular movement, headache, visual defects (diplopia), photophobia, decreased visual acuity

B. MEDICAL AND SURGICAL INTERVENTIONS

1. Supportive care of the unconscious individual

a. Maintain airway, administer oxygen, and provide ventilation

b. Anticonvulsant therapy
   (1) Prophylactically—for moderate to severe head injuries, phenytoin (Dilantin) or Tegretol is given
   (2) If seizure occurs, usually focal or grand mal, manage initially with diazepam (Valium) I.V.; later, change to phenytoin, I.V. or P.O., or Tegretol, P.O.

Table 20.2

Cranial nerve assessment and findings

Cranial Nerve and Function	*Assessment*	*Deficits*
I Olfactory Sense of smell	Have patient close eyes; assess sense of smell in each nostril, independently, by presenting patient with familiar substance; occlude one nostril and ask patient to sniff with the other	Absence of smell (anosmia), unilateral or bilateral
II Optic Vision	Assess visual acuity in each eye	Loss of visual acuity
	Fundoscopic examination	Papilledema; optic atrophy
	Test visual fields with confrontation testing; examiner wiggles one finger of hand, simultaneously, in all temporal quadrants (nasal, temporal, upward, and downward fields)	Patient does not see object in visual field Observe patient's activities for areas of neglect
III Oculomotor Pupillary constriction; elevation of upper eyelid; eye movement in most directions	Inspect eyelids for ptosis (drooping)	Ptosis
	Examine shape and size of pupils; look for pupil equality and position	Irregular, asymmetric pupil Pinpoint or dilated pupil
	Assess pupil reflexes (light); direct reaction or indirect reaction	Nonreactive pupil Nonconsensual response
	Test for accommodation	No pupil constriction as object moves closer
	Test for ocular movements (follows objects with eyes)	Restricted eye movement Ophthalmoplegia Dysconjugate movement Photophobia Strabismus Absent oculomotor or oculocephalic response Diplopia common with head injury
	Check for nystagmus; have patient watch object, and observe patient's field of gaze for jerky eye movements	Nystagmus secondary to cerebellar lesions, vestibular deficits, or medication toxicity
IV Trochlear Downward and inward movement of eye	Assess eye movement inward and downward	Muscle entrapment possible with orbital fracture Restricted eye movements

(Continued)

Table 20.2 continued

Cranial Nerve and Function	Assessment	Deficits
V Trigeminal Sensory—three divisions 1. Ophthalmic 2. Maxillary 3. Mandibular	Assess sensation to face (forehead, cheeks, and jaw on each side); check sharp/dull sensation; temperature; light touch	Diminished or absent touch, pain, or temperature sensations
	Assess corneal and blink reflexes; note tears	Sensory portion controlled by CN V; absence of blink response
Motor—temporal and masseter muscles (jaw clenching and lateral movement of jaw)	Assess strength and symmetry of masseter and temporal muscles during jaw clenching and lateral jaw movements	Differences in muscle tone and/or atrophy
	Assess muscle integrity of the face, as well as the sensory component of the tongue	
	Assess jaw reflex; tap middle of chin with reflex hammer while jaw slightly ajar	Failure of mouth to close after tap on chin
VI Abducens Lateral movement of the eye	Assess lateral eye movement	Restricted eye movement
VII Facial Sensory—taste on anterior two-thirds of tongue	Assess sense of taste to anterior two-thirds of the tongue; test each side separately	Failure to identify sweet, salty, sour, or bitter substances
Motor—muscles of the face	Assess symmetry of the face at rest and during deliberate facial movements (smiling; pursing lips, puffing out cheeks, wrinkling nose/forehead, and raising eyebrows)	Spasms, atrophy, or tremors Check for weakness of muscles of entire face, or only lower portion of face; if entire face is affected, peripheral nerves are involved; if only lower portion is affected, central nervous system is involved
	Corneal reflex	Absence of blink response
VIII Vestibulocochlear Hearing and balance	Assess patient's sense of hearing in both ears; include data from audiologist's evaluation	Hearing loss Failure to turn to disturbance Tinnitus
	Weber test assesses bone conduction	Bone conduction is faster than air conduction
	Rinne test assesses bone vs air conduction	

Cranial Nerve and Function	*Assessment*	*Deficits*
	Check for lateralization	Hearing is better on one side than the other
	Observe for nystagmus	Vestibular component must be evaluated to recognize high level balance abnormalities
	If patient is unresponsive and tympanic membrane is intact, assess oculovestibular response for vertigo, tinnitus, or balance problems	Vertigo Disequilibrium
IX Glossopharyngeal	Test CN IX and CN X together	
Motor—pharynx	Assess upward movement of the soft palate and uvula	Failure of soft palate/uvula to rise as patient says "Ah"
Sensory—taste on posterior one-third of tongue	Check gag reflex Observe swallowing and feeding	Hoarseness, nasal voice quality Aspiration, gagging
X Vagus Motor—palate and larynx Sensory—pharynx, larynx	Assess palatal reflex	Failure of soft palate/uvula to rise as patient says "Ah" Palate and uvula deviate from paralyzed side in vagal lesion
	Assess gag reflex	Aspiration, dysphagia, coughing
	Assess voice quality	Hoarseness, nasal voice quality
XI (Spinal) Accessory	Assess trapezius and sternocleidomastoid muscles	
	Ask patient to shrug shoulders	Drooping of shoulder
	Ask patient to turn chin against hand	Weakness/paralysis of muscle group
XII Hypoglossal Tongue	Assess movement and strength of tongue	Note asymmetry, deviation, or atrophy
	Ask patient to stick out tongue	Fasciculations and atrophy Tongue deviates to paralyzed side

c. Tetanus prophylaxis and antibiotic therapy for open wound; continue antibiotics for 7 to 10 days for high suspicion of meningitis or wound infection
d. Fluid management is controversial
   (1) Dehydration has been advocated to decrease cerebral volume and cerebral edema
   (2) Dehydration is problematic in multiinjured patients who have increased fluid requirements to achieve hemodynamic stability
   (3) Normohydration, replacing insensible and urinary losses with 5% dextrose and .45% normal saline I.V., is often recommended
e. Decompress stomach
f. Urinary catheter to straight drainage
g. Maintain blood pressure within therapeutic range

2. Insert a device (e.g., subarachnoid screw, ventriculostomy) to monitor intracranial pressure

3. Control intracranial pressure

a. Maintain $PaCO_2$ level at 25 to 30 mm Hg to constrict cerebral vessels
b. Hypothermia may be indicated
c. Corticosteroid therapy (controversial)
d. Barbiturate therapy (coma) may be indicated to reduce cerebral metabolism
e. Osmotic and loop diuretics
f. Calcium channel blockers (Nimodipine)
g. Drain CSF via ventricular catheter

4. Surgical care of wound

a. Control bleeding
b. Debride and repair scalp lacerations, avulsions, and penetrating wounds, as needed
c. Elevate and debride depressed fractures
d. Resect large contused areas and/or perform decompressive craniectomy to control intracranial hypertension and prevent herniation, if necessary
e. Evacuate epidural and acute subdural hematomas
f. Repair site of CSF leak if spontaneous closure does not occur in 7 to 10 days
g. Reconstruct skull defects (cranioplasty)

C. NURSING ASSESSMENT

1. Interview patient and/or family regarding mechanism of injury, history of head trauma; note loss of consciousness and/or seizure activity (see Module 19—Nursing Assessment—for detailed information)

2. Physical examination—document baseline and observe frequently for changes and trends

a. Neurological signs
   (1) Level of consciousness (LOC)—to provide consistency in evaluation, describe the patient's response in specific behavioral terms
      (a) Awake and alert; oriented/disoriented to person, place, and time
      (b) Short-term memory ability; shortened attention span; difficulty following simple/complex commands
      (c) Restless, agitated, irritable
      (d) Audio or visual hallucinations
      (e) Responsiveness
         i) Appropriate when stimulated, otherwise drowsy
         ii) Generally unresponsive; aroused only after repeated noxious stimuli are applied, and withdraws appropriately
         iii) No spontaneous movement; unarousable; elementary attempts to respond to noxious stimuli
         iv) Unarousable; nonpurposeful response to painful stimuli with flexion or extension of the extremities
         v) Unarousable and unresponsive to all stimuli

(2) Pupillary check
  (a) Shape, e.g., round, oval, keyhole, irregular
  (b) Size—normal range is 3 to 7 mm
  (c) Response to light
    i) Direct—light shone directly into the eye should cause pupil to immediately constrict
    ii) Consensual—light shone into one pupil should cause similar, simultaneous constriction to occur in the other pupil
    iii) Accommodation—the pupil should constrict when the focus changes from a distant object to a nearby object
(3) Brain stem reflexes
  (a) Corneal
    i) Lightly brush a wisp of cotton from the lateral side of the eye across the corneal surface; repeat for the other eye, but use a new wisp of cotton
    ii) Normally, both eyes close when either eye is brushed
  (b) Oculocephalic or doll's eyes phenomenon—NOTE: done only after cervical spine injury has been ruled out
    i) Rapidly turn patient's head from one side to another
    ii) Normally, the eyes deviate in the direction opposite to the way the head is turned
    iii) Record as positive (normal response), abnormal (dysconjugate or asymmetrical eye movement), or negative (no movement of either eye)
(4) Cranial nerve function (see Table 20.2)
(5) Motor response
  (a) Function
    i) 5 = normal muscle strength
    ii) 4 = normal range of motion against some resistance
    iii) 3 = normal range of motion against gravity only
    iv) 2 = weak contraction; unable to overcome gravity
    v) 1 = slight muscle contraction; no joint movement
    vi) 0 = complete paralysis
  (b) Posturing (1)
    i) Decorticate—upper arms held tightly to sides; elbows, wrists, and fingers flexed; legs extended and internally rotated; feet plantar flexed
    ii) Decerebrate—jaws clenched and neck extended; arms adducted and extended at elbows; forearms pronated; wrists and fingers flexed; legs extended at knees; feet plantar flexed
  (c) Deep tendon reflexes
    i) Babinski—plantar response
      a) Test by using a sharp object to stroke lateral sole of foot and across ball of foot
      b) Normal response is plantar flexion of all toes
      c) Abnormal (positive) response is dorsiflexion of the great toe with or without fanning of the other toes
    ii) Other reflexes—biceps, triceps, brachioradial, patellar, Achilles
      a) Test by lightly tapping with a reflex hammer over site of tendon insertion into a specific muscle; response occurs due to muscle contraction when tendon is suddenly stretched

b) Grading scale

0 (0)	absent
1 (+)	diminished
2 (++)	normal
3 (+++)	brisker than normal
4 (++++)	hyperactive (clonus)

c) All reflexes may be diminished in cerebral shock

(6) Sensory function
- (a) Superficial touch
- (b) Superficial and deep pressure and pain
- (c) Sensitivity to heat and cold
- (d) Sensitivity to vibration
- (e) Sensitivity to position (proprioception)

(7) Respiratory pattern (2)
- (a) Normal rate and depth
- (b) Cheyne-Stokes—rhythmic waxing and waning of respiratory rate and depth; alternates with brief apneic periods
- (c) Central neurogenic hyperventilation—regular, sustained hyperpnea with forced inspiration and expiration; often associated with respiratory alkalosis
- (d) Apneustic breathing—prolonged, gasping inspiration followed by inefficient, brief expiration
- (e) Cluster breathing—periods of irregular breathing alternating with apneic periods
- (f) Ataxic breathing—completely irregular breathing, which often progresses to apnea

b. Glasgow Coma Scale for eye opening, motor, and verbal response (see Module 19—Nursing Assessment)
- (1) GCS score 13 to 15 = minor head injury
- (2) GCS score 9 to 12 = moderate head injury
- (3) GCS score 3 to 8 = severe head injury

c. Palpate skull and scalp for lacerations, hematomas, and/or fractures

d. Examine for facial fractures

e. Examine nostrils and external auditory canals for presence of blood or CSF

f. Observe for Battle's sign 24 to 36 hrs after injury

g. Observe for signs of increasing intracranial pressure

(1) Early signs
- (a) Deterioration in LOC, i.e., confusion, restlessness, lethargy
- (b) Pupillary dysfunction
- (c) Motor weakness, e.g., monoparesis, hemiparesis
- (d) Headache

(2) Late findings
- (a) Continued deterioration in LOC, i.e., coma
- (b) Possible vomiting
- (c) Hemiplegia or abnormal posturing, decorticate or decerebrate
- (d) Increased blood pressure, decreased pulse, widening pulse pressure
- (e) Respiratory irregularities
- (f) Impaired brain stem reflexes

(g) Measure ICP and calculate cerebral perfusion pressure (CPP)
i) CPP is mean systemic arterial pressure minus ICP
ii) Average adult CPP range is 80 to 100 mm Hg; 60 to 150 is within normal range
iii) CPP greater than or equal to 60 is necessary to provide sufficient blood supply to brain

3. Laboratory studies
a. Trauma profile for blood and urine
b. Urine electrolytes
c. Serum osmolarity—diagnoses injury to hypothalamus which may cause diabetes insipidus (DI), as indicated by serum osmolarity greater than 295 mOsm/kg, or syndrome of inappropriate antidiuretic hormone secretion (SIADH), serum osmolarity less than 280 mOsm/kg

4. Radiologic studies
a. SSF
b. Chest x-ray
c. Computerized axial tomography (CAT scan)
d. Cerebral angiography
e. Cervical spine film
f. Brain scan
g. Echoencephalogram
h. Magnetic resonance imaging (MRI)

5. Other studies
a. Lumbar puncture
b. Electroencephalogram (EEG)
c. Evoked potentials—visual, brain stem auditory, and somatosensory

D. NURSING DIAGNOSES, EXPECTED OUTCOMES, AND INTERVENTIONS

1. Potential for alteration in cerebral tissue perfusion related to head trauma, possible seizure activity
a. Expected outcome—adequate brain perfusion as evidenced by
(1) GCS 9 or higher
(2) Absence of progressive motor/sensory deficit
(3) ICP below 15 mm Hg
(4) Reflexes and EOMs intact
(5) Normothermia
(6) Stable vital signs
b. Nursing interventions
(1) Obtain baseline and ongoing neurological assessment; report changes to physician
(2) Monitor for signs and symptoms of increased ICP; include LOC, pupils, respiratory pattern, vital signs, motor, function, and ICP monitor readings
(3) Control intracranial pressure

(a) Elevate head of bed 30°, if no cervical spine injury
(b) Maintain patient's neck in neutral position to allow unrestricted venous blood flow
(c) Assist patient to hyperventilate using Ambu bag or ventilator setup
(d) Space nursing activities to allow rest periods for patient
(e) Monitor ICP
i) Calculate CPP; report deviations from normal
ii) Drain CSF, as prescribed, if ventricular catheter is in place
(f) Maintain fluid restriction
(g) Administer and maintain barbiturate coma

2. Potential for physical injury related to seizure activity

a. Expected outcomes—patient incurs no additional injuries; airway patent
b. Nursing interventions
(1) Observe for seizures
(2) Place on seizure precautions
(3) Administer anticonvulsants; monitor for therapeutic levels
(4) Document onset, progression, and duration of seizure
(5) Provide for patient safety; protect patient from falling and self-injury

3. Potential for infection related to open wounds, CSF leak, and/or invasive monitoring

a. Expected outcomes—no infectious process incurred; normal WBC and body temperature
b. Nursing interventions
(1) Observe for otorrhea or rhinorrhea; note halo signs from blood-tinged fluid, and positive glucose on clear, watery fluid
(2) Instruct patient not to blow nose or cough
(3) Do not suction patient nasally if anterior fossa fracture is present, or if basilar fracture has not been ruled out
(4) Do not insert nasogastric tube if cribriform plate fracture is suspected
(5) Observe for and report signs of meningitis
(6) Obtain CSF specimen for culture
(7) Cleanse and dress wounds using aseptic technique
(8) Observe suture lines and catheter insertion sites for signs of local infection
(9) Monitor temperature and WBC
(10) Administer antibiotics as prescribed
(11) Maintain patency of urinary catheter; change to external device or urinal, as soon as possible

4. Potential for impaired gas exchange related to impaired central regulation of breathing, obstruction, absent gag reflex, or aspiration

a. Expected outcomes
(1) Normal ABGs—PaO_2 greater than 90 mm Hg and pCO_2 between 35 and 45 mm Hg
(2) Regular respiratory rate, 12 to 20/min, and pattern
(3) Clear, bilateral breath sounds and chest x-ray
b. Nursing interventions
(1) Maintain a patent airway
(2) Provide high flow humidifed oxygen
(3) Assist with and maintain endotracheal intubation, or tracheostomy and mechanical ventilation

(4) Monitor ABGs
(5) Monitor serial chest x-rays
(6) Assess breath sounds every one or two hours
(7) Hyperventilate before and after each tracheal suctioning

5. Impaired physical mobility related to depressed level of consciousness, and motor, sensory, and/or proprioceptive defects

a. Expected outcomes
(1) Normal range of joint motion; no contractures
(2) Skin intact
(3) Eyes free of irritation
(4) Mobility at optimal level consistent with neurologic status

b. Nursing interventions
(1) Prevent complications of immobility (see Module 16—Medical Sequelae)
(2) Reposition patient at least every two hours
(3) Assess patient's skin condition frequently and institute measures to prevent pressure sores
(4) Provide range of motion exercises at least every eight hours
(5) Maintain functional alignment of patient's extremities and head
(6) Check patient's corneal reflex and instill artificial tears if absent or diminished; eyes may be taped shut at night

6. Potential for fluid volume deficit related to diuretic therapy, fluid restriction, possible diabetes insipidus

a. Expected outcomes
(1) Patient in fluid balance
(2) Normal skin turgor
(3) Urine output greater than 30 ml and less than 200 ml/hr
(4) Urine-specific gravity 1.015 to 1.025
(5) Serum electrolytes within normal limits
(6) Serum osmolarity within normal limits (280–295 mOsm/kg)
(7) No significant weight fluctuations

b. Nursing interventions
(1) Maintain strict record of fluid intake and output
(2) Monitor urine specific gravity
(3) Monitor serum electrolytes
(4) Weigh patient and monitor changes
(5) Assess skin turgor and other physical parameters of hydration
(6) Monitor hemodynamic status
(7) Provide adequate fluid intake via oral, gastric, or intravenous routes

7. Alteration in thought processes, transient or long-term, secondary to head injury

a. Expected outcomes
(1) Patient incurs no additional injury
(2) Patient is oriented to time, place, person
(3) Patient recognizes visual and tactile stimuli
(4) Patient responds appropriately to requests
(5) Memory appears similar to premorbid state

b. Nursing interventions
(1) Provide a safe environment

(a) Keep side rails up, bed in low position, and controls locked at all times
(b) Frequently observe patient
(c) Sedate patient, as needed, to facilitate treatment
(d) Use restraints as a last resort

(2) Provide appropriate stimulation and reality orientation
(a) Address patient by name
(b) Identify yourself each time you approach patient
(c) At least daily, repeat information that helps orient patient, e.g., time, place, reason for being in hospital
(d) Provide simple explanations for procedures
(e) Keep personal, familiar patient possessions within sight and reach, e.g., family photos
(f) Keep a calendar and clock within sight
(g) Redirect patient's attention from internal to external environment
(h) Assist with early evaluation of the patient by neuropsychologist and integrate recommendations into plan of care
i) Collaborate with other team members, including occupational therapist and psychologist, in implementing coma stimulation protocol

(3) Prevent overstimulation
(a) Allow patient time to process each piece of information
(b) Provide clear, precise explanations in terms familiar to patient
(c) Eliminate unnecessary stimuli
(d) Use an unhurried approach
(e) Provide frequent scheduled rest periods

(4) Additional interventions (see Module 17—Rehabilitation)

8. Knowledge deficit of family/significant others regarding consequences of head injury

a. Expected outcomes
(1) Family/significant others express understanding of all aspects of care given to patient
(2) Family/significant others identify useful strategies to deal with problems and behaviors caused by patient's neurological deficits
(3) Family/significant others appropriately utilize medical/nursing staff and support groups for support and assistance

b. Nursing interventions
(1) Explain to family/significant others the possible behavioral states that the patient may demonstrate, including
(a) Disorientation to time, place, person
(b) Agitation due to inability to process stimuli
(c) Emotional lability such as inappropriate laughter, tears, anger
(d) Lack of motivation
(e) Inability to concentrate
(f) Poor short-term memory
(g) Altered libido
(h) Speech impairments including receptive or expressive dysphasia
(2) Teach family/significant others coping strategies that medical/nursing staff have found successful in relating to the patient

(3) Provide a comforting and trusting environment for the family/significant others to encourage them to relate their fears and anxieties
(4) Refer family/significant others to local support groups and the National Head Injury Foundation
(5) Encourage family/significant others to spend time with patient and participate in care

9. **Additional nursing diagnoses**

a. Potential for fluid overload related to altered central regulation of thirst and SIADH
b. Altered nutrition, less than body requirements, related to depressed level of consciousness, absent gag reflex, immobility
c. Alteration in elimination, bowel and bladder, related to depressed level of consciousness, dehydration, indwelling catheter, sedation
d. Potential for impaired skin integrity related to immobility
e. Impaired skin integrity related to scalp injuries and catheter insertion sites
f. Potential for impaired home maintenance management related to functional deficits caused by patient's head injury

References

1. Hickey, J. V. (1986). *The clinical practice of neurological and neurosurgical nursing* (2nd ed., pp. 133, 347, 581). Philadelphia: J. B. Lippincott Co.
2. Davis J., Fagerness, A., Richmond, T., & Stewart, C. (1984). Nurse's clinical library: Neurological disorders. In H. K. Hamilton (Ed.), *Nursing '84 Books* (p. 61). Springhouse, PA: Springhouse Corp.

Suggested Readings

Ammons, A. M. (1990). Cerebral injuries and intracranial hemorrhage as a result of trauma. *Nursing Clinics of North America, 25*(1), 23–33.

Cardona, V. D. (Ed.). (1985). *Trauma nursing.* Oradell, NJ: Medical Economics Co.

Fink, M. E. (1987). Emergency management of the head-injured patient. *Emergency Medicine Clinics of North America, 5*(4), 783–795.

Franco, L. M. (1984). Cerebral contusion: A prototype for head injury. *Journal of Neurosurgical Nursing, 16*(1), 45–48.

Gardner, D. (1986). Acute management of the head-injured adult. *Nursing Clinics of North America, 21*(4), 555–562.

Gennarelli, T. A. (1984). Emergency department management of head injuries. *Emergency Medicine Clinics of North America, 2*(4), 751–752.

Harmon, A. R. (Ed.). (1985). *Nursing care of the adult trauma patient.* New York: Wiley Medical Publications.

Knezevich, B. A. (1986). *Trauma nursing: Principles and practice.* Norwalk, CT: Appleton-Century-Crofts.

Mason, P. J. (1989). Cognitive assessment parameters and tools for the critically injured adult. *Critical Care Nursing Clinics of North America, 1*(1), 45–53.

Ricci, M. (Ed.). (1984). *Core curriculum for neuroscience nursing.* Park Ridge, IL: American Association of Neuroscience Nurses.

Richmond, T. S. (Ed.). (1989). Brain resuscitation. *Critical Care Nursing Clinics of North America, 1*(1).

Walleck, C. A. (1989). Controversies in the management of the head-injured patient. *Critical Care Nursing Clinics of North America, 1*(1), 45–53.

Section IV
Systematic Approach to Trauma Nursing

MODULE 21
SPINAL CORD INJURY

Julia C. Mahon, RN, CNRN, CCRN

Prerequisite

Review anatomy and physiology of the spinal cord, its supporting structures, blood supply, and associated innervations of various levels within the spinal column.

Objectives

1.0 Describe major types of spinal injuries.
1.1 Identify mechanisms that cause spinal cord injuries.
1.2 Briefly describe characteristic loss of function associated with each level of spinal cord injury.
1.3 Differentiate complete and incomplete spinal cord injuries.
2.0 Describe initial assessment for possible spinal cord injury.
2.1 Identify initial immobilization steps at the scene.
2.2 Identify assessment priorities in the prehospital and emergent phase.
2.3 Describe neurological examination of both sensory and motor functions.
2.4 Describe laboratory and radiologic studies commonly required to assess spinal cord injury.
2.5 Identify preinjury history that affects potential rehabilitative outcome.
3.0 Anticipate and assist with appropriate medical-surgical interventions for spinal cord injury.
3.1 Describe pharmacologic agents commonly utilized.
3.2 Identify types of immobilization devices.
3.3 Given specific patient data, identify which medical-surgical interventions may be necessary.

4.0 Develop nursing diagnoses based on assessment data.
4.1 List common nursing diagnoses with specific etiologic factors related to spinal cord injury.
4.2 Identify signs and symptoms that validate each nursing diagnosis.
5.0 Identify nursing interventions and rationale for each nursing diagnosis related to spinal cord injury.
5.1 Given a patient scenario, prioritize nursing interventions.
5.2 Identify goals that promote optimal rehabilitative outcome.
6.0 Evaluate patient response to medical and nursing intervention.
6.1 Define desirable rehabilitative outcomes with measurable criteria for the various levels of spinal cord injury.
6.2 Identify nursing activities required to monitor and evaluate patient status.
6.3 List types of data to include in documentation.
6.4 Identify trends in patient assessment which require priority interventions by the nurse or physician.
7.0 Given a specific case history, formulate a plan of care for the patient with spinal cord injury who requires care throughout the trauma continuum.

A. PATTERNS OF INJURY: PATHOPHYSIOLOGY RESULTING FROM SPECIFIC MECHANISMS

1. **Axial loading—vertical compression due to falling from height and landing on feet or buttocks, or head in diving injuries; causes burst or explosive fractures**
2. **Flexion**
   a. Hyperflexion of head and neck, as seen with sudden deceleration in head-on collision; greatest stress at C5, C6
   b. Lateral flexion is associated with varying degrees of posterior ligament damage and overriding of facet joints; requires reduction with weights
3. **Hyperextension**
   a. Backward and downward movement of head and neck, as in rear-end collisions, which are most common cause
      (1) Causes extreme cord stretch as head arcs
      (2) May not cause vertebral fracture; "whiplash" is a minor form of hyperextension injury
   b. Seen in elderly who fall and strike chin/head
4. **Penetrating wounds cause cord injuries as a direct result of tissue destruction; usually do not cause fractures**

B. CLASSIFICATION OF TISSUE INJURY

1. **Concussion—shaking of cord; usually accompanied by transient deficits lasting 24 to 48 hrs; rare**
2. **Contusion**
   a. Bruising of cord tissue caused by fracture, dislocation, or direct trauma

b. Patient may have edema, necrosis, and temporary loss of function due to compression

3. Laceration—tearing of cord substance from knife or bone projecting into spinal cord; permanent injury results due to neural tissue damage

4. Hemorrhage

a. Bleeding in or around cord as supplying vessels are torn/stretched

b. Bleeding alters neurochemistry, which further increases cord damage

5. Vascular interruption

a. Ischemia of primary spinal cord vessels—two posterior spinal arteries and one anterior spinal artery

b. May be temporary; necrosis from prolonged ischemia leads to permanent loss of function

6. Transection

a. True transection is rarely seen; "physiologic" transection due to vascular interruption is common

b. Cord necroses quickly; may occur within four hours after traumatic insult

7. Fractures

a. Caused by direct and indirect forces
   (1) Cervical and lumbar segments are most frequently injured, since they are areas of high spinal mobility
   (2) Lumbar fractures from seat belts are common
   (3) Thoracic spine injuries are less common, since spine is more rigid

b. Specific fractures
   (1) Simple fracture—involves spinous/transverse process; alignment intact; some cord compression
   (2) Compression fracture—body of vertebra wedged/compressed anteriorly; usually from hyperflexion; cord compression possible
   (3) Comminuted fracture (burst fracture)—body of vertebra shatters and may be driven into cord
   (4) Teardrop fracture—small bone fragment breaks from anterior edge of vertebra and lodges within cord
      (a) Intervention necessary to remove fragments
      (b) Cord damage present if fragment has penetrated cord substance
   (5) Cervical fractures involving the first cervical vertebra (atlas), and the second cervical vertebra (axis)
      (a) Odontoid (dens) fractures—severe vertical compression at C2 level, e.g., falling on head or being thrown through windshield
         i) Result in both anterior and posterior displacement; cord damage possible; spinal canal widens in this area, which allows for a great degree of mobility
         ii) May be missed on plain films; take open mouth views, if suspected; cervical magnetic resonance imaging (MRI) or tomograms may be necessary
         iii) Treated with immobility (halo) and, in some cases, bed rest
      (b) Atlantooccipital dislocation—rare avulsion of C1 body from occipital bone; immediately fatal
      (c) Jefferson's fracture—rare fracture of C1 where body splits into several parts

i) Immediate cord damage may not occur
ii) Fracture segments can migrate; fatal injuries can occur
(d) Hangman's fracture—avulsion fracture through arch of C2 with body of C2 separated from supporting posterior elements; immobilization necessary; patient usually asymptomatic
(e) Dislocations—overriding of vertebra with some damage to ligaments and supporting structures
i) Disrupted alignment; considered "unstable" due to malalignment and potential for worsening cord injury
ii) Spinal cord injury possible
(f) Subluxation—partial/incomplete dislocation of one vertebra over another
i) Initial trauma may cause subluxation, then vertebra can realign spontaneously due to repelling forces of the trauma
ii) Patient sustains cord injury with initial subluxation or may have transient deficits
iii) Complete spinal cord injury possible with spontaneously resolved subluxation

c. Stable vs unstable fractures
(1) Fractures are more stable if there is limited damage to supporting structures, or bony alignment is preserved
(2) Any injury, even with transient spinal cord injury, is treated as unstable with the potential for worsening deficits
(3) Specific instructions for patient movement (usually under direct supervision of orthopaedic surgeon or neurosurgeon) should be clearly stated, especially if patient is not in an immobilization device (collar, halo, tongs, and/or traction)
(4) Stable injuries usually pose no immediate spinal cord compromise, but potential for deficit remains; many spinal cord injury centers now perform early spinal fusion

C. SPINAL CORD SYNDROMES

1. **Complete injury—no preserved sensorimotor function below level of injury**
2. **Incomplete injury—preservation of some sensorimotor fibers below level of lesion with varying degrees of function**

a. Anterior cord syndrome
(1) Occurs with flexion injuries or fractures that cause spinothalamic and corticospinal tract injuries
(2) Characterized by loss of pain, temperature, and motor function below level of lesion
(3) Light touch, position, and vibration are preserved

b. Brown-Séquard syndrome
(1) Common with knife or bullet wounds that cause transverse hemisection of cord
(2) Characterized by ipsilateral loss of motor, touch, position, pressure, vibration
(3) Contralateral loss of pain and temperature

c. Central cord syndrome
   (1) Hyperextension injury causes damage and/or edema to central cervical segments of cord; usually no fracture
   (2) Upper extremity deficits worse than lower; varying sensory deficits
d. Posterior cord syndrome involves posterior columns and affects proprioception and vibration senses; rare
e. Root syndromes can involve any body area; compression occurs due to disc herniation or subluxation of vertebral body
f. Horner's syndrome
   (1) Seen with high cervical lesions; involves paralysis of cervical portion of sympathetic chain
   (2) Characterized by pupillary constriction, anhidrosis (inability to sweat) on affected side of face, ptosis of affected eyelid
g. Sacral sparing
   (1) Damage to major cord substance, but radicular arteries preserve outer circumference of cord
   (2) Sensation to sacral area preserved; positive prognostic indicator for possible functional return and for bowel/bladder function

3. Manifestations of spinal cord injury

a. Upper motor neuron lesion
   (1) Damage to upper motor neurons
      (a) Originate in brain and transverse tracts within the cord
      (b) Upper motor neurons terminate at each segmental level throughout cord
      (c) Synapse with lower motor neurons arising in the spinal cord and connecting to muscle or organ
   (2) Upper motor neurons inhibit lower motor neurons; prevent hyperactive response to local stimulation
   (3) Reflex arc is intact; therefore, patients experience spastic paralysis and increased muscle tone
b. Lower motor neuron lesion
   (1) Destruction of reflex arc with interruption of communication pathway to upper motor neurons
   (2) Occurs at any cord segment; most serious in sacral portion where lower motor neurons control bowel, bladder, and sexual functioning
   (3) Decreased muscle tone and loss of reflexes, therefore, flaccid paralysis
c. Spinal shock
   (1) Occurs immediately after spinal cord injury
   (2) Characterized by flaccid paralysis, absent reflexes, loss of all pain, temperature, touch, proprioception, and pressure below the level of the lesion; absent/impaired thermoregulation
   (3) Subsides in hours or weeks, depending on individual
   (4) Severe pain may be present just above the level of injury due to zone of heightened sensitivity
   (5) Absent somatic/visceral sensations below the lesion; bowel distension and loss of peristalsis
   (6) Marked hemodynamic effects, especially in high cervical injuries
      (a) Bradycardia and hypotension due to absent/impaired sympathetic nervous system innervation

(b) Venous pooling in lower extremities makes patient extremely sensitive to sudden position changes

(7) May see varying degrees of spinal shock; acute spinal cord injury does not always mean complete functional loss

(8) Period of spinal shock ends as spinal neurons regain some excitability; perianal reflexes return

(a) Anal reflex—anal sphincter puckers upon rectal examination

(b) Bulbocavernosus reflex—muscle contraction occurs as the glans penis is squeezed or the urinary catheter is pulled

D. COMPLICATIONS OF SPINAL CORD INJURIES

1. **Deep vein thrombosis**
2. **Pulmonary embolus**
3. **Respiratory arrest (due to level of injury or to ascending injury)**
4. **Respiratory insufficiency**
5. **Bronchial obstruction**
6. **Adult respiratory distress syndrome**
7. **Pneumonia**
8. **Aspiration**
9. **Atelectasis**
10. **Tension pneumothorax**

E. LEVELS OF SPINAL INJURY

Table 21.1

Levels of spinal cord injury and landmarks of assessment

Location	*Motor*	*Sensory*
Cervical		
C2, C3 injuries may be rapidly fatal due to respiratory paralysis	Total quadriplegia with absent/impaired diaphragm function; absent intercostal muscle function	Loss of all sensory function from neck down
C4	Total quadriplegia with absent/impaired diaphragm function; this level is associated with phrenic nerve innervation; may include hemidiaphragm injury	Sensory level at clavicle and above
C5	Quadriplegia with deltoid and biceps function; biceps weak, if present	Sensation intact to head, shoulders, deltoid area, part of forearms (lateral aspect of arm)

Location	Motor	Sensory
C6	Quadriplegia with deltoid and biceps function strong; shoulder rotators also functional but may be weak	Sensation in forearms, palms, and thumbs intact
C7	Quadriplegia (incomplete); much increased arm strength; wrist extensors functional; triceps functional	Sensation intact to middle finger
C8	Quadriplegia with strong triceps; wrist, and finger extensors stronger; may develop finger flexors	Sensation in midchest; positive arm, hand, and finger sensation
Thoracic		
T1 to T5	Paraplegia; loss of all muscles below midchest	Sensation intact to midchest; includes arms and hands
(T1, T2 supply inner arm; T4 landmark is nipple line)		
T6 to T12	Paraplegia; intact trunk muscles for torso support	Intact chest sensation
(T10 landmark is umbilicus; T12 landmark is groin)		
Lumbosacral		
L1 to L5	Paraplegia; loss of muscle function of pelvis, legs	
L1 to L3	Hip rotation and flexion; may have some flexion of legs	Sensation intact in knees; some sensation in inner thighs and anterior surface of thigh (L3)
L3 to L4	More control of extension of knees	Sensory level extends to upper legs
L4 to L5	Dorsiflexion of ankles; includes S1	
L5 to S1	Eversion of feet	
L4 to S1	Internal rotation of hip and abductors, inversion of feet	
L4 to S2	Flexion of knees	
S1 to S2	Plantar flexion of feet	
S2 to S5	Control of bowel and bladder function may or may not be lost	

F. MEDICAL AND SURGICAL INTERVENTIONS

1. **Prehospital management**
   a. Assess and maintain patient's airway, breathing, and circulation; open airway with modified jaw thrust in any suspected cervical spine injury
   b. Immobilize patient's head and neck in neutral position with collar and cervical immobilization devices, and long board
   c. Extricate patient from vehicle or site while maintaining spinal immobilization
   d. Triage to appropriate facility, i.e., regional spinal cord injury center or trauma center
2. **Emergency department**
   a. Primary survey—triage assessment of ABCs

(1) Evaluate airway and level of respiratory function
(2) Intubate without cervical hyperextension (blind nasal)
(3) Evaluate circulatory system; spinal shock is responsible for early bradycardia and hypotension in cervical injuries

b. Secondary survey for obvious/occult injuries to other systems
(1) Chest/abdominal trauma is associated with cervical spine injuries
(2) Evaluate for aortic tear, since this may cause paraplegia due to interrupted vascular supply
(3) Suspect long bone injuries in all cases of spinal cord injury
(4) Suspect closed head injury in all cases of traumatic spinal cord injury
(5) Initiate fluid therapy, urinary catheter, nasogastric tube, and hemodynamic lines, as needed

c. Neurological assessment allows quick estimation of cord involvement
(1) Conduct exam systematically to identify highest level of preserved function
(2) Assessment landmarks
(a) Assess motor and sensory functions
(b) Assess spinal cord functions (see Table 21.2)
(3) Deep tendon reflexes (DTR)
(a) Test bicep, supinator, tricep, knee, and ankle reflexes

Table 21.2

Brief assessment of spinal cord function

Cord Level	*Motor Examination*	*Sensory Landmark*
C1 to C4	For phrenic nerve function, look for spontaneous inspiratory effort, respiration, movement of diaphragm	Back of head (C2); neck and clavicle (C3, C4)
C5	Ask patient to shrug shoulders, take a deep breath; biceps—ask patient to bend arm at elbow	Anterior surface of arms
C6	Wrist extensors—ask patient to bend wrist up	Forearms
C7	Triceps—ask patient to extend arm at elbow	Fingers
C8	Check finger-thumb apposition	Fingers
T1 to T7	Chest muscles—ask patient to cough	Nipple line (T4)
T8 to T12	Ask patient to tighten muscles of abdomen	Umbilicus (T10)
L1 to L3	Ask patient to flex hips	Hips (L2)
L2 to L4	Ask patient to straighten legs	Anterior surface of knees (L3) and lower legs (L4, L5)
L5	Ask patient to bend and straighten toes	Posterior thighs
S1		Ankles; posterior lower legs
S2 to S4	Ask patient to tighten sphincter around examiner's finger	Posterior thighs (S2); buttocks (S3)

(b) Preserved DTRs below injury level can be a good prognostic sign
i) Temporary areflexia below the level of injury is common during spinal shock
ii) Once cord reorganization begins, evaluate bulbocavernosus reflex (external anal sphincter function); main indicator of future bowel, bladder, sexual functioning

d. Laboratory studies—trauma profile for baseline evaluation

e. Radiographic evaluation
(1) Use caution during initial films; limit excessive motion of spine
(2) Treat all patients as if their spines are "unstable" until proven otherwise
(3) Plain radiographs
(a) Take lateral and anterior-posterior views
(b) Physician may need to pull down on the wrists to fully view C7 to T1, especially in obese or muscled individuals
(c) Swimmer's view (arms above the head) may be needed to see all cervical vertebrae
(d) C1 to C2 level may require films taken with the patient's mouth open
(4) Physician is responsible for maintaining spinal alignment and applying or removing collar/traction device when moving patient
(5) Use serial radiographs for closed reduction attempts; physician should supervise all films
(6) Computerized axial tomography (CAT scan) outlines spine clearly
(7) Tomography useful to obtain longitudinal cross-sections of vertebral column
(8) MRI used to determine injury to surrounding support structures
(9) Myelography

f. General considerations
(1) Common injury sites are the most mobile joints of the spine, e.g., cervical area and thoracolumbar junction
(2) Severity of bony injury does not predict neurological damage; a severe fracture in one individual could produce little damage, while in another it could produce paralysis
(3) The key to assessment is a consistent method of sensorimotor evaluation and the comparison of serial data

3. Nonsurgical management

a. Immobilize spinal/vertebral column
(1) Cervical spine
(a) Base treatment on injury type and spinal stability
(b) Use temporary immobilization devices until spine is aligned and autofusion has begun
i) Tongs, e.g., Gardner-Wells, Vinke, Crutchfield
ii) Skeletal traction with patient on bed with bed board
iii) Skeletal traction with Roto-Rest kinetic treatment table, Stryker frame, or Foster frame
(c) For long-term use, immobilize cervical spine with
i) Foam collar—provides mild support in very stable injuries in a compliant patient
ii) Hard collar—provides firm support to neck; removable but provides anterior-posterior brace
iii) Sternal-occipital-mandibular immobilizer (SOMI) brace—partially removable brace that provides full support to chin and posterior neck; skin care is problematic

iv) Halo vest—provides permanent traction/immobilization for full duration of healing process (eight weeks minimum)
   a) Pins are inserted into skull and can be adjusted for angle of traction; provides safe patient mobility
   b) Some patients are initially immobilized with halo brace before surgical intervention
   c) Halo brace then can be converted to vest for permanent traction

(2) Thoracic or lumbar spine
   (a) Initial traction may include skeletal pins in both tibias; countered with equal pull from tongs inserted into skull (Halo-femoral traction)
   (b) Body cast or fiberglass jacket may be used for several months while healing occurs
   (c) Other jackets include canvas, corset-like brace, Jewett brace, Knight-Taylor brace; remove braces for skin assessment or when patient is flat in bed
   (d) Trend is toward early spinal fusion to prevent complications of prolonged bed rest

(3) Sacral or coccygeal spine injuries are treated with bed rest and girdle-like braces

b. Specific pharmacological interventions
   (1) Steroid therapy (controversial)
      (a) May reduce spinal cord edema
      (b) Doses vary from a one-time loading dose (dexamethasone, 25 mg), immediately postinjury, to a loading dose (20 to 40 mg) with several days of tapered therapy (4 to 6 mg every 4 to 6 hrs); Solu-Medrol also may be used with bolus dose followed by continuous IV therapy for 24 hrs
   (2) Osmotic diuretics (mannitol) are used to reduce edema; may be given in combination with plasma expanders (dextran) to support capillary blood flow to cord
   (3) Sodium bicarbonate is used to maintain normal pH of cerebrospinal fluid (CSF); may be acidotic from tissue ischemia
   (4) Cautious fluid management
      (a) Expect hypotension during spinal shock
      (b) Treat patient only if symptomatic from hypoperfusion, e.g., ECG changes in older population, decreased level of consciousness, or decreased urinary output
   (5) Gastric antacids and/or histamine (H_2) blockers to prevent gastric ulcers
   (6) Atropine for symptomatic severe bradycardia in cases of unopposed parasympathetic stimulation (high cervical injuries)

c. Respiratory management
   (1) High flow humidified oxygen
   (2) Continuous positive airway pressure (CPAP)
   (3) Intubation/tracheostomy
   (4) Mechanical ventilation
      (a) Positive pressure ventilation
      (b) Negative pressure ventilation
   (5) Phrenic nerve pacing—diaphragmatic pacing
      (a) Used for ventilator-dependent patients who demonstrate some diaphragm function; able to take even a few breaths on their own

(b) Electrodes surgically implanted over phrenic nerve; provide innervation to diaphragm
(c) Patient develops tolerance to pacer which allows him/her to stay off the ventilator for increasing periods of time

4. Surgical management

a. Efficacy of early surgical intervention remains controversial (1); early surgery may be indicated for
(1) Evidence of cord compression
(2) Progressive deficits
(3) Compound fracture of the vertebra
(4) Penetrating wounds of spinal cord or the surrounding structures
(5) Bone fragments in the canal

b. Surgical procedures
(1) Anterior-posterior fusion using banked bone, grafted bone from patient, wires, rods, or plates
(a) Fusion stabilizes injury area and may prevent further injury to nerve roots or spinal cord
(b) Metal rods, e.g., Harrington or Lugue, placed along vertebral column increase the stability of thoracic or lumbar spine
(2) Decompressive laminectomy is used to relieve pressure on spinal cord and nerve roots; anterior or posterior approach may be used

c. Postoperative concerns
(1) Cervical (anterior approach)—patient may experience difficulty swallowing
(a) Monitor for signs of neck swelling, which impedes respiratory effort
(b) Avoid pillows that may hyperflex the head even if brace/collar is in place
(2) Thoracic (anterolateral approach)
(a) Patient will have chest tubes from thoracotomy
(b) Potential for pulmonary compromise, especially if patient experienced complete neurologic deficits at upper thoracic levels preoperatively
(3) Spinal fusion results in firm union of bone; some mobility permanently lost

5. Goals of spinal cord injury treatment

a. Decision to operate is based on consultation between patient, orthopaedic surgeon, neurosurgeon, and other consultants

b. Treatment may include period of nonsurgical observation/traction followed by operative fusion
(1) Realignment of bony structure for optimal functioning of all supporting structures
(2) Decompression of cord/nerves prevents pain, loss of function, further compromise of function, and aids the natural healing process

G. NURSING ASSESSMENT

1. Interview (see Module 19–Nursing Assessment)

a. Mechanism of injury

b. Reports of pain, weakness, paralysis

c. In assessing mental status, consider head injury or hypothermia as source of decreased level of consciousness

2. **Physical examination**
a. Neurological assessment
   (1) Level of consciousness using Glasgow Coma Scale
   (2) Sensorimotor function (see Table 21.2)
      (a) Have all team members observe first exam to establish baseline
      (b) Conduct sensorimotor exam every two hours during acute phase when reducing fracture or adjusting traction, and when serial films are being done
   (3) Monitor for possible ascending injury, e.g., worsening deficits, small decreases in motor skills, or altered patterns of respiration, especially cervical injuries
   (4) Cranial nerve assessment for high cervical injuries (see Module 20—Head Injury)
      (a) Assess cranial nerves 9 (glossopharyngeal), 10 (vagus), 11 (accessory), and 12 (hypoglossal)
      (b) In high cervical injuries (C2, 3, 4) traction effect is possible on these nerves, so function may be diminished or absent
      (c) Accessory muscle function can be confused with shoulder shrug ability
   (5) Assess pain; dysesthesias or paresthesias at zone of injury may occur
   (6) Assess body temperature; quadriplegics may be poikilothermic (body temperature assumes external environmental temperature) due to absent input from periphery for temperature control
   (7) Monitor for signs of autonomic dysreflexia—**a neurologic emergency**
      (a) Seen in patients with injuries above T6 level once spinal shock has subsided and reflex activity has resumed
      (b) Signs and symptoms
         i) Severe hypertension—as high as 300 mm Hg systolic
         ii) Nasal congestion
         iii) Severe "pounding" headache
         iv) Flushing and sweating above lesion
         v) Cool, vasoconstricted extremities below level of injury
      (c) Triggered by noxious stimulus
         i) Distended bladder or bowel, pressure sore, labor in the pregnant patient, any acute abdominal process, e.g., appendicitis, prolonged positioning in one area, or tight shoes
         ii) Elicits sympathetic discharges below level of lesion
         iii) Reflex stimulation of sympathetic nervous system causes spasm of pelvic arterioles and produces vasoconstriction below injury level
         iv) Hypertension sensed by baroreceptors in the carotid sinus and aortic arch; results in vasodilation above lesion
      (d) May result in cerebral vascular accident, seizures, or death from paroxysmal hypertension
      (e) Treatment
         i) Relieve hypertension; elevate head of bed
         ii) Relieve trigger mechanism; usually effective in lowering blood pressure and providing relief from symptoms
         iii) Pharmacological intervention may be necessary; drugs of choice include diazoxide (Hyperstat), hydralazine (Apresoline), or sodium nitroprusside (Nipride)

(f) Prevent dysreflexia by recognizing trigger mechanisms, i.e., noxious stimuli
  i) Look for cause—urinary catheter most frequent trigger mechanism
  ii) Trigger mechanisms may be different for each patient
  iii) Patient, family, significant other must be fully aware of causes and treatment of autonomic dysreflexia

b. Cardiovascular system
 (1) Assess heart rate, blood pressure, and patient tolerance to vital sign changes
  (a) Bradycardia and hypotension associated with spinal shock may occur due to vasomotor collapse
  (b) Orthostatic hypotension may occur and is usually self-limiting
  (c) Assess tolerance of bradycardia or hypotension through level of consciousness, signs of hypoxia, feelings of dizziness, shortness of breath, decreased urine output, presence of ectopic beats (junctional or ventricular escape beats)
 (2) Continuously monitor cardiac rhythm for severe bradycardia may require a pacemaker for patients with acute cervical injury
 (3) Assess for presence of deep vein thrombosis (DVT) or pulmonary embolism
  (a) Assess leg size, color, and temperature at least every eight hours
  (b) Monitor body temperature; deep vein thrombosis may cause unexplained fever
   i) Approximately 15 to 20% of spinal cord injured patients develop DVT
   ii) Of these, 5 to 15% develop pulmonary emboli—a leading cause of death
  (c) Apply sequential compression boots
  (d) Screen lower extremities with noninvasive device (Doppler) to detect flow pattern changes

c. Respiratory system
 (1) Assess rate, rhythm, symmetry of chest wall movement, breath sounds, and use of accessory muscles to breathe; retraction of neck muscles is a visible sign of poor oxygenation and may indicate respiratory decompensation
 (2) Assess muscular ability with vital capacity, negative inspiratory force, minute volumes on admission and routine; partial paralysis of the diaphragm can occur in cervical injury; one side may be affected
 (3) Assess oxygenation with arterial blood gases, pulse oximetry, skin color, altered level of consciousness due to hypoxia
 (4) Other assessments include pulmonary function studies, ventilator settings; rising inspiratory pressures indicate decreasing lung compliance

d. Gastrointestinal system
 (1) Measure abdominal girth, auscultate bowel sounds, and palpate the abdomen
  (a) Anticipate paralytic ileus in acute stage
  (b) Severe distension interferes with adequacy of respirations
 (2) Determine gastric pH and hematest stools
 (3) Pay careful attention to abdominal assessment, since patient may be insensate to pain/distension

e. Genitourinary system
 (1) Assess urine color, clarity, character, and amount
 (2) Monitor renal function and urinalysis

(a) Urinary tract infection (UTI) is a serious complication that can lead to renal disease
(b) Assess urine pH—alkaline urine predisposes patient to renal stone formation as calcium exits the body

(3) Sexuality assessment
(a) Females—pattern of menses; sensation during intercourse
(b) Males—ability to achieve erection; ability to ejaculate
(c) Usually a major concern, but patient is often reluctant to discuss

f. Integumentary system
(1) Assess all skin surfaces at least every four hours
(a) Inspect areas under braces, splints, and/or traction devices
(b) Bony prominences prone to develop pressure sores
(2) Skin lesions can develop in just a few hours in the paralyzed patient

g. Musculoskeletal system
(1) Assess joint range of motion (ROM) for stiffness, decreased mobility, and/or shortening of ligaments
(2) Monitor for signs of developing spasticity, i.e., flexor/extensor spasms which occur after spinal shock
(3) Monitor for heterotopic ossification; most common in quadriplegia and spastic paralysis (see Module 17—Rehabilitation)

H. NURSING DIAGNOSES, EXPECTED OUTCOMES, AND INTERVENTIONS

1. **Impaired physical mobility related to paralysis**

a. Expected outcomes
(1) Neuromuscular deficit does not increase
(2) Patient positions self or directs others to perform positioning for comfort
(3) Proper body alignment is maintained
(4) Normal joint range of motion
(5) Additional outcomes (see Figure 21.1)

b. Nursing interventions
(1) Within safe limits, maintain full ROM in all of patient's joints, especially if fracture site is unstable
(2) Gradually increase patient's tolerance to an upright position once brace is placed or fusion is done
(3) Have patient use all functional muscle groups whenever possible; alter physical environment to allow maximum, functional muscle use
(4) Collaborate with physical therapist and occupational therapist to develop plan of care that preserves muscle mass and function
(5) Turn patient every two to four hours; build skin tolerance gradually

2. **Self-care deficits: feeding, bathing/hygiene, dressing/grooming, and toileting related to muscular paralysis and immobilization devices**

a. Expected outcomes
(1) Patient directs his/her care

Figure 21.1

Sequelae of spinal cord injury and rehabilitation challenges. The vertebrae are numbered on the left side of the drawing and the spinal nerves are numbered on the right. From L. S. Brunner & D. S. Suddarth (Eds.), *Textbook of medical surgical nursing* (6th ed.). Philadelphia: J. B. Lippincott Company, 1988, p. 1505. Reprinted with permission.

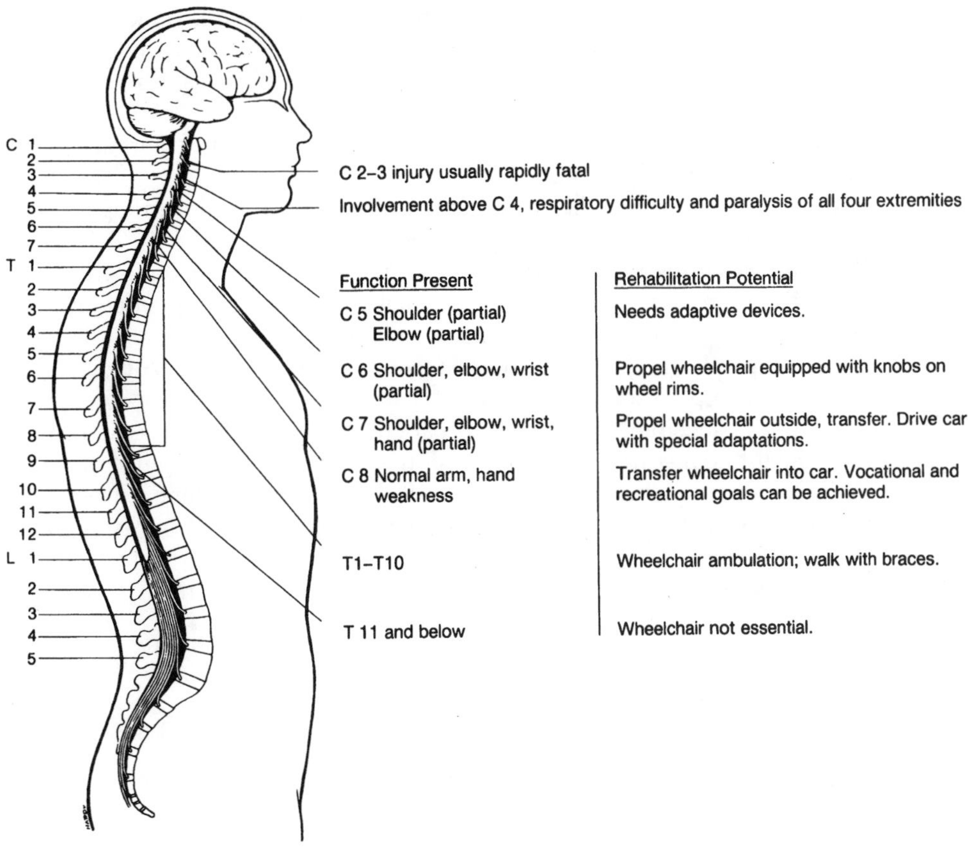

(2) Patient expresses satisfaction with level of control over daily care
(3) Activities of daily living are accomplished

b. Nursing interventions
   (1) Assist/encourage patient to perform any task within his/her ability; incorporate family and friends into treatment goals
   (2) Teach patient to use assistive devices, as needed, such as built-up utensils, mouth call systems, prism glasses
   (3) Communicate with physical therapist and occupational therapist daily to follow progress regarding patient's self-care changes

3. **Sensory-perceptual deficits: visual, kinesthetic, and tactile related to absent/abnormal input from periphery, and limited field of vision within immobilization device**

a. Expected outcomes

(1) Patient identifies unusual sensory experiences
(2) Patient/family recognize and manage perceptual deficits or alterations, i.e., paresthesias/dysethesias
(3) Patient makes maximum use of innervated skin surface

b. Interventions
(1) Monitor for changes in sensory level; mark level on skin in the acute phase
(2) Prepare patient for unusual sensory experiences common in spinal cord injury, e.g., phantom pains, limbs "floating," hot skin, feet twisted or moving, burning pains in arms; reassure patient that unusual sensory experiences are common
(3) Maintain awareness of immobilized person's field of vision; communicate this to other health care providers
(4) Reorient as necessary; utilize contact with the outside world through visitors, TV, staged stimulation with radio or videotape
(5) Provide comforting visual symbols, including items from home, in the patient's immediate environment; since patient's view may be of ceiling or floor while in traction, place objects on ceiling or floor
(6) Position mirrors and prism glasses to increase amount of area visualized from patient's position
(7) Avoid use of specific time frames, as patient may have altered sense of time
(8) Use touch to convey concern; pay attention to actual sensory level of the patient; many patients report a strong need for touch in intact sensory zones

4. Pain related to fracture, dysesthesias, or paresthesias at site of injury

a. Expected outcomes
(1) Patient/family verbalize and use methods that minimize paresthesias/ dysesthesias
(2) Patient reports comfort within limits of traction/bracing

b. Nursing interventions
(1) Position patient for comfort
(2) Administer analgesics as needed; avoid the use of narcotics
(3) Desensitize areas of dysesthesias with ice or touch
(4) Work through range of motion as able; work through pain by using exercise to increase patient's tolerance

5. Decreased cardiac output related to spinal shock

a. Expected outcomes
(1) Adequate cardiac output maintained
(2) Heart rate and blood pressure adequate to provide perfusion as noted by level of consciousness, urine output of 0.5 to 1.0 ml/kg/hr, and tissue oxygenation

b. Nursing interventions
(1) Monitor heart rate and blood pressure continuously in acute injuries
(2) Use caution in sudden patient movement, especially when raising the head of the bed
(3) Gradually reorient patient to upright position once spinal shock stabilizes
(4) Assist with insertion of transvenous or external pacemaker for the patient intolerant of extreme bradycardias
(5) Use abdominal binder to increase venous return to the heart if patient sits or stands

(6) Maintain adequate hydration

6. **Potential fluid volume deficit related to use of osmotic diuretics, spinal shock, or ileus**
   a. Expected outcomes
      (1) Adequate vascular volume maintained
      (2) Heart rate and blood pressure adequate to provide perfusion as noted by level of consciousness, urine output of 0.5 to 1.0 ml/kg/hr, or tissue oxygenation
   b. Nursing interventions
      (1) Measure vital signs and intake and output
      (2) Administer I.V. fluids; titrate fluid intake carefully in acute phase to assure adequate vascular volume without overload; fluid quickly accumulates in hypoperfused lungs
      (3) Carefully monitor response to vasopressors; response may be less than expected, since the sympathetic nervous system is compromised
7. **Potential altered tissue perfusion related to vasovagal episodes**
   a. Expected outcomes
      (1) Absence of vasovagal episodes
      (2) Organs and periphery adequately perfused
      (3) Patient/family recognize causative factors and avoid them when possible
   b. Nursing interventions
      (1) Avoid nursing actions that prolong vagal stimulation, e.g., suctioning
      (2) Hyperoxygenate prior to suctioning
      (3) Closely monitor heart rate and rhythm
      (4) Note causal pattern of bradycardic episodes
      (5) Administer atropine in extreme symptomatic bradycardia; avoid repeated use
      (6) Keep temporary pacemaker at bedside for the patient with repeated, severe episodes
      (7) Use caution when turning patient to prone position, especially the first time; cervical spine injured patients are particularly sensitive to this and may have asystole or bradycardia
8. **Potential altered tissue perfusion related to poikilothermia**
   a. Expected outcomes
      (1) Skin warm, dry, with normal color
      (2) Adequate peripheral pulses
   b. Nursing interventions
      (1) Monitor core temperatures every two to four hours
      (2) Avoid extremes in room temperature; alter environment to keep patient normothermic
      (3) Instruct family members about need for careful temperature regulation
9. **Ineffective breathing pattern related to muscular paralysis and/or gastric distension secondary to ileus**
   a. Expected outcomes
      (1) Adequate tidal volume and respiratory rate
      (2) Arterial blood gases within normal limits
   b. Nursing interventions
      (1) Assist with tracheal intubation—do not hyperextend the neck; blind nasal or fiberoptic intubation preferred

(2) Maintain patient with prescribed tidal volume, rate, FiO_2; negative pressure ventilator may be indicated
(3) Monitor chest excursion
(4) Monitor patient response to diaphragmatic pacing
(5) Develop and implement weaning protocol as soon as possible
(a) Assess for hypoxia, fatigue
(b) Trend vital capacity (VC), negative inspiratory force (NIF), rate and minute volumes
(c) Initiate tracheal plugging
(d) Utilize T-piece trials
(6) Insert and maintain patency of nasogastric tube
(7) Avoid overdistension of bowel, which can impede ventilation

10. Ineffective airway clearance related to impaired/absent cough

a. Expected outcomes
(1) Patent airway
(2) Lung sounds clear

b. Nursing interventions
(1) Evaluate breath sounds every two hours
(2) Monitor vital capacity, negative inspiratory force, O_2 saturation, pulse oximetry, sequential arterial blood gases to identify early signs of respiratory compromise
(3) Provide chest physiotherapy and postural drainage
(4) Administer respiratory inhalants, intermittent positive-pressure breathing (IPPB), bronchodilators
(5) Encourage frequent incentive spirometry to build muscular reserves
(6) Suction trachea p.r.n.
(7) Note color, odor, amount of pulmonary secretions
(8) Obtain bacterial culture when indicated
(9) Assist the cervical injured patient to "quad" cough; provide upward thrusts on diaphragm as patient takes a deep breath

11. Impaired gas exchange related to lung injury, absent intercostal muscle functions, diaphragm function, or impaired level of consciousness

a. Expected outcomes
(1) Normal tidal volume, respiratory rate, and PaO_2
(2) Arterial blood gases within normal limits

b. Nursing interventions
(1) Monitor respiratory rate, tidal volume, arterial blood gases, SaO_2
(2) Provide high flow humidified oxygen via ventilator, mask, or nasal cannula
(3) Sedate patient, as needed, to decrease airway resistance and improve ventilation
(4) Monitor for signs and symptoms of ascending paralysis related to cord edema
(5) Perform chest physiotherapy at least three to four times each day; encourage patient to use incentive spirometry, which can be adapted for tracheostomy use
(6) Instruct patient/family about activities that promote health and foster optimal lung function, i.e., avoid people with upper respiratory tract infection; avoid smoking

12. **Altered patterns of urinary elimination: retention or incontinence related to absent innervation to urinary bladder**
  a. Expected outcomes
    (1) Urine remains free of infection
    (2) Bladder empties completely
    (3) Patient/family perform catheterization, if necessary
  b. Nursing interventions
    (1) Promote urinary voiding if neuromuscular function is adequate
      (a) Stimulate trigger zones to facilitate voiding, i.e., tap the bladder: apply suprapubic pressure (Credé's method) every two to four hours
      (b) Develop regular schedule for toileting
      (c) Utilize upright position if possible
    (2) Insert urinary catheter and maintain closed urinary drainage system
      (a) Maintain catheter patency; blockages and resultant overdistension may trigger autonomic dysreflexia
      (b) Anticipate atonic bladder in initial stage; bladder becomes spastic as spinal shock subsides and reflex function returns
      (c) Provide catheter care every eight hours
      (d) Tape catheter to abdomen for males and to inner thigh for females
      (e) Remove catheter as soon as possible
      (f) Institute intermittent catheterization program (see Module 17—Rehabilitation)
    (3) Evaluate bladder function by cystometric studies
    (4) Obtain urine specimens for culture and sensitivity, weekly, or if urine character changes
    (5) Ensure adequate fluid intake; during rehabilitation phase, provide 3 liters/day
13. **Sexual dysfunction related to injury**
  a. Expected outcomes
    (1) Patient/family utilize counseling services as needed
    (2) Patient/family demonstrate knowledge of cause of sexual dysfunction and techniques to maintain sexual functioning
    (3) Patient identifies methods of sexual satisfaction
    (4) Patient discusses sexual concerns with partner
  b. Nursing interventions
    (1) Address questions about sexuality honestly—seek out appropriate consultation for detailed explanation of facts
      (a) S2 to S4 spinal levels control innervation to genitals
      (b) Females
        i) Lack sensation during intercourse
        ii) Most continue menstrual cycles and are able to become pregnant
        iii) May deliver vaginally, but autonomic hyperreflexia can occur, which requires cesarean section
      (c) Males
        i) Upper motor neuron lesions—60 to 70% with complete lesions can achieve erection but are unable to ejaculate or have orgasm
        ii) Lower motor neuron lesions
          a) Complete lesions—unable to achieve erection

b) Incomplete lesions—most can achieve erection and may ejaculate
iii) Some centers are experimenting with early sperm removal in males concerned about fathering children
(2) Refer to urologist/gynecologist for the patient concerned about long-term reproductive potential
(3) Confront patient about behaviors with sexual content; use as a forum for patient to express his/her concerns
(4) Provide privacy for patient/partner
(5) Teach patient and partner techniques for dealing with problems, e.g., catheters, incontinence, lack of vaginal lubrication

14. **Actual/potential impairment of skin integrity related to pressure from immobilization devices and lack of voluntary movement**
a. Expected outcomes
(1) Skin surfaces remain intact
(2) Patient and family become adept at skin assessments and care
b. Nursing interventions
(1) Turn patient and examine skin every two hours in the acute phase; reinforce importance of examining skin with both patient and family
(2) Stress importance of skin assessment as a long-term need of the patient; elicit help of family/significant others to assure good skin care
(3) Document skin condition every eight hours with particular attention to reddened areas or skin disruptions
(4) Avoid pressure on reddened areas—prevent decubiti through pressure relief, turning, gel pads under braces or bony prominences

15. **Powerlessness related to sudden loss of independence and/or mobility**
a. Expected outcomes
(1) Patient effectively directs his/her care
(2) Patient expresses satisfaction with level of control over his/her daily care
(3) Patient makes choices regarding treatment options
b. Nursing interventions
(1) Recognize the impact of permanent injury on the individual's psychological well-being
(2) Enhance patient power by providing opportunities for choices whenever possible
(3) Encourage patient to move toward self-advocacy in decisionmaking; start with small tasks
(4) Reinforce behaviors that promote patient power—this includes reinforcement among staff members
(5) Identify one staff member with whom patient is best able to talk about his/her concerns
(6) Help patient realize that he/she will need to direct others about his/her care in the future
(7) Identify and seek familial supports of patient; elicit their aid in health maintenance of the patient and in encouraging patient's self-advocacy
(8) Confront your own feelings about permanent disability and quality of life

16. **Additional nursing diagnoses**
a. Constipation related to decreased bowel motility, areflexia, and perceptual impairment (see Module 17—Rehabilitation)

b. Potential for alteration in tissue perfusion related to venous pooling in the extremities (see Module 16—Medical Sequelae)
c. Alteration in nutrition—less than body requirements (see Module 11—Nutrition)
d. Disturbance in self-concept related to changes in body image, self-esteem, role performance, and/or personal identity
e. Sleep pattern disturbance related to anxiety/fear
f. Grieving related to loss
g. Impaired verbal communication related to need for mechanical ventilation (see Module 17—Rehabilitation)
h. Knowledge deficit related to injury and its implications, and required self-care
i. Altered thought process related to stress/trauma

I. NURSING SKILLS

1. **Emergency removal of halo brace front for CPR**
2. **Manipulation of halo brace, tongs, Philadelphia collar, soft cervical collar, body jacket and their care**
3. **Assisted "quad" coughing**
4. **Use of Olympic Trach Talk for verbalization**
5. **Use of negative pressure ventilation**
6. **Trigger voiding mechanisms, e.g., Credé's, stroking inner thigh, digital stimulation to anus/rectum**

Reference

1. Youmans, J. R. (Ed.). (1982). *Neurological surgery* (2nd ed.). Philadelphia: W. B. Saunders Co.

Suggested Readings

Adelstein, W., & Watson, P. (1983). Cervical spine injuries. *Journal of Neurosurgical Nursing, 15*(2), 65–71.

Alspach, J. G. (Ed.). (1991). *Core curriculum for critical care nursing* (4th ed.). Philadelphia: W. B. Saunders Co.

Bartol, G. (1978). Psychological needs of the spinal cord injured person. *Journal of Neurosurgical Nursing, 10*(4), 171–175.

Buchanan, L. (1982). Emergency: First aid for spinal cord injury. *Nursing, 12*(8), 68–75.

Buchanan, L., & Nawoczenski, D. (Eds.). (1987). *Spinal cord injury: Concepts and management approaches.* Baltimore: Williams & Wilkins.

Dijans, W. T. (1987). Radiology of acute spinal trauma. *Critical Care Clinician,* 3(3), 495–518.

Hanak, M., & Scott, A. (1983). *Spinal cord injury: An illustrated guide for health care professionals.* New York: Springer Publishing Co.

Hickey, J. V. (1986). *The clinical practice of neurological and neurosurgical nursing* (2nd ed.). Philadelphia: J. B. Lippincott.

Nikas, D. L. (1982). *The critically ill neurosurgical patient.* New York: Churchill Livingstone.

Reed, M. A. (1987). Nursing considerations in acute spinal cord injury. *Critical Care Clinician,* 3(3), 679–691.

Richmond, T. S. (1990). Spinal cord injury. *Nursing Clinics of North America,* 25(1), 57–69.

Stanton, G. M. (1984). A needs assessment of significant others following spinal cord injury. *Journal of Neurosurgical Nursing,* 16(5), 253–256.

Walleck, C. A. (Ed.). (1990). Spinal cord injury. *Trauma Quarterly,* 4(3).

Worth, M. H. (Ed.). (1982). *Principles and practices of trauma care.* Baltimore: Williams & Wilkins.

Zejdlik, C. (1983). *Management of spinal cord injury.* Monterey, CA: Wadsworth Health Sciences Division.

Section IV
Systematic Approach to Trauma Nursing

MODULE 22
CARDIOTHORACIC TRAUMA

Sharon G. Smith, MSN, RN, CCRN

Prerequisite

Review anatomy and physiology of pulmonary and cardiovascular systems.

Objectives

1.0 Describe common cardiothoracic injuries.
1.1 Briefly describe pathophysiology and major defining characteristics of each major type of cardiothoracic injury.
1.2 Describe frequent mechanisms of injury for each cardiothoracic injury.
2.0 Describe the initial assessment for possible cardiothoracic injury.
2.1 Identify types of prehospital information that give clues to diagnosis.
2.2 Identify important items in the patient interview that relate to cardiothoracic trauma.
2.3 Identify steps in physical examination of the chest.
2.4 List laboratory studies used in suspected chest injury.
2.5 List radiologic studies commonly required for definitive diagnosis.
3.0 Develop nursing diagnoses based on assessment data.
3.1 List common nursing diagnoses and specific etiologic factors related to cardiothoracic trauma.
3.2 Identify signs and symptoms that validate the specific nursing diagnoses.

4.0 Anticipate and assist with appropriate medical-surgical interventions for cardiothoracic injury.

4.1 Given specific patient data, recognize medical-surgical interventions that might be required.

4.2 Given specific patient data, state the equipment to be obtained to assist with medical interventions.

4.3 Describe pharmacologic agents likely to be used for the patient with cardiothoracic injury and the rationale for each agent.

5.0 Identify nursing interventions required for the patient with chest injury.

5.1 List common nursing interventions, and their rationale, for patients with cardiothoracic trauma.

5.2 Given a patient scenario, prioritize nursing interventions.

6.0 Evaluate patient response to medical and nursing interventions.

6.1 Define desirable outcomes with measurable criteria for the patient with cardiothoracic trauma.

6.2 List nursing activities required for continuous monitoring and evaluation of patient status.

6.3 List types of data to include in nursing documentation.

6.4 Cite trends in patient status that may require priority interventions from nurse or physician.

7.0 Given a specific case history, formulate a plan of nursing care for a patient who experiences cardiothoracic injury and requires care throughout the trauma continuum.

A. PATTERNS OF INJURY: PATHOPHYSIOLOGY

1. **Bony structures**

a. Rib fracture

(1) Etiology—usually blunt trauma from motor vehicle crashes (MVCs), falls, assaults

(2) Cause decreased minute ventilation due to splinting from pain, and pulmonary shunting from atelectasis and hypoxia

(3) May be associated with concomitant injuries

(a) First and second rib fractures associated with fractures of clavicle and scapula

(b) First rib fractures seen with lacerations of subclavian artery or vein, and aortic rupture

(c) Left lower rib fracture associated with splenic injury

(d) Right lower rib fracture associated with liver injury

(e) Sternal fracture associated with pulmonary contusion and/or cardiac contusion

(4) Cartilaginous injuries are similar, but often more painful, and take longer to heal

(5) Diagnostic indicators

(a) Chest wall pain aggravated by deep breathing, coughing

(b) Localized tenderness
(c) Shallow respiratory effort
(d) Movement, crepitus at fracture site
(e) Upright PA chest film may show rib fractures
(6) Complications
(a) Pneumo/hemothorax
(b) Pneumomediastinum
(c) Tension pneumothorax
(d) Nonunion of fracture

b. Flail chest
(1) Fracture of two or more ribs and/or cartilage on both sides of impact point results in "floating" segment
(a) Anterior, lateral, posterior, or sternal
(b) Subatmospheric, intrathoracic pressure during inspiration causes segment to go inward (paradoxic movement)
(c) Underlying alveolar tissue compressed; causes pulmonary physiologic shunting and venous admixture, resulting in decreased PaO_2
(d) Mortality rates range from 5 to 50%
(2) Etiology—blunt trauma, e.g., steering wheel
(3) May not be seen initially as patient splints chest wall and muscle spasms occur; seen as patient tires, usually within first 24 hrs
(4) Chest wall stable at about two to three weeks after injury
(5) Diagnostic indicators
(a) Rapid and labored breathing
(b) Paradoxical chest wall movement
(c) Palpation of crepitus, fracture
(d) Pain on inspiration or palpation
(e) Hypoxia
(f) Absent or decreased breath sounds on affected side
(g) Dyspnea, tachypnea, respiratory failure
(h) Abrasion, laceration, or ecchymosis
(i) Chest x-ray may show rib or sternal fractures
(3) Related injuries are pulmonary contusion or pneumothorax

c. Sternal fracture
(1) Require enormous force to fracture; therefore, look for cardiopulmonary injuries
(2) Mortality—25 to 45% (1)
(3) Diagnostic indicators
(a) Often unstable; look for flail sternum
(b) Palpable "step-off" deformity
(c) Mediastinal air under sternum; "crunch" felt with palpation
(d) Pain that increases with deep breath
(e) Local tenderness, crepitus, or deformity
(f) ECG abnormalities from cardiac contusion

2. Pleural spaces

a. Pneumothorax
(1) Air in pleural space due to rupture of air sacs
(a) Loss of intrapulmonary/intrapleural subatmospheric pressure

(b) Elastic recoil leads to collapse; causes decreased area for ventilation/perfusion and hypoxemia

(2) Etiology—blunt, penetrating, or iatrogenic trauma; pneumothorax is the most common chest injury

(3) Diagnostic indicators
- (a) Frequently asymptomatic
- (b) Shortness of breath; respiratory distress
- (c) Sudden, sharp, pleuritic pain
- (d) Hyperresonance on percussion
- (e) Decreased or absent breath sounds
- (f) Chest x-ray shows pneumothorax

b. Open pneumothorax

(1) Equilibrium established between the pleural space and atmospheric pressure
- (a) If opening is two-thirds the tracheal diameter, air flows through the pleural opening rather than the normal airway, since air follows the path of least resistance
- (b) Mediastinal "to and fro" motion with inspiration and expiration

(2) Etiology—penetrating trauma, e.g., GSW, impalement; large chest wall defect

(3) Diagnostic indicators
- (a) Visible defect
- (b) Restlessness
- (c) Dyspnea, tachypnea, cyanosis
- (d) Asymmetrical chest expansion
- (e) Gas bubbles at wound site; subcutaneous emphysema
- (f) Sucking sound
- (g) Hypoxia
- (h) Reduced venous return

c. Tension pneumothorax

(1) One-way valve created, so air enters pleural space on inspiration but cannot escape on expiration
- (a) Positive pressure builds in pleural space causing collapse of affected lung
- (b) Mediastinal shift away from affected lung

(2) Etiology—blunt or penetrating trauma
- (a) Open chest wound
- (b) Damage to lung parenchyma
- (c) Barotrauma
- (d) Fractured ribs
- (e) Tracheobronchial tree injuries

(3) Diagnostic indicators
- (a) Restlessness; extreme agitation
- (b) Severe air hunger, dyspnea, tachypnea, retractions
- (c) Hypoxia
- (d) Decreased or absent breath sounds on affected side
- (e) Tracheal deviation from affected side
- (f) Hypertympany to percussion
- (g) Decrease in cardiac output from impaired venous return, increased intrathoracic pressure, and kinking of great vessels
- (h) Tachycardia

(i) Distended neck veins; hypovolemia will prevent this sign
(j) Upright PA chest film
(4) Complications
(a) Decreased cardiac output
(b) Upper airway obstruction
(c) Pneumomediastinum or subcutaneous emphysema

d. Hemothorax
(1) Blood in pleural space
(2) Etiology—blunt, penetrating, or iatrogenic injury
(3) Diagnostic indicators
(a) Dyspnea; shortness of breath
(b) Decreased breath sounds on side of hemothorax
(c) Dull percussion note
(d) Chest x-ray shows increased density or haziness
(4) Complications
(a) Decreased cardiac output
(b) Fibrosis
(c) Empyema

e. Massive hemothorax
(1) Accumulation of 1.5 to 4 liters of blood in pleural space; pleural space can hold entire blood volume
(2) Etiology—blunt or penetrating trauma
(a) Bleeding sources on left side, in decreasing order of frequency; left is most common side for bleeding sources
i) Rib fracture
ii) Pulmonary parenchyma
iii) Aortic isthmus
iv) Spleen
v) Heart
vi) Intercostal artery
vii) Supraaortic vessel
viii) Major pulmonary vessel
ix) Diaphragm
(b) Bleeding sources on right side, in decreasing order of frequency
i) Rib fracture
ii) Pulmonary parenchyma
iii) Liver
iv) Intercostal/internal mammary artery
v) Supraaortic vessel
vi) Pulmonary vessel
vii) Aortic isthmus
viii) Heart
ix) Diaphragm
(3) Diagnostic indicators
(a) Shock symptoms
(b) Lack of breath sounds on affected side
(c) Tracheal deviation toward unaffected side
(d) Hypoxia

(e) Flat neck veins
(f) Mediastinal shift
(g) Decrease in cardiac output
(h) Dullness to percussion
(i) Upright PA chest film
(4) Complication—exsanguination leading to cardiac arrest

3. Thoracic tissues

a. Upper airway obstruction
(1) Aspiration of foreign bodies, blood, and teeth; maxillofacial trauma; edema; tongue prolapse; prolonged, severe compression to chest
(2) Etiology—blunt and penetrating trauma; burns; traumatic asphyxia
(3) Diagnostic indicators
(a) Inability to talk or "get enough air"
(b) Restlessness, anxiety, unresponsiveness
(c) Hypoxia
(d) Hypercarbia
(e) Use of accessory muscles in neck and abdomen; retractions
(f) Tachycardia
(g) Cyanosis
(h) Large or expanding hematoma
(i) Massive edema
(j) Chest/neck radiographs
(k) Bronchoscopy

b. Ruptured larynx or trachea
(1) Infrequent injuries that can be rapidly fatal; extravasation of blood into laryngeal tissues results in airway edema and asphyxia due to obstruction
(2) Larynx is composed of unpaired cartilage (cricoid, thyroid, and epiglottic) and paired cartilage (arytenoid, cuneiform, and corniculate); latter play major role in phonation
(3) After age 40, thyroid cartilage loses much of its elasticity, so severe force often shatters cartilage
(4) Mechanism of injury—blunt (most common), or penetrating injury; usually caused by deceleration with upward and backward force to neck by steering wheel, clothesline, or strangulation
(5) Associated injuries
(a) Cervical spine injuries
(b) Recurrent laryngeal nerve injuries
(c) Carotid or jugular vein injuries
(d) Esophageal injuries
(e) Oral injuries; facial fractures
(f) Chest injuries
(g) Closed head injuries
(6) Injuries include soft tissue contusion and laceration, avulsion of vocal cords, fracture of thyroid and cricoid cartilage, subluxation of arytenoid joint, or laryngotracheal disruption (2)
(7) Diagnostic indicators
(a) One-third of patients have no symptoms (2)
(b) Airway distress; stridor

(c) Dysphonia, hoarseness, aphonia
(d) Hemoptysis
(e) External signs of trauma; wound proximity
(f) Crepitus; palpable fracture
(g) Subcutaneous emphysema
(h) Distortion of cartilaginous landmarks
(i) Pain with neck motion, coughing, or swallowing (dysphagia)
(j) Cough
(k) Extreme agitation
(l) Inability to make high-pitched "e" sound, which requires mobile cricoarytenoid joints, normal tense cords, and functional intrinsic laryngeal neuromuscular mechanisms (3)
(m) Local wound exploration
(n) Free air in neck on plain film of neck
(o) Laryngeal CAT scan
(p) Indirect or direct laryngoscopy

(8) Complications
(a) Airway obstruction
(b) Aspiration
(c) Cellulitis or abscess
(d) Superior laryngeal nerve injury
(e) Permanent voice changes
(f) Stenosis caused by exaggerated healing, especially in cricoid injuries
(g) Posttraumatic fibrosis of cricoarytenoid joint, which severely impairs vocalization; minimized with fine surgical techniques

c. Ruptured bronchus
(1) Injury may occur at any level; most occur within one inch of the carina
(a) Pneumothorax on affected side
(b) Causes decreased ventilation, hypoxia, mediastinal emphysema with possible cardiac decompensation

(2) Etiology
(a) Blunt trauma—impact creates sudden, increased pressure in airway against closed glottis
(b) Penetrating trauma—seen in association with carotid, esophageal, or jugular trauma

(3) Diagnostic indicators
(a) Dyspnea, respiratory distress
(b) Tension pneumothorax, usually on right side
(c) Mediastinal and subcutaneous air
(d) Air leak and inability of lung to reexpand despite chest tube insertion; may be due to tension pneumothorax
(e) Hemoptysis
(f) Chest x-ray shows pneumomediastinum, pneumothorax, subcutaneous emphysema, upper rib fractures
(g) Bronchoscopy for definitive diagnosis

(4) Complications
(a) Massive subcutaneous emphysema with possible obstruction of remaining bronchus

(b) Aspiration of blood causing pneumonia or chemical pneumonitis
(c) Infection, bronchiectasis

d. Inhalation injury
   (1) Results in a variety of abnormalities, including tracheobronchitis, airway obstruction, injury to alveolar epithelium, increased capillary permeability, pulmonary edema, impaired gas exchange, and/or pulmonary insufficiency
   (2) Major types and etiologies
      (a) Carbon monoxide poisoning—by-product of combustion; CO is liberated in great amounts during a fire and has an affinity for hemoglobin 200 times greater than that of oxygen
      (b) Lower airway injury—primarily a result of the effects of chemicals, rather than heat, on respiratory passages
         i) Smoke is composed of a unique mixture of solid and liquid particles in gases
         ii) Gases, e.g., nitrous oxide and sulfur dioxide, combine with lung water to generate corrosive acids and alkalis
      (c) Upper airway injury—due to effects of direct heat on oral cavity, nasopharynx, pharynx, and vocal cords
         i) Generally, a blast of hot gas causes reflex closure of epiglottis and vocal cords, which prevents heat damage to lower airway
         ii) Inflammatory response causes edema and potential obstruction of upper airway
      (d) Restrictive abnormalities
         i) May result from decreased chest excursion due to restrictive effect of circumferential chest burns
         ii) Noncardiogenic pulmonary edema may result from increased extravasation into pulmonary parenchyma as a consequence of generalized burn edema, or inflammatory response to smoke inhalation
   (3) May be associated with concomitant cutaneous burns; increases mortality 30 to 40% compared to patients with similar burn area and no inhalation component
   (4) Diagnostic indicators
      (a) Pulmonary abnormalities are not always apparent; maintain high index of suspicion, particularly if victim is found in a closed space
      (b) History of injury scenario; length of exposure, type of burning/chemical material, condition of patient when rescued
      (c) Elevated carboxyhemoglobin; neurologic symptoms of carbon monoxide poisoning, including fatigue, dizziness, ataxia, headache, confusion, combativeness, seizures, hallucinations, or coma
      (d) Tachycardia, cardiac dysrhythmia, and/or ischemic changes on ECG
      (e) Tachypnea, cough, hoarseness, stridor, dyspnea, sternal retractions, wheezing, sooty sputum, chest pain or tightness, rales, and rhonchi
      (f) Cutaneous burns of face and neck, burns or sooty nares and nasal vibrissae, erythema, blisters, and/or edema of lips, buccal, and pharyngeal mucosa areas
      (g) Fiberoptic bronchoscopy
      (h) Serial chest x-rays often normal, initially
      (i) Pulmonary function studies

(j) Xenon-133 lung scan
(5) Complications
(a) Pulmonary edema
(b) Bronchopneumonia
(c) Respiratory insufficiency, ARDS
(d) Bronchial or tracheal stenosis
(e) Bronchial obliterans, bronchiectasis
(f) Chronic bronchitis
(g) Neurologic sequelae of carbon monoxide poisoning, e.g., personality changes and memory impairment

e. Pulmonary contusion
(1) Bruising of lung causes
(a) Capillary hemorrhage
(b) Leukocyte and platelet aggregation in pulmonary vasculature; leads to release of vasoactive substances
(c) Loss of pulmonary capillary integrity; extravasation of water and plasma proteins into alveolar and interstitial spaces; congestive atelectasis
(d) Surfactant dilution resulting in decreased lung compliance
(e) Decreased functional residual capacity due to pulmonary physiologic shunt, which causes venous admixture and hypoxemia
(2) Etiology—blunt trauma (deceleration), or high-velocity missile
(3) Diagnostic indicators
(a) Hemoptysis
(b) Fever
(c) Tachycardia
(d) Hypoxia, hypercarbia
(e) Wheezing, rales, tachypnea
(f) Decrease in pulmonary compliance
(g) Increase in airway pressure
(h) Nonsegmental whiteout on chest x-ray
(4) Complications
(a) Irreversible hypoxia and acidosis
(b) Pleural effusion
(c) Infection

f. Ruptured esophagus
(1) Etiology—penetrating injury is primary cause; in blunt trauma; rupture occurs due to blow to upper abdomen or ingestion of caustic substance
(2) Diagnostic indicators
(a) Shock out of proportion to injury
(b) Particulate matter in chest tube
(c) Subcutaneous and/or mediastinal air noted on palpation or chest x-ray
(d) Gastrografin swallow and/or esophagoscopy for definitive diagnosis
(3) Complications
(a) Mediastinitis
(b) Vascular erosion, from esophageal juices, which leads to hemorrhage
(c) Esophageal stricture
(d) Mechanical tracheal obstruction
(e) Pneumothorax

(f) Pulmonary effusion
(g) Empyema
(h) Malnutrition

g. Ruptured diaphragm
(1) Hole in diaphragm; abdominal contents may herniate through diaphragm; ruptures are more common on left side
(2) Etiology—blunt or penetrating trauma
(3) Diagnostic indicators
(a) Range from no symptoms to profuse shock
(b) Require high index of suspicion; no specific external signs
(c) Severe pain may be referred to shoulder
(d) Dyspnea; decreased breath sounds
(e) If abdominal contents herniate
i) Bowel sounds in chest
ii) Decreased breath sounds on side with compressed lung
iii) Shock
iv) Upright PA chest film may show nasogastric tube (NGT) in left chest
v) Contrast studies of esophagus and/or stomach
(f) If not diagnosed, patient may have days to decades of positional dyspnea, dyspnea upon exertion, chest pain, intermittent, cramping epigastric pain, distress after heavy meals or when lying supine
(4) Complications—bowel necrosis; atelectasis

4. Cardiovascular tissues

a. Cardiac contusion
(1) Bruising of heart; small to large area of hemorrhage that can rupture at any time
(a) Capillary hemorrhage causing disruption or separation of myocardial fibers
(b) Decreased cardiac output and decreased inotropic effect
(2) Etiology—blunt trauma
(3) Diagnostic indicators
(a) High index of suspicion based on mechanism of injury
(b) Precordial pain
(c) External signs of trauma, i.e., contusions, lacerations
(d) Tachycardia most common sign
(e) Arrhythmias—multiple premature ventricular contractions (PVCs), ventricular tachycardia, atrial fibrillation, or conduction blocks
(f) ECG changes indicative of ischemia
(g) Serial creatine phosphokinase isoenzymes (CPK-MB) fractions; more than 5% of total CPK indicates damage
(4) Complications
(a) Cardiac tamponade
(b) Cardiogenic shock if contusion involves more than 40% of ventricular surface
(c) Myocardial rupture
(d) Fibrosis with or without ventricular aneurysm
(e) Valve injuries
(f) Constrictive pericarditis is common
i) Findings include pericardial friction rub, fatigue, complaints of chest pain

ii) Treat with nonsteroidal antiinflammatory drugs (NSAIDs)

b. Cardiac tamponade
  (1) Accumulation of blood in the tough, nondistensible pericardium
  (2) Etiology—blunt and penetrating trauma; penetrating trauma is most common
  (3) Diagnostic indicators
    (a) Beck's triad
      i) Decrease in systolic BP
      ii) Venous pressure elevation; distended neck veins not seen with severe hypovolemia; elevated central venous pressure
      iii) Muffled heart sounds
    (b) Narrowing pulse pressure
    (c) Paradoxical pulse (pulsus paradoxus)—systolic BP decreases more than 10 mm Hg with inspiration
    (d) Agitation
    (e) Air hunger; respiratory distress
    (f) Pericardiocentesis provides diagnosis and initial treatment

c. Aorta or great vessel rupture/transection
  (1) Description
    (a) Complete transection often results in immediate death
    (b) Incomplete transections require high index of suspicion for rapid diagnosis and intervention
      i) Intimal tears and thrombosis possible
      ii) Common anatomic sites that are susceptible to shearing injuries
        a) Ligamentum arteriosum, distal to the origin of left subclavian artery
        b) Root of the aorta above aortic valve
        c) Aortic hiatus at diaphragm
        d) Innominate artery
      iii) High risk of early rupture; therefore, time is of the essence
  (2) Etiology—blunt (acceleration/deceleration) and penetrating trauma
  (3) Diagnostic indicators
    (a) Restlessness; dyspnea
    (b) Hoarseness from hematoma-induced laryngeal complications
    (c) Dysphagia from hematoma-induced esophageal complications
    (d) Stridor
    (e) Retrosternal, interscapular pain
    (f) Upper extremity hypertension
    (g) Pulse and blood pressure difference between arms
    (h) Palpable difference in pulse amplitude between upper and lower extremities
    (i) Decreased or absent femoral pulses
    (j) Tachycardia
    (k) Hypotension
    (l) Pallor
    (m) Unrelenting shock
    (n) Chest x-ray findings
      i) Widened mediastinum
      ii) Obliteration of aortic knob
      iii) Pleural capping

iv) Deviation of NGT to the right
v) Fracture of first or second rib
(o) CAT scan or MRI
(p) Arteriogram—definitive diagnostic modality
(4) Complications
(a) Paraplegia
(b) Bowel ischemia
(c) Renal failure
(d) Anoxia
(e) Brain injury
(f) Left ventricular failure
(g) Complications related to aortic cross-clamping; massive hypertension or left recurrent laryngeal nerve injury

d. Other cardiac injuries
(1) Description
(a) Lacerations of heart chambers
(b) Lacerations of valve leaflets
(c) Penetrating injuries of coronary arteries or veins; injuries to the left anterior descending coronary vessels are most common
(d) Thrombosis of coronary artery
(e) Perforation of cardiac septum usually fatal
(2) Etiology
(a) Blunt trauma—rapid deceleration of heart against anterior chest wall or crushing injury; anterior wall of right ventricle is most frequently involved
(b) Penetrating trauma
(3) Diagnostic indicators
(a) Arrhythmias
(b) Murmurs
(c) Pericardiocentesis
(d) Congestive failure
(e) CPK-MB fraction greater than 5% of total CPK
(f) 12-lead ECG
(g) 2-D echocardiogram
(h) Cardiac catheterization once patient is stable

B. MEDICAL AND SURGICAL INTERVENTIONS

1. General interventions

a. Open airway; relieve obstruction

b. Intubate airway—listed in preferred order
(1) Oro- or nasopharyngeal airway
(2) Endotracheal tube
(3) Cricothyroidotomy for obstructed airway
(4) Tracheostomy for obstructed airway

c. Correct hypoxemia with high flow humidified oxygen—100% nonrebreathing mask preferred

d. Occlude sucking chest wound with sterile dressing; secure on only three sides to prevent development of a tension pneumothorax
e. Convert tension pneumothorax to open pneumothorax with needle decompression at second intercostal space, midclavicular line (MCL)
f. Utilize mechanical ventilation
   (1) Positive end-expiratory pressure (PEEP)
   (2) Independent lung ventilation
   (3) Pressure support ventilation
   (4) High frequency jet ventilation
g. Provide continuous positive airway pressure (CPAP)
h. Control bleeding by direct external pressure, operative intervention, or radiographic embolization
i. Apply pneumatic antishock garment
j. Administer warmed I.V. fluids, blood, and blood components; autotransfusion
k. Administer antibiotics as prescribed
l. Treat acidosis
m. Insert thoracostomy tube
n. Perform pericardiocentesis
o. Perform thoracotomy
p. Utilize cardiopulmonary bypass
q. Surgically repair specific injuries
r. Bronchoscopy to remove foreign bodies

2. Specific injury treatment

a. Rib fractures
   (1) Alleviate pain with prescribed pain medications, nerve blocks, epidural medications, or TENS unit
   (2) Avoid rib binders, as they may increase atelectasis
   (3) Initiate operative fixation in severe cases
b. Flail chest
   (1) Stabilize flail segment with sandbags, or tape and pads; initially, turn patient onto affected side
   (2) Intubate and ventilate; PEEP often required
   (3) Perform open reducation internal fixation if massive flail
   (4) Control pain to allow full lung expansion
   (5) Prevent hypoxemia; correct respiratory acidosis
c. Sternal fractures
   (1) Treatment of fractures rarely needed; treat associated injuries
   (2) Surgical repair may be required
   (3) Manage pain
d. Pneumothorax—allow lung reexpansion with chest tube and waterseal drainage
e. Open pneumothorax
   (1) Close defect with occlusive dressing; anchor on three sides only to prevent tension pneumothorax
   (2) Surgical repair of defect
f. Tension pneumothorax
   (1) Immediately decompress affected cavity; use at least a 14-gauge needle, inserted above rib margin at second intercostal space in midclavicular line (MCL); avoid internal mammary and intercostal arteries
   (2) Establish waterseal drainage

g. Hemothorax
   (1) Insert large bore closed chest tube drainage
   (2) Monitor drainage amount and replace blood loss
   (3) Repair surgically, if necessary
   (4) Prevent infection (empyema)
h. Massive hemothorax
   (1) Resuscitate with fluid prior to thoracostomy; chest tube may release tamponade of bleeding vessels
   (2) Insert chest tube and monitor drainage
   (3) Replace blood loss; initiate autotransfusion
i. Upper airway obstruction—provide patent airway and/or relieve obstruction
j. Ruptured larynx or bronchus
   (1) Obtain/maintain airway—airway obstruction is most common cause of death
      (a) Intubation
         i) Blind or hasty intubation may cause mucosal stripping and bleeding, displacement of fractured cartilage into airway lumen, or laryngeal obstruction
         ii) In gaping wounds, can intubate directly through wound and do formal tracheotomy in operating room
         iii) Utilize fiberoptic bronchoscope to help intubation
      (b) Immediate cricothyroidotomy or tracheostomy
      (c) Operative repair possibilities
         i) Suture or wire lacerations
         ii) Replace tissue defects with mucosal grafts from cheek, fascial flap, or synthetic patch
         iii) Reduce/repair cartilage fractures
         iv) Place stents to support repair for six to eight weeks
         v) Laryngotomy for fracture, collapse, or separation of hyoid and cricoid cartilage (2)
      (d) Antibiotics should be prescribed
      (e) Maintain tracheostomy until healing is complete and edema is gone (four to eight days)
   (2) Observe patient if no airway obstruction
      (a) Edema/hemorrhage may occlude or obstruct airway in next 48 hrs
      (b) Place patient on bed rest, stabilize neck, and keep head of bed at 30° angle
      (c) Provide humidified oxygen to keep airway moist
      (d) Prophylactic antibiotics
      (e) Minimize analgesics and sedation, which may depress respiration and increase possiblity of airway obstruction
      (f) Observe for progressive subcutaneous emphysema; treatment is needed if it does occur
      (g) Keep NPO for about 48 hrs; swallowing is painful and often causes pharyngeal spasm and/or aspiration
k. Ruptured bronchus
   (1) Maintain airway; insert endotracheal tube past laceration or insert bifurcated tube
   (2) Synchronous independent lung ventilation (SILV)
   (3) Perform immediate operative repair to prevent stricture
l. Inhalation injury

(1) Prophylactic intubation
(2) Continuous positive airway pressure
(3) High flow (100% initially) humidified oxygen
(4) Pharmacologic agents—bronchodilators, steroids (controversial), antibiotics
(5) Fluid replacement; avoid overload
(6) Mechanical ventilation with PEEP
(7) Hyperbaric oxygenation may be useful in treatment of severe carbon monoxide poisoning

m. Pulmonary contusion
(1) Decrease pulmonary shunt
(a) Administer O_2; use lowest FiO_2 possible
(b) Increase FRC with PEEP
(2) Increase effective compliance with diuretics
(3) Treat unilateral contusion with SILV, if indicated

n. Ruptured esophagus
(1) Control airway bleeding
(2) Reconstruct surgically
(3) Prevent infection with adequate drainage and antibiotics
(4) Maintain nutrition
(5) Intubate stomach to decrease possible aspiration and promote drainage

o. Ruptured diaphragm
(1) Often overlooked; diagnose early
(2) Repair operatively

p. Cardiac contusion
(1) Relieve myocardial ischemia; treatment is similar to that for a patient with myocardial infarction
(2) Monitor cardiac output and cardiovascular status
(3) Intraaortic balloon pump (IABP) may be used in cardiogenic shock
(4) Monitor for life-threatening cardiac arrhythmias for first 48 to 72 hrs

q. Cardiac tamponade
(1) Perform pericardiocentesis—removal of 15 to 20 ml of fluid may relieve tamponade
(2) Open thoracotomy if pericardiocentesis does not relieve tamponade
(3) Definitive operative intervention needed; must identify pathology and prevent rebleeding

r. Aortic or great vessel rupture/transection
(1) Maintain adequate circulating volume
(2) Cardiopulmonary bypass or vessel clamping
(3) Operative resection and grafting

C. NURSING ASSESSMENT

1. Interview (see Module 19—Nursing Assessment)

a. Mechanism of injury

b. Subjective complaints
(1) Dyspnea; shortness of breath
(2) Pain related to respiration

c. History of pulmonary and/or cardiac disease

2. Physical examination

a. Inspection
   (1) Chest symmetry
   (2) Tracheal position
   (3) Neck vein distension
   (4) Respiratory rate and rhythm
   (5) Color of lips, conjunctivae, distal extremities
   (6) Lacerations, contusions, abrasions

b. Palpation
   (1) Carotid and peripheral pulses
   (2) Subcutaneous emphysema
   (3) Tracheal position
   (4) Fractures of ribs, clavicles, sternum, and/or thoracic spine

c. Percussion
   (1) Dull tones frequently found with hemothorax
   (2) Hypertympany found with pneumothorax

d. Auscultation
   (1) Breath sounds
   (2) Heart sounds for loudness, muffling, murmurs, extra sounds
   (3) Blood pressure in both arms

3. Laboratory studies

a. Trauma profile
b. Arterial blood gases
c. Cardiac enzymes and isoenzymes

4. Radiologic studies

a. Chest x-ray
b. Computerized axial tomography (CAT) scan
c. Arteriography
d. Fluoroscopy
e. Magnetic resonance imaging
f. Gastrografin or barium swallow

5. Other studies

a. Electrocardiogram
b. Nuclear scans
c. Fiberoptic bronchoscopy
d. Echocardiogram

D. NURSING DIAGNOSES, EXPECTED OUTCOMES, AND INTERVENTIONS

1. Ineffective breathing pattern related to pain of injuries or surgical interventions

a. Expected outcomes
   (1) Respiratory rate regular at 12 to 20/min
   (2) Tidal volume of at least 10 ml/kg

(3) Arterial blood gases in normal range
(4) Patient takes deep breath without pain

b. Nursing interventions
(1) Monitor breathing pattern, rate, tidal volume, and signs and symptoms of respiratory distress
(2) Teach patient to splint chest prior to moving or coughing; avoid rib binders as they prevent patient from taking a deep breath and thus ensure atelectasis
(3) Position patient to promote optimal lung expansion
(4) Administer analgesia as prescribed; utilize continuous infusions or patient-controlled analgesia for more consistent pain relief
(5) Assist with intercostal nerve blocks
(6) Assist with Marcaine infusions into chest tube
(7) Assist with transcutaneous electrical nerve stimulation (TENS) unit
(8) Monitor epidural infusions of narcotics

2. Ineffective breathing pattern related to unstable chest wall segment, loss of thoracic bellows, lung collapse, or open pneumothorax

a. Expected outcomes
(1) Respiratory rate 12 to 20/min
(2) PaO_2 greater than 80 mm Hg on room air
(3) Clear chest x-ray
(4) Tidal volume at least 10 ml/kg

b. Nursing interventions
(1) Monitor flail segment; effective treatment should eliminate or minimize defect
(2) Defect may not be immediately obvious
(3) Stabilize flail with sandbags, dressings, and tape, or by turning patient to affected side before intubation
(4) Provide high flow humidified oxygen
(5) Assist with intubation and monitor ventilation
(6) Maintain mechanical ventilation until patient is able to breathe effectively without support; three weeks required for start of bony union
(7) May require sedation and/or paralysis to allow for control of ventilation
(8) Apply sterile nonocclusive dressing at end of exhalation; tape on three sides; check for tension
(9) Prepare patient for, and assist with, chest tube insertion
(10) Additional interventions (see 1.b. above)

3. Impaired gas exchange related to decrease in functioning lung tissue, pulmonary contusion, aspiration of foreign body, smoke inhalation, air leak from tracheobronchial tree rupture

a. Expected outcomes
(1) PaO_2 greater than 80 mm Hg on room air
(2) SVO_2 is 70 to 75%
(3) Oxygen saturation greater than 98%
(4) Respiratory rate regular and 12 to 20/min

b. Nursing interventions
(1) Maintain patent airway; assist with intubation
(2) Administer humidified oxygen
(3) Auscultate breath sounds

(4) Monitor I.V. fluids; avoid fluid overload in patients with pulmonary contusion
(5) Monitor breathing pattern and signs and symptoms of respiratory distress
(6) Monitor ABGs, SVO_2, chest x-rays, and pulse oximetry
(7) Assist with bronchoscopy to remove foreign body or diagnose tracheal rupture
(8) Position patient to enhance perfusion of healthy lung tissue
(9) Provide pulmonary toilet
(10) Relieve tension pneumothorax or hemothorax
(11) Assess and maintain closed chest drainage system
(12) Monitor chest tube drainage for continuous air leaks (tracheoesophageal fistula, PEEP, CPAP)
(13) Increase functional residual capacity
(14) Change inspiratory-expiratory (I:E) ratio to increase inspiratory time
(15) Maintain SILV

4. Ineffective airway clearance related to impaired cough and/or increased, thick secretions or obstruction

a. Expected outcomes—patent airway
b. Nursing interventions
(1) Provide adequate hydration
(2) Assess airway
(3) Manually remove debris or obstruction
(4) Open airway; position oropharyngeal airway
(5) Assist with intubation and maintain mechanical ventilation
(6) Prepare patient for cricothyroidotomy
(7) Assess for dysphonia, stridor, subcutaneous emphysema, hemoptysis, dyspnea, accessory muscle use
(8) Teach patient splinting techniques for coughing
(9) Ultrasonic nebulization

5. Decreased cardiac output related to alterations in intrapleural pressures, i.e., tension pneumothorax, hemothorax, open pneumothorax

a. Expected outcomes
(1) Apical pulse rate 60 to 100/min; normal sinus rhythm
(2) Cardiac output at 4 l to 8 l/min
(3) SVO_2 is 70 to 75%
(4) Able to walk distance typical of preinjury status
(5) Urine output greater than 0.5 to 1.0 ml/kg/hr
(6) Normal movement of extremities
(7) Peripheral pulses intact
b. Nursing interventions
(1) Monitor ABGs, SVO_2, pulse oximetry, cardiac output, cardiac index, systemic vascular resistance, shunt fraction ratio
(2) Position patient to enhance perfusion of healthy lung tissue and enhance cardiac output
(3) Set up, monitor, and maintain closed chest drainage; notify physician if initial pleural drainage is more than 1500 ml blood, or hourly output is more than 200 ml/hr, for four hours, in patient without coagulopathy
(4) Set up, monitor, and maintain autotransfusion system

(5) Inspect and redress chest tube insertion site as needed
(6) Document character and amount of chest drainage
(7) Perform or assist with needle decompression for tension pneumothorax

6. **Decrease in cardiac output and myocardial perfusion related to direct cardiac injury**

a. Expected outcomes
(1) Apical pulse rate 60 to 100/min; normal sinus rhythm
(2) Cardiac output at 4 l to 8 l/min
(3) SVO_2 is 70 to 75%
(4) Able to walk distance typical of preinjury status
(5) Urine output greater than 0.5 to 1.0 ml/kg/hr
(6) Normal movement of extremities
(7) Peripheral pulses intact

b. Nursing interventions
(1) Initiate two large bore peripheral I.V.s and infuse warmed, lactated Ringer's solution
(2) Apply direct pressure to bleeding sites
(3) Protect patient from hypothermia
(4) Set up, monitor, and maintain autotransfusion system
(5) Note new onset of murmurs, emboli, or arrhythmias
(6) Treat congestive heart failure
(7) Use IABP to assist ventricular function as necessary
(8) Monitor cardiac enzymes
(9) Prepare patient for diagnostic studies to determine degree of injury

7. **Additional nursing diagnoses**

a. Fluid volume deficit related to massive hemothorax or aortic rupture
b. Fear related to feelings of suffocation, etc.
c. Potential for infection related to foreign body, vascular graft insertion, or leakage from esophagus
d. Potential for infection related to pulmonary stasis, wound contamination, and inadequate wound drainage (see Module 16—Medical Sequelae—and Module 12—Infection)
e. Altered nutritional status related to altered GI anatomy

References

1. Rutherford, R. B., & Campbell, D. N. (1985). Thoracic injuries. In G. D. Zuidema, R. B. Rutherford & W. F. Ballinger (Eds.), *The management of trauma* (4th ed., pp. 391–448). Philadelphia: W.B. Saunders Co.
2. Howell, E., Sherer, C. & Leyden, A. (1988). Face and neck trauma. In E. Howell, L. Widra & M. G. Hill (Eds.), *Comprehensive trauma nursing: Theory and practice* (pp. 470–494). Boston: Scott, Foresman & Co.
3. Walton, R. L., Bunker, J., & Borath, G. L. (1986). Maxillofacial trauma. In D. D. Trunkey & F. R. Lewis (Eds.), *Current therapy of trauma* (pp. 181–223). Philadelphia: B. C. Decker.

Suggested Readings

American College of Surgeons, Committee on Trauma. (1989). *Advanced trauma life support student manual.* Chicago: Author.

Balliot, R., Dontigny, L., Verdant, A., Page, P., Page, A., Mercer, C., & Cossetti, R. (1987). Penetrating chest trauma: A 20-year experience. *The Journal of Trauma,* 27(9), 994–997.

Beresky, R., Klinger, R., & Peake, J. (1988). Myocardial contusion: When does it have clinical significance? *The Journal of Trauma,* 28(1), 64–68.

Boggs, R. L. (1988). Cardiovascular trauma. *Trauma Quarterly,* 4(2), 81–89.

Del Rossi, A. J. (Ed.). (1990). Blunt thoracic trauma. *Trauma Quarterly,* 6(3).

Hammond, S. C. (1990). Chest injuries in the trauma patient. *Nursing Clinics of North America,* 25(1), 35–43.

Hurn, P. D. (1988). Thoracic injuries. In V. D. Cardona, P. D. Hurn, P. J. Mason, A. M. Scanlon-Schilpp & S. W. Veise-Berry (Eds.), *Trauma nursing: From resuscitation through rehabilitation* (pp. 449–490). Philadelphia: W. B. Saunders Co.

Kulshrestha, P., Iyer, K. S., Das, B., Baltram, A., Kumar, A. S., Sharma, M. I., Ran, I. M., & Venogupal, P. (1988). Chest injuries: A clinical and autopsy profile. *The Journal of Trauma,* 28(6), 844–847.

Mann, J. K., & Oakes, A. R. (Eds.). (1980). *Critical care nursing of the multiinjured patient.* Philadelphia: W. B. Saunders Co.

Mattox, K. L., Moore, E. E., & Feliciano, D. V. (Eds.). (1988). *Trauma.* East Norwalk, CT: Appleton & Lange.

Sharma, O. P. (1989). Traumatic diaphragmatic rupture: Not an uncommon entity—Personal experience with collective review of the 1980s. *The Journal of Trauma,* 29(5), 678–682.

Strange, J. M. (Ed.). (1987). *Shock trauma care plans.* Springhouse, PA: Springhouse Corp.

Turner, J. T. (1990). Cardiovascular trauma. *Nursing Clinics of North America,* 25(1), 119–130.

Von Rueden, K. T. (1989). Cardiopulmonary assessment of the critically ill trauma patient. *Critical Care Clinics of North America,* 1(1), 33–34.

Weil, P. H., & Margolis, I. B. (1981). Systematic approach to traumatic hemothorax. *American Journal of Surgery,* 142(6), 692–694.

Section IV
Systematic Approach to Trauma Nursing

MODULE 23
ABDOMINAL AND GENITOURINARY INJURY

Donna Wivell Dorozinsky, MSN, RN

Prerequisite

Review anatomy and physiology of liver, spleen, gastrointestinal system, pancreas, and genitourinary system.

Objectives

1.0 Describe common abdominal and genitourinary injuries.
1.1 Briefly describe pathophysiology and major defining characteristics of each injury.
1.2 State frequent mechanisms of injury associated with abdominal and genitourinary trauma.
1.3 State diagnostic indicators for each injury.
1.4 State selected management for each injury.
2.0 Describe the initial assessment for suspected abdominal and genitourinary injuries.
2.1 Identify important items in the patient interview that relate to abdominal and genitourinary trauma.
2.2 Identify steps in the physical examination of the abdomen and genitourinary system.

2.3 List common laboratory studies in the assessment of suspected abdominal and genitourinary injuries.
2.4 List common radiological studies required for definitive diagnosis of abdominal and genitourinary trauma.
3.0 Develop nursing diagnoses based on assessment data.
3.1 List common nursing diagnoses related to abdominal and genitourinary trauma.
3.2 Identify common etiologic factors related to each diagnosis.
3.3 Identify signs and symptoms that validate these diagnoses.
4.0 Anticipate and assist with appropriate medical-surgical interventions for abdominal and genitourinary injuries.
4.1 Given specific patient data, anticipate medical-surgical interventions that may be required.
4.2 Given specific patient data, state the equipment to be obtained to assist with medical interventions.
4.3 Describe pharmacological agents likely to be required for the patient with abdominal and genitourinary injuries; include rationale for each.
4.4 List essential preparations for operative interventions in the patient with abdominal and genitourinary trauma.
5.0 Identify nursing interventions required for the patient with abdominal and genitourinary injuries.
5.1 Relate interventions to specific nursing diagnoses.
5.2 Identify the rationale for each intervention.
5.3 Given a patient scenario, prioritize nursing interventions.
6.0 Evaluate patient's response to medical and nursing interventions.
6.1 Define desirable outcomes with measureable criteria for the patient with abdominal and genitourinary trauma.
6.2 List nursing activities required for continuous monitoring and evaluation of patient status.
6.3 List types of data to be included in nursing documentation.

A. PATTERNS OF INJURY

1. Common etiologies of abdominal injury

a. Blunt abdominal injury is greatest diagnostic challenge
   (1) Mechanisms of injury—MVC, falls, assaults
   (2) Usually in population below 50 years old
   (3) Mortality of 23 to 46% is related to high frequency of associated injuries, e.g., head and thorax (1)
   (4) Organs most commonly injured are liver and spleen; pancreas, stomach, kidneys, and bladder are less likely to be injured

b. Penetrating injury—usually associated with violent crime
   (1) Gunshot wounds (GSW) and stab wounds most common; GSWs are most serious type
   (2) Other penetrating agents include sharp objects, such as metal or glass, found in industry, on farms, and at recreational sites
   (3) Usual population is urban

(4) Mortality (2)
  (a) Stab wounds—1 to 2%
  (b) GSW—5 to 15%; major cause of death is exsanguination prior to definitive treatment
(5) Wound evisceration often accompanies penetrating injury

2. Liver injury

a. Etiology—blunt or penetrating trauma
  (1) Most often caused by vehicular injury
  (2) Mortality rate 10 to 20% (3); usually due to hemorrhage
b. May be associated with left lower rib fractures
c. Diagnostic indicators
  (1) Abdominal guarding
  (2) Profound shock; not responsive to fluid replacement
  (3) Positive abdominal CAT scan
  (4) Positive peritoneal lavage
  (5) Pain in right upper quadrant (RUQ)
  (6) Laboratory studies
    (a) Elevated WBC
    (b) Decreased hematocrit (Hct) and hemoglobin (Hgb)
    (c) Elevated liver enzymes (SGPT, SGOT, and alkaline phosphatase)
    (d) Abnormal coagulation studies, including increased clotting and prothrombin times
d. Grading liver injuries provides a way of identifying extent of injuries (4)
  (1) Grade I—simple injuries; nonbleeding
  (2) Grade II—simple injuries managed by superficial sutures or observation
  (3) Grade III—major intraparenchymal injury with active bleeding but not requiring inflow occlusion to control hemorrhage
  (4) Grade IV—extensive intraparenchymal injury with major active bleeding requiring inflow occlusion
  (5) Grade V—juxtahepatic venous injury, i.e., injury to retrohepatic cava or main hepatic vein
e. Selective management
  (1) Conservative treatment—observation for Grade I injuries
  (2) Operative treatment
    (a) Hemostatic agents, e.g., Gelfoam, Avitene used for Grades I and II
    (b) Drainage
      i) Often bleeding has ceased spontaneously by the time the abdomen is opened; wounds are not sutured
      ii) Drain wounds with large Penrose drains; often several are used
      iii) Drains are brought out through abdominal stab wounds
      iv) Wounds are commonly drained by dependent gravity rather than suction
      v) Drains are required for 5 to 10 days
    (c) Suturing
      i) Provides hemostasis of bleeding injuries
      ii) Ligation of major portions of the hepatic artery also may be needed
    (d) Resection—Grade III and above
      i) Used to control bleeding in severe liver injuries

ii) Resection done 2 to 3 cm beyond the point of injury
iii) Lobectomy reserved for patients who are unstable, despite hepatic resection and/or occlusion of hepatic artery
(e) Transplant—Grade V only

f. Complications of hepatic injury
(1) Disseminated intravascular coagulation (DIC) and clotting abnormalities
(2) Sepsis
(3) Pulmonary—pneumonia and atelectasis
(4) Liver failure

3. Splenic injury

a. Etiology—blunt or penetrating trauma
(1) Often seen with penetrating lower left chest injuries
(2) Most are caused by blunt trauma from MVCs
(3) Deceleration injuries can cause the mobile stomach and colon to transfer the force to the fixed spleen
(4) Assault also accounts for a portion of urban injuries

b. Associated injuries
(1) Vascular disruptions
(2) Left lower rib fractures
(3) Thoracic injuries

c. Diagnostic indicators
(1) Kehr's sign—palpation of left upper quadrant (LUQ) elicits referred left shoulder pain; caused by blood in the peritoneum irritating the diaphragm
(2) Positive peritoneal lavage
(3) Positive CAT scan
(4) Shock; not responsive to fluid replacement
(5) Laboratory studies
(a) Elevated WBC
(b) Decreased Hgb/Hct

d. Selective management
(1) Conservative management—observation
(a) Indications
i) Blunt injuries when no other abdominal injury is suspected
ii) Patient hemodynamically stable
iii) Patient alert and oriented
iv) No coagulopathy present
(b) Treatment
i) Bed rest
ii) Monitor laboratory values frequently
iii) Monitor vital signs closely
iv) Assess abdomen frequently, including abdominal girth; consistent examiner preferred
v) Replace blood components as needed
(2) Splenorrhaphy (splenic repair) preferred, whenever possible, due to complication of overwhelming postsplenectomy infection
(3) Partial splenectomy
(4) Total splenectomy indicated for patients who remain in shock or have associated life-threatening injuries

e. Grading of splenic injury (5)
   (1) Grade I—simple capsular tear and/or subcapsular hematoma; nonsurgical management and suture repair
   (2) Grade II—single or multiple capsular disruptions with parenchymal injury that does not extend into hilum or involve major vessels; minor suture repair and topical hemostatic agent, or splenectomy
   (3) Grade III—deep fractures, single or multiple, that extend into hilum and/or involve major vessels; major suture repair or splenectomy
   (4) Grade IV—injuries that have completely shattered or fragmented the spleen, or avulsed the organ from its blood supply; partial splenic debridement with major suture repair or splenectomy
f. Complications
   (1) Overwhelming postsplenectomy infection (OPSI) or fulminant pneumococcal bacteremia (pneumococcemia); may be prevented by postoperative vaccination (Pneumovax)
   (2) Wound infection
   (3) Subdiaphragmatic abscess
   (4) Pulmonary complications
   (5) Hypovolemic shock

4. Pancreatic injury

a. Relatively uncommon; seen in about 2% of all abdominal trauma (6)
b. Etiology—penetrating or blunt trauma
c. Morbidity/mortality
   (1) Morbidity rate of 36% (7)
   (2) Mortality rate of 8% in stab wounds, 25% in GSWs, and 50% in blunt injuries (6)
      (a) 3 to 9% of deaths due to pancreatic injury alone (8)
      (b) Injury to head of pancreas has twice the mortality of the body/tail injury
   (3) Delay in diagnosis is most frequent cause of morbidity or mortality
      (a) Late signs of injury may develop 12 to 36 hrs after injury
      (b) Symptoms include epigastric pain, tenderness, and guarding
      (c) Injury may occur during clamping of splenic artery for splenectomy
d. Other associated injuries
   (1) Abdominal injuries
   (2) Liver or splenic injuries
   (3) Major abdominal vascular injuries
e. Diagnostic indicators—signs of injury may not be seen immediately
   (1) Local wound exploration to determine penetration of the peritoneum
   (2) Peritoneal lavage may be positive or negative if bleeding is retroperitoneal
   (3) Elevated serum amylase, in most cases
   (4) Positive abdominal CAT scan
   (5) Grey-Turner's sign (ecchymosis in flank area) seen with retroperitoneal organ injuries, e.g., pancreas, kidney
f. Specific management
   (1) Goal is to control bleeding, control pancreatic secretion, and preserve function
   (2) Drainage—hallmark of treatment
      (a) Used for contusions and minor lacerations

(b) Drains are in place 8 to 14 days
(c) Drainage is highly irritating to normal tissue; prevent skin damage
(3) Suture and drain lacerations without ductal injury
(4) Distal pancreatectomy (resection) for major ductal disruptions of the neck, body, or tail of pancreas
(5) Roux-en-Y procedure for crush injuries or injuries to head of pancreas
(6) Closure of proximal end with limb to the jejunum for repair of complete transection
(7) Pancreatoduodenectomy for combination injuries to duodenum, pancreatic head, or common bile duct

g. Metabolic considerations
(1) Impaired exocrine function alters production of fluid and enzymes; may affect digestion of fat and fat-soluble substances
(2) Altered glucose metabolism possible; glucose intolerance if more than 80% of pancreas is removed
(3) Calcium binds with fatty acids released from fat necrosis after injury; hypocalcemia may occur
(4) Use Demerol for pain management; causes less spasm of pancreatic sphincter than morphine

h. Complications and management (8)
(1) Cutaneous or enteric fistula—19% incidence
(a) Maintain drainage system; protect skin from drainage
(b) Replace fluid volume lost; replace bicarbonate if necessary
(c) Usually heals spontaneously with early total parenteral nutrition (TPN)
(2) Pancreatic pseudocyst
(a) 12% incidence; seen several weeks to months after injury
(b) More common with blunt injury; may be due to inadequate drainage
(c) Eventually releases fluid, enzymes, and necrotic tissue
(d) Signs and symptoms include pain, nausea, vomiting, abdominal mass on palpation, and/or increase in serum amylase
(e) Can cause bacterial contamination or abscess formation
(3) Abscess
(4) Delayed hemorrhage
(5) Diabetes/pancreatic insufficiency
(6) Traumatic pancreatitis
(a) Normally enzymes are not activated until they reach duodenum; after trauma, enzymes are activated, which results in an autodigestive state
(b) Signs and symptoms
i) Severe pain radiating toward back
ii) Fever
iii) Vomiting; distension
iv) Weakness
v) Dyspnea
vi) Peritonitis
vii) Increased amylase
a) Serum—elevates within 12 hrs of onset and decreases within 72 hrs
b) Urinary—elevates within 72 to 120 hrs of onset

(c) Complications from vasodilation with release of kinins include shock, adult respiratory distress syndrome (ARDS), ileus, DIC, and/or acute renal failure
(d) Management
i) Hemodynamic stabilization
ii) Reduce pancreatic stress
a) No oral feedings
b) TPN or jejunal feedings
c) Nasogastric suction decreases hydrochloric acid (HCl) secretion, which stimulates enzyme release
iii) Surgery for pseudocyst, abscess, or common duct obstruction

5. Stomach, mesentery, and small bowel injuries

a. Etiology
(1) Penetrating trauma is the most frequent cause of mesentery and small bowel injuries; 80% of abdominal GSWs result in intestinal penetration (1)
(2) Blunt trauma usually results in perforation or small mesenteric tears (9)
(a) Gastric injury—1 to 2% incidence
(b) Small bowel injury—5 to 15% incidence; due to increasing seat belt use, small bowel injury is no longer rare
(c) Frequent causes of bowel trauma
i) Handlebars and seat belts
ii) Direct blows that crush organs between object and spinal column
iii) Shearing forces causing violent torsion, e.g., MVC, fall, jump
(d) Specific injuries may include perforation, rupture, transection, or intramural hematoma
(e) Isolated stomach, mesentery, or small bowel injuries are rare

b. Common associated injuries
(1) Thoracic
(2) Renal
(3) Other abdominal organ injuries

c. Diagnostic indicators
(1) Nausea, vomiting
(2) Positive peritoneal lavage
(3) Stomach injuries may show bloody gastric drainage
(4) Duodenal injuries—specific indicators
(a) Fever
(b) Jaundice
(c) High intestinal obstruction
(d) Fluid loss
(e) Pain in epigastrium or right lower quadrant (RLQ)
(f) Mild epigastric or right side tenderness
(5) Patients with mesentery and small intestine injuries may show no symptoms; small bowel pH is neutral and, therefore, causes less peritoneal irritation
(6) Selected laboratory studies
(7) Flatplate x-ray of the abdomen
(8) Abdominal CAT Scan
(9) Signs are often subtle and require frequent assessment with early diagnosis and intervention

d. Selective management
 (1) Stomach—primary closure; simple closure with rare resection
 (2) Duodenum
  (a) Simple lacerations—primary closure
  (b) Duodenal dysfunctionalization and repair for severe injury, i.e., gastrojejunostomy or duodenojejunostomy
  (c) Vagotomy, antrectomy, and gastrojejunostomy if first part of duodenum is injured
  (d) Treat upper GI obstruction from intramural hematoma with nasogastric suction and I.V. fluids; usually resolves in five days
 (3) Mesentery and small intestine
  (a) Evacuate hematomas and ligate bleeders
  (b) Suture small contusions or perforations
  (c) Resect
   i) Large or irregular wounds
   ii) Infarcted or crushed areas
   iii) Bowel with mesentery injury
   iv) Bowel with large hematomas at mesenteric border
   v) Large intramural hematomas
   vi) Avulsion of mesentery
   vii) Large transverse tears of mesentery
   viii) Long linear lacerations of bowel
   ix) Short bowel segment with multiple perforations
  (d) Repair main mesenteric vessels to prevent bowel infarctions
  (e) Ileostomy
e. Complications
 (1) Ileus
 (2) Peritonitis
 (3) Pulmonary complications
 (4) Ischemic bowel syndrome

6. Large bowel and rectal injuries

a. Occurrence—5% of all abdominal injuries (6)
b. Etiology—penetrating, 85%, or blunt trauma (10)
c. Mortality rate 3 to 9%; higher with delayed diagnosis (11)
d. Diagnostic indicators
 (1) Positive peritoneal lavage; high WBC; presence of fecal fiber
 (2) Significant injuries may produce minimal symptoms; signs of peritonitis may appear late
 (3) Pain and tenderness upon rectal exam
 (4) Flatplate x-ray of the abdomen
 (5) Radiologic dye studies of abdomen
e. Selective treatment
 (1) Goals include
  (a) Divert fecal stream via colostomy
  (b) Debride if needed
  (c) Drain area
 (2) Treatment options based on extent of injury
  (a) Close primarily if little tissue destruction, e.g., small puncture wounds

(b) Resect and anastomose
(c) Close primarily with proximal colostomy
(d) Resect with colostomy
(e) Exteriorize wound
(3) Irrigate abdomen with saline or antibiotics to remove fecal material

f. Complications
(1) Incisional infection
(2) Abscess
(3) Intestinal obstruction
(4) Colocutaneous fistula
(5) Bowel ischemia

7. **Vascular injury**

a. Etiology
(1) Blunt deceleration injuries—MVC
(a) Avulsions of major vessel branches, e.g., intestinal branches from mesenteric artery
(b) Intimal tear resulting in thrombosis, e.g., renal artery thrombosis
(2) Penetrating injuries
(a) Intimal flap injury with thrombosis
(b) Vessel wall defect
(c) Hematomas
(d) Complete transection

b. Mortality of aortic injuries is greater than 50% due to exsanguination (12)

c. Diagnostic indicators
(1) Hemodynamic instability
(2) Hematuria
(3) Abdominal distension
(4) Flatplate of abdomen
(5) Intravenous pyelogram (IVP)
(6) Arteriogram

d. Selective management
(1) Control bleeding
(2) Replace fluid and blood components
(3) Inferior vena cava injuries
(a) Difficult to identify and repair
(b) If below renal veins, ligate; if suprarenal, repair
(c) Factors adversely affecting survival
i) Preoperative hypotension
ii) Superior location of injury
iii) Associated vascular or visceral injury
(d) Mortality usually from hemorrhage; sepsis also possible
(4) Portal vein
(a) Lateral repair, end-to-end anastomosis, or portacaval shunt
(b) Ligation causes hepatic necrosis
(5) Aorta
(a) Suprarenal area is difficult to reach; therefore aortic injuries are the most lethal
(b) Clamp vessel to allow operative repair; clamping may impair circulation to spinal cord (paraplegia) or kidney

(c) Close primarily with patch or graft
(d) Repair is associated with high failure and infection rates
(6) Repair proximal superior mesenteric artery injuries to prevent bowel necrosis
(7) Repair renal artery injuries; perform nephrectomy or transplant kidney
(8) Ligate celiac, gastric, splenic, and inferior mesenteric arteries, if necessary

e. Complications
(1) Thrombosis
(2) Dehiscence—failed anastomosis
(3) Infection
(4) Vascular—enteric fistulas, particularly with anterior aortic repairs, aortic grafts, or grafts to mesenteric artery

8. **Kidney injuries**

a. Occurrence—10 to 15% of all abdominal trauma (13)
b. Etiology—blunt or penetrating; blunt force sets kidney in motion, causing dissection of renal arteries and pedicles
c. Associated injuries—lower rib fractures or severe injuries of other abdominal organs
d. Diagnostic indicators
(1) Previous history of renal disease predisposes patient to renal injury compliance
(2) Urinalysis for hematuria is required for all patients; however, severe kidney injuries may not always reveal hematuria
(3) Radiographic studies
(a) Kidneys, ureters, bladder study (KUB)—identification of a lower rib fracture indicates possible kidney damage
(b) Intravenous pyelogram (IVP)—single view technique may be used in emergency departments prior to full IVP, or with operative urgency
(c) CAT scan
(d) Renal angiography
i) Used when IVP or CAT scan is inconclusive
ii) Used to determine renal injury associated with ruptured aorta

e. Specific kidney injuries
(1) Renal contusions—most common type of renal trauma
(a) Indications
i) Bruising at 11th or 12th rib
ii) Hematuria
iii) Flank pain
iv) Visible hematoma on IVP
(b) Selective management
i) Generally conservative
ii) Bed rest
iii) Monitor serial vital signs, urinalysis, and urine ouptut
(2) Renal laceration—includes fragmentation and laceration of the renal pedicles and renal system; results in severe bleeding and possible urine extravasation
(a) Indications
i) Profuse hematuria

ii) Hemodynamic instability
iii) Other severe injuries
(b) NOTE: assure proper functioning of the other kidney prior to nephrectomy
(c) Perform angiogram prior to surgery if patient is stable
(3) Renal pedicle trauma—most serious of renal injuries
(a) Hematuria may be profuse or absent
(b) Other indications include hemodynamic instability and other serious injuries
(c) Perform preoperative angiogram to determine exact location of injury
(d) Nephrectomy commonly required

9. Ureteral injury
a. Etiology—penetrating injury most common; usually a result of GSW
b. Diagnostic indicators
(1) Maintain high index of suspicion
(2) Perform IVP if injury is suspected, even if hematuria is absent
c. Selective management—surgical repair and/or urinary diversion procedure, e.g., nephrostomy tubes, ureterostomy
d. Complications
(1) Retroperitoneal urinoma seen with delayed treatment
(2) Infection
(3) Fistulas rare

10. Bladder injury
a. Etiology
(1) Any trauma to pelvic region should produce high index of suspicion of bladder injury
(2) High incidence in individuals with a full bladder who are injured in MVCs (ruptured bladder syndrome)
(3) Acceleration-deceleration injury of empty bladder may cause contusions
b. Almost always associated with pelvic fracture
c. Diagnostic indicators
(1) Gross hematuria
(2) Radiographic studies
(a) Cystography very accurate; rupture indicated by extravasation of contrast material
(b) CAT scan shows extravasation; as accurate as cystography
d. Selective management
(1) Manage nonoperatively if injury is minor; drain bladder via urinary catheter or suprapubic tube until urine extravasation is absent on cystography
(2) Repair serious injuries operatively
e. Complications
(1) Infection
(2) Urinary frequency or urgency; usually subsides over time

11. Urethral injury
a. Etiology
(1) Female—associated with pelvic fracture; however, female urethral injury is rare
(2) Male—fairly common and more severe than female injury

b. Associated injuries include pelvic fracture or other GU injuries
c. Diagnostic indicators
   (1) Blood at the meatus
      (a) DO NOT insert urinary catheter through urethra
      (b) Perform suprapubic tap to achieve urine drainage
   (2) High-riding prostate, pushed superiorly, on rectal exam is usually caused by hematoma
   (3) Radiographic study—retrograde urethrogram indicates complete or partial tear
d. Selective management
   (1) Suprapubic cystostomy for urinary diversion
   (2) Stable patients with incomplete tears may be managed with a urinary catheter acting as a stent (splint)
e. Complications include impotence, stricture, or incontinence

12. Genital injuries
a. Occurrence—fairly uncommon but psychologically devastating
b. Etiology—blunt or penetrating trauma
   (1) Female—usually caused by pelvic fracture or rape; also caused by waterskiing accidents
   (2) Male—causes include missiles or explosions, avulsions from industrial equipment, self-instrumentation, or deceleration injuries
c. Associated with renal or pelvic injuries
d. Specific injuries
   (1) Testicular/scrotal injuries
      (a) Diagnostic indicators
         i) Large scrotal hematoma
         ii) Inability to transilluminate light through scrotum
         iii) Pain radiating into flank or groin
         iv) Scrotal edema
      (b) Management
         i) Immediate surgical repair
         ii) Treat degloving injuries by implanting testicles in thigh to allow time for healing
   (2) Penile injuries
      (a) Blunt force results in fracture of erect penis
      (b) Penetrating injury commonly results from a laceration occurring in an industrial or recreational accident
      (c) Management
         i) Usually requires immediate surgical repair
         ii) Blunt penile injuries may be managed conservatively
            a) Scrotal support, ice, and hospitalization
            b) Require longer recovery period than with surgical repair
   (3) Female reproductive tract injuries
      (a) Enlarged uterus is prone to increased injury, e.g., pregnancy, postpartum, or uterine tumors
      (b) Injury to fallopian tube or ovary is usually treated with excision
      (c) Penetrating injuries to lower aspect of uterus are usually treated with hysterectomy
   (4) Female external genitalia injuries

(a) Vaginal bleeding is most common clinical finding
(b) Perform speculum exam in all females with pelvic injury
(c) Vaginal tears caused by pelvic fractures often are complicated with pelvic abscess

B. MEDICAL AND SURGICAL INTERVENTIONS

1. **Maintain airway and breathing; administer high flow humidified oxygen**
2. **Support circulation**
a. Control bleeding of abdominal wounds
b. Replace fluids and blood components
c. Apply pneumatic antishock garment (PASG) to temporarily tamponade bleeding
3. **Insert nasogastric tube (NGT) to decompress and drain stomach; reduces risk of aspiration and gastric distension**
4. **Insert bladder catheter to decompress bladder, measure urinary output, or stent an injury**
5. **Peritoneal lavage**
a. Indications
   (1) Persistent abdominal pain with no obvious cause
   (2) Cerebral deficit caused by head injury or intoxication
   (3) Hypotension; not responsive to fluid replacement
   (4) Spinal cord injury
   (5) Pelvic fractures
b. Procedure
   (1) Insert urinary catheter and nasogastric tube (NGT)
   (2) Inject local anesthesia
   (3) Introduce the catheter using open (3 to 5 cm incision), semiopen (1 cm incision), or trocar technique
   (4) Attempt aspiration; if more than 10 ml of frank blood is aspirated, patient needs immediate laparotomy
   (5) If no blood is aspirated, infuse 500 to 1000 ml of warmed lactated Ringer's or normal saline solution
   (6) Drain fluid by gravity; reverse Trendelenburg can facilitate drainage
   (7) Suture or pack wound; apply dressing
c. Interpretation of results
   (1) Unless gross blood is aspirated, obtain sample of lavage fluid for quantitative analysis
   (2) Positive results
      (a) WBC count above 500/mm^3
      (b) Bile, bacteria, or feces present
      (c) RBC count above 100,000/mm^3 in blunt trauma, or above 5000/mm^3 in penetrating trauma
6. **Laparotomy to control bleeding and repair organs**
a. Once surgery is indicated, move patient to operating room (OR) as soon as possible
b. Prescribe preoperative antibiotics
c. Debride entrance and exit sites of GSWs and shotgun wounds
d. Insert chest tube to prevent pneumothorax

7. **Prescribe antibiotics and tetanus prophylaxis**
8. **Provide nutritional support; enteral route preferred; TPN if necessary (see Module 11—Nutrition)**

C. NURSING ASSESSMENT

1. **Interview (see Module 19—Nursing Assessment)**
2. **Physical examination—sequential examination by the same nurse is imperative to determine minor changes in patient's condition**

a. Inspect
   (1) Presence and location of wound; DO NOT remove impaled objects
   (2) Position of legs; patients with peritoneal irritation are often more comfortable with legs bent
   (3) Presence of abdominal distension; same examiner, preferably, should consistently measure abdominal girth
   (4) Discoloration—abdominal or retroperitoneal
   (5) Blood at the meatus

b. Auscultate for presence/absence of bowel sounds, or bruits of abdominal aorta, renal, and femoral arteries

c. Percuss all quadrants

d. Palpate for guarding and tenderness

e. Perform physical assessment throughout trauma continuum; may detect late signs of injury, or presence of complications such as ileus or abscess

3. **Laboratory studies**

a. Trauma profile
b. Lipase
c. Peritoneal lavage fluid analysis
d. Bilirubin
e. Pregnancy test

4. **Radiologic studies**

a. Chest x-ray, abdominal flatplate, KUB
b. CAT scan
c. Arteriogram
d. Cystogram; retrograde urethrogram
e. Intravenous pyelogram (IVP)

D. NURSING DIAGNOSES, EXPECTED OUTCOMES, AND INTERVENTIONS

1. **Actual/potential fluid volume deficit related to diarrhea, drainage, or hemorrhage**

a. Expected outcomes
   (1) Urinary output greater than 0.5 to 1.0 ml/kg/hr
   (2) Serum BUN below 20; serum creatinine 1.5 or less
   (3) Vital signs within normal range

b. Nursing interventions
  (1) Control bleeding
  (2) Monitor vital signs frequently
  (3) Ensure adequate venous access
  (4) Administer fluids and blood components as prescribed
  (5) Measure intake and output accurately
  (6) Obtain baseline laboratory studies; monitor serial results
  (7) Observe for signs and symptoms of electrolyte imbalance; administer supplements as prescribed

2. Potential for infection related to splenectomy, penetrating abdominal injury, spilling of bowel contents, or invasive procedure

a. Expected outcomes
  (1) Absence or rapid detection of infection
  (2) Normal WBC; afebrile
  (3) Satisfactory wound closure
  (4) Patient demonstrates self-care to reduce infection risk

b. Nursing interventions
  (1) Monitor vital signs including body temperature
  (2) Monitor WBC and differential
  (3) Ensure sterile technique is maintained appropriately
  (4) Administer antibiotics and Pneumovax as prescribed
  (5) Assess wound site for signs of infection and provide wound care as prescribed
  (6) Apply sterile dressing to open wounds
  (7) Encourage coughing, deep breathing, and use of incentive spirometry
  (8) Ensure patency of drainage tubes
  (9) Educate patient regarding increased risk of infection due to loss of splenic function; antibiotic prophylaxis is needed for early signs of infection
  (10) Provide nutritional support to enhance immune response

3. Altered bowel elimination related to paralytic ileus, loss of gastrointestinal integrity, or ostomy

a. Expected outcomes
  (1) Patient achieves normal bowel patterns and stools
  (2) Patient adapts to bowel diversion
  (3) Patient achieves gastric motility
  (4) Ileus is absent

b. Nursing interventions
  (1) Administer pain medications as ordered and assess for side effects
  (2) Insert nasogastric tube; monitor quality and amount of drainage
  (3) Insert rectal tube as needed
  (4) Ausculate bowel sounds
  (5) Determine usual pattern of elimination; note current pattern
  (6) Note amount, color, frequency, and consistency of stool
  (7) Administer stool softeners, antiflatulents, bowel stimulants, or bulk forming laxatives, as prescribed
  (8) Provide adequate fluid intake
  (9) Advance oral feedings slowly; monitor patient response
  (10) Mobilize patient rapidly to promote bowel function

(11) Provide colostomy or ileostomy care
(12) Provide appropriate nutritional support
(13) Observe for abdominal distension; serial measurements of abdominal girth

4. **Alteration in urinary patterns related to genitourinary injury or surgical diversion**

a. Expected outcomes
(1) Normal urinary pattern; bladder emptied adequately
(2) Normal urine output
(3) Patient adapts to urinary diversion

b. Nursing interventions
(1) Assess pain related to urination; administer pain medications as prescribed
(2) Monitor accurate intake and output; note urine color, amount, frequency, incontinence, and/or retention
(3) Maintain patency of closed urine drainage systems or tubes
(4) Encourage adequate fluid intake
(5) Observe for signs of urinary infection
(6) Test urine for blood and protein
(7) Reassure patient and provide adequate information to allay anxiety concerning urinary function
(8) Provide catheter care per protocol
(9) Prevent tension on urinary drainage devices, e.g., tape catheter

5. **Potential/actual altered nutrition; less than body requirements related to inadequate dietary intake, abdominal cramping or pain, anorexia, and/or malabsorption**

a. Expected outcomes
(1) Adequate nutrient and caloric intake
(2) Weight approaches premorbid level
(3) Patient is able to maintain oral intake

b. Nursing interventions
(1) Initiate enteral feedings, as soon as possible, to maintain gastrointestinal integrity
(2) Administer I.V. nutrients as prescribed
(3) Document nutrient and calorie intake
(4) Refer patient to a nutritionist (see Module 11—Nutrition)

6. **Altered skin integrity related to local trauma, gastrointestinal drainage, surgical incision, or evisceration**

a. Expected outcomes
(1) Intact skin
(2) Adequate wound healing

b. Nursing interventions
(1) Assess wound site for signs of irritation, excoriation, or infection
(2) Keep skin around drainage site dry and protected; bag drainage and use protective skin barriers as indicated
(3) Cleanse, debride, and protect open wounds
(4) Reduce tension on healing wounds by positioning, splinting when coughing, abdominal binders, use of overbed trapeze, etc.
(5) Provide optimum nutrition and increase protein intake

(6) Instruct patient about self-care of wounds and healing skin
(7) Treat evisceration
(a) Allay patient anxiety
(b) Apply wet saline sterile dressing
(c) Notify physician
(d) Administer prescribed medications, e.g., analgesics, sedatives, muscle relaxants
(e) Prepare patient for OR
(8) Additional interventions (see Module 13—Wound Healing)

7. **Body image disturbance related to altered gastrointestinal or genitourinary structure or function**

a. Expected outcomes
(1) Patient verbalizes self-acceptance
(2) Patient is able to reconstruct his body image
(3) Patient manages self-care and premorbid activities of daily living
(4) Patient understands body changes

b. Nursing interventions
(1) Allow patient to verbalize feelings and concerns
(2) Assess patient's and significant other's level of knowledge about structure or function of gastrointestinal or genitourinary tracts
(3) Discuss the meaning of alterations to patient and significant other
(4) Observe interactions of patient and significant other; evaluate supportive resources
(5) Refer to appropriate counselors
(6) Provide accurate information about changes in body structure/function
(7) Refer to support groups as needed, e.g., ostomy clubs
(8) Assist patient to master self-care
(9) Involve famiy/significant others in patient care
(10) Reinforce positive views of self-concept

8. **Potential for ineffective breathing pattern related to decreased respiratory effort secondary to abdominal pain**

a. Expected outcomes
(1) Pulmonary function within normal limits
(a) Respiratory rate 12 to 20/min
(b) PaO_2 80 to 100 mm Hg on room air
(c) Normal respiratory pattern; tidal volume above 10 to 15 ml/kg
(2) Patient is free of pulmonary complications

b. Nursing interventions
(1) Ausculate breath sounds frequently
(2) Monitor rate, rhythm, and depth of respirations
(3) Position patient to enhance optimal chest excursion
(4) Monitor arterial blood gases, if available
(5) Provide adequate analgesia
(6) Teach patient to splint incision prior to coughing and moving
(7) Encourage coughing, turning, deep breathing, and use of incentive spirometry
(8) Assist and encourage ambulation, as soon as possible

E. ADDITIONAL NURSING DIAGNOSES

1. **Pain related to distension, incision, tubes, intestinal gas; secondary to abdominal or genitourinary injury or repair**
2. **Constipation related to abdominal injury and anatomical diversion**
3. **Altered tissue perfusion related to vascular injury or vascular thrombosis**
4. **Altered sexual functioning related to changes in gastrointestinal or genitourinary structure/function**

References

1. Gibson, D. E. (1987). Abdominal trauma. *Trauma Quarterly, 4*(1), 11–25.
2. Cayten, C. G. (1984). Abdominal trauma. *Emergency Medicine Clinics of North America,* 2(4), 799–821.
3. Shaftan, G. W. (1982). Injuries to the liver and spleen. In M. H. Worth (Ed.), *Principles and practices of trauma care* (pp. 172–188). Baltimore: Williams & Wilkins.
4. Pachter, H. L., Liang, H. G., & Hofstetter, S. R. (1987). Injury to the liver and biliary tract. In K. L. Mattox, E. E. Moore & D. V. Feliciano (Eds.), *Trauma* (pp. 429–442). Norwalk, CT: Appleton & Lange.
5. Buntain, W. L. (1987). Splenic trauma. In J. M. Hurst (Ed.), *Common problems in trauma* (p. 81). Chicago: Year Book Medical Publishers.
6. Mason, P. J. (1988). Abdominal trauma. In V. D. Cardona, P. D. Hurn, P. J. Mason, A. M. Scanlon-Schilpp & S. W. Veise-Berry (Eds.), *Trauma nursing: From resuscitation through rehabilitation* (p. 511). Philadelphia: W. B. Saunders Co.
7. Rea, R. E., Bourg, P. W., Parker, J. G., & Rushing, D. (1987). *Emergency nursing core curriculum.* Philadelphia: W. B. Saunders Co.
8. Anderson, C. B., & Ballinger, W. F. (1985). Abdominal injuries. In G. D. Zuidema, R. B. Rutherford & W. F. Ballinger (Eds.), *The management of trauma* (4th ed.). Philadelphia: W. B. Saunders Co.
9. Schwab, C. W., Shaikh, K. A., & Talucci, R. C. (1988). Injury to the stomach and small bowel. In K. L. Mattox, E. E. Moore & D. V. Feliciano (Eds.), *Trauma* (pp. 459–472). Norwalk, CT: Appleton & Lange.
10. Crass, R. A. (1986). Duodenum, small intestine, and colon. In D. D. Trunkey & F. R. Lewis (Eds.), *Current therapy of trauma—2* (p. 294). Philadelphia: B. C. Decker.
11. Thal, E. R., McClelland, R. N., & Shires, G. T. (1985). Abdominal trauma. In G. T. Shires (Ed.), *Principles of trauma care* (3rd ed., pp. 291–344). New York: McGraw-Hill.
12. Myles, R., & Yellin, A. (1979). Traumatic injury to the abdominal aorta. *American Journal of Surgery, 138*(2), 273–277.
13. McAninch, J. W. (1988). Genitourinary trauma. In K. L. Mattox, E. E. Moore, & D. V. Feliciano (Eds.), *Trauma* (pp. 537–552). Norwalk, CT: Appleton & Lange.

Suggested Readings

American College of Surgeons, Committee on Trauma. (1989). *Advanced trauma life support student manual.* Chicago: Author.

Doenges, M. E., & Moorhouse, M. F. (1985). *Nurse's pocket guide: Nursing diagnoses with interventions.* Philadelphia: F. A. Davis Co.

Dunham, C. M., & Cowley, R. A. (1986). *Shock/trauma critical care handbook.* Rockville, MD: Aspen Publishers.

Feliciano, D. V., Bitondo, C., Mattox, K., Rumisek, J. D., Burch, J. M., & Jordan, G. L., Jr. (1985). A four year experience with splenectomy versus splenorrhaphy. *Annals of Surgery, 201*(5), 568–575.

Jacobs, L. M., & Bennett, B. R. (Eds.). (1988). Abdominal trauma. *Emergency Care Quarterly,* 3(4).

McSwain, N. E., & Kerstein, M. D. (Eds.). (1989). *Evaluation & management of trauma.* Norwalk, CT: Appleton-Century-Crofts.

Semonin-Holleran, R. (1987). Critical nursing care for abdominal trauma. *Critical Care Nurse,* 8(3), 48–56.

Shires, G. T. (Ed.). (1979). *Care of the trauma patient* (2nd ed.). New York: McGraw-Hill.

Strange, J. M. (Ed.). (1987). *Shock trauma care plans.* Springhouse PA: Springhouse Corp.

Swearingen, P. L., Sommers, M. S., & Miller, K. (Eds.). (1988). *Manual on critical care: Applying nursing diagnosis to adult critical illness.* St. Louis: C. V. Mosby Co.

Wagner, M. M. (1990). The patient with abdominal injuries. *Nursing Clinics of North America,* 25(1), 45–55.

Section IV
Systematic Approach to Trauma Nursing

MODULE 24
MUSCULOSKELETAL INJURY

Mary Bailey, RN, CEN

Prerequisite

Review anatomy and physiology of the musculoskeletal system.

Objectives

1.0 Describe common musculoskeletal injuries.
1.1 List major types of musculoskeletal injuries.
1.2 Briefly describe pathophysiology and major characteristics of each type of injury.
1.3 State frequent mechanisms of injury for each problem.
2.0 Describe the assessment for possible musculoskeletal injuries.
2.1 Identify the types of information obtained from the prehospital setting that give clues to diagnosis.
2.2 Identify important items in the patient interview that relate to musculoskeletal injuries.
2.3 Identify steps in physical assessment of musculoskeletal injuries.
2.4 List radiologic studies commonly required for definitive diagnosis.
3.0 Develop nursing diagnoses based on assessment data.
3.1 List common nursing diagnoses with specific etiologic factors related to musculoskeletal trauma.

3.2 Identify signs and symptoms that validate the specific nursing diagnosis.

4.0 Anticipate and assist with appropriate medical-surgical interventions for musculoskeletal trauma.

4.1 Given specific patient data, recognize which medical-surgical interventions might be required.

4.2 Given specific patient data, state the equipment to be obtained to assist with medical-surgical interventions.

4.3 Describe pharmacologic agents likely to be required for the patient with musculoskeletal injury and discuss the rationale for each.

4.4 Identify treatment goals related to optimal function during rehabilitation.

5.0 Identify nursing interventions required for the patient with musculoskeletal injury.

5.1 List common nursing interventions, including rationale, required for patients with musculoskeletal injury.

5.2 Given a patient scenario, set priorities for nursing interventions.

5.3 Relate interventions to specific nursing diagnoses.

6.0 Evaluate patient's response to medical-surgical and nursing interventions.

6.1 Define desirable outcomes with measurable criteria for the patient with musculoskeletal injury.

6.2 List nursing activities required for continuous monitoring and evaluation of patient status.

6.3 List types of data to include in nursing documentation.

6.4 Cite trends in patient status that may require priority interventions from nurse or physician.

7.0 Given a specific case history, formulate a plan of care for a patient who experiences musculoskeletal injury and requires care at specific points in the trauma continuum.

A. PATHOPHYSIOLOGY

1. Musculoskeletal injuries are the most common form of trauma; rarely life-threatening but may result in long-term disability

2. Functions of the musculoskeletal system

a. Supports the skeleton and soft tissue

b. Protects the internal structures

c. Allows movement and leverage

d. Stores mineral salts and fats

e. Hematopoiesis

3. Fractures

a. Classified by cause

(1) Pathologic—minor trauma in diseased bone

(2) Stress/fatigue—unaccustomed or repeated trauma; usually seen in the lower extremities

(3) Traumatic—impact of a force upon the body

b. Classified by type (see Figure 24.1)
    (1) Closed—intact skin over site
    (2) Open/compound—open wound over fracture site
        (a) Grade I—small wounds less than 1 cm caused by low-velocity trauma such as protrusion of a fragment of bone, or by low-velocity bullet with minimal damage to soft tissue.
        (b) Grade II—wounds extensive in length and width, but with little or no avascular or devitalized soft tissue, and relatively little foreign material
        (c) Grade III—wounds of moderate or massive size, with considerable devitalized soft tissue and foreign material, or traumatic amputation (1)

Figure 24.1

Types of fractures. From D. S. Suddarth. (Ed.), *The Lippincott manual of nursing practice* (5th ed.). Philadelphia: J. B. Lippincott Co., 1991, p. 767. Reprinted with permission.

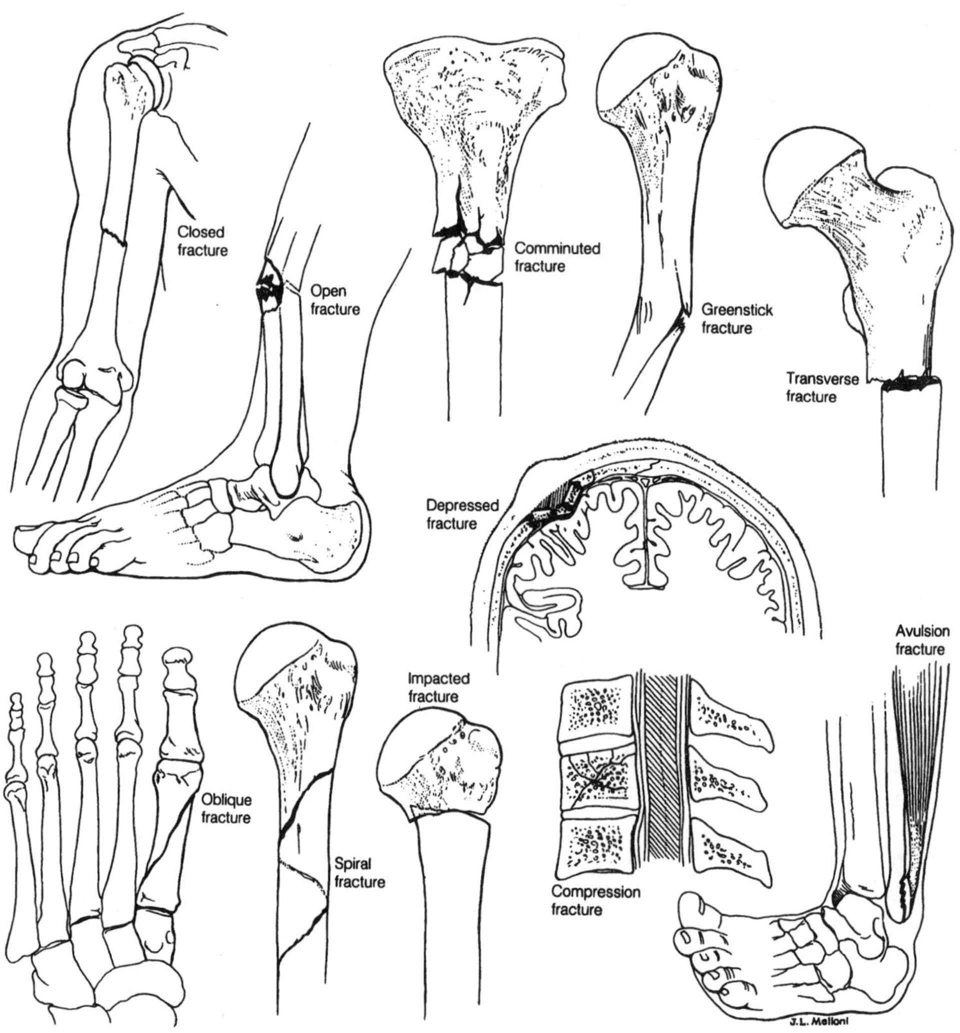

        (d) Grade IIIA—wounds with extensive soft tissue lacerations or flaps, or wounds of high-energy trauma but with adequate soft tissue to cover the fractured bone (1)
        (e) Grade IIIB—wounds with extensive soft tissue injury or loss, periosteal stripping, and bone exposure (1)
        (f) Grade IIIC—open fractures associated with arterial injury that requires repair (1)
    (3) Complete—break that extends through entire bone
    (4) Incomplete—partial break through bone, e.g., greenstick fracture seen in children
    (5) Displaced—bone fragments separate from fracture line
    (6) Comminuted—three or more fragments at fracture line
    (7) Impacted—fracture line that has been compressed or telescoped into itself
    (8) Overriding—complete fracture with distal and proximal ends of the bone overriding each other

c. Anatomic site of fracture
    (1) Epiphyseal—end of bone; acts as a growth plate to provide longitudinal bone growth; not fused in children
    (2) Metaphyseal—wider end of long bone shaft next to epiphyseal plate
    (3) Diaphyseal—shaft of a long bone
    (4) Salter-Harris classification of epiphyseal plate fractures (2)
        (a) Type I—complete epiphyseal separation without fracture; most common in younger children with thick epiphyseal plates
        (b) Type II—most common epiphyseal fracture; separation of epiphyseal plate with a fracture through the metaphysis which produces a triangular fragment
        (c) Type III—fracture through part of the epiphysis and extending into the joint
        (d) Type IV—fracture completely through the epiphyseal plate and extending through a portion of the metaphysis
        (e) Type V—crush injury to an area of the epiphyseal plate that is nondisplaced, and no fracture line is visible on x-rays

d. Fracture planes (see Figure 24.1)
    (1) Longitudinal—fracture line that extends in the same direction as the long bone axis
    (2) Transverse—fracture line forms a 90° angle across shaft of bone; caused by angulation or direct trauma
    (3) Oblique—fracture line forms a 45° angle across shaft of bone; caused by a twisting motion
    (4) Spiral—similar to oblique but has a longer fracture line and climbing appearance; caused by twisting force with planted distal portion (e.g., foot)
    (5) Compression—crush-type fracture from severe force to head or heels; vertebrae are forced together
    (6) Avulsion—chip fracture caused by forceful contractions of a muscle; bone breaks off at insertion
    (7) Depressed—fracture area lower than surrounding bone; fracture usually involves a flat bone and large amount of soft tissue injury

e. Healing of fractures

(1) Local factors in healing
  (a) Contact between bones is necessary for healing
  (b) Bone movement slows healing
  (c) Severity of trauma
  (d) Amount of bone lost
  (e) Type of bone injured—flat, cancellous bone heals faster
  (f) Presence or absence of infection
  (g) Intraarticular fracture—free synovial fluid can destroy hematoma and prolong healing
  (h) Blood supply to area—diminished blood supply may lead to avascular necrosis
(2) Systemic factors in healing include age, nutritional status, or preexisting disease

B. PATTERNS/MECHANISMS OF INJURY

1. Injury forces and motions (see Figure 24.2)

a. Direct trauma—energy absorbed at impact site
  (1) Tapping fractures
    (a) Deceleration force applied over small area, e.g., nightstick, kick
    (b) Transverse fracture of one bone with minimal soft tissue damage
  (2) Crush fractures
    (a) Comminuted fractures, transverse fractures, or both
    (b) Extensive soft tissue, vascular, and nerve damage
  (3) Penetrating injuries
    (a) Projectiles of various velocities
      i) High-velocity—extensive soft tissue damage; bone disintegrates and bone fragments become secondary missiles
      ii) Low-velocity—may splinter bone shaft; little soft tissue damage
    (b) Impalement injuries
    (c) Patient is highly susceptible to infection due to contamination at time of injury

b. Indirect trauma—impact causes damage at a distance from point of impact
  (1) Angulated fractures—result from forces that cause bone bending
  (2) Rotational fractures—result from twisting forces and may result in spiral fractures

2. Mechanisms of Injury

a. Falls—injuries can occur even from a standing position; height of fall helps estimate energy force

b. Sports injuries—impalement, equipment, body contact, and poor conditioning

c. Assaults—fists, body contact, and implements, e.g., bats, hammers

d. Motor vehicles—impact with the vehicle's interior and other occupants, and deceleration forces

3. Patterns of injury (see Module 2—Mechanisms of Injury)

a. Pedestrian vs motor vehicle

Figure 24.2

Classification of fractures according to the mechanism. From J. W. Harkess, W. C. Ramsey, & B. Ahmadi, Principles of fractures and dislocations. In D. A. Rockwood & D. P. Green, (Eds.), *Fractures in adults,* Vol. I. Philadelphia: J. B. Lippincott Company, 1984, p. 10. Reprinted with permission.

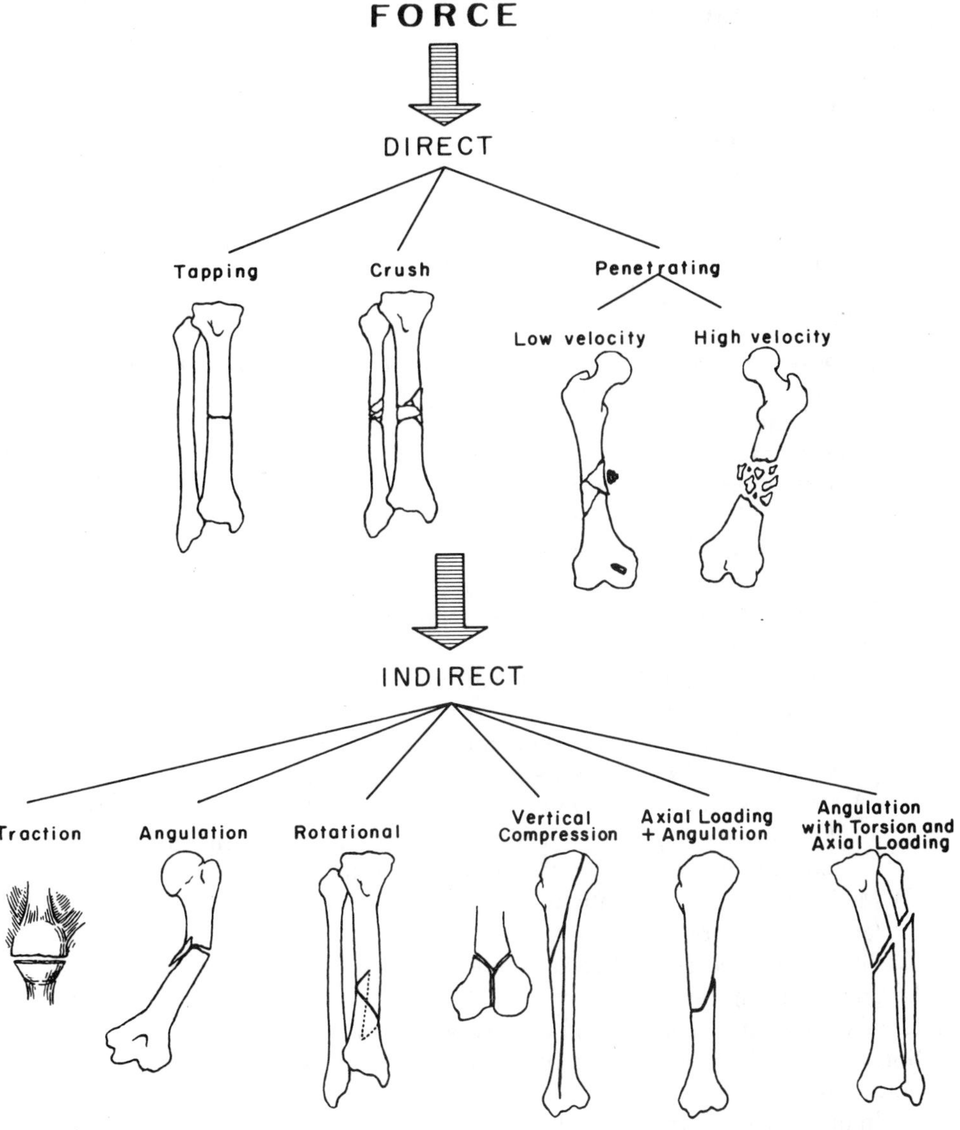

b. Motorcycle crashes (MCC)
c. Don Juan injury—jump from balcony or height
d. Motor vehicle crashes (MVC)

C. SPECIFIC INJURIES

1. **Musculotendinous injuries**
a. Tendons are relatively avascular, so infection is problematic
b. Strain—weakening or overstretching of muscle where it attaches to tendon
   (1) Injury severity and symptoms may be mild, moderate, or severe
   (2) Signs and symptoms
      (a) Mild—local pain and point tenderness
      (b) Moderate—(a) with swelling, discoloration, and inability to use joint for long periods of time
      (c) Severe—(a), (b), and patient may have heard snapping sound; severely restricted range of motion (ROM)
   (3) Rare neurovascular compromise
   (4) X-rays negative
   (5) Medical-surgical interventions
      (a) Immobilize injured area with elastic compression bandage, i.e., Ace wrap
      (b) Apply cold to injured area
      (c) Elevate injured area
      (d) Patient should not bear weight for up to 48 hrs
c. Achilles tendon rupture
   (1) Usually seen in athletes over 30 years old involved in start-and-stop sports
   (2) Signs and symptoms
      (a) Sharp pain extends from heel into the back of the leg
      (b) Sudden inability to use the foot
      (c) Deformity of calf develops
      (d) Thompson's Test—compression of the calf muscle with patient prone and foot free results in ankle flexion if tendon intact
   (3) Medical-surgical interventions
      (a) Elastic compression bandage, i.e., Ace
      (b) Surgery necessary to repair tendon
2. **Ligamentous injuries**
a. Ligaments connect bones together; relatively avascular
b. Sprain—tearing of ligamentous fibers; usually occurs when joint exceeds its normal ROM
   (1) Injuries range from first to third degree
      (a) First degree—minor tear of ligament fiber
      (b) Second degree—partial tear of ligament
      (c) Third degree—complete tear of ligament
   (2) Signs and symptoms
      (a) First degree—mildly tender, ecchymotic, and slightly decreased ROM
      (b) Second degree—(a) with point tenderness and swelling

(c) Third degree—(a), (b), with pain, loss of function, abnormal motion, possible deformity

(3) Neurovascular compromise may occur with unstable joint

(4) Diagnostic studies
  (a) X-rays negative; stress views may be ordered for third degree sprains
  (b) Arthrography—x-ray dye study that demonstrates third degree tears
  (c) Arthroscopy

(5) Medical and surgical interventions
  (a) Conservative treatment most common—rest, ice, compression wrap, elevation
  (b) Surgical repair if unstable third degree injury

(6) Knee injury
  (a) Involves anterior or posterior cruciate ligaments, medial and lateral collateral ligaments, or any combination
  (b) Etiology
    i) Weight bearing with foot fixed
    ii) Direct lateral blow injuries—medial collateral, medial meniscus, anterior and posterior cruciate ligaments, and potential fractures
    iii) Direct medial blow injuries—lateral collateral, iliotibial, and biceps femoris
    iv) Direct anterior blow injuries—hyperextended knee caused by tearing the posterior cruciate and capsule
  (c) Characteristics
    i) Pinpoint pain and tenderness
    ii) Swelling
    iii) Hemarthrosis
    iv) Limitation of motion
    v) Difficulty bearing weight
    vi) Instability with varus and valgus stress, or anterior and posterior "drawer sign"
  (d) Diagnostic indicators
    i) Clinical diagnosis
    ii) Knee radiographs
    iii) Arthroscopy and arthrogram
    iv) MRI and CAT scan
  (e) No specific neurovascular compromise
  (f) Medical and surgical interventions
    i) Analgesia
    ii) Cold packs
    iii) Elevation
    iv) Crutches
    v) Aspiration of hemarthrosis
    vi) Arthroscopic repair
    vii) Physical therapy

3. Nerve damage may be partial or complete; partial injuries usually cause temporary loss of function

4. Vascular injuries

a. Injuries include contusions, lacerations, vessel kinking, and traumatic false aneurysms

b. Also caused by thrombosis at site of injury; risk higher with hypotensive episodes
c. Difficult to diagnose due to swelling and deformity

5. Joint injuries

a. Contusion—causes inflammatory response with edema, exudate, and decreased ROM
b. Subluxation (incomplete dislocation)—some articular contact remains
c. Dislocations
   (1) Separation of two articular surfaces in joint capsule; damages joint capsule and usually tears ligament
   (2) Signs and symptoms common to ALL dislocations
      (a) Severe pain
      (b) Deformity at joint
      (c) Swelling
      (d) Point tenderness
      (e) Significant decrease in range of motion
   (3) X-ray pre- and postreduction in most cases
   (4) Medical and surgical interventions
      (a) Careful palpation of joint
      (b) Splint in position found
      (c) Do not relocate joint in prehospital environment unless severe neurovascular compromise or prolonged transport time
      (d) Rapid transport—the longer the joint is dislocated, the harder it is to relocate
      (e) Assess for associated fractures
d. Specific injuries
   (1) Sternoclavicular dislocations
      (a) Mechanisms of injury
         i) Significant direct or indirect force required for this uncommon injury
         ii) Dislocation can be anterior or posterior
      (b) Signs and symptoms
         i) Deformity more prominent with anterior dislocations; depression in posterior
         ii) Pain increases with abduction
         iii) Swelling in anterior dislocations
         iv) Tachypnea, jugular venous distension, and decreased arm pulses in posterior due to vessel compression
      (c) Diagnosed by sternoclavicular x-rays and CAT scan; tomograms needed in rare cases
      (d) Medical and surgical interventions
         i) Posterior—place sandbag between scapula
         ii) Towel clip traction as an emergency measure in posterior
         iii) Surgical repair more common in posterior
         iv) Sling, figure-of-eight splint for anterior
   (2) Acromioclavicular (AC) dislocations
      (a) Caused by fall or force applied to point of shoulder
      (b) Results in disruption of synovial joint and tear of relatively weak capsular ligaments
      (c) Severity classification from first to third degree (complete) joint dislocation
      (d) Additional signs and symptoms

i) Unable to raise arm or bring arm across chest
ii) Hematoma
iii) Deformity, primarily third degree
iv) No specific neurovascular compromise
(e) Diagnosed with bilateral x-rays for comparison; add 5 to 10 lbs of weight to diagnose complete tear
(f) Medical and surgical interventions
i) Sling and swathe or A-C strap after reduction
ii) Surgical removal of distal segment when recurrence or limited motion in adults or coracoclavicular fixation
(3) Shoulder dislocation—most common dislocation
(a) Anterior dislocations—90% (3)
i) Usually from fall on extended arm that is abducted and externally rotated
ii) Can be described as subclavicular, subcoracoid, or subglenoid
(b) Posterior—rare
i) Usually seen after severe muscle contractions, e.g., seizure or electrical shock
ii) Arm abducted and internally rotated
(c) Additional signs and symptoms
i) Severe muscle spasm
ii) Inability to move arm
iii) Deformity, e.g., flat deltoid
iv) Lowered axilla
v) Prominence of acromion process
(d) 55 to 60% of dislocations are recurrent; highest risk within two years of first episode, especially if patient is under 25 years old
(e) Complications
i) Above age 40—rotator cuff tear often seen with dislocations
ii) Brachial plexus injury
iii) Axillary artery or vein injury rare
iv) Associated fractures
v) Axillary nerve damage
(f) Medical and surgical interventions
i) Muscle relaxants and analgesia
ii) Sling and swathe for one to six weeks, depending on age; immobilize younger patients for longer periods of time
iii) Closed reduction under local analgesia and muscle relaxants
iv) Surgery for multiple recurrences
(4) Elbow dislocation
(a) From fall on hyperextended arm or point of elbow
(b) Posterior dislocation most common
(c) Additional signs and symptoms
i) Deformity—elongated olecranon and palpable olecranon fossa
ii) Ecchymosis
iii) "Locked" elbow
(d) Complications
i) Rare neurovascular compromise

a) Avulsion of medial epicondyle with ulnar nerve injury
b) Ulnar or median injury possible; ulnar most common
ii) Volkmann's ischemic contracture
a) Compression of brachial artery due to swelling or disruption
b) Ulnar nerve paresthesias
iii) Myositis ossificans with improper reduction or immobilization
iv) Compartment syndrome
v) Vascular congestion
(e) Medical and surgical interventions
i) Prompt reduction
ii) Immobilize with posterior splint
iii) Cast and sling
iv) Open reduction internal fixation (ORIF) if neurovascular compromise
(5) Hip dislocations
(a) Anterior dislocation—more common type; caused by MVCs, falls
(b) Posterior dislocation—unusual in falls; caused from impact of knee against dashboard in MVCs
(c) Signs and symptoms
i) Shortened leg
ii) External rotation (anterior) or internal rotation (posterior, often called pelican position, with knee and hip flexion)
iii) Palpable femoral head in groin (anterior)
iv) Inability to move leg
(d) Complications
i) Femoral artery compromise
ii) Sciatic nerve injury, particularly in posterior dislocations
iii) Avascular necrosis of femoral head
a) Increased risk if not reduced in less than 24 hrs
b) Symptoms appear 17 to 24 months after injury
iv) Fractured acetabulum in posterior
(e) Medical and surgical interventions
i) Rule out femoral head, pelvic, and acetabulum fractures
ii) Early closed reduction under general anesthesia
iii) Bed rest for three to six weeks
iv) Traction may be used
v) Nonweight-bearing for two to four weeks
(6) Knee dislocations—A MEDICAL EMERGENCY
(a) Patterns of injury
i) Direct force applied with knee in flexion (dashboard) causes posterior dislocations
ii) Violent abduction force on tibia vs femur causes lateral dislocations
iii) Violent adduction force on the tibia against the femur causes medial dislocations
iv) Direct force applied with knee in hyperextension
(b) Additional signs and symptoms
i) Instability from ligamentous injury
ii) Inability to bear weight
iii) Joint effusion

iv) Deformity

(c) Complications

i) High incidence of vascular injury; arteriogram frequently required

ii) Popliteal artery injury requires immediate treatment to preserve limb

iii) Severe capsule damage usually present

iv) Peroneal nerve injury possible

v) Popliteal and tibial nerve damage with fractured tibia

(d) Medical and surgical interventions

i) Immediate closed reduction to prevent popliteal artery occlusion

ii) If displaced, internal fixation

iii) If pulse absent, open reduction

iv) Immobilize after surgery with 15° flexion

(7) Patellar dislocations

(a) Mechanisms of injury

i) Direct blow to medial/superior area causes lateral dislocation

ii) Quadriceps contraction with sudden flexion and external rotation

iii) Rapid rotation on planted foot

(b) Signs and symptoms

i) Lateral deformity

ii) Hemarthrosis possible

iii) Knee held in flexion position

(c) Medical and surgical interventions

i) Early closed reduction

ii) Knee immobilizer

(8) Ankle dislocations

(a) Commonly associated with fracture from lateral stress motion with ROM of ankle exceeded

(b) Signs—inability to move joint, swelling, and deformity

(c) Vascular compromise possible

(d) Medical and surgical interventions—relocate by closed or open reduction

(9) Foot—tarsal and metatarsal

(a) Rare injuries; seen with MVCs and MCCs

(b) Open injuries common

(c) Sign—inability to use foot

(d) Medical and surgical interventions—cast; no weight bearing on foot

6. Fractures—breaks in continuity of bone

a. General considerations

(1) Signs and symptoms for ALL fractures

(a) Pain

(b) Point tenderness

(c) Deformity

(d) Swelling

(e) Ecchymosis

(2) Diagnostic studies

(a) Plain radiographs for ALL fractures

i) Anterior-posterior and lateral views at a minimum

ii) Include joint above and below injury

iii) Comparison views of other side, especially in children

(b) Arteriogram/angiogram
i) Used for fractures/dislocations associated with potential vascular injury
a) Pelvic fractures
b) First and second rib fractures
c) Scapular fractures
d) Sternal fractures
e) Knee fractures/dislocations
ii) Digital subtraction angiography preferred
(c) Computerized axial tomography (CAT) most useful for pelvic fractures
(d) Bone scan most useful for stress fractures
(e) Arthrogram most useful for knee injuries
(f) Urethrogram/cystogram most useful for pelvic fractures with blood at the urinary meatus
(3) Medical and surgical interventions for ALL fractures
(a) Control bleeding; replace fluid loss
(b) Immobilize fractures, as found, unless vascular compromise
(c) Stabilize fractures
i) Closed reduction and splint, bandage, or cast
ii) Open reduction internal fixation (ORIF) with plates, screws, and/or rods for open fracture
iii) External fixator used in open fractures, especially Grades III, IIIA, or IIIC
(4) Complications for ALL fractures
(a) Osteomyelitis—may be late sequelae
i) Signs and symptoms
a) Pain and guarding
b) Muscle spasms around joint, in septic arthritis
c) Swelling of affected area
d) Tenderness upon palpation
e) Involved area red and warm
f) Low-grade fever
g) Foul-smelling drainage, if open lesion
ii) Treat with long-term antibiotics
(b) Fat emboli (see Module 16—Medical Sequelae)
(c) Venous thrombosis and emboli (see Module 16—Medical Sequelae)
b. Clavicle fractures
(1) Mechanisms of injury
(a) Fall on outstretched arm/shoulder
(b) Direct lateral trauma to shoulder such as contact injury in sports
(c) Fracture usually in outer or middle third of clavicle
(2) Additional signs and symptoms
(a) Crepitus
(b) Patient tilts head to injured side
(3) Complications
(a) Rare neurovascular compromise
(b) If clavicle displaced, subclavian artery or vein injury is possible
(4) Medical and surgical interventions
(a) Figure-of-eight splint

(b) ORIF, if badly comminuted fracture or neurovascular compromise

c. Scapula fractures
 (1) Mechanisms of injury
  (a) Violent, direct trauma or severe muscle contraction
  (b) Requires significant force
 (2) Additional signs and symptoms
  (a) Pain that increases with abduction
  (b) Ecchymosis
 (3) Complications
  (a) Axillary artery or nerve injury
  (b) Brachial plexus injury
  (c) Rare neurovascular compromise
  (d) Pneumothorax
  (e) Pulmonary contusion
  (f) Clavicle or rib fractures
 (4) Medical and surgical interventions
  (a) Treat associated injuries
  (b) Sling, or sling and swathe
  (c) Physical therapy for early joint rotation

d. Shoulder fractures
 (1) Encompasses glenoid, humeral head, or humeral neck
 (2) Humerus has four divisions—greater tuberosity, lesser tuberosity, surgical neck, and anatomical neck
 (3) Mechanisms of injury
  (a) Caused by fall on outstretched arm in abduction
  (b) Direct shoulder trauma
  (c) Fractures usually occur in elderly; in young, a dislocation will occur
 (4) Additional signs and symptoms
  (a) Unable to move arm
  (b) Arm held in adduction
  (c) Gross swelling and discoloration
 (5) Complications
  (a) Brachial plexus injury possible
  (b) Axillary nerve injury possible
  (c) Arterial injury rare
  (d) Higher incidence of neurovascular compromise in abduction presentations
 (6) Medical and surgical interventions
  (a) Reduce fracture; ORIF possible
  (b) Conservative treatment with sling and swathe (immobilization risks frozen shoulder)
  (c) Shoulder immobilizer used for a few days, then early arm exercises, e.g., Codman routine, to prevent frozen shoulder and increase ROM

e. Humerus—midshaft fractures
 (1) Mechanisms of injury
  (a) Caused by direct force from fall or blow
  (b) Indirect cause via fall on elbow or outstretched arm
  (c) Usually occurs in those above 50 years old and in children
  (d) Common in motor vehicle injuries

(2) Additional signs and symptoms
  (a) Abnormal mobility; shortening
  (b) Crepitus
  (c) Ecchymosis
(3) Complications
  (a) Radial nerve injury common in midshaft fractures
  (b) Brachial artery injury possible
  (c) Ulnar and median nerves may also be injured
  (d) Hemorrhage
(4) Medical and surgical interventions
  (a) U-shaped splint from axilla to elbow (sugar tong)
  (b) Collar and cuff, or sling and swathe
  (c) Apply mild, steady, downward traction, if neurovascular compromise
  (d) Open reduction, if neurovascular compromise is present
  (e) Early hand exercises
  (f) Check for commonly associated chest trauma

f. Humerus—supracondylar fractures
(1) Mechanisms of injury
  (a) Common in young children and athletes
  (b) Extension injuries due to fall on extended elbow; stable only in significant flexion
  (c) Flexion injuries due to fall on flexed elbow; relatively stable in extension
(2) Additional signs—unable to move elbow; deformity
(3) Diagnostic studies
  (a) X-rays show posterior fat pad sign in children or adolescents
  (b) Anterior fat pad sign may also indicate fracture
(4) Complications
  (a) Vascular compromise (frequent)
  (b) Brachial artery laceration
  (c) Median and radial nerve damage
  (d) Volkmann's ischemic contracture
    i) Due to ischemia of muscles and nerves
    ii) Signs and symptoms
      a) Inability to move fingers
      b) Pain on passive motion of fingers
      c) Severe forearm pain after reduction
      d) Swollen, cyanotic, and cold extremity
      e) Decreased sensation
    iii) Remove cast and extend forearm
(5) Medical and surgical interventions
  (a) Sling/swathe
  (b) Closed reduction or pins/plaster in OR
  (c) Dunlap's traction—skin traction with arm and traction hanging off of the bed at right angle, and hand waving at ceiling; counter traction over distal humerus (4)
  (d) Physical therapy

g. Elbow fractures—olecranon, proximal radius
(1) Mechanisms of injury

(a) Fall on point of elbow (olecranon)
(b) Fall on outstretched hand with elbow flexed and triceps contracted (proximal radius)
(c) Common in children
(2) Additional signs and syptoms
(a) Ecchymosis
(b) Decreased ROM, especially with radial head/neck fracture
(c) Pain on pronation and supination
(d) Joint effusion; may be hemorrhagic
(3) Medical and surgical interventions
(a) Type I (nondisplaced)—immobilize break; may aspirate hemarthrosis to decrease pain and increase ROM
(b) Type II (displaced)—may be impacted, depressed, or angulated; treatment is controversial; remove radial head (adults only), especially if depressed more than 3 mm
(c) Type III (comminuted)—fracture of entire radial head; excise radial head in adults

h. Radial or ulnar shaft fractures
(1) Mechanisms of injury
(a) Direct blow or fall on extended arm
(b) Radius and ulna are connected by thick interosseous membrane and often fractured together; open fractures common
(2) Complications
(a) Malunion or nonunion
(b) Infection
(c) Volkmann's contracture
(d) Compartment syndrome
(e) Radial, ulnar, or median nerve compromise
(3) Medical and surgical interventions
(a) Nondisplaced fractures in children can be treated by closed reduction
(b) Simple, nondisplaced ulna fractures can be treated by closed reduction
(c) Usually need ORIF
(d) General anesthesia often required
(e) Cast and sling

i. Distal forearm fractures—Colles' type
(1) Mechanisms of injury
(a) Fall on outstretched hand
(b) Fall from height
(c) Very common, especially in middle-aged or older females
(2) Additional signs and symptoms
(a) "Silver fork" deformity—dorsal angulation
(b) Ecchymosis
(3) Complications
(a) Median and ulnar nerve stretch, contusion, or compression
(b) Compartment syndrome
(c) Carpal tunnel syndrome
(d) Aseptic necrosis is a rare complication
(e) Loss of some palmar flexion and dorsiflexion common

(f) Decreased rotation and finger stiffness
(g) Malunion common
(4) Medical and surgical interventions
(a) Closed reduction
(b) Cast and sling
(c) External fixator for severe comminution
(d) Maintain ROM of thumb, fingers, elbow, and shoulder

j. Distal forearm fractures—Smith's type
(1) Distal radius fracture with volar displacement of distal fragment
(2) Transverse fracture of distal radius carpal tunnel row displaced volarly (reverse Colles')
(3) Mechanisms of injury
(a) Usually blow on dorsum of wrist in pronation
(b) Backward fall on hand with forearm in supination
(4) Additional signs and symptoms
(a) Ecchymosis
(b) "Garden spade" deformity—volar angulation
(c) Lower end of radius protrudes
(5) Complications—radial artery injury or possible median nerve injury
(6) Medical and surgical interventions
(a) Closed reduction in most cases
(b) Cast and sling
(c) Immobilize injured area for six to eight weeks

k. Scaphoid/navicular fractures
(1) Mechanism of injury—fall on outstretched hand
(2) Additional symptom—point tenderness in anatomic snuffbox
(3) Diagnostic indicators—navicular views on x-rays or bone scan may be needed to diagnose
(4) Complications
(a) Avascular necrosis
(b) Delayed union
(c) Nonunion
(5) Medical and surgical interventions
(a) Sling
(b) Cast with gauntlet-type cast, which includes thumb

l. Hand/metacarpal fractures
(1) Boxer's fracture—fracture of the fifth metacarpal
(2) Bennett's fracture—first metacarpal subluxation or dislocation
(3) Mechanisms of injury
(a) Usually contact injuries, e.g., sports, fighting
(b) Axial force on partially flexed metacarpal
(c) Avulsion fracture—extensor tendon tears off bone, e.g., catching a ball
(d) Crush injuries
(4) Additional signs and symptoms
(a) Severe swelling
(b) Inability to use
(c) Boxer's—decreased prominence of fifth metacarpal
(d) Frequently open fracture

(5) Medical and surgical interventions
  (a) Bennett's—usually requires ORIF
  (b) Boxer's—usually requires closed reduction and gutter splint
  (c) Splint in functional position

m. Finger/phalangeal fractures
  (1) Mechanism of injury is direct injury or hyperflexion
  (2) Additional signs and symptoms
    (a) Subungual hematoma—severe throbbing pain
    (b) Mallet finger—inability to extend finger
  (3) Medical and surgical interventions
    (a) Closed reduction—use local anesthesia without epinephrine
    (b) Splint in position of function; however, for mallet, splint with hyperextension at distal interphalangeal joint
    (c) Open reduction, if open fracture
    (d) Release subungual hematoma—trephine nail

n. Pelvic fractures
  (1) Represents 3% of all fractures (5); second most common cause of death associated with trauma (6); mortality rate 8 to 50% (5); open fractures—greater than 50% mortality (7)
  (2) Mechanisms of injury
    (a) Direct crush or impact
    (b) Indirect transmission of forces through femur, e.g., dashboard vs knee
    (c) Fall from height
    (d) Categorized according to injury and stability
  (3) Additional signs and symptoms
    (a) Crepitus
    (b) Tender over symphysis pubis, anterior spines, iliac crests, sacrum, or coccyx
    (c) Inability to bear weight
    (d) Shock from otherwise unexplained source
    (e) Ecchymosis in perineum, groin, suprapubic area, or flanks
    (f) Instability or pain of pelvic ring with manual pressure over symphysis, femoral heads, or iliac crests
    (g) Bleeding from urethra, rectum, or vagina
    (h) Spinous process muscle spasm
    (i) Hematuria
  (4) Diagnostic studies
    (a) Diagnose with x-rays or CAT scans
    (b) Retrograde urethrogram and/or cystogram to rule out genitourinary injuries
    (c) Arteriogram may be needed to identify bleeding site
  (5) Complications
    (a) Retroperitoneal hemorrhage
    (b) Fat emboli
    (c) Bladder, urethral, vaginal, or bowel injuries
    (d) Sciatic nerve injury possible
    (e) Two-thirds are complicated by other fractures and soft tissue injuries (8)
  (6) Medical and surgical interventions

(a) Replace fluid and blood loss
(b) Immobilize pelvis with PASG, external fixation, or internal fixation
(c) Embolize bleeding vessel, via arteriogram, if unable to control bleeding with PASG or external fixation
(d) Monitor for shock or internal injuries
(e) Stable pelvic fractures, e.g., pubic rami, ischial tuberosity, or anterior iliac spine, usually require nonoperative treatment, analgesia, and bed rest for two weeks
(f) Unstable fractures, e.g., Malgaigne fractures, straddle fractures, crush injuries, usually require external fixation, possible ORIF, and internal soft tissue repair

o. Acetabulum fractures
(1) Mechanisms of injury—require considerable force
(a) Auto-pedestrian
(b) Fall from height
(c) Contact with unmovable object, e.g., knee against dashboard
(2) Additional signs and symptoms
(a) Tenderness with movement
(b) Unable to bear weight
(3) Complications—sciatic nerve injury (foot drop) or missed injury
(4) Medical and surgical interventions
(a) Two weeks of bed rest
(b) Six weeks nonweight bearing on crutches if fracture is only minimally displaced
(c) If displaced, use closed reduction and traction
(d) ORIF for severe injuries

p. Hip fractures
(1) Types of fracture
(a) Intracapsular—femoral head
(b) Intertrochanteric fractures—femoral neck
(c) Subtrochanteric fractures—below lesser trochanter and above middle third of femur
(2) Mechanisms of injury
(a) Osteoporosis is a significant contributing factor
(b) Direct force from fall
(c) Stress fractures from overuse
(d) Indirect force from neck of femur over posterior acetabulum, or pull of iliopsoas muscle
(3) Additional signs and symptoms
(a) External rotation and limb shortening
(b) Inability to bear weight
(4) Complications
(a) Blood loss greater than three units
(b) Avascular necrosis
(c) Fixation failure
(d) Nonunion
(5) Medical and surgical interventions
(a) Bed rest

(b) Closed reduction possible in trochanteric fractures
(c) Early ORIF is usual treatment
(d) Possible prosthetic hip replacement

q. Femoral shaft fractures
(1) Mechanisms of injury
(a) Indirect injury from transmission of force, e.g., knee into dashboard
(b) Direct injury, e.g., pedestrian vs MVC, MVC vs MVC, or MCC
(c) Other fractures in same extremity common
(2) Additional signs and symptoms
(a) Inability to bear weight
(b) Limb shortening from muscle spasm
(3) Complications
(a) Blood loss greater than four units
(b) Peroneal palsy
(c) Fat emboli
(d) Associated knee and/or hip fractures
(e) Nerve and artery injuries occur more frequently during manipulation than at impact
(f) Malunion or nonunion
(g) Refracture and/or implant failure
(4) Medical and surgical interventions
(a) Splint with Thomas half ring, Hare, Sager, etc.
(b) Skeletal traction
(c) Spica cast for children
(d) External fixation
(e) ORIF with rod or plate; treatment of choice to allow early mobilization in multiple trauma
(f) Replace blood and fluid loss

r. Patella fractures
(1) Mechanisms of injury
(a) Direct injury from fall on knee
(b) Quadriceps contraction during fall
(c) Chondral fracture possible
(d) "Clipping" in football
(e) Considered open fracture if accompanied by abrasions
(2) Additional signs and symptoms
(a) Hemarthrosis
(b) Crepitus
(c) If fracture displaced, deformity results
(3) Medical and surgical interventions
(a) Knee immobilizer
(b) Cast
(c) ORIF if displaced
(d) Patellectomy rare
(e) Arthroscopy to check for osteochondral fracture
(f) Aspiration of hemarthrosis if nondisplaced

s. Tibia/fibula fractures
(1) Mechanisms of injury

(a) Direct injury from MVC, pedestrian impact with bumper of vehicle, or fall
(b) Indirect injury from rotary and compression forces, e.g., skiing or falling
(c) Associated soft tissue injury
(2) Additional sign—inability to bear weight
(3) Complications
(a) Tibial compartment syndrome
(b) Peroneal nerve injury
(c) Infection, especially pin tracts
(d) Knee/ankle stiffness
(e) Malunion or nonunion, especially if comminuted
(f) Osteomyelitis
(g) Circulatory damage
(4) Medical and surgical interventions
(a) Closed reduction and cast
(b) If displaced or comminuted fractures, use ORIF or external fixation
(c) If open wounds, external fixation
(d) Immobilize fractures at least six weeks
(e) Fasciotomy for compartment syndrome

t. Ankle fractures
(1) Mechanisms of injury
(a) Inversion injury causes fracture of lateral malleolus
(b) Eversion injury causes fracture of medial malleolus, often with fibular head fractures
(c) Fall from height, or deceleration, can cause impaction and posterior dislocation
(2) Additional symptom—unable to bear weight
(3) Complications
(a) Compartment syndrome
(b) Vascular problem with dislocation or trimalleolar fracture
(c) Joint stiffness
(d) Peroneal nerve injury
(4) Medical and surgical interventions
(a) Immobilize with posterior splint
(b) Cast when swelling has decreased
(c) ORIF for medial or posterior malleolus fractures

u. Foot fractures—tarsal and metatarsal
(1) Mechanisms of injury
(a) Common injuries
(b) Inversion injuries tear base of metatarsal; fifth metatarsal most commonly injured
(c) Direct force, or forceful flexion or extension
(d) Stress fracture, usually distal second or third metatarsal
(2) Additional symptom—unable to bear weight
(3) Complications—rare
(a) Avascular necrosis—talus has tenuous blood supply
(b) Malunion
(c) Osteomyelitis

(d) Arthritis
(4) Medical and surgical interventions
(a) Nonweight bearing
(b) Immobilize with splint, shoe, or cast
(c) ORIF
(d) Compression dressing and soft splint
(e) Arthrodesis may be necessary in severe or comminuted fractures

v. Calcaneus fractures—os calcis
(1) Mechanisms of injury
(a) Direct heel strike, or jump from height (Don Juan injury)
(b) Associated injuries—bilateral calcaneus injuries, T12/L1 compression fractures, and bilateral Colles' fractures
(2) Additional signs and symptoms
(a) Inability to bear weight
(b) Back pain possible
(3) Complications—tibial nerve injury
(4) Medical and surgical interventions
(a) Splint
(b) Cast and crutches
(c) External fixation
(d) Operative repair
(e) If nondisplaced fracture, rest, ice, elevation, no weight bearing

w. Toe (metatarsal and phalangeal) fractures
(1) Mechanisms of injury
(a) Direct injury from fall or stubbed toe
(b) Heavy object dropped on foot
(2) Additional symptoms—unable to bear weight
(3) Medical and surgical interventions
(a) Dry cotton or Webril between toes
(b) Buddy tape to other larger toes
(c) Splint
(d) Cast if great toe injury
(e) Closed reduction with local anesthesia and without epinephrine

7. **Amputations**

a. Mechanisms of injury
(1) Saws, knives, or hatchets cause a guillotine (complete) injury with clean-cut edge
(2) Machines may cause partial or incomplete amputation, e.g., industrial machines, meat grinders, power mowers, MVCs

b. Medical and surgical interventions
(1) Monitor ABCs and control bleeding
(2) Administer tetanus and antibiotics
(3) Irrigate thoroughly, but gently, with saline
(4) Moist sterile dressing with plain mesh gauze
(5) Preserve part for possible replantation
(a) Place wrapped part in sterile bag and place bag in ice
(b) Transfer patient to most appropriate facility for replantation, if possible
(6) Consider psychiatric consultation to assist patient with body image and role concerns

D. NURSING ASSESSMENT

1. Interview (see Module 19—Nursing Assessment)

a. Mechanism of injury (see Module 2—Mechanisms of Injury)
b. Pain (see Module 14—Pain)
c. Paresthesias
  (1) Diminished sensation
  (2) Burning sensation
  (3) Pins and needles sensation
d. Paralysis—musculoskeletal function
  (1) Weight-bearing ability
  (2) Mobility of injured part; assess extension, flexion, abduction, adduction, supination, and pronation
e. Prior treatment
f. Previous orthopaedic problems

2. Physical assessment

a. Always compare injured part to analogous part
b. Inspection
  (1) Skin color
  (2) Position of extremity—anatomically aligned or deformed
  (3) Open or closed fractures
  (4) Bleeding—estimate amount
  (5) Skin defects—abrasion, laceration, or avulsion
  (6) Swelling and ecchymosis
c. Palpation
  (1) Skin temperature and capillary refill
  (2) Pulse rate, symmetry, and quality
  (3) Tenderness at specific point
  (4) Limited or abnormal joint motion—check joint above and below injury
  (5) Grade motor strength using a standard scale
  (6) Grade pulses distal to injury using a standard scale
  (7) Crepitus may be felt but is never tested
  (8) Peripheral nerve assessment (9)
    (a) Most are mixed motor and sensory nerves
    (b) Test against resistance for motor portion
    (c) Axillary
      i) Motor—abduction of upper arm
      ii) Sensory—specific area over deltoid area, i.e., military patch
    (d) Radial
      i) Motor—extend wrist or thumb
      ii) Sensory—dorsum of thumb
    (e) Ulnar
      i) Motor—fan out extended fingers
      ii) Sensory—tip of small finger
    (f) Median
      i) Motor—touch thumb to little finger base
      ii) Sensory—tip of index finger

(g) Peroneal
i) Motor—dorsiflexion of foot and extension of toes
ii) Sensory—dorsal web space between first and second toe
(h) Tibial
i) Motor—plantar flexion of ankle and toes
ii) Sensory—medial lateral aspect of sole of the foot

d. Percussion—check deep tendon reflexes
e. Auscultation
(1) Vital signs—fractures can cause significant blood loss
(2) Breath sounds—especially with scapula, first rib, or sternal fractures
(3) Bowel sounds for suspected pelvic fracture
(4) Bruit over injured area
f. Laboratory studies
(1) Trauma profile
(2) Urine myoglobin—crush injuries

E. NURSING DIAGNOSES, EXPECTED OUTCOMES, AND INTERVENTIONS

1. **Pain related to muscle spasm, ischemia, nerve injury, edema, or fracture movement**
a. Expected outcome—pain relieved or diminished
b. Nursing interventions
(1) Immobilize suspected injuries, including the joint above and below injury
(2) Splint injury as found and elevate extremity
(3) Apply ice to injured area for prescribed time period
(4) Administer analgesia and muscle relaxants, as needed
(5) Assess patient for development of long-term pain syndromes
(a) Phantom limb pain
i) Seen after amputation
ii) Explain phenomenon to patient
iii) Increase activity of patient
iv) Analgesics and distraction
(b) Arthritis
(c) Causalgia (see Module 14—Pain)

2. **Alteration in peripheral tissue perfusion related to injury, swelling, or vascular damage**
a. Expected outcome—adequate tissue perfusion
(1) Presence and symmetry of pulse
(2) Rapid capillary refill
(3) Normal skin color
(4) Temperature remains normal; deviations detected early
b. Nursing interventions

(1) Monitor neurovascular/motor status on injured extremity at frequent intervals
(2) Elevate and cool extremity to decrease swelling
(3) Ensure adequate fluid volume to prevent venous sludging
(4) Deep vein thrombosis prophylaxis—most common fatal complication of orthopaedic surgery; usually seen in lower extremity injuries (see Module 16—Medical Sequelae)
(5) Assess for signs and symptoms of compartment syndrome; i.e., increased pressure within a muscle compartment that compromises the circulation to the contents of the compartment
  (a) Commonly seen in lower leg and forearm
  (b) Check for paresthesias with two-point discrimination and light touch; frequently described as burning sensation
  (c) Check for pain on passive movement (dorsiflexion) and pain out of proportion to the injury
  (d) Tenseness of palpation
  (e) Diminished power on motor exam
  (f) Diminished pulse is a late sign
(6) Monitor tissue compartment pressures; notify physician if pressure is greater than 40 mm Hg
(7) Notify physician immediately if compartment syndrome suspected
  (a) Prepare for cast bivalving at early signs and symptoms
  (b) Assist with fasciotomy
    i) Monitor distal extremity neurovascular status every hour
    ii) Maintain sterile dressings to fasciotomy sites
    iii) Prepare patient for probable skin grafting to fasciotomy sites
(8) Observe patient for signs of avascular necrosis
  (a) Maintain a high index of suspicion for necrosis around the femoral head and neck, carpus (scaphoid), and talus
  (b) Educate patient about the need to immobilize fracture and maintain nonweight bearing since compression increases risk of necrosis

3. Potential fluid volume deficit related to blood loss

a. Expected outcomes
  (1) Normovolemia with urine output of 0.5 to 1.0 ml/kg/hour
  (2) Hematocrit and hemoglobin within normal limits
b. Nursing interventions
  (1) Control bleeding by direct pressure, compression, or splinting
  (2) Immobilize suspected fracture to prevent vessel injury
  (3) Assess distal extremities for pulses, capillary refill, and temperature
  (4) Predict adult blood loss by fracture sites (8)
    (a) Humerus—1.0 to 2.0 units
    (b) Elbow—0.5 to 1.5 units
    (c) Forearm—0.5 to 1.0 units
    (d) Pelvis—1.5 to 4.5 units
    (e) Hip—1.5 to 2.5 units
    (f) Femur—1.0 to 2.0 units
    (g) Knee—1.0 to 1.5 units
    (h) Tibia—0.5 to 1.5 units

(i) Ankle—0.5 to 1.5 units
(5) Administer I.V. fluids and/or blood, as ordered
(6) Prepare patient for arteriogram to rule out artery injury, if indicated
(7) Utilize tourniquets only in extremely life-threatening situations

4. Potential for infection related to open fractures and soft tissue injury

a. Expected outcomes—absence of infection as evidenced by normal body temperature, WBC, and negative wound cultures
b. Nursing interventions
(1) Monitor vital signs and temperature
(2) Meticulous aseptic technique when dressing wounds and injury sites
(3) Monitor wound drainage at least every shift
(4) Perform pin care to remove crusted exudate
(a) Cleanse with soap and water and apply antimicrobial ointment, or
(b) Wrap pin sites with povidone iodine-soaked gauze, or
(c) Cleanse with half-strength hydrogen peroxide and apply antimicrobial ointment
(5) Administer antibiotics as prescribed; usually for open fractures and soft tissue injuries
(6) Provide tetanus immunization
(7) Assist with debridement of devitalized tissue
(8) Prevent skin breakdown, particularly at cast edges, splints, or braces
(9) Observe for signs and symptoms of osteomyelitis
(10) Observe patients for signs and symptoms of gas gangrene; high index of suspicion in patients with history of shock, hypotension, vascular impairment, or with edema, tight casts, or bandages (see Module 12—Infection)

5. Immobility related to orthopaedic interventions, devices, or healing requirements

a. Expected outcomes
(1) Mobility is restored to maximum potential
(2) Skin integrity is maintained
b. Nursing interventions
(1) Monitor urine output and urinalysis; bone demineralization promotes renal calculi
(2) Limit milk intake to decrease calcium levels in urine
(3) Provide adequate hydration
(4) Perform exercises that transmit forces along the bone shaft, e.g., foot against footboard
(5) Use continuous passive motion machines if long-term immobility anticipated
(6) Additional interventions (see Module 16—Medical Sequelae)

6. Self-care deficit related to immobility and care requirements

a. Expected outcomes
(1) Patient ambulates safely in hospital and home environments
(2) Patient demonstrates cast care, pin care, external fixator care
(3) Patient uses adaptive equipment safely, e.g., braces, canes, walkers, or crutches
(4) Patient verbalizes understanding of procedures
b. Nursing interventions

(1) Teach patient techniques for use of equipment at home
(2) Promote patient's safety during ambulation
(3) Procure adaptive equipment as necessary
(4) Provide home care consultation and referral as needed
(5) Explain all procedures to patient

7. **Additional nursing diagnoses**

a. Potential alteration in gas exchange related to embolic phenomena
b. Powerlessness
c. Alteration in body image
d. Ineffective individual coping
e. Diversional activity deficit
f. Alteration in tissue integrity
g. Dysfunctional grieving associated with physical loss
h. Alteration in renal function secondary to myoglobin released from damaged muscle

F. NURSING SKILLS LIST

1. **Assist with closed reduction**
2. **Assist with aspiration/injection of joint or fracture**
3. **Teach crutch walking and use of adaptive equipment**
4. **Use of continuous passive motion machines**

References

1. Gustilo, R. B., Mendoza, R. M., & Williams, D. N. (1984). Problems in the management of type III (severe) open fractures: A new classification of type III open fractures. *The Journal of Trauma, 24*(8), 742–746.
2. Joy, C. (1989). Musculoskeletal trauma. In C. Joy (Ed.), *Pediatric trauma nursing* (p. 124). Rockville, MD: Aspen.
3. Knezevich, B. A. (1986). Orthopaedic trauma. In B. A. Knezevich (Ed.), *Trauma nursing: Principles and practice* (p. 144). Norwalk, CT: Appleton-Century-Crofts.
4. Simon, R. R., & Koenigsknecht, S. J. (1982). *Orthopaedics in emergency medicine: The extremities* (p. 437). New York: Appleton-Century-Crofts.
5. Thomas, C. L. (1985). Fractures of the pelvis and hip. In G. D. Zuidema, R. B. Rutherford & W. F. Ballinger (Eds.), *The management of trauma* (4th ed., pp. 668–680). Philadelphia: W. B. Saunders Co.
6. Iverson, L. D., & Clawson, D. K. (1977). *Manual of acute orthopaedic therapeutics.* Boston: Little, Brown & Co.
7. American College of Surgeons, Committee on Trauma. (1989). *Advanced trauma life support instructor manual.* Chicago: Author.
8. Iverson, L. D., & Clawson, D. K. (1987). *Manual of acute orthopaedic therapeutics* (3rd ed., pp. 3, 171). Boston: Little, Brown & Co.

9. Urbanski, P. A. (1984). The orthopaedic patient: Identifying neurovascular injury. *AORN Journal, 40*(5), 707–711.

Suggested Readings

Bailey, M. (1982). Emergency: First aid for fractures. *Nursing, 12*(11), 72–81.

Benson, D., Riggins, R. S., Lawrence, R. M., Hoeprich, P. D., Huston, A. C., & Harrison, J. A., III. (1983). Treatment of open fractures: A prospective study. *Journal of Trauma, 23*(1), 25–30.

Berquist, T. H. (1985). *Diagnostic imaging of the acutely injured patient.* Baltimore: Urban & Schwarzenberg.

Bucholz, R. W., Lippert, F. G., Wenger, D. R., & Ezaki, M. Z. (1984). *Orthopaedic decision making.* Philadelphia: B. C. Decker.

Cardona, V. D. (Ed.). (1985). *Trauma reference manual.* Bowie, MD: Brady Communications Co.

Desiderio, V., & Hyatt, G. (1980). Peripheral nerve injuries secondary to fractures and dislocations. *Current Concepts in Trauma Care, 3*(4), 4–7.

Eichelberg, M. R., & Pratsch, G. L. (1988). *Pediatric trauma care.* Rockville, MD: Aspen.

Halpern, J. (1982). Patterns of trauma. *Journal of Emergency Nursing, 8*(8), 170–175.

Halpern, J. S. (1989). Lower extremity peripheral nerve assessment. *Journal of Emergency Nursing, 15*(4), 333–337.

McSwain, N. (1980). Kinematics of orthopaedic injury secondary to trauma. *Current Concepts in Trauma Care, 3*(4), 14–16.

Nahum, A. M., & Mebain, J. (Eds.). (1985). *The biomechanics of trauma.* Norwalk, CT: Appleton-Century-Crofts.

Neff, J. (1985). Standardized care plans: Abdominal pain, gastrointestinal bleeding, and orthopaedic injury. *Journal of Emergency Nursing, 11*(6), 339–344.

Peter, N. K. (1988). Care of patient with traumatic pelvic fractures. *Critical Care Nurse, 8*(3), 62–77.

Proehl, J. N. (1988). Compartment syndrome. *Journal of Emergency Nursing, 14*(5), 283–292.

Redheffer, G. M., & Bailey, M. (1989). Assessing and splinting fractures. *Nursing, 19*(6), 51–59.

Strange, J. M. (Ed.). (1987). *Shock trauma care plans.* Springhouse, PA: Springhouse Corp.

Strange, J. M., & Kelly, P. M. (1988). Musculoskeletal trauma. In V. D. Cardona, P. D. Hurn, P. J. Mason, A. M. Scanlon-Schilpp & S. W. Veise-Berry (Eds.), *Trauma nursing: From resuscitation to rehabilitation* (pp. 525–569). Philadelphia: W. B. Saunders Co.

Suarez, R. S., & Kimbrough, E. E. (1985). Fractures of the tibia. *Current Concepts in Trauma, 8*(4), 4–9.

Section IV
Systematic Approach to Trauma Nursing

MODULE 25
MAXILLOFACIAL AND EYE, EAR, NOSE, AND THROAT INJURY

Susan W. Somerson, MSN, RN, CEN

Prerequisite

Review facial anatomy and Module 13 (Wound Healing).

Objectives

1.0 Describe maxillofacial, eye, ear, nose, and throat (MEENT) injuries that occur frequently and/or are associated with significant morbidity and mortality.

1.1 Describe three mechanisms of injury associated with maxillofacial injuries.

1.2 List pathophysiology characteristic of each injury.

1.3 List other body system injuries frequently associated with each specific MEENT injury.

2.0 Describe the initial assessment for possible MEENT injury.

2.1 List desirable data to include in the history of the injury.

2.2 Describe subjective findings that should be evaluated/elicited.

2.3 Describe the physical examination of the face, eyes, ears, and nose.

3.0 List common nursing diagnoses for a patient with MEENT injury.

4.0 Anticipate and assist health care team with interventions that limit patient morbidity and mortality.

4.1 Identify emergent interventions, equipment, and nursing roles needed to reestablish/maintain the ABCs.

4.2 Identify interventions, equipment, and nursing roles in reestablishment of normal physiological structure/function in MEENT injuries.

5.0 List nursing interventions, with rationale for each nursing diagnosis, applicable to the patient with MEENT trauma.

6.0 Evaluate patient response to medical and nursing interventions.

6.1 Define desirable outcomes with measurable criteria for the patient with MEENT trauma.

6.2 List key indicators used to monitor and evaluate a patient's response to therapeutic interventions.

6.3 List indicators that demand emergent interventions by the health care team.

6.4 List types of data to include in nursing documentation.

7.0 Given a specific case history, formulate a plan of care for a patient who experiences MEENT injury and requires care throughout the trauma continuum.

A. PATTERNS OF INJURY: PATHOPHYSIOLOGY

1. **Mechanisms of injury**
a. Blunt trauma
   (1) Unrestrained passenger in rapid deceleration situations, e.g., motor vehicle crashes (MVC) or motorcycle crashes (MCC)
   (2) Other rapid decelerations, e.g., falls
   (3) Assaults, interpersonal violence
   (4) Sports injuries
   (5) Industrial injuries
b. Penetrating trauma, e.g., gunshot wounds (GSWs), stab wounds, blasts, and other projectiles
c. Toxic exposures, e.g., acid and alkali
d. May be associated with closed head injury, cervical spine injury, and/or vascular injury
2. **Bony structures (see Figure 25.1)**
a. Nasal fracture—fracture through nasal bone(s); may be displaced, involve nasal septum, or be accompanied by epistaxis
   (1) Etiology—blunt force
   (2) Diagnostic indicators
      (a) Edema
      (b) Obvious deformity at dorsum of nose
      (c) Ecchymosis
      (d) Epistaxis
      (e) Pain on palpation
      (f) Crepitus on palpation

Figure 25.1

Bones of the middle facial skeleton. From S. L. Deli & T. C. Bower, Maxillofacial and soft tissue injuries. In V. D. Cardona, P. D. Hurn, P. J. B. Mason, A. M. Scanlon-Schilpp & S. W. Veise-Berry (Eds.), *Trauma nursing: From resuscitation through rehabilitation.* Philadelphia: W. B. Saunders Company, 1988, p. 576. Reprinted with permission.

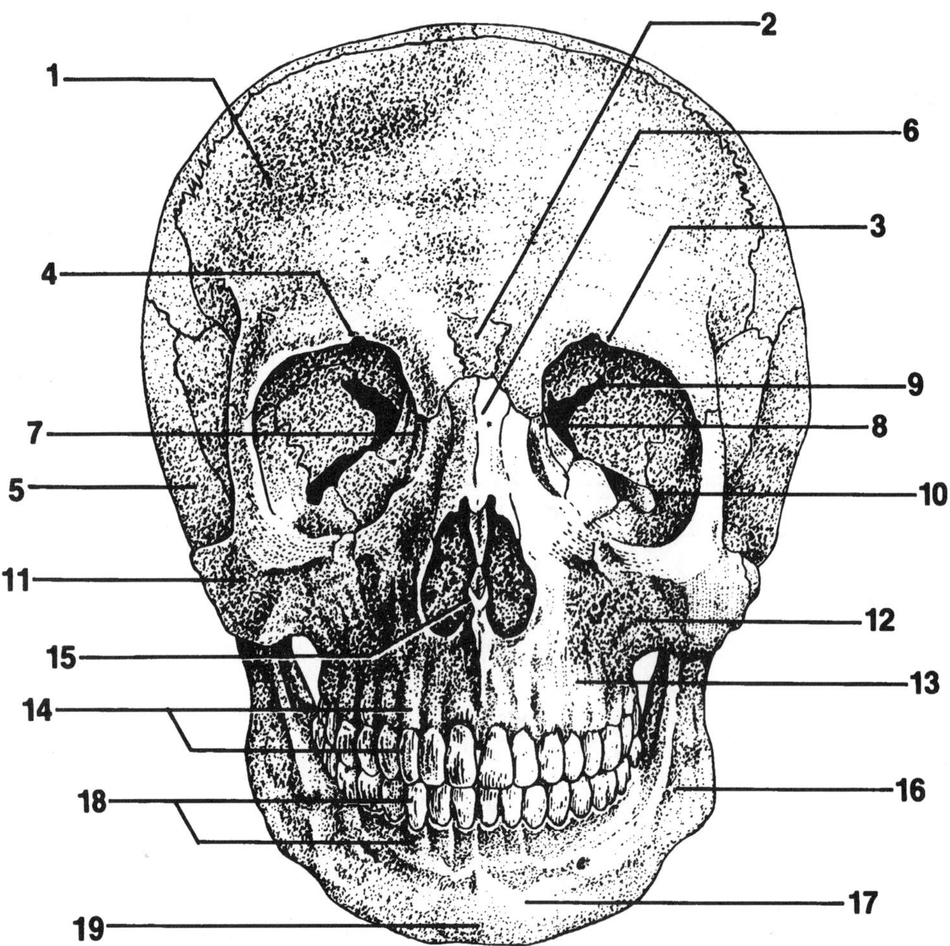

BONES OF UPPER THIRD	BONES OF MIDDLE THIRD	BONES OF LOWER THIRD
1. Frontal bone	9. Superior orbital fissure	16. Body of mandible
2. Glabella	10. Inferior orbital fissure	17. Base of mandible
3. Supraorbital margin	11. Zygomatic bone	18. Alveolar part with teeth
4. Supraorbital notch	12. Zygomatic process	19. Mental protuberance
5. Temporal bone	13. Body of maxilla	
6. Nasal bone	14. Alveolar process with teeth	
7. Lacrimal bone	15. Nasal septum, vomer	
8. Ethmoid bone		

(3) Associated injuries—nasoethmoid/orbit complex fractures

b. Nasoethmoid/orbit complex fractures—fracture through nasal bone, ethmoid, and medial orbit
   (1) Fractures tend to be complex, with fragmentation and/or crumbling of ethmoid sinus
   (2) Fracture of cribriform plate attached to ethmoid results in violation of cranial vault with potential CSF leak
   (3) Fracture line can impinge on optic canal; causes optic nerve injury and blindness
   (4) Etiology—blunt, high-energy force applied to dorsum of nose, which causes the complex to telescope inward
   (5) Diagnostic indicators
      (a) Edema
      (b) Obvious saddle deformity at dorsum of nose
      (c) Medial periorbital ecchymosis
      (d) Medial subconjunctival hemorrhage
      (e) Subcutaneous emphysema if ethmoid sinus violated
      (f) CSF leak if fracture of cribriform plate or ethmoid sinus
      (g) Telecanthus—widening of intercanthal space (distance between medial canthi of eyes)
      (h) Epistaxis
      (i) Evidence of pneumocranium on x-ray
   (6) Associated injuries
      (a) Open or closed head injuries
      (b) C-spine injuries, especially C5 to C7
      (c) Ocular injuries, especially lacrimal apparatus

c. Mandible fractures
   (1) Defining characteristics
      (a) May involve alveolar body (insertion for teeth); would be an open fracture
      (b) Occurrence varies with mechanism of injury and area of mandible (1)
         i) Symphysis—7.1%
         ii) Parasymphysis—body, 41.5%, or angle, 23.7%
         iii) Ramus—3%
         iv) Coronoid process—0.4%
         v) Condyloid process—23.1%
         vi) Alveolar process—1.2%
   (2) Etiology
      (a) Blunt trauma—fracture at contact site
         i) Arc shape of mandible transmits force along structure; more than 50% result in second fracture distant from initial contact point
         ii) Tendency to fracture increases in endentulous patients; teeth add strength and substance to bone
      (b) Penetrating trauma—industrial injuries, e.g., chain saw, or gunshot wounds and blast injuries
   (3) Diagnostic indicators depend on fracture location
      (a) Malocclusion, cross-bite, open bite (objective or subjective)
      (b) Pain on palpation or jaw motion
      (c) Deformity of dental arch; palpable defect of curvilinear arch, or deviation in height of adjacent teeth

(d) Limited range of motion when opening mouth
(e) Trismus (spasm of the muscles used for chewing)
(f) Anesthesia or hypesthesia over area innervated by mandibular branch of trigeminal nerve
(g) External ecchymosis
(h) Mucosal lacerations, gingival lacerations, hematomas in soft tissues, especially floor of mouth and buccal gutters near fracture site, and/or bleeding tooth sockets
(i) Airway obstruction secondary to collapse of tongue against posterior pharynx, with symphyseal or bilateral body fractures, as the support base for tongue is lost
(j) Loose, missing teeth; malalignment of adjacent teeth

(4) Associated injuries
(a) Intraoral, dental injuries
(b) C-spine injuries, especially C1 to C4
(c) Injury to major vasculature in face and neck
(d) Injury to trachea, esophagus, or hypopharynx
(e) Injuries to ear canal, e.g., with condylar fractures

d. Zygomaxillary complex fractures
(1) Defined by one of two fracture patterns
(a) Tripod fracture—fracture through three suture lines where zygoma attaches to facial skeleton
i) Medial maxilla/infraorbital rim generally violates maxillary sinus
ii) Frontozygomatic suture
iii) Zygomatic arch
iv) Displacement causes depressed inferior lateral orbital rim with ocular implications
(b) Zygomatic arch fracture—no interference with function unless displacement impinges on coronoid of mandible
(2) Etiology—blunt force
(3) Diagnostic indicators
(a) Tenderness on palpation of sites
(b) Step deformity of inferior lateral orbital rim
(c) Periorbital ecchymosis
(d) Subconjunctival hemorrhage
(e) Anesthesia or hypesthesia over distribution of infraorbital branch of trigeminal nerve
(f) Unilateral epistaxis
(g) Subcutaneous emphysema if maxillary sinus violated
(h) Depressed malar eminence; edema can obscure
(i) Trismus
(j) Enophthalmos (sunken globe); causes diplopia
(k) Limitation in extraocular movements (EOMs) from periorbital edema (transient) or entrapment of periorbital contents and musculature (permanent, usually requires surgical intervention)
(l) Bony support is lost in involved orbit; contents sit lower resulting in structurally caused diplopia
(m) Ecchymosis, hematoma of upper buccal sulcus

(n) Limited mandible movement if zygoma or arch impinges on coronoid processes
(o) Air-fluid levels on maxillary sinus x-ray
(4) Associated injury—ocular/orbital injury
e. Midface fractures—LeFort I (horizontal fracture)
(1) Defining characteristics
(a) Separation of maxillary alveolar ridge and hard palate from remainder of maxilla
(b) Unilateral, bilateral, or hemicombination with other LeFort fracture (see Figure 25.2)
(2) Etiology—blunt trauma to midface just below nose
(3) Diagnostic indicators
(a) Maxilla moves independently; not mobile if fracture is impacted
(b) Epistaxis
(c) Malocclusion, e.g., cross-bite, open bite
(4) Associated injuries
(a) Dental/alveolar injuries
(b) Vascular injuries
f. Midface fractures—LeFort II (pyramidal fracture)
(1) Defining characteristics

Figure 25.2

LeFort fractures of the maxilla. From D. D. S. Helfrick, Pathogenesis and evaluation of maxillary fractures. In R. H. Mathog, *Maxillofacial trauma.* Baltimore: Williams and Wilkins, ©1984, p. 225. Reprinted with permission.

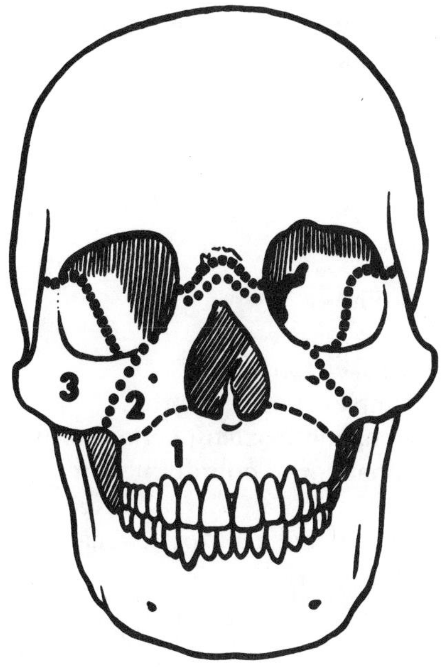

LeFort fractures of the maxilla (front view).

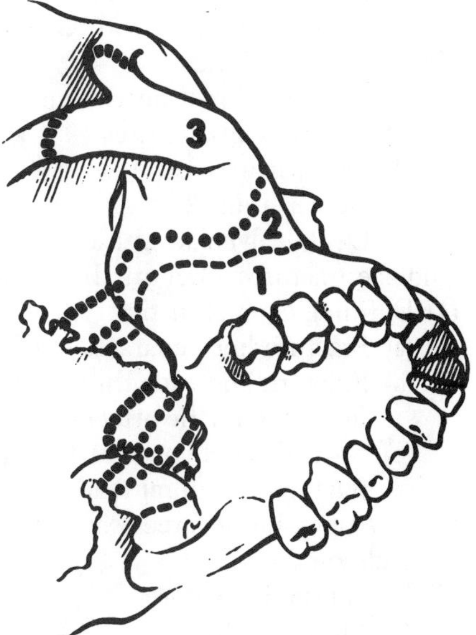

Lateral view of LeFort fractures.

(a) Pyramid-shaped midface fracture segment; segment displaced downward and backward
(b) Fracture segment starts at dorsum of nose with obvious nasal or nasoethmoid fracture; medial and infraorbital rims fractured
(c) Fracture line extends inferior and lateral through maxilla, generally passing medial to zygoma
(d) Fracture line passes through maxillary sinus
(e) Unilateral, bilateral, or hemicombination with other LeFort fracture

(2) Etiology—blunt trauma aimed at midface
(3) Diagnostic indicators
(a) Midface telescoped (caved) in
(b) Elongation between eyes and upper lip
(c) Obvious nasal fracture
(d) Free-floating maxilla; immobile if impacted
(e) Telecanthus (widening between eyes)
(f) Periorbital ecchymosis
(g) Medial inferior subconjunctival hemorrhage
(h) Epistaxis
(i) Anesthesia or hypesthesia in area innervated by infraorbital branch of trigeminal nerve
(j) Malocclusion (open bite) from impingement of molars if maxilla is displaced downward and backward
(k) Airway obstruction if maxilla is displaced downward into oropharynx
(l) Early onset of massive edema in two to three hours
(m) CSF leak (rhinorrhea) possible; perform halo test
i) Allow a drop of bloody drainage to fall on white bed sheet
ii) If CSF fluid is in drainage, it migrates outward from original spot and presents as clear to yellowish halo
iii) CSF does not crust when dried on sheet; mucous drainage crusts
iv) Alert patients with CSF leak may report salty or sweet taste

(4) Associated injuries
(a) Open or closed head injuries
(b) Basilar skull fractures
(c) Vascular injuries
(d) Ocular injuries
(e) Dental/alveolar injuries

g. Midface fractures—LeFort III (craniofacial disjunction)
(1) Defining characteristics
(a) Fracture line separates midface from cranial skeleton
(b) Fracture line runs through nasoethmoid complex, posterior orbit, frontozygomatic attachments, zygomatic arch, and maxillosphenoid suture
(c) Nasoethmoid complex fracture predisposes patient to cribriform plate fracture and dural tear

(2) Etiology—blunt force results in separation of entire midface from cranial skeleton
(3) Diagnostic indicators
(a) Elongated face

(b) Early onset of massive edema (within two to three hours)
(c) Telecanthus
(d) Bilateral periorbital ecchymosis
(e) Bilateral subconjunctival ecchymosis
(f) Bilateral epistaxis
(g) CSF leak—rhinorrhea, otorrhea (see LeFort II)
(h) Pain, crepitus over fracture sites
(i) Battle's sign if basilar fracture
(j) Malocclusion (open bite) secondary to face displaced downward and backward; results in impingement of posterior teeth
(k) Airway obstruction if fracture segments are displaced inferiorly and posteriorly
(l) Rocking face: movement of maxilla moves entire face separately from cranium
(m) Unilateral, bilateral, or hemicombination with other LeFort fracture

(4) Associated injuries
(a) Basilar skull fractures
(b) Dural tear may manifest as CSF leak (CSF rhinorrhea, CSF otorrhea)
(c) Ocular injury
(d) Open or closed head injury

h. Orbital fractures—blow-out fractures
(1) Sudden increase in intraorbital pressure causes fracture at weakest point of orbital box; generally floor of orbit, which sits above porous maxillary sinus
(2) Periorbital contents (fat, muscle) may herniate downward and become incarcerated
(3) Etiology—blunt trauma
(a) Projectile with small surface area delivered with high force to anterior globe, e.g., squash ball, tennis ball
(b) Objects with larger surface areas tend to impact on, and be absorbed by, orbital rim; globe spared from compression and increased intraorbital pressure; orbital rim fractured rather than orbital wall; fracture may extend through walls of orbit
(4) Less frequently, may involve superior, lateral, or posterior walls
(5) Diagnostic indicators
(a) Pain on palpation of orbital rim, if fracture line is through orbital rim
(b) Palpable stepoff from orbital rim, if fracture line is through orbital rim
(c) Loss of bony support results in structurally caused diplopia
(d) Limited EOMs if rectus muscle is entrapped; limitation depends on structure or apparatus entrapped
(e) Edema
(f) Periorbital ecchymosis
(g) Subconjunctival hemorrhage
(h) Retained malar prominence; in pure blow-out fracture, zygomatic portion of orbital rim is not involved
(i) Enophthalmos; edema may initially obscure
(j) Infraorbital anesthesia
(6) Associated injuries—sinus injury or ocular injury

3. Soft tissue trauma

a. Laceration, avulsion, abrasion (see Module 26—Integumentary and Soft Tissue Injury)
   (1) Suspect potential injuries to other structures, e.g., globes, nerves, fractures, ducts, until proven otherwise
   (2) Due to high vascularity of facial area, there is greater potential for viability of injured tissue than in other areas of the body

b. Contusion, hematoma
   (1) Suspect fracture at site of hematoma or contusion, until proven otherwise
   (2) Edema or hematoma, particularly intraoral, may impinge on available airway space
   (3) Nasal septal hematomas can result in septal perforation or fistula if not drained
   (4) Diagnostic indicators
      (a) Septal hematoma; bulging, dark mass on speculum exam
      (b) Intraoral hematomas, sublingual or in gingival-buccal gutters

4. Injuries to accessory structures

a. Parotid gland and Stensen's duct—parotid is one of the glands responsible for production of saliva; Stensen's duct carries saliva from gland and empties into oral cavity at a point opposite the second maxillary bicuspid
   (1) Laceration or transection of parotid gland and/or duct
   (2) Etiology—penetrating trauma in area between tragus of ear and maxillary molars
      (a) Parotid duct parallels facial nerve tract
      (b) Suspect duct laceration if facial nerve dysfunction (motor deficit)
   (3) Diagnostic indicators
      (a) Clear fluid in wound after hemostasis is achieved by pressure
      (b) Obvious gland tissue noted in wound

b. Lacrimal apparatus injury—tear glands and ducts
   (1) Laceration or transection of lacrimal glands and ducts
   (2) Etiology—laceration or transection of lacrimal glands and ducts from primary injury, or secondary to fracture segments of nasoethmoid complex
   (3) Diagnostic indicators
      (a) Telecanthus
      (b) Failure of fluorescein, instilled in conjunctival sac, to appear in nostrils
      (c) Lack of tearing

c. Injury to facial nerve
   (1) Laceration or contusion causing dysfunction of facial nerve (primarily motor deficits); may be temporary if nerve is contused
   (2) Etiology
      (a) Penetrating trauma—lacerations where facial nerve root is seated, from tragus of ear to midpupillary line
      (b) May result from secondary trauma inflicted by surrounding injuries
      (c) Facial nerve path parallels parotid duct; suspect injury to facial nerve if evidence of parotid duct injury
   (3) Diagnostic indicators
      (a) Facial flattening on affected side
      (b) Inability to close eyelid on affected side
      (c) Inability to perform exaggerated facial movements on affected side

d. Ear injury
  (1) Defined by
    (a) Obvious laceration or rupture of structures, e.g., pinna, canal, tympanic membrane
    (b) Structural changes interfering with normal transmission of sound
  (2) Etiology
    (a) Penetrating—lacerations or missile injuries
    (b) Blunt—primary or secondary injuries
      i) Canal laceration may result from mandibular condyle fracture fragment forced upward and backward
      ii) Injuries from pressure changes, e.g., being struck on ear with flat hand, increases pressure in canal and ruptures tympanic membrane (TM)
  (3) Diagnostic indicators
    (a) Bleeding from external structures or canal
    (b) Decreased hearing
    (c) Ruptured TM on otoscopic examination
    (d) Suspect basilar skull fracture if hemotympanum, CSF otorrhea, Battle's sign
  (4) Associated injuries—temporal skull injuries, e.g., basilar skull fracture, temporal artery epidural hematoma

5. Ocular trauma

a. Globe rupture, penetrating, and perforating injuries
  (1) Defining characteristics
    (a) Globe rupture—rupture in globe integrity due to increased hydrostatic pressure when force applied to globe sitting in bony box; ruptures at weakest junction (limbus)
    (b) Globe perforation—through-and-through violation of entire globe wall due to perforating object; may involve extrusion of intraocular fluids or tissue; projectile may rest in anterior or posterior chamber (retained foreign body), or pass through opposite wall of globe
    (c) Globe penetration—partial-thickness violation of globe wall, e.g., superficial laceration of conjunctiva or impaled object that rests in outer layers of sclera
  (2) Etiology
    (a) Penetrating, perforating injuries
      i) Industrial accidents; failure to wear protective eyewear
      ii) Stab wounds, gunshot wounds
      iii) Blast injuries with projectiles
      iv) Lacerated eyelid may have a globe injury beneath
      v) Entry site may be small and obscured by subconjunctival hemorrhage
    (b) Blunt injury by relatively small surface area objects, e.g., ball, fist; large surface area objects spare globe by impacting on, and being absorbed by, bony orbit
  (3) Diagnostic indicators
    (a) Globe perforation or rupture
      i) Small, shrunken eyeball
      ii) Irregularly shaped pupil; "teardrop pupil" may point in direction of perforation

iii) Visual evidence of prolapsed contents on exterior eyeball
iv) Decreased visual acuity
v) Sticky substance (vitreous fluid) noted on eyeball
vi) May be able to visualize foreign bodies, e.g., metal fragments, on fundoscopic exam or x-ray
vii) Associated with hyphema

(b) Penetrating injury
i) Foreign object may remain imbedded in eye
ii) Lacerations of external layers of globe

b. Retinal injury
(1) Separation of retina from choroid; loss of nutrient channel results in death of retinal tissue
(2) Etiology—blunt or penetrating force to globe
(a) Blunt trauma—hemorrhage or trauma within globe results in scarring and traction on retina with subsequent detachment
(b) Penetrating trauma to retina—creates fistula between vitreous and choroid of posterior globe; vitreous leaks behind retina and increased pressure results in detachment
(3) Diagnostic indicators
(a) Changes in vision—gradual or sudden
i) Flashes of light
ii) Cloudy, gray vision
iii) Curtain falling in front of eyes
iv) Floaters in field of vision
(b) Generally no complaints of pain
(c) Fundoscopic exam
i) Generally negative findings; detachment usually in periphery, which requires specialized equipment to visualize
ii) May find wrinkled retina, gray retina, or change of red reflex to black

c. Chemical injuries—acid and alkali
(1) Defined by
(a) Acid solutions—generally cause epithelial damage only; proteins in eye act as barrier to further penetration
(b) Alkali solutions—combine with cellular lipids and move deeply into eye; damage continues over several hours
(2) Etiology—accidental contact with acid or alkali; determine nature of contaminant as quickly as possible
(3) Diagnostic indicators
(a) History of exposure
(b) Pain—no pain in severe injury
(c) Presence of facial skin burns
(d) Loss of vision
(e) Changes in globe noted during treatment
i) Opacification, whitening of cornea
ii) Fragments, filaments of tissue floating in irrigation pathway

d. Hyphema
(1) Defined by blood in anterior chamber
(a) Due to stretching of iris vessels, which bleed into anterior chamber
(b) Rebleeding usually within five days of initial injury

(2) Etiology—generally blunt trauma
(a) Blunt force applied to globe decreases anterioposterior length and increases circumferential length, which tears iris vessels
(b) Force required to cause hyphema is capable of producing more serious intraocular injuries, e.g., retinal detachment, retinal tear, vitreous hemorrhage
(c) Penetrating or perforating trauma may rupture blood vessels, which bleed into anterior chamber
(3) Diagnostic indicators
(a) Blood in anterior chamber on lateral or frontal visualization; may obscure entire chamber or present as small meniscus in lower aspect of anterior chamber
(b) Patients with hyphema tend to demonstrate sleepiness or lethargy

e. Vitreous hemorrhage
(1) Defined by
(a) Rupture of small vessels of uvea or retina results in bleeding into vitreous
(b) Facilitates scar tissue formation with resultant deformities in vitreous bands; leads to changes in tension on intraocular structures
(2) Etiology—blunt or penetrating trauma
(3) Diagnostic indicators
(a) Visual changes, e.g., patient can only see shadows
(b) Red reflex becomes black
(c) Inability to visualize retina
(d) Patient complains only of floaters in brief, small episodes of bleeding

f. Injury by metallic foreign bodies (FB)
(1) Defining characteristics
(a) Perforating FBs containing iron cause siderosis
i) Chronic, degeneration of retina; may lead to blindness
ii) Onset months to years postinjury
iii) Severity dependent on iron content
iv) Once siderosis has started, prognosis is poor; object should be removed early
(b) Metallic fragment visible on globe and surrounded by rust ring if iron present; formation begins within hours
(2) Etiology—penetrating trauma; often industrial accident from failure to wear protective devices (goggles); metal fragments penetrate or perforate globe
(3) Diagnostic indicators
(a) Metal fragment seen on fundoscopic exam
(b) Metal fragment on x-ray, CAT scan, ultrasound
(c) If onset of siderosis, night blindness and narrowing of visual fields
(d) Metal fragment or rust ring visible on globe; complaint of FB sensation

B. MEDICAL AND SURGICAL INTERVENTIONS

1. Maintain airway

a. Recognize impending airway obstruction and treat or secure airway before problematic

b. Suction blood, vomitus, FBs, avulsed teeth
c. Tongue may obstruct, especially in patients with flail mandible (base of tongue attachment lost); grasp tongue and pull anteriorly to open airway
d. Use padded ring forceps to hold tongue forward, if airway obstruction is due to loss of bony support
e. Manually reduce fractures obstructing airway
f. Esophageal obturators (EOA, EGTA) are generally impractical; facial fractures prohibit seal necessary for effective functioning
g. Endotracheal intubation—prophylactic in injuries likely to progress to massive edema
   (1) Avoid nasal intubation in midface fractures
   (2) Oral intubation with in-line C-spine stabilization unless spine cleared
   (3) Creation of surgical airway needed for upper airway obstruction, due to massive edema or structural changes, and/or when intubation is impossible, e.g., anatomic distortion or edema obscures landmarks
   (4) Percutaneous transtracheal jet ventilation (TTJV, needle cricothyroidotomy)
      (a) Uses high flow oxygen, O_2 source 50 psi, via large bore catheter inserted through cricothyroid membrane
      (b) Special attachments, e.g., toggle switches, permit intermittent insufflation
      (c) Adequate for short-term oxygen delivery; inadequate for expiration of CO_2
         i) Not used for more than 30 to 60 minutes
         ii) Convert to cricothyroidotomy or tracheostomy
      (d) Does not completely protect airway from aspiration
   (5) Cricothyroidotomy
      (a) Surgical opening through cricothyroid membrane; allows passage of curved tracheostomy tube 5.0 to 7.0 mm
      (b) Used in prehospital or admitting areas until a tracheostomy is performed under controlled conditions
   (6) Tracheostomy—indicated for LeFort II and III, or maxillofacial trauma with concurrent chest or intracranial pathology

2. Maintain breathing—provide humidified oxygen and mechanical ventilation as needed

3. Support circulation

a. Manually reduce excessively bleeding fractures
b. Insert nasal packing if cranial vault is intact
c. Apply pressure to accessible bleeding points; firm posterior structure required for pressure to tamponade bleeding; otherwise, occult bleeding may continue
d. Replace fluids
e. Ligate or embolize at angiography, if major vessel bleeding is uncontrolled by usual measures
f. Consider coagulopathies and treat as needed

4. Minimize functional morbidity of specialized senses

a. Begin early identification and treatment
b. Obtain immediate ophthalmologic consultation
c. Chemical exposure, especially alkali, to eyes
   (1) Immediate, copious irrigation with normal saline solution (NSS) or water (up to 6 liters and over several hours for alkali exposure); continue until ocular fluid pH is between 7.3 and 7.7

(2) Remove contact lenses prior to irrigation; chemical solutions remain under lenses and are absorbed by contact lenses
(3) Sweep out solid material with moist cotton tip applicator; sweep out folds and corners of eye

d. Penetration, perforation, or rupture of globe
(1) Prevent application of pressure to globe with careful examination; rest fingers on bony orbits ONLY; do not force eyelids apart
(2) Defer examination for ophthalmologist if attempts to observe globe cause pressure to globe or patient to struggle, which increases intraocular pressure
(3) Apply Foxx shield or similar rigid device

e. Intraocular injury—limit activities and drugs that increase intraocular pressure

5. Restoration of structural integrity

a. Skin and mucous membranes
(1) Consider plastic surgery consultation for optimal cosmetic outcome
(2) Primary repair performed up to 24 hrs postinjury, generally within 6 to 12 hrs
(3) Primary closure vs secondary closure or graft based on tissue defect and degree of contamination
(4) Removal of debris (tattooing) may require general anesthesia and can be done concurrently with other scheduled surgery; must be done within 12 hrs postinjury
(5) Do not shave patient's eyebrows
(6) Drain nasal septal hematomas; if undrained, a nasal septal fistula may result
(7) Suture large lacerations in mucous membranes; smaller ones may heal by secondary intention
(8) Lidocaine, a local anesthetic, may produce tissue deformity leading to less satisfactory results; lidocaine with epinephrine not used in areas of limited vascularity, e.g., tip of nose, ear
(9) Avulsions of ear and nose tip can be replanted; handle as any amputated tissue
(10) Light compressive bandage after ear repair or drainage of ear hematoma to prevent "cauliflower ear"

b. Bony structures—fracture reduction may be delayed depending upon specific bones involved
(1) Delayed reduction allows edema to subside and yields better cosmetic repair
(2) Reduction methods (open vs closed reduction, repair vs observation) depend on surgeon's preference, displacement of fracture, amount of damage, and subsequent effect on surrounding structures, morbidity, direction of fracture line
(a) Manual reduction and splinting or packing for nasal fracture
(b) Manual reduction and monitoring for some zygomaxillary complex fractures
(c) Monitoring only, for nondisplaced zygomaxillary complex fractures
(d) Open or closed reduction with packing
i) Some nasal fractures
ii) Some zygomaxillary complex fractures
(e) Closed reduction with external stabilization; arch bars, or stents in edentulous patients, with or without intermaxillary fixation (IMF)

i) Mandible fractures
ii) LeFort I fractures
iii) Alveolar body fractures

(f) Open reduction and fixation; wiring, plating, arch bars, and IMF; suspension wiring of arch bars to a point above highest fracture; grafting or prosthesis
i) Mandible fractures
ii) LeFort I, II, III
iii) Zygomaxillary complex fractures
iv) Nasoethmoid fractures
v) Orbital fractures
vi) May place arch bars, but defer IMF until nasal obstruction is relieved, or danger of postanesthesia vomiting has passed

(g) Open reduction with wiring and external fixation is reserved for severely comminuted mandibular fractures with large tissue defects

c. Auditory structures—drain pinna hematomas; follow with light compressive bandage

d. Nasal septum—drain hematomas and pack

6. **Restoration of functional integrity**

a. Soft tissue structures
(1) Parotid duct and gland—surgical repair using stent
(2) Facial nerve repair—surgical repair if morbidity noted, e.g., inability to close eyelid, interference with speech
(3) Eyelid repair—preferably done by ophthalmologist for optimal lid function and long-term corneal integrity

b. Intraoral structures
(1) Consider oromaxillofacial surgery consultation
(2) Handle avulsed teeth properly
(a) DO NOT ATTEMPT TO "CLEAN"; leave attached tissue intact
(b) Place in cold, whole milk or, if patient is alert, in patient's cheek; optimal medium is Hank's solution
(3) Replace viable teeth in sockets as soon as possible; stabilize with arch bars or wiring to adjacent teeth

c. Ocular structure
(1) Surgical release of entrapped extraocular muscles
(2) Surgical repair of avulsed lens, perforated globe, detached retina, and lacrimal apparatus
(3) Surgical removal of intraocular blood and superficial foreign bodies, including rust ring
(4) Antibiotic therapy
(5) Drug therapy to control intraocular pressure
(6) Patching to prevent eye movement
(7) Cycloplegic eyedrops
(8) Position patient to facilitate reattachment of structures
(9) Utilize contact lenses to seal small, superficial lacerations
(10) Hospitalization and bed rest for hyphema
(11) Monitor intraocular pressure
(12) Monitor visual acuity through examination

d. Auditory structures—repair ruptured TM

7. **Prevention of infection**

a. Antibiotics for contamination from intraoral pathogens, or in case of dural tear and CSF leak or sinus violation

b. Irrigate lacerations with copious amounts of normal saline

c. Tetanus prophylaxis (see Module 26—Integumentary and Soft Tissue Injury)

d. Limit use of nasal tubes to prevent sinusitis

8. **Maintenance of nutritional intake using supplemental oral feedings, enteral feedings, or total parenteral nutrition**

9. **Consultation with specialty support services including speech pathologist, nutritionist, psychologist, and/or audiologist**

C. NURSING ASSESSMENT

1. **Interview**

a. Mechanisms of injury, including characteristics of foreign bodies (FBs)

b. Use of protective adjuncts, e.g., goggles

c. Precipitating events

d. Subjective complaints

(1) Respiratory distress

(2) Feeling of nasal obstruction

(3) Changes in vision, e.g., diplopia, decreased acuity, shadows, flashes of light

(4) Changes in hearing

(5) Change in surface area sensation; hypesthesia or anesthesia

(6) Pain at rest or upon specific movements

(7) Drainage felt in oropharynx

(8) Alteration in taste; sweet or salty taste suggests CSF drainage

(9) Feeling of "teeth not fitting right"

(10) Limitation of jaw excursion

2. **Physical examination specific to MEENT injury**

a. Evaluate ventilatory effort

(1) Use of accessory muscles

(2) Auscultate upper airway for noisy respiration or airway compromise, e.g., stridor, laryngospasm

(3) Signs of hypoxia, agitation, tachycardia, tachypnea

b. Obvious occult hemorrhage; check oropharynx

c. Inspect face from top to bottom

(1) Overall face—inspect full frontal view, profile, quarter profile, and superior to inferior views

(a) Obvious deformities, facial symmetry at rest, facial flattening; compare right to left

(b) Symmetry of motor function, especially facial nerve distribution, e.g., patient demonstrates an exaggerated smile, raises eyebrows, scrunches eyelids (defer until globe perforation or penetration ruled out)

(c) Lacerations, contusions, bruising, tissue defect; note ecchymosis around eyes (raccoon's eyes), or mastoid process (Battle's sign)
(d) Drainage from nose or ears
(2) Intraoral
(a) Hematomas, contusions, lacerations on floor of mouth, gums, gutters of upper and lower jaws, posterior oropharynx, tongue
(b) Blood draining from nasopharynx down back of throat
(c) Missing teeth
(d) Deformities of bony structure and dental arch; malocclusion
(3) Intranasal
(a) Septal deviation
(b) Lacerations
(c) Hematomas
(d) Hemorrhage or drainage; check by using halo test
(4) Ocular examination
(a) Visual acuity—perform prior to ANY manipulation of eye and orbit; ONLY exception is chemical exposure
i) Use Snellen chart or other reading material; check right (OD), left (OS), and both eyes (OU)
ii) Document if patient uses corrective lenses
iii) Document if patient can read print
iv) Document if patient can see gross movements, e.g., fingers
v) Document if patient perceives light only
(b) Physical examination
i) NOTE: do not force swollen lids apart until globe rupture or perforation is ruled out
ii) In retracting lids, rest fingers on bony orbit only; do not place any pressure on globe
iii) Apply protective shield and refer to ophthalmologist if difficulty is encountered
(c) Check for presence of contact lenses
(d) Globe
i) Subconjunctival hemorrhage
ii) Pupil size and shape
iii) Obvious perforations with extrusion of globe contents
iv) Appearance of turgor; shrunken globe
(e) Cornea
i) Lateral view for irregularities in corneal surface; evaluate depth of anterior chamber
ii) Anterior and lateral views for clarity of cornea and anterior chamber; check inferior aspect for hyphema
(f) Eye position and movement
i) Eyes lying in different planes, e.g., tripod or blow-out fracture; affected eye sits a few centimeters lower than the non-involved eye
ii) Eyeball sunken or recessed in orbit (enophthalmos)
iii) Limitation of extraocular movements
iv) Telecanthus
(g) Fundoscopic examination

(5) Ear examination
(a) Lacerations, contusions, hematomas
(b) Blood or drainage from ear canal
(c) Otoscopic examination of TM and ear canal; defer if there is bleeding or CSF drainage
(d) Gross assessment of hearing

d. Palpation—orderly and systematic from top to bottom; search for obvious deformities, pain on palpation, crepitus, subcutaneous emphysema, abnormal mobility, stepoffs
(1) Frontal forehead area
(2) Supraorbital ridges
(3) Nasal bridge
(4) Infraorbital ridges
(5) Maxilla mobility assessed by physician
(6) Zygomatic complex and arch
(7) TMJ functioning—patient opens and closes mouth while examiner palpates TMJ
(8) Mandible—symphysis, body, angle, ramus
(9) Intraoral palpation of soft tissues, e.g., sublingual, buccal gutters, gingiva, for edema, hematoma, stepoffs
(10) Palpation for loose teeth

3. Laboratory studies

a. Trauma profile
b. Salivary amylase for parotid injuries

4. Radiologic studies

a. C-spine
b. Facial series
(1) Lateral and anteroposterior views of skull—sinuses, roof of orbits, frontal bone, nasoethmoid area, and zygomaticofrontal area
(2) Water's view—maxilla, zygoma, orbits, and nasal bones
(3) Towne's view—rami, condyles of mandible
(4) Jug handle view—zygomatic arches
c. Mandible films—PA, lateral oblique
d. Panorex—tomograms of the mandible
e. Sinus films
f. Craniofacial CAT scan

D. NURSING DIAGNOSES, EXPECTED OUTCOMES, AND INTERVENTIONS

1. Ineffective airway clearance related to debris, structural changes, edema, surgical intervention

a. Expected outcome—patent airway
b. Nursing interventions
(1) Suction intraoral debris, blood, vomitus, foreign bodies, and teeth

(2) Perform jaw thrust while maintaining C-spine stabilization
(3) Assist with oro- or nasotracheal intubation
(4) Assist with establishment of surgical airway
(5) Pull tongue forward to open airway in instances of flail fracture of mandible (clamps may be needed)
(6) Monitor airway status; watch for obstruction from increasing edema or intraoral hematomas
(7) Monitor for hypoxemia and respiratory distress
    (a) Agitation, restlessness
    (b) Tachycardia, tachypnea
    (c) Use of accessory muscles
    (d) Stridor
(8) Suction oropharynx and trachea p.r.n.
(9) Encourage patient to cough and deep breathe
(10) Maintain patent tracheostomy during periods of massive facial edema
(11) Keep wire cutters immediately available for intermaxillary fixation; use to cut *vertical* wires
(12) Elevate head of bed to 30° once C-spine is cleared, to minimize edema
(13) Use lightweight ice packs or chilled compresses for 48 hrs to minimize edema

2. Potential for infection related to disruption of normal barriers: skin, mucous membranes, bony compartments

a. Expected outcomes
(1) Absence or rapid detection of infection
(2) Normal WBC; afebrile
(3) Satisfactory wound healing

b. Nursing interventions
(1) Assess rhinorrhea and otorrhea for CSF (halo test)
(2) Assist with irrigation and closure of lacerations; conservative debridement of devitalized tissue only
(3) Intraoral care as per physician preference
(4) No water or FBs in ear if ruptured TM
(5) Administer antibiotics as prescribed
(6) Avoid nasal tubes if possible, e.g., NGT, nasotracheal intubation, or suctioning
(7) Prevent meningitis if CSF leak
    (a) Elevate head of bed after C-spine is cleared
    (b) Instruct patient not to blow nose if CSF leak
    (c) No instrumentation for cleaning nares and auditory canals, if CSF otorrhea or rhinorrhea
(8) Aseptic eye care as prescribed; wipe eyes with moistened, sterile 2 × 2s from inner canthus to outer canthus
(9) Suture line care as per physician preference; may include
    (a) Weak hydrogen peroxide and NSS solution, and ointment to limit crusting
    (b) Dry sterile dressing over nonadherent medium, initially; may be left open thereafter
(10) Monitor for local infection and cellulitis (see Module 12—Infection)

(11) Monitor for signs of meningitis
  (a) Meningeal signs, e.g., nuchal rigidity
  (b) Irritability; change in level of consciousness
  (c) Fever; elevated WBC
(12) Monitor for signs and symptoms of toxic shock syndrome if nasal packing is in place
  (a) Fever of 40°C (102°F) or greater
  (b) Diffuse macular erythema; desquamation in one to two weeks
  (c) Hypotension
  (d) Multisystem involvement with laboratory derangements or physical examination; at least three systems involved
    i) GI, e.g., vomiting, diarrhea
    ii) Muscular
    iii) Mucous membranes
    iv) Renal
    v) Hepatic
    vi) Hematological
    vii) CNS
  (e) Rule out Rocky Mountain spotted fever, leptospirosis, rubeola, and infections of blood, throat, or CSF

c. Monitor for signs and symptoms of sinusitis, e.g., pain, pressure over sinuses

3. Altered oral mucous membrane integrity related to maxillofacial trauma or therapy

a. Expected outcomes
  (1) Prevent further intraoral trauma
  (2) Mucous membranes intact and free from irritation

b. Nursing interventions
  (1) Consider wax over IMF protuberances
  (2) Intraoral care per physician preference; based on procedure performed and suture material used; possible care regimens include
    (a) No intraoral manipulations in first 24 hrs
    (b) Intraoral irrigation with warm NSS and suction catheter
    (c) Intraoral irrigation with hydrogen peroxide and NSS mix
      i) If patient is awake and IMF is in place, begin with weak solution; sudden foaming may panic patient who feels unable to control secretions
      ii) Gradually increase to 50% mixture
      iii) May be limited to seven days' use
    (d) Avoid mouthwashes due to high sugar content
    (e) Use small, soft toothbrush for stimulation hygiene to gums
  (3) Apply lubricants or moisturizers to lips
  (4) Use gentle suctioning technique
  (5) Monitor for intraoral irritation from devices, edema, pain, and friability of gums

4. Altered nutrition: less than body requirements related to loss of teeth, loss of ability to smell or chew, or surgical intervention, e.g., intermaxillary fixation

a. Expected outcomes
  (1) Patient attains and maintains optimal nutritional status

(2) Weight six weeks postinjury is within range for height and body frame
(3) Patient masticates and swallows solid food following removal of therapeutic devices
(4) Patient describes strategies to modify food intake within constraints of patient/injury/therapeutic plan

b. Nursing interventions
(1) Additional nursing interventions (see Module 11—Nutrition)
(2) Avoid very hot or cold foods
(3) Blenderize foods; avoid bland baby foods; add seasonings to taste
(4) Have suction available when patient eats or drinks
(5) Teach patient to use straw or soft tubing attached to syringe for feeding; instill small amounts of liquid in buccal pouch
(6) For swallowing difficulty, obtain speech therapy consultation; consider adding thickening agents (Thickit) to food

5. Body image disturbance related to temporary (edema) or permanent (scars, tissue defects) changes in face appearance

a. Expected outcomes
(1) Optimal cosmetic outcome one year postinjury
(a) Patient acts to prevent excessive scar formation or discoloration
(b) Patient maintains moisture in suture lines and prevents crusting with ointment
(c) Patient demonstrates suture line care to prevent infection
(d) Patient avoids bright sunlight for one year
(2) Suture line demonstrates minimal inflammation; no evidence of hyperpigmentation

b. Nursing interventions
(1) Provide and teach optimal conditions for satisfactory cosmetic results
(a) Teach patient to avoid direct sunlight and use sunblock for one year to minimize hyperpigmentation in scar
(b) Additional interventions (see Module 13—Wound Healing)
(2) Support patient in adjusting to limitations; be realistic, and do not make any guarantees
(a) Refer patient to community-based support groups
(b) Refer patient to hospital-based psychologist, if major adjustments are required, or maladaptive adjustment is noted
(3) Reinforce that scar maturation takes one year, and decisions about revision are made then

6. Knowledge deficit related to home care needs

a. Expected outcomes
(1) Patient verbalizes and/or demonstrates knowledge and skills necessary for home care, prior to discharge
(a) Identifies proper wires to be cut from IMF
(b) Demonstrates proper mouth care
(c) Demonstrates proper suture line care and dressing change
(d) Ability to relate and demonstrate what foods are appropriate and appropriate methods of preparation
(2) Patient verbalizes and demonstrates strategies to perform ADL in a manner that will prevent further injury, if deficits are present at time of discharge

(a) Visual deficit
(b) Tactile deficit
(c) Auditory deficit

(3) Patient verbalizes signs, symptoms, and situations when he/she must call physician or return to hospital
(4) Patient demonstrates eye care, e.g., cleansing, medication administration, use of protective devices

b. Nursing interventions

(1) Teach strategies to prevent further intraoral trauma and identify early signs and symptoms of irritation (see Nursing interventions, 3.b. above)
(2) Teach strategies to promote optimal oral nutrition (Nursing interventions, 4.b. above)
(3) Teach activity limits; depends on type of injury and therapy

(a) Patients discharged with IMF

i) No alcohol or fizzing drinks; alcohol dulls responses, including gag; fizzing drinks may create feeling of fullness and a sense of inability to control oral contents
ii) No swimming or water sports; patient may not be able to quickly expel water
iii) No activities that cause patient to grit teeth, e.g., lifting, pulling, straining, pushing
iv) Verbalize when and how to cut IMF wires; wire cutters immediately available at all times

(b) Patients discharged after ocular injury

i) Use protective devices as ordered by physician
 a) Glasses or rigid eye shield
 b) Use at all times or only during sleep
ii) Instill eyedrops and perform aseptic eye care
iii) Teach activities to avoid
 a) Sudden jerky movements of the eye, e.g., reading, walking in crowds where prone to be bumped or jostled
 b) Increased intraocular pressure, e.g., vomiting, straining, lifting, pushing, or bending over
iv) Safety in activities of daily living
 a) No driving until cleared by physician
 b) Use articles with high contrast colors at home, e.g., buy red toothbrush for a yellow bathroom
 c) Caution in performing high-risk activities, e.g., when pouring hot liquid, move slowly and make physical contact between objects
 d) Use low glare lighting
 e) Use adjuncts as prescribed, e.g., magnifiers, telescopes, colored glasses
 f) Maneuvers for mobility, e.g., use cane to detect steps or curbs; feel for chair with back of legs or hands before sitting down

(c) Patients with ruptured TM—no swimming or water in ears until cleared by physician
(d) Situations in which patients should contact physican and/or return to emergency department

i) If IMF wires are cut
ii) Signs and symptoms of infection or oral irritation
iii) Reinjury of traumatized area
iv) Changes in vision or other specialized senses

(e) Provide information on required equipment procurement and usage

7. **Sensory/perceptual alterations: visual, related to edema, structural changes, injury to ocular structures**

a. Expected outcomes
(1) Vision—returns to preinjury status; ability to maneuver and work with adjuncts as needed, e.g., magnifiers, telescopes
(2) Patient verbalizes and/or demonstrates knowledge and skills needed for home care, e.g., applies shield, instills eyedrops, and performs aseptic care
(3) Patient verbalizes and/or demonstrates strategies to perform ADL that prevent further injury, if visual deficits are present at time of discharge

b. Nursing interventions
(1) Initiate therapy to halt injury
(a) Remove caustic agents by immediate copious eye irrigation with saline or water; remove contact lenses
(b) Prevent increased intraocular pressure
i) Bed rest with head of bed elevated
ii) On physician order, bilateral eye patches to limit eye movement; Foxx shield if there is evidence of perforation, penetration, or rupture
iii) Administer antiemetics; limit noxious stimuli to prevent vomiting
iv) Instruct patient to avoid increases in intraocular pressure, e.g., no bending, straining, coughing
(c) Prevent ocular damage from dryness or corneal abrasion, if facial nerve deficit is present
i) Use ointment and artificial tears for lubrication; patch as ordered
ii) Use Foxx shield during sleep
iii) Use adjuncts to prevent drying, e.g., sterilized square of plastic wrap applied to surrounding bony prominences with petroleum jelly
(2) Modify environment and patient's behavior if loss of vision or depth perception
(a) Side rails up
(b) Call bell is accessible and placed consistently in agreed-upon location
(c) Provide escort when ambulating; allow patient to grasp your upper arm as you walk slightly ahead
(d) Provide assistance with activities of daily living
(e) Orient patient to immediate surroundings; describe room using patient's bed as focal point
(f) Identify yourself upon entering the room; speak to patient before touching him/her; describe to patient your actions before performing them
(g) Do not move articles in patient's immediate area without consulting patient
(h) Modify lighting for patient's comfort; use diffused lighting to decrease glare

(3) If patient's eyes are swollen shut, tell patient this to dispel fears of permanent blindness

8. **Social isolation related to loss of use of sense organs, cosmetic defects or surgical therapies**

a. Expected outcomes

(1) Demonstrates ongoing use of positive coping mechanisms in dealing with changes in body image; verbalizes and accepts changes in body image one year following final surgical interventions

(a) Establishes community support system

(b) Verbalizes realistic outcome expectations

(c) Returns to work or school; seeks other social opportunities

(2) Patient communicates effectively in social interactions

b. Nursing interventions

(1) Announce presence on entering room; speak to patient before touching; describe actions before performing them

(2) Use touch, particularly when a number of sense organs are impacted, e.g., intubated patient with swollen eyes, in a noisy ED or ICU environment

(3) Utilize alternate mechanisms for communication, e.g., chalkboard, pencil and paper; instruct patients with IMF not to open mouth

(4) Encourage patient to take in stimuli within limits of deficits, e.g., radio, TV, followed by questions about information presented

(5) Schedule brief five-minute visits with patient on a hourly basis; alternate staff assigned to visit

9. **Potential for aspiration related to obstruction of normal exits for oral and nasal secretions**

a. Expected outcomes

(1) Prevention of aspiration

(2) Patient verbalizes and/or demonstrates knowledge and skills, listed below, necessary to prevent aspiration, e.g., cutting wires of IMF

b. Nursing interventions

(1) Instruct alert patients to lean forward for oral care; allows secretions to drain out of mouth

(2) Use fingers and/or a mirror to direct catheter for suctioning and feeding, if there are sensory changes in patient's lips

(3) Instruct patients in IMF that emesis and secretions should be able to drain through IMF, and to position themselves (forward tilt) to facilitate this process

(4) Identify wires holding arch bars in place (horizontal wires), and wires holding arch bars and teeth in occlusion (vertical wires); teach patient that *vertical* wires are to be cut, if usual measures (suction, position) are ineffective and release of IMF becomes imperative

(5) Use antiemetics as ordered, p.r.n.

(6) Suction for blood, secretions, vomitus, teeth, or foreign bodies

(7) Anticipate tracheal intubation for protection of patients with inability to control secretions

(8) Swallowed blood is a GI irritant; anticipate vomiting and have suction ready

(9) Maintain balloon seal of endotracheal tube; suction well prior to deflation

(10) Cautious oral hygiene in patients with changes in level of consciousness, even if trachea is intubated
 (a) Begin oral care as per physician preference
 (b) Position patient to facilitate drainage of irrigation fluids into cheek, e.g., lateral position with bed flat
 (c) Use small amounts of irrigant; place suction catheter in cheek before starting
 (d) Avoid high pressure irrigations
(11) Use antiemetics as prescribed

10. **Additional nursing diagnoses**
 a. Fluid volume deficit related to blood loss at injury sites
 b. Sensory/perceptual alterations, tactile, related to nerve injury
 c. Sensory/perceptual alterations, gustatory, related to intraoral injury to receptors, or injury to olfactory structures
 d. Sensory/perceptual alterations, olfactory, related to edema, nasal obstruction, or injury to olfactory structures
 e. Sensory/perceptual alterations, auditory, related to injury to conduction structures or nerve paths
 f. Potential for trauma related to injury to nervous innervation, or loss of sense organ function
 g. Fear related to unknown environment and procedures, sudden changes in life-style, and possibility of permanent changes in appearance or function
 h. Impaired skin integrity related to tissue defects or lacerations
 i. Impaired verbal communication related to maxillofacial injury or therapy, e.g., intubation, IMF
 j. Pain related to distraction of fracture lines, edema, lacerations, contusions, hematoma

E. SPECIALIZED NURSING SKILLS

1. **Open the airway with anterior displacement of tongue via clamp**
2. **Assist with insertion of nasal packing**
3. **Assist with placement and care of arch bars and IMF**
4. **Irrigate eyes and instill eye medications**
5. **Apply eye patch, Foxx shield, or rigid device**

Reference

1. Bochlogyros, P. N. (1985). A retrospective study of 1,521 mandibular fractures. *Journal of Oral and Maxillofacial Surgery, 43*(8), 597–599.

Suggested Readings

Arnet, G. F., & Basehore, L. M. (1984). Dentofacial reconstruction. *American Journal of Nursing, 84*(12), 1488–1490.

Black, J. M., & Arnold, P. G. (1982). Facial fractures. *American Journal of Nursing, 82*(7), 1086–1088.

Brown-Stewart, P. (1989). Maxillofacial trauma: Implications for trauma care. *Critical Care Nurse, 9*(6), 44–57.

Cardona, V. D. (Ed.). (1985). *Trauma reference manual.* Bowie, MD: Brady Communications Co.

Cinotti, A. (Ed.). (1985). *Handbook of ophthalmologic emergencies.* New York: Elsevier Science Publishing Co.

Fincke, M. K., & Lanros, N. E. (Eds.). (1986). *Emergency nursing: A comprehensive review.* Rockville, MD: Aspen Publishers.

Krekorian, E. A. (1988). Maxillofacial and mandibular injuries. In K. L. Mattox, E. E. Moore & D. V. Feliciano (Eds.), *Trauma* (pp. 269–288). East Norwalk, CT: Appleton & Lange.

Lower, J. (1986). Maxillofacial trauma. *Nursing Clinics of North America, 21*(4), 610–628.

Manson, P. N. (1984). Maxillofacial injuries. *Emergency Medicine Clinics of North America,* 2(4), 761–781.

Parke, D. W., & Hamill, M. B. (1988). Injury to the eye. In K. L. Mattox, E. E. Moore & D. V. Feliciano (Eds.), *Trauma* (pp. 289–299). East Norwalk, CT: Appleton & Lange.

Pavan-Langston, D. (1985). *Manual of ocular diagnosis and therapy.* Boston: Little, Brown & Co.

Tumulty, G., & Fesler, M. (1984). Eye trauma. *American Journal of Nursing, 84*(6), 740–744.

Section IV
Systematic Approach to Trauma Nursing

MODULE 26
INTEGUMENTARY AND SOFT TISSUE INJURY

Betsy L. Musser, MSN, RN, CEN
Elizabeth W. Bayley, MS, PhD, RN

Prerequisite

Review anatomy and physiology of the skin; review Module 2 (Mechanisms of Injury) and Module 13 (Wound Healing).

Objectives

1.0 Describe common integumentary and soft tissue injuries.
1.1 List major types of integumentary and soft tissue injuries.
1.2 Briefly describe pathophysiology and major defining characteristics of each type of injury.
1.3 State frequent mechanisms of injury for each type.
1.4 List common complications of integumentary and soft tissue injury.
2.0 List laboratory and radiologic studies frequently used in the diagnosis of integumentary and soft tissue injuries.
3.0 Anticipate and assist with appropriate medical-surgical interventions for integumentary and soft tissue injuries.
3.1 Given specific patient data, recognize which medical-surgical interventions might be required.
3.2 Given specific patient data, state the equipment to be obtained to assist with medical interventions.
3.3 Describe the pharmacologic agents most likely to be required for the patient with integumentary and soft tissue injuries, and the rationale for each.
3.4 List essential preparations for operative interventions in the patient with integumentary and soft tissue injuries.
3.5 Identify treatment goals related to optimal function during rehabilitation.

4.0 Describe initial nursing assessment for integumentary and soft tissue injuries.
4.1 List essential content of the patient interview, including prehospital factors that are essential to meaningful nursing diagnoses and interventions.
4.2 Identify steps in the physical examination of integumentary and soft tissue injuries.
5.0 Develop nursing diagnoses based on assessment data.
5.1 List common nursing diagnoses related to integumentary and soft tissue injuries.
5.2 Identify specific etiologic factors related to each diagnosis.
5.3 Identify signs and symptoms that validate the specific nursing diagnoses.
6.0 Identify nursing interventions required for the patient with integumentary and soft tissue injuries.
6.1 List common nursing interventions required in patients with integumentary and soft tissue injuries.
6.2 Given a patient scenario, prioritize nursing interventions.
6.3 Relate interventions to specific nursing diagnoses.
6.4 Identify the rationale for nursing interventions.
7.0 Evaluate patient response to medical and nursing interventions.
7.1 Define desirable outcomes with measurable criteria for the patient with integumentary and soft tissue injuries.
7.2 List nursing activities required for continuous monitoring and evaluation of patient status.
7.3 List types of data to be included in nursing documentation.
7.4 Cite trends in patient status that may require priority interventions from nurse or physician.
8.0 Given a specific case history, formulate a plan of nursing care for a patient who experiences integumentary and/or soft tissue injuries, and requires care in various phases of the trauma continuum.

A. PATTERNS OF INJURY AND PATHOPHYSIOLOGY

1. **Thermal burns**
   a. Etiology (see Module 2—Mechanisms of Injury)
   b. Severity is primarily dependent on depth and extent
   c. Burn depth classification
      (1) Superficial partial-thickness (first degree)
         (a) Damage to epidermis and superficial dermis
         (b) Red, dry, and painful
         (c) Common sunburned appearance
      (2) Deep partial-thickness (second degree)
         (a) Epidermis destroyed and dermis damaged
         (b) Blisters or moist surface
         (c) Red to mottled white
         (d) Painful
         (e) Prone to scars if deep dermis damaged
         (f) Capable of spontaneous reepithelialization
      (3) Full-thickness (third degree)

(a) Epidermis and dermis destroyed
(b) Subcutaneous structures may be involved
(c) Color varies widely; may be white, beeswax, dark red, brown, charred
(d) Dry and leathery
(e) Little to no pain
(f) Destruction of hair follicle permits hair to be pulled out easily
(g) Usually requires skin graft for wound closure

d. Extent of burn injury
(1) Estimated by Rule of Nines—divides body surface into areas, each representing 9% or a multiple of 9% of body surface area (BSA)
(a) Each upper extremity and the head is assigned a value of 9% BSA
(b) Each lower extremity, the anterior trunk, and the posterior trunk comprise 18% BSA each
(c) Provides quick estimate in prehospital setting; reasonably accurate in individuals over nine years of age (1)
(2) Lund and Browder chart and its modifications—recognizes that the proportion of body surface covering specific body parts changes with age, e.g., the head and neck of an infant constitute 20% BSA compared with 9% in an adult (2)
(a) Provides most reliable estimate of extent of injury
(b) Used in emergent and acute phases of injury to determine treatment and prognosis, and as a guide to appropriate patient referrals and planning for wound closure

e. Modified American Burn Association Injury Severity Grading System (1)
(1) Minor burns
(a) <15% BSA partial-thickness in adults
(b) <10% BSA partial-thickness in children
(c) <2% BSA full-thickness not involving eyes, ears, face, hands, feet, or perineum
(d) <1% BSA full-thickness on above body areas
(e) Does not include electrical burns, or burns accompanied by inhalation or other injury
(2) Moderate burns
(a) 15 to 25% BSA partial-thickness in adults
(b) 10 to 20% BSA partial-thickness in children
(c) 2 to 10% BSA full-thickness not involving eyes, ears, face, hands, feet, or perineum
(d) Does not include electrical burns, or burns accompanied by inhalation or other injury
(3) Major burns
(a) >25% BSA partial-thickness in adults
(b) >20% BSA partial-thickness in children
(c) >10% BSA full-thickness
(d) All burns of the face, eyes, ears, feet, hands, or perineum; although these burns may involve small areas, they may present potential cosmetic or functional impairment
(e) All high-voltage electrical burns
(f) All burns involving inhalation injury or additional major trauma

f. Burn center transfer criteria
   (1) Transfer from receiving hospital to a regional burn center is indicated for all patients with major burns
   (2) Other high-risk patients who may require specialized care include young children, the elderly, and individuals with significant preexisting health and social problems that may compromise their ability to respond to treatment
g. Localized changes due to burn injury
   (1) Loss of skin barrier
   (2) Evaporative fluid loss from wound surface
   (3) Loss of body temperature control due to damaged skin microcirculation and inability to regulate body heat peripherally
   (4) Altered inflammatory response due to vascular damage
   (5) Edema
h. Systemic changes
   (1) Cardiovascular
      (a) Increased capillary permeability
      (b) Hypovolemia due to plasma leakage from vascular compartment to interstitial tissue
      (c) Decreased cardiac output due to hypovolemia
   (2) Renal
      (a) Decreased glomerular filtration rate due to hypovolemia
      (b) With deep burns, myoglobin from muscle damage may lead to acute tubular necrosis
      (c) Inadequate fluid resuscitation may lead to renal failure
   (3) Pulmonary—associated with concomitant inhalation injury (see Module 22—Cardiothoracic Trauma)
      (a) Decreased oxygenation due to carbon monoxide poisoning
      (b) Upper airway edema from heat or toxic chemicals produced by combustion
      (c) Lower airway irritation and edema from inhaled chemical products of combustion
      (d) Restrictive defects of thorax due to circumferential chest burns
      (e) Noncardiogenic pulmonary edema from effects of fluid shifts into lung parenchyma
   (4) Gastrointestinal
      (a) Paralytic ileus
      (b) Gastric erosion and Curling's ulcer
   (5) Hematologic
      (a) Hemolysis of damaged red blood cells
      (b) Initially, increased hemoglobin and hematocrit, with increased blood viscosity
      (c) Thrombocytopenia
      (d) Anemia (after initial stage)
   (6) Immunologic
      (a) Loss of skin barrier to infection
      (b) Decreased serum immunoglobulins
      (c) Abnormal neutrophil function
      (d) Altered cellular immunity and lymphocytopenia

(e) Rapid colonization of wound surfaces may lead to burn wound sepsis
(f) Susceptible to potentially fatal septicemia

(7) Metabolic alterations (see Module 11—Nutrition)
(a) Decreased cardiac output, oxygen consumption, and resting energy expenditure in early shock phase
(b) Within hours to days, hypermetabolic phase occurs with increased cardiac output, oxygen consumption, and metabolic rate
(c) Increased catecholamine, cortisol, and glucagon production
(d) Increased core body temperature
(e) Caloric expenditure and protein catabolism is greater in burn injury than in any other type of trauma

2. Chemical burns

a. Etiology and severity (see Module 2—Mechanisms of Injury)
b. Local effects are similar to thermal injury; may have a splatter pattern
c. Systemic response, particular to a specific chemical, can occur if chemicals are absorbed through skin or inhaled; otherwise, body systems are affected similarly to thermal burns

3. Electrical burns

a. Etiology and severity (see Module 2—Mechanisms of Injury)
b. Local effects
(1) Entry wound—may be charred, centrally depressed, and leathery; surrounded by reddened area
(2) Exit wound—smaller, dry, circumscribed; "explosion" appearance
(3) Similar to iceberg, i.e., surface wound represents only a small portion of total tissue destruction; subcutaneous fat, fascia, muscle, and bone may be damaged or destroyed

c. Systemic effects—every organ system can be damaged directly by the passage of current, or indirectly by stress and damage of other structures (3)
(1) Cardiovascular
(a) Vascular thrombosis with vessel collapse
(b) Delayed vessel aneurysm or rupture due to vessel wall injury and necrosis
(c) Dysrhythmias and conduction disturbances due to coronary artery spasm, coronary endarteritis, or diffuse myocardial damage (3)

(2) Renal failure may occur due to direct kidney injury from electrical current, release of myoglobin from damaged muscle, and poor renal perfusion from hypovolemia

(3) Neurological
(a) Headache, intraventricular hemorrhage, cerebral edema, and seizures may occur if entry site is the head
(b) Motor nerves are affected more often than sensory
(c) Quadriplegia, hemiplegia, ascending paralysis, amyotrophic lateral sclerosis, or transverse myelitis due to direct neuronal or vascular injury, or demyelination may occur days to two years after injury
(d) Short-term memory may be absent or diminished for four to six weeks after injury

(4) Pulmonary
(a) Respiratory arrest, due to skeletal muscle contractions, may occur initially

(b) Effusion and pneumonitis result from direct thoracic injury
(5) Gastrointestinal
(a) Visceral damage with bowel necrosis and perforation may occur; symptoms usually develop two to three weeks after injury
(b) Other abdominal organs may also be damaged, resulting in symptoms of organ dysfunction
(c) Ileus and Curling's ulcer may occur, as in other types of burns
(6) Associated injuries
(a) Cataracts evident three months to two years after injury
(b) Vertebal compression, dislocations, and fractures, and long bone fractures may occur due to tetanic contractions or falls
(c) Compartment syndrome due to muscle damage; edema and increased pressure in fascial compartment result in decreased tissue perfusion, ischemia, and neurovascular compromise

4. Ionizing radiation

a. Etiology and severity (see Module 2—Mechanisms of Injury)
b. Local (skin) effects are similar to partial-thickness thermal burns; may be superficial or deep
c. Systemic effects
(1) Rapidly dividing cells are most sensitive to effects of radiation
(2) Exposure to less than 100 rads usually produces no symptoms; exposure to more than 1000 rads may be fatal within 24 hrs (4)
(3) Individual tolerance varies
(4) Acute radiation syndrome (5)
(a) Prodromal phase
i) Tissue necrosis due to release of histamine and bradykinin
ii) Anorexia, vomiting, and diarrhea
(b) Latent phase
i) Feelings of well-being; symptom-free
ii) Length of phase is inversely related to exposure dose
(c) Manifest illness stage
i) Hematopoietic alterations due to depressed bone marrow activity (200 to 700 rads)
a) Lymphocytes disappear within 24 hrs
b) Granulocytes disappear within days
c) Platelets decrease within 10 days
d) Death from hemorrhage and infection may ensue
ii) Gastrointestinal effects of 700 to 1000 rads
a) Bacteria enter vascular compartment through denuded villi, causing infection
b) Increased cell permeability occurs with bleeding into gut
iii) Central nervous system
a) Increased intracranial pressure with more than 1000 rads
b) Effects are caused by nonbacterial inflammatory foci or radiation-induced toxic products
(d) Recovery phase
i) Probable if only 100 to 200 rad dose with good response to treatment
ii) Possible if 500 or less rad dose with positive response to hematopoietic treatment

iii) Improbable if greater than 700 rad dose with multisystem complications

5. Cold injury (frostbite)

a. Etiology, severity, and factors affecting susceptibility (see Module 2—Mechanisms of Injury)

b. Classifications of cold injury (6)

(1) First degree—mild

(a) Involves epidermis

(b) Appears red to slightly cyanotic

(c) Edematous

(d) Painful; itches and "burns"

(2) Second degree—superficial

(a) Involves epidermis and dermis

(b) Characterized by blisters with yellow fluid and by deep tissue edema

(c) Skin cold but pliable

(d) Severe "burning" pain

(3) Third degree—deep

(a) Involves skin and subcutaneous tissue

(b) Skin is nonpliable

(c) Characterized by blood-filled blisters and severe edema

(d) Skin appears waxy or cyanotic

(4) Fourth degree—deep complete

(a) Involves skin, subcutaneous tissue, muscle, and bone

(b) Anesthetic

(c) Minimal edema in frostbitten area, which is surrounded by red, painful, edematous tissue

(d) Persistently cold and numb

c. Frostbite may be associated with hypothermia and its sequelae, e.g., anoxia, cerebral edema, metabolic acidosis, cardiac dysrhythmias

d. Complications

(1) Compartment syndrome may occur in two to four hours

(2) Necrosis requiring amputation may develop; line of demarcation is clear; allow ample time to assess viable tissue before amputation

6. Laceration

a. A full-thickness skin tear

b. Caused by penetrating trauma, e.g., tearing, cutting, or pressure splitting

c. Integumentary injury may be accompanied by damage to underlying nerves, tendons, vessels, fasciae, or muscles

d. Jagged edges predispose patient to potential scar formation

7. Abrasion

a. A loss of partial-thickness skin with minimal bleeding

b. Caused by scrapes to the epidermis and dermis from friction, e.g., in falls and bicycle crashes

c. Tatooing from embedded foreign material, e.g., roadbed gravel, may occur

8. Avulsion

a. Full-thicknesses loss of tissue, which prevents wound approximation

b. Types include partial (flap), complete, or degloving

c. Caused by penetrating trauma (tearing, cutting, or pressure splitting)

d. Compromised circulation may slow healing
e. Extensive scarring with disability, disfigurement, and loss of skin function in affected area may occur

9. **Amputation**
   a. A shearing or crush injury, resulting in partial or complete amputation, with disruption of the neurovascular supply
   b. Caused by penetrating trauma from power saws, lawn mowers, snow blowers, etc., or major crush injury (see Module 24—Musculoskeletal Injury—for more information)
10. **Crush injury**
    a. Tissue, nerve, and vascular damage, with or without fractures, due to extreme external pressure
    b. Caused by blunt trauma from a wringer, machinery, or heavy weight applied to a body part
    c. Related complications include anaerobic infection, subungual hematoma, compartment syndrome, myoglobinuria, acute tubular necrosis, potential degloving injury
11. **Blast injury**
    a. A pressure, shearing, or penetrating injury resulting in damage to gas-containing organs
    b. Involves partial or full-thickness skin disruption, with or without fractures, nerve, and/or vascular damage (see Module 2—Mechanisms of Injury—for classification and examples)
12. **Puncture**
    a. A small, penetrating wound that bleeds minimally before sealing off
    b. Caused by sharp objects, e.g., nails, needles, glass shards, knives, animal, human, or insect bites
    c. Related complications include damage to underlying structures, damage from enzymes such as venom, and infections from anaerobic microbes, e.g., *Clostridium tetani,* and rabies
    d. Injury variations include imbedded foreign body, impaled foreign body, and injection injury from high pressure paint or grease gun (prone to compartment syndrome)

B. DIAGNOSTIC STUDIES

1. **Wound biopsy for histologic and microbiologic analysis**
2. **Wound culture**
3. **Fluorescein dye injection to determine burn wound depth, and wound edge viability in lacerations and avulsions**
4. **Triphasic technetium-99m stannous pyrophosphate scintigraphy postfrostbite to determine prognosis for tissue salvage (7)**
5. **Monitor tissue pressure in crush and burn injuries**
6. **CAT, MRI, arteriogram, and other radiologic studies, as indicated, to determine soft tissue and bone status**

7. **ECG and serum potassium when extensive tissue damage occurs, as in burns or crush injury**
8. **Evaluate hearing, if injury from explosive force**
9. **Surgical exploration to determine tissue viability, e.g., electrical burns**

C. MEDICAL AND SURGICAL INTERVENTIONS FOR ALL INTEGUMENTARY INJURIES

1. **Maintain airway and breathing; support circulation; immobilize cervical spine**
2. **Provide narcotic analgesia prior to painful wound exploration, cleansing, and/ or debridement**
3. **Provide anesthesia for wound care procedures**

a. Topical—e.g, 4% Xylocaine for cleansing and debridement of abrasions; use caution in instance of large body surface wound due to absorption and systemic vascular effects

b. Local
   (1) 1 to 2% Xylocaine for cleansing and suturing lacerations
   (2) 1 to 2% Xylocaine with 1:200,000 epinephrine for hemostasis of face and scalp lacerations; never used on toes, ears, fingers, penis, nose, or with elderly patients

c. Regional—1% Xylocaine for cleansing, debridement, suturing, or reconstruction of lacerations and amputations

d. Systemic—ketamine for burn wound care; Valium, Pentothal, Versed, or Brevital for surgical exploration in reconstruction of laceration or amputation

4. **Cleanse wound (see Module 13—Wound Healing—for additional information)**

a. Use bacteriocidal solution and water, and gentle technique, for lacerations and abrasions

b. May use hydrotherapy for burns and frostbite

c. Irrigate deep lacerations and avulsions with sterile saline

d. Use jet irrigation for punctures (except wood)

5. **Tetanus prophylaxis**

a. Tetanus-prone wounds generally have at least one of the following characteristics: over six hours old; contaminated; over 1 cm in depth; infected; contain devitalized tissue, burns, or crush injuries

b. To provide active immunity, administer tetanus toxoid, DT, or DPT (for children under seven years), if no prior tetanus immunization, incomplete or uncertain immunization series, or over 5 to 10 years have passed since last booster

c. To provide passive immunity, tetanus immune globulin may be prescribed for extensive, contaminated wounds and some moderate wounds, if no prior tetanus immunization, incomplete or uncertain immunization series, or over 5 to 10 years have passed since last booster

d. Dosage information (see latest Centers for Disease Control guidelines) (8)

6. **Wound debridement**

a. Mechanical—use scissors and forceps, or wet-to-dry dressings

b. Surgical—operative excision of devitalized tissues

c. Enzymatic—e.g., Travase or Elase to soften and dissolve burn eschar

7. **Surgical exploration of wound—particularly important where deep muscle, nerve, tendon, or visceral damage has occurred, e.g., bullet wound, electrical burn**

D. MEDICAL AND SURGICAL INTERVENTIONS FOR SPECIFIC INJURIES

1. **Burns**

a. Stop the burning process
   (1) Rescuer must protect self from fire, chemicals, electricity, radiation
   (2) Remove source of heat; turn current off
   (3) Flush chemicals with copious amounts of water for at least 15 to 30 min; irrigate patient's eyes (saline preferred) and remove contact lenses
   (4) Allow the wound to cool to normal temperature; do not apply ice
   (5) Follow radiation decontamination protocol for radiation injury

b. Provide fluid resuscitation
   (1) For thermal and chemical burns, estimate fluid replacement using a standard formula, e.g., Parkland formula: 4 ml lactated Ringer's solution/kg/% BSA given over first 24 hrs postburn; administer half of estimated 24-hr requirement in first 8 hrs, and second half over next 16 hrs
      (a) Formula provides an estimate of patient requirements; patient response, including urine output and vital signs, is ultimate guideline
      (b) Goal is to provide adequate volume to perfuse vital organs without overloading vascular compartment; careful titration of fluids, based on prescribed intake and urine output, is essential
   (2) Desirable urine output is 0.5 to 1.0 ml/kg/hr; for electrical burns, increase fluid intake to provide urine output of 1.5 to 2.0 ml/kg/hr
   (3) Colloids, e.g., albumin, are added at physician's discretion, usually after the first 24 hrs

c. Prevent hypothermia, particularly during transport, wound care, and operative procedures

d. Treat hyperthermia with antipyretics if patient's core temperature is above 39°C (103°F)

e. Monitor cardiac rhythm in all patients with electrical burns and other major or moderate burns

f. Initiate topical antibacterial therapy—prevents burn wound sepsis but generally inhibits eschar separation; prescribed agent may need to be varied over long term due to development of resistant microbial strains
   (1) Sulfamylon cream (mafenide acetate 10%)
      (a) Wide spectrum bacteriostatic against Gram-negative and Gram-positive organisms
      (b) Penetrates thick eschar and therefore is useful for electrical burns
      (c) Active against resistant organisms; ineffective against fungus
      (d) Painful for one to two hours after application

(e) May cause allergic reaction (rash), metabolic acidosis, hyperpnea; contraindicated in respiratory insufficiency

(2) Silvadene (silver sulfadiazine 1%)
- (a) Wide spectrum bacteriostatic
- (b) Ineffective against fungus
- (c) Depresses granulocyte function
- (d) Minimal pain upon application
- (e) May cause allergic reaction (rash, pruritis)

(3) Cerous nitrate solution 1%
- (a) Bacteriocidal
- (b) Often used in combination with silver sulfadiazine
- (c) Not systemically absorbed
- (d) May inhibit wound healing
- (e) Rewet every four hours to maintain therapeutic concentration

(4) Betadine liquid or ointment
- (a) Broad spectrum bacteriocidal
- (b) Fungistatic
- (c) May increase systemic iodide level or cause metabolic acidosis
- (d) Mildly irritating

(5) Other topical antibacterials include Furacin, Polysporin, Garamycin cream (gentamicin sulfate), Neomycin (neomycin sulfate), and silver nitrate 5% solution

g. Prescribe oral and intravenous systemic antibiotics based on clinical indication, and culture and sensitivity reports

h. Apply gauze and biological dressings (see Module 13—Wound Healing)

i. Perform escharotomy—incision into the burned skin down to subcutaneous fat
- (1) Relieves constricting effects of circumferential full-thickness burns; allows tissue expansion, restores adequate blood supply, and decreases neurovascular compression
- (2) May be needed for extremities or trunk during first 6 to 24 hrs after injury

j. Fasciotomy—incision through full-thickness burn into underlying subcutaneous fat and fascia to relieve edema and compartment syndrome; used in electrical and deep thermal burns involving muscle

k. Debride and excise burn eschar in operating room
- (1) Tangential—sequential "shaving" of burned layers down to viable tissue
- (2) Fascial—primary removal of burned skin and underlying fat to level of fascia or muscle
- (3) May be accompanied by large blood loss

l. Autografting (see Module 13—Wound Healing)

m. Release of contractures

n. Reconstructive (plastic) surgery; includes tissue expansion techniques to improve cosmetic deformities

2. Cold injuries

a. Treat general hypothermia—core body temperature below 35°C (95°F)
- (1) Goal is to warm core first, or core and extremities together, to avoid after-drop and rewarming shock
- (2) Internal warming—provide warm humidified oxygen, warm irrigations, e.g., gastric or peritoneal lavage, enemas, and warm I.V. solutions; cardiopulmonary bypass or peritoneal or hemodialysis

(3) External warming—immerse in tub of 40°C (104°F) water; use warmed blankets and heat shield

b. Rapidly rewarm affected part with water bath 40° to 42°C (104° to 108°F)
c. Immobilize extremities until warmed, then increase range of motion to decrease edema
d. McCauley's protocol—prevents microvascular changes (9)
   (1) Debride superficial blisters; debride deep blisters
   (2) Apply topical antithromboxane
   (3) Administer systemic antiprostaglandin, e.g., ibuprofen or aspirin
e. Penicillin during edema phase
f. No smoking
g. Local debridement and/or amputation
h. Grafting of viable, noninfected tissue
i. Prevent refreezing of affected areas

3. Lacerations, abrasions, avulsions

a. Monitor closely for hypovolemia with large scalp or facial avulsion due to high vascularity of scalp and face
b. Suture and dress as indicated
c. May require microvascular or flap graft repair

4. Amputation

a. Control hemorrhage
   (1) Pressure is preferred method
      (a) Use direct pressure or pressure dressing
      (b) Apply pressure to specific pressure points to decrease blood flow to an area when other control measures fail, e.g., shoulder or groin
      (c) Elevate part above heart level
   (2) Apply tourniquet
      (a) Use only for uncontrollable bleeding and probable exsanguination
      (b) Write application time on patient's forehead
   (3) Vascular clamps may be used when an artery is readily accessible
b. Preserve amputated part for potential replantation; NOTE: protocols vary
   (1) Rinse the part with sterile normal saline or lactated Ringer's solution
   (2) Roll subcutaneous fat to the inside
   (3) Wrap in saline-moistened (not wet) gauze
   (4) Place in a plastic bag
   (5) Seal and place on ice, or in a second bag of iced water or iced saline
c. Place sterile dressing, moistened with saline, on stump
d. Replant amputated part, or form functional stump using skin or flap graft

5. Crush injury

a. Prescribe osmotic diuretics to maintain kidney perfusion and prevent tubular necrosis, due to presence of large amounts of hemoglobin and myoglobin from muscle destruction
b. Treat for hyperkalemia, e.g., Kayexalate
c. Perform fasciotomy and muscle decompression for compartment syndrome
d. Perform operative repair of underlying structures, including blood vessels, nerves, and bones
e. Amputate extremity if not salvageable

6. **Blast injury**
a. Monitor function of all organs closely; blast effects can be widespread and remote from site of obvious injury
b. Explore wound surgically to determine pathway of missiles
c. In operating room, debride and remove embedded foreign bodies, e.g., shell, bullet, shrapnel
7. **Puncture wound**
a. Initiate meticulous wound cleansing and remove foreign substance
b. Explore wound, debride, and perform fasciotomy as needed
c. For animal bites, rabies prophylaxis may be needed (see Module 12—Infection)
d. For insect and snake bites, antivenom may be needed
e. Observe and treat for anaphylaxis from animal toxins, e.g., sting ray
f. Observe and treat for anaerobic infection; hyperbaric oxygen may be indicated

E. NURSING ASSESSMENT

1. **Interview**
a. Prehospital information, including mechanisms of injury, possible contaminants, and time of injury; wound is considered contaminated if over six hours old
b. Location when found, e.g., if burn victim is found in closed space, suspect inhalation injury
c. Weather conditions; duration of exposure to agent causing injury, e.g., heat, cold
d. Estimated blood loss
e. Past medical history, particularly conditions that affect healing, e.g., diabetes, prior splenectomy
f. Current medications with implications for wound healing, e.g., steroids, aspirin
g. Allergies, and manifestation, particularly to tetanus toxoid, Xylocaine, epinephrine, antibiotics
h. Tetanus immunization history
2. **Physical examination**
a. Inspection
   (1) Depth and extent—use Rule of Nines, or Lund and Browder, or Berkow charts for burns; use millimeter ruler for other wounds
   (2) Appearance of wound edges, presence of foreign bodies, debris, contaminants, bleeding, and circulatory adequacy
   (3) For burn injury or injury accompanied by extensive bleeding, observe urine output including amount, color, quality
   (4) Motor function of nerves distal to injury
      (a) Radial—wrist hyperextension
      (b) Median—thumb to little finger opposition
      (c) Ulnar—abduct all fingers; thumb and index finger in perfect "O"
      (d) Femoral—extend knee or flex hip against resistance
      (e) Peroneal—dorsiflexion of foot
      (f) Tibial—plantar flexion

(5) Look for possible injuries to underlying tissues
(a) Exposed or dysfunctional tendons
(b) Fractured bones
(c) Torn blood vessels
(d) Ischemic muscles
(6) Edema
b. Palpation
(1) Sensory function of nerves distal to injury
(a) Radial—dorsal web surface of thumb
(b) Median—index finger
(c) Ulnar—little finger
(d) Femoral—anterior thigh and medial lower leg
(e) Peroneal—anterior and lateral lower leg
(f) Tibial—medial and lateral sole
(2) Motor strength in involved body part
(3) Pain (point tenderness)
(4) Skin turgor
(5) Circulatory adequacy
(a) Peripheral pulses
(b) Skin temperature
(c) Capillary refill
(6) Related injuries (may be less obvious)
c. Auscultation
(1) Blood pressure with burn, crush, or rapidly bleeding wound
(2) Breath sounds when inhalation injury accompanies burns
(3) Peripheral pulses using Doppler
(4) Bowel sounds in crush injury or major to moderate burn injuries

3. Laboratory studies
a. Trauma profile
b. Culture and sensitivities of wound exudate
c. Quantitative wound biopsy (burns)
d. Carboxyhemoglobin and arterial blood gases, if inhalation injury accompanies burns

4. Radiologic studies
a. Chest x-ray for visceral or inhalation injuries
b. Xenon lung scan for inhalation injury
c. Arteriogram for electrical burn, avulsion, laceration, amputation, frostbite, crush or blast injury
d. Venogram for electrical burns or crush injuries
e. Nuclear scans for blast injuries and electrical or radiation burns
f. CAT scan for blast injuries and electrical or radiation burns

5. Other studies
a. Electrocardiogram for inhalation, electrical, moderate or major thermal burns, blast and crush injuries, hypothermia
b. Bronchoscopy for burns with inhalation injury
c. Fluorescein dye to determine wound depth and/or assess wound edge viability for burns and cold injuries, avulsions, lacerations, and abrasions

F. NURSING DIAGNOSES, EXPECTED OUTCOMES, AND INTERVENTIONS

1. **Impairment of skin integrity related to thermal, chemical, electrical, radiation, or mechanical trauma**
a. Expected outcome—wound heals with optimal function and cosmetic appearance
b. Nursing interventions
   (1) Control bleeding
   (2) Cleanse, debride, and/or irrigate wound as prescribed
   (3) Apply topical agents as prescribed
   (4) Apply wound dressings by using aseptic techniques
      (a) Apply dressings distal to proximal
      (b) Ensure that no two wound surfaces touch, e.g., wrap burned fingers separately
   (5) Prepare patient for operative procedures to debride or graft wound
   (6) Provide appropriate care to donor and graft sites, using protocols that protect wound and enhance healing
2. **Potential for infection related to open wound, wound contamination, or poor wound healing**
a. Expected outcomes
   (1) Absence of local or systemic signs of infection such as local warmth, redness, and pain surrounding wound or fever, decreased bowel signs, or hyperpnea
   (2) Wound exudate cultures are negative
   (3) Wound heals normally
b. Nursing interventions
   (1) Wash hands meticulously before and after wound care activities; use clean or sterile gloves appropriately
   (2) Implement CDC universal, and wound and skin precautions as needed; don mask, gown, and sterile gloves for major burns or extensive open wounds
   (3) Provide tetanus prophylaxis
      (a) Administer tetanus toxoid and human immune globulin I.M. in opposite deltoids
      (b) Instruct patient about possible side effects (redness, pain, slightly increased temperature) and measures to alleviate discomfort (warm compresses, antipyretics, analgesics
      (c) Instruct patient to continue with basic follow-up series
   (4) Observe wound site closely and report signs of infection to physician
   (5) Obtain wound cultures as required
   (6) Assess body temperature every four hours
   (7) Assist patient with hygiene to keep unaffected skin and hair clean; shave or clip hair adjacent to wound, if indicated by physician
   (8) Maintain integrity of clean blisters or follow physician's directive for care
   (9) Ban live plants, cut flowers, or water pitchers from immunosuppressed patient's area, e.g., major burns, to eliminate reservoirs of infection
   (10) Administer antibiotics as prescribed and observe patient's response
   (11) Administer antivenom or rabies prophylaxis, if indicated

3. **Pain related to tissue destruction, edema, and medical-surgical interventions for wound care**
   a. Expected outcomes
      (1) Patient states that wound discomfort is tolerable during wound manipulations
      (2) Patient is able to rest and/or concentrate on diversions and participate in care appropriately
      (3) Patient exhibits relaxed facial muscles and body position
      (4) Patient verbalizes need for pain relief and responds to appropriate measures for increased comfort
   b. Nursing interventions (see Module 14—Pain)
      (1) Use intravenous route for analgesics for patients with moderate to major burns or patients with decreased tissue perfusion
      (2) Administer analgesia approximately 30 min prior to painful procedures, i.e., dressing changes and mechanical debridement
      (3) Instruct patient in use of patient-controlled analgesia and/or encourage patient to request analgesics before pain becomes severe
      (4) Evaluate response and notify physician if pain relief is inadequate and/or prohibits patient's participation in care, e.g., exercise
   c. Provide diversional activities, relaxation exercises, and audio or visual imagery
   d. Provide frequent rest periods for patient during long, painful procedures that are gauged to patient's tolerance
   e. Position patient to promote comfort; prevent potential contractures
4. **Potential alteration in peripheral tissue perfusion related to edema or circulatory impairment**
   a. Expected outcomes—adequate perfusion of peripheral tissues as evidenced by warmth, color, capillary refill less than three seconds, presence of peripheral pulses, healing of peripheral wounds
   b. Nursing interventions
      (1) Palpate distal pulses or auscultate with Doppler, and check for capillary refill hourly; compare to normal limb
      (2) Monitor for edema, color, or temperature change
      (3) Position patient to allow for adequate blood flow and to minimize dependent edema; elevate extremities
      (4) Do not massage frostbitten area
      (5) Monitor tissue pressure; notify physician of elevation above 30 mm Hg
      (6) Assess for signs of compartment syndrome, including pain disproportionate to injury, pain on passive movement, or numbness; notify physician, if indicated
      (7) Remove all jewelry on affected extremities
      (8) Maintain intermittent cold applications to reduce edema of selected wounds
      (9) Prepare for rapid rewarming of frostbitten area
5. **Knowledge deficit regarding self-care of wound**
   a. Expected outcomes
      (1) Patient and family verbalize wound care instructions and potential wound-related problems
      (2) Patient and family demonstrate and participate in wound care procedures, including activities that prevent infection, deformity, and scarring
   b. Nursing interventions
      (1) Explain sequence of normal healing of integumentary injuries and rationale for treatments and diagnostic measures

(2) Teach patient to
  (a) Protect wound from infection and additional trauma from mechanical forces, heat, cold, or sun
  (b) Observe wound for signs of infection
  (c) Implement dressing changes by using appropriate supplies and techniques
  (d) Use massage, lubricants, and pressure garments to soften skin and reduce scars
(3) Stress importance of following discharge instructions for optimal wound healing, scar reduction, and follow-up care
(4) Refer patient to cosmetologist, if indicated
(5) Include family in instructions and have both patient and family demonstrate wound care procedures
(6) Refer patient to home health agency, as needed

6. Impaired physical mobility related to tissue loss, decreased range of joint motion, and wound contracture

a. Expected outcomes
  (1) Patient's muscle strength and joint mobility are optimal
  (2) Patient participates in prescribed exercise and splinting programs
  (3) Patient ambulates and accomplishes activities of daily living
b. Nursing interventions
  (1) Instruct patient in use of assistive devices, as needed
  (2) Consult with physical and occupational therapists to develop an exercise program and appropriate splinting and positioning techniques
  (3) Assist with range of motion exercises every four to eight hours
  (4) Administer analgesics 30 min prior to scheduled exercise
  (4) Maintain extremities and head in functional position when patient is at rest
  (5) Apply splints and elastic garments, as needed
  (6) Involve family with exercises and other modalities that encourage patient's physical mobility and functional wound healing

7. Hypothermia related to exposure to cold ambient environment, and loss of skin microcirculation and protective subcutaneous tissue

a. Expected outcome—core body temperature within normal range; patient reports comfort with ambient temperature
b. Nursing interventions
  (1) Maintain ambient temperature in patient care area at 25° to 28°C (76° to 82°F); particularly important for patients with extensive wounds and burns
  (2) Use warmed solutions for wound cleansing and topical therapy
  (3) Assess body temperature every two to four hours
  (4) Cover patient with dressings and bath blankets to prevent evaporative heat loss; use heat shields and other warming devices p.r.n.

8. Body image disturbance related to actual changes in body appearance, loss of body parts, and/or loss of function

a. Expected outcomes
  (1) Patient adapts to altered appearance and function
  (2) Patient's expectations about body appearance and function after wound healing are consistent with reality
b. Nursing interventions
  (1) Acknowledge normalcy of emotional response to wounded integument

(2) Maintain a calm, unhurried manner to encourage patient to verbalize; listen to patient's concerns regarding body image
(3) Prepare patient and significant others for changes in patient's appearance and stages of wound healing and scar maturation
(4) Support patient in identifying strengths and positive aspects of self-concept and in maintaining unique identity
(5) Acknowledge patient losses and support grieving process in patient and significant others
(6) Allow liberal visiting; provide privacy for patient to express feelings to family, friends, and trauma team members who can help patient plan for reintegration with society and a meaningful occupation
(7) Promote effective coping strategies
(8) Arrange visit from another individual who has adjusted to a similar injury or disfigurement
(9) Assist patient with maintenance of appearance and encourage consultation with cosmetologist, plastic surgeon, counseling services, and support groups

9. **Additional nursing diagnoses**

a. Alteration in nutrition: less than body requirements, related to decreased caloric intake and increased protein and caloric needs, due to hypermetabolic state (see Module 11—Nutrition)
b. Potential fluid volume deficit related to hemorrhage, inadequate fluid resuscitation, evaporative fluid loss (see Module 10—Shock)
c. Potential alteration in renal tissue perfusion related to fluid loss and acute tubular necrosis from myoglobinuria, secondary to crush or burn injury (see Module 16—Medical Sequelae)
d. Anxiety related to anticipation of pain with wound manipulation (see Module 14—Pain—and Module 15—Psychosocial Response)
e. Ineffective patient and/or family coping related to altered self-concept resulting from changes in body appearance and/or function (see Modules 15—Psychosocial Response—and Module 17—Rehabilitation)

References

1. Warden, G. D. (1987). Outpatient care of thermal injuries. *Surgical Clinics of North America, 67*(1), 147–157.
2. Bayley, E. W. (1990). Wound healing in the patient with burns. *Nursing Clinics of North America, 25*(1), 205–222.
3. Bingham, H. (1986). Electrical burns. *Clinics in Plastic Surgery, 13*(1), 75–85.
4. Martin, M. T. (1988). Radiation. In E. Howell, L. Widra & M. G. Hill. (Eds.), *Comprehensive trauma nursing: Theory and practice* (pp. 809–817). Glenview, IL: Scott, Foresman & Co.
5. Welsh, M. D. (1986). Acute radiation syndrome. *Dimensions of Critical Care Nursing, 5*(5), 277–283.
6. Knezevich, B. A. (Ed.). (1986). *Trauma nursing: Principles and practice* (pp. 247–248). Norwalk, CT: Appleton-Century-Crofts.
7. Gottlieb, L. J. (1990, March). Surgical treatment of frostbite injury. In D. M.

Smith, Jr. (Chair), *Electrical, nonthermal injuries, and pain management.* Symposium conducted at the Annual Meeting of the American Burn Association, Las Vegas.

8. Centers for Disease Control, Advisory Committee on Immunization Practices. (1985). Diphtheria, tetanus, and pertussis guidelines for vaccine prophylaxis and other preventive measures. *Morbidity and Mortality Weekly Report, 34*(27), 405–423.
9. Robson, M. C. (1990, March). Epidemiology, pathophysiology, and management of frostbite. In D. M. Smith, Jr. (Chair), *Electrical, nonthermal injuries, and pain management.* Symposium conducted at the Annual Meeting of the American Burn Association, Las Vegas.

Suggested Readings

Bayley, E. W., & Smith, G. (1987). The three degrees of burn care. *Nursing '87, 17*(3), 34–41.

Butman, A., Paturas, J., McSwain, N., & Dineen, J. (Eds.). (1986). *Prehospital trauma life support.* Akron, OH: Education Direction, Inc.

Callahan, J. (1985). Compartment syndrome. *Orthopedic Nursing, 4*(4), 11–15.

Cardona, V. D., Hurn, P. D., Mason, P. J. B., Scanlon-Schilpp, A. M., & Veise-Berry, S. W. (Eds.). (1988). *Trauma nursing: From resuscitation through rehabilitation.* Philadelphia: W. B. Saunders Co.

Dyer, C., & Roberts, D. (1990). Thermal trauma. *Nursing Clinics of North America, 25*(1), 85–117.

Howell, E., Widra, L., & Hill, M. G. (Eds.). (1988). *Comprehensive trauma nursing: Theory and practice.* Glenview, IL: Scott, Foresman & Co.

Lanros, N. E. (1988). *Assessment and intervention in emergency nursing.* Norwalk, CT: Appleton & Lange.

O'Hara, M. (1987). Emergency care of the patient with a traumatic amputation. *Journal of Emergency Nursing, 13*(5), 272–277.

Rea, R. E., Bourg, P. W., Parker, J. G., & Rushing, D. (1987). *Emergency nursing core curriculum* (3rd ed.). Philadelphia: W. B. Saunders Co.

Robertson, K. E., Cross, P. J., & Terry, J. C. (1985). Burn care. *American Journal of Nursing, 85*(1), 29–47.

Seward, P. (1987). Electrical injuries: Trauma with a difference. *Emergency Medicine, 19*(9), 66–80.

Sinclair, C. (1981). Management of radiation accident victims: A suggested protocol. *Journal of Emergency Nursing, 7*(3), 87–91.

MODULE 27
PERIPHERAL VASCULAR INJURY

Paula Crawford Gamble, MSN, RN
Susan A. Turcke, MSN, RN, CEN

Objectives

1.0 Describe common peripheral vascular injuries.
1.1 Briefly describe pathophysiology and major defining characteristics for each major type of peripheral vascular injury.
1.2 Describe frequent mechanisms of injury for each peripheral vascular injury.
2.0 Describe the assessment for possible peripheral vascular injury.
2.1 Identify important information to obtain from the prehospital providers.
2.2 List essential data to obtain during the patient interview in peripheral vascular injury.
2.3 List hard and soft signs of vascular injury and the influence of these signs on treatment decisions.
2.4 List radiologic studies commonly needed to diagnose peripheral vascular injury.
3.0 Develop nursing diagnoses based on assessment data.
3.1 List common nursing diagnoses and specific etiologic factors related to peripheral vascular trauma.
3.2 Identify signs and symptoms that validate specific nursing diagnoses.
4.0 Identify nursing interventions required for the patient with peripheral vascular injury.
4.1 List common interventions, including rationale required, for the patient with peripheral vascular trauma.
4.2 Given a patient scenario, prioritize nursing interventions.

5.0 Evaluate patient response to medical and nursing interventions.
5.1 Define desirable outcomes with measurable criteria for the patient with peripheral vascular trauma.
5.2 List nursing activities required for continuous monitoring and evaluation of patient status.
5.3 List types of data to include in nursing documentation.
5.4 Cite trends in patient status which may require priority interventions from nurse or physician.

A. PATTERNS OF INJURY

1. Introduction
a. Incidence of peripheral vascular injury has increased in recent years due to urban violence
b. Improved prehospital care has decreased mortality from early exsanguination
c. Injuries may be arterial, venous, or combined
 (1) Arterial injuries are most critical due to ischemia and/or hemorrhage
  (a) Associated with multiple injuries and varying degrees of shock
  (b) Frequently associated with nerve, vein, and bone injuries
 (2) Clot usually forms in venous injuries as surrounding tissues tamponade this low pressure system; isolated venous injuries are rare
 (3) Combination injuries usually require repair of both arterial and venous injuries

2. Mechanisms of injury
a. Penetrating trauma causes unpredictable injuries including transection, laceration, and intimal injury
 (1) Gunshot wounds (GSWs) most common
 (2) Also caused by sharp instruments or stab wounds
 (3) Shotgun pellets fired less than 10 feet from victim act as high-velocity missiles
b. Blunt injuries
 (1) Usual injuries are contusion with spasm, localized hematoma, or intimal disruption from vessel stretching
 (2) Fracture movement or joint dislocation can perforate vessel
 (3) Blunt injuries are less obvious than penetrating and may be overlooked; maintain high index of suspicion

3. Signs and symptoms of vascular injury
a. Hard signs of arterial injury indicate significant injury and/or impending limb loss and require immediate surgery (1)
 (1) Massive external bleeding
 (2) Rapidly expanding hematoma
 (3) Palpable thrill or audible bruit over a hematoma
 (4) Any classic sign of arterial occlusion
  (a) Distal pulselessness
  (b) Pallor
  (c) Paresthesia

(d) Pain
(e) Paralysis
(f) Poikilothermia—body temperature, e.g., injured limb, varies with environmental temperature
(5) External bleeding

b. Soft signs indicate possible vascular injury (1)
(1) Questionable history of arterial bleeding at the scene
(2) Proximity of the wound to artery and vein
(3) Diminished unilateral distal pulse
(4) Abnormal ankle-brachial pressure index; ankle pressure should be equal to or greater than brachial systolic pressure (2)
(5) Abnormal flow velocity wave form on Doppler ultrasonography
(6) Small nonpulsatile hematoma
(7) Neurological deficit

4. **Injuries/pathology**

a. Wall defect, laceration
(1) Wound produced by tearing of vessel; ranges from simple puncture to nearly complete transection
(2) Etiology—penetrating (most common) or blunt trauma
(3) Diagnostic indicators
(a) Signs and symptoms usually do not appear until thrombosis is present
(b) Distal pulses remain, in most cases
(c) Systolic bruit with tangential injury
(d) Greater hemorrhage than with complete transection; exsanguination may occur

b. Complete vessel transection
(1) Complete cut or tear across vessel; injuries range from simple transection to loss of vessel substance
(a) Transected intima curls inward; divided media contracts and pulls adventitia over vessel ends
(b) Ends retract and bleeding may stop due to spasm, clot, or thrombosis
(c) Exsanguination can occur but is more common with partial transection
(2) Etiology—high-velocity injuries, e.g., hunting or assault rifles, shotguns at point-blank range
(3) Diagnostic indicators—loss of pulse and peripheral ischemia

c. Contusion, intimal flap, or disruption
(1) Injury to vessel lining which initiates minor bleeding or progressive thrombus formation leading to vessel occlusion or distal emboli
(a) Injuries range from trivial hemorrhage in adventitia to diffuse fragmentation and hematoma throughout arterial wall
(b) Intimal disruption is most severe injury
(c) Some heal spontaneously and others lead to distal ischemia
(2) Etiology—blunt or penetrating trauma with stretching of vessel (deceleration injuries) (1)

d. Crush injury
(1) Composite injury involving soft tissue, blood vessels, and bones
(2) Etiology—great force applied to specific body area
(3) Diagnostic indicators

(a) Crushed area swollen and tense with skin vesicles
(b) Elevated hemoglobin and hematocrit from plasma leakage into interstitial tissue
(c) Hyperkalemia due to potassium leakage from injured cells; may cause lethal cardiac arrhythmia
(d) Oliguria and renal failure from decreased intravascular volume, diminished renal perfusion, and release of myoglobin and toxins from damaged muscle

(4) Compartment syndrome possible (see Module 24—Musculoskeletal Injury)
(5) Staphylococci and Gram-negative infection common; septicemia is major cause of death

5. Specific injuries (3)

a. Subclavian artery
(1) Caused by penetrating trauma, iatrogenic injury, or fracture of the first rib or clavicle
(2) One arm characteristically cool, pale, and pulseless
(3) May cause intrapleural hematoma or widening of the mediastinum
(4) Intubate early to prevent airway obstruction from expanding hematoma
(5) Operative treatment necessary via trapdoor incision or supraclavicular incision
(6) Complications of injury include phrenic nerve injury, recurrent laryngeal nerve injury, thoracic duct, vagus nerve, and brachial plexus injuries

b. Axillary arteries
(1) Usually due to penetrating trauma but can be caused by dislocation of shoulder or fracture
(2) Diagnostic indicators—bleeding, hematoma, pulse deficits, brachial plexus injury, or arteriovenous (AV) fistula
(3) Expose through supraclavicular or infraclavicular incision

c. Brachial artery
(1) From penetrating trauma, bone fracture, elbow dislocation, or iatrogenic injury
(2) Common; occurs in 20% of all peripheral vascular injuries (often iatrogenic) and 50% of all upper extremity vascular injuries
(3) Extensive injury requires saphenous vein graft

d. Iliac artery injuries do not tamponade easily; 40% mortality

e. Femoral artery
(1) Most commonly injured vessel in lower extremity
(2) 40% associated with venous injury; 20% associated with femoral or sciatic nerve injury
(3) May be caused by midshaft femur fractures
(4) Diagnostic indicators—large hematoma and thigh swelling
(5) 2 to 5% mortality; complication rate 20%, usually from thrombosis of vascular or operative repair or DVT
(6) Requires wide mobilization and end-to-end anastomosis
(7) Synthetic grafts found to be superior to saphenous vein grafts
(8) Restore profunda femoral, as soon as possible, since it will become primary source of blood supply; highly susceptible to atherosclerosis

f. Popliteal arteries

- (1) Posterior knee dislocations or proximal tibia fractures can injure popliteal artery
- (2) 30 to 40% amputation rate even after repair due to
  - (a) Failure of repair and gangrene of extremity
  - (b) Invasive infection
  - (c) Massive continuous edema and myonecrosis that continues despite adequate arterial repair
  - (d) Severe pain in a functionless limb, or chronic osteomyelitis with progressive loss and nonunion (late cause) (4)
- (3) Particularly susceptible to distal ischemia
- (4) Repair popliteal vein in all cases of popliteal artery injury to prevent obstructed venous outflow with very high risk of thrombus

g. Tibial arteries
- (1) Distal tibia/fibula fractures or ankle dislocations can lacerate posterior or anterior tibial artery
- (2) Identifying arterial injury is difficult, unless two of the three arteries are injured

h. Venous injuries
- (1) Repair at least these injuries (5)
  - (a) Popliteal injuries to prevent loss of leg after arterial repair
  - (b) Massive soft tissue injury
  - (c) Large veins to prevent chronic venous insufficiency
- (2) Repair to protect arterial repair and prevent late phlebitis, if time permits
  - (a) Repairs often occlude in one to two weeks, but this allows growth of collateral circulation
  - (b) Patency, even for 24 to 72 hrs, may allow establishment of collateral venous return
  - (c) Recannulation within four to six weeks is possible, even if early thrombosis of vein graft occurs
- (3) Difficult to repair because muscle layer is thin, and clamp can easily tear vessel; prosthetic grafts work poorly
- (4) Acute venous insufficiency after arterial repair occurs in first 12 to 24 hrs
  - (a) Extremity appears cool, bluish, and has massive edema
  - (b) Elevation and elastic compression wraps to extremity are indicated

6. Complications

a. Spasm
- (1) Sustained contraction of smooth muscle in vessel; lumen partially occluded without apparent damage
- (2) Mechanical myogenic response not mediated by neural stimuli; generally of short duration
- (3) Causes severe pain
- (4) Treat with simple mechanical or hydraulic dilation
- (5) Topical magnesium sulfate, local anesthetics, and/or papaverine may relieve spasm (2)

b. Failure of early repair
- (1) Manifested by poor color and decreased or absent pulses about two hours after repair
- (2) Diagnose via angiogram

(3) Venous repair decreases incidence

c. Thrombosis of repair
   (1) In arterial injuries, thrombosis occurs in early postoperative period
      (a) Characterized by loss of distal arterial pulsations, sudden coolness of distal extremity, and severe pain distal to repair
      (b) Requires immediate return to the operating room (OR) to remove clot and instill regional heparin
      (c) Vascular repair may need to be constructed
   (2) Venous repairs occlude gradually over first one to two weeks after injury; collateral circulation will develop
d. Infection in soft tissue
   (1) May expose vascular repair or disrupt graft/repair
   (2) Cleanse and debride; cover repair with porcine xenograft and pack wound with fine mesh gauze (FMG)
   (3) If infection resolves, close wound with split-thickness skin graft (STSG) or myocutaneous flap
   (4) If vascular repair fails, resect vessel and use extraanatomic bypass graft
e. Loss of extremity due to prolonged ischemia; maximum time before irreversible muscle damage occurs is estimated to be four to six hours
f. Rebleeding
   (1) Early—usually due to technical problem, diathesis from shock, or depleted clotting factors
   (2) Late—usually signifies infection
   (3) Manifested by secondary hemorrhage—bright red blood from wound; may be trivial but **always** heralds catastrophic hemorrhage
   (4) Return patient to OR immediately
   (5) Usually related to sepsis
   (6) If bleeding occurs with prosthetic graft, ligate and resect; reexplore four to eight weeks later and insert vein graft
g. Acute complications—edema, emboli, disseminated intravascular coagulation (DIC)
h. Delayed complications—pain; decreased functioning; contractures (Volkmann's) due to delay in fasciotomy or prolonged ischemia
i. Missed injuries, e.g., with multiple arterial injuries; distal arterial injury may be overlooked
j. Stenosis from technical problems or intimal hyperplasia at suture line weeks or months later; may lead to occlusion
k. Arteriovenous fistulae
   (1) Communication between lacerated artery and vein which permits arterial flow into hematoma
   (2) Etiology—arterial blood forms hematoma between vessels; hematoma contracts over time and is reabsorbed, permitting direct arteriovenous blood flow
   (3) Usually found three to five weeks after injury but sometimes identified immediately
   (4) Diagnostic indicators depend on location and size of fistula
      (a) Continuous bruit over fistula
      (b) Local temperature elevation with dilated and possibly pulsatile veins

(c) Occlusion of fistula results in slowed heart rate due to reduced flow to atrium (Nicaladoni-Branham sign) (6)
(d) Extremity ischemic if large shunt occurs
(5) Complications—heart failure, intraarterial infections, and distal gangrene (6)
(6) Present in 10% of patients with lower extremity vascular injury (1)
(7) Spontaneous closure is possible but rare

l. Pseudoaneurysm
(1) Partially lacerated artery temporarily sealed by clot
(a) Lining communicates with lumen of artery
(b) Clot liquifies and hematoma begins to pulsate and enlarge
(c) Hematoma continues to increase causing compression and eventual destruction of peripheral nerves
(d) Resulting hematoma does not completely occlude lumen but forms cavity in continuity with arterial lumen
(e) Appears to be an aneurysm but does not have all layers of arterial wall
(2) Diagnostic indicators—intense pain; progressively increases in size until rupture
(3) Manifested as a late complication, three to five weeks after injury, because missed initially
(4) Classic error to confuse hematoma of false aneurysm with an abscess

B. MEDICAL AND SURGICAL INTERVENTIONS

1. **Maintain airway and breathing**
2. **Control hemorrhage**
   a. Apply direct pressure over injury
   b. Apply pressure dressing directly to area of injury
   c. Use automatic orthopaedic inflatable tourniquet intermittently for vascular control; place pressure cuff proximal to injury and inflate above systolic pressure; closely observe to prevent additional injury
   d. Keep compression dressing and/or blood pressure cuff in place until patient is prepared and draped in the OR
   e. Direct vascular control with clamps should be done by surgeon only
3. **Support circulation**
4. **Splint fractures to prevent additional injuries to neurovascular structures**
5. **Determine nature and extent of injury; angiogram is the gold standard for diagnosis and delineation of anatomy and magnitude of injury**
   a. Urgent repair may be needed without preoperative angiography; angiogram may be done in the OR
   b. Angiogram is of limited benefit in penetrating injury; perform immediate exploration in the OR
6. **If angiogram is negative, continue observation or explore in the OR; observation alone for injuries with soft signs of vascular injury is controversial but is currently used in some centers (7)**
7. **Minimize delay from time of injury to repair; generally repair should be attempted within 6 to 12 hrs to minimize ischemia**

8. **Prepare skin and drape all potential surgical areas proximal and distal to vascular control, before operative intervention**
9. **Prevent infection and further injury**
   a. Administer broad-spectrum antibiotics immediately; continue for three to five days
   b. Irrigate wound with saline or antibiotic solutions; debride devitalized tissue and foreign material
10. **Operative repair of vessels**
   a. Incise to provide easy access proximally and distally
   b. If hemorrhage is present, gain proximal and distal control through the application of small angio-access clamps, bulldog clamps, umbilical tapes, or rubber tapes
   c. Techniques for repair
      (1) Ligation may be used in veins and small arteries, noncritical main arteries below the elbow or knee, and distal profunda femoral artery
         (a) Exception—superficial femoral vein in distal thigh or popliteal vein injuries
         (b) Ligation is usually well tolerated, but may seriously impair arterial inflow and result in secondary ischemia and subsequent amputation
      (2) Lateral arteriorrhaphy or venorrhaphy is used for small lacerations or punctures, pellet or missile wounds
      (3) Patch angioplasty for wall defects is used infrequently
      (4) Segmental resection and end-to-end anastomosis used for through-and-through injury or extensive wall disruption
      (5) Interposition graft used when end-to-end anastomosis not possible; saphenous vein graft is conduit of choice
      (6) If both nonvascular and vascular injuries, sequence of repair is determined by surgeon
         (a) Arteries are usually repaired prior to stabilization of adjacent fractures
         (b) Exceptions are made when fracture is segmented, or extremity cannot be moved to expose vascular injury
      (7) Care of soft tissue wound is easier, and risk of suture line "blowouts" is decreased by tunneling bypass through uninjured tissue
      (8) Coagulopathy after a vascular repair, massive edema, or extensive contamination of soft tissue over vascular repair may preclude immediate wound closure
         (a) Cover vascular repair with porcine xenograft under antibiotic-soaked gauze
         (b) Return patient to OR in one to three days for delayed primary closure
   d. Postoperative evaluation and care
      (1) Palpation of normal distal pulses in an arterial repair of the upper extremity is acceptable evidence of adequate repair
      (2) When an end-to-end anastomosis or interposition graft is done in lower extremity, completion angiography is necessary to rule out embolus, thrombosis, or technical problems
      (3) If major vein is ligated in either lower extremity, apply elastic wraps and elevate extremity above the level of the heart for first postoperative week

11. **Indications for fasciotomy** (8)
   a. Early postoperative edema, compartment pain, and tension
   b. Combined arterial and venous injuries
   c. Massive soft tissue damage
   d. Delay between wounding and definitive repair
   e. Prolonged hypotension
   f. Swelling of extremity
   g. Venous ligation in the popliteal and femoral area
   h. Tissue pressure of more than 35 to 45 mm Hg

C. NURSING ASSESSMENT

1. **Interview**
a. Mechanism of injury and accident scenario
b. Length of wound exposure and type of contamination
c. Blood loss—estimate amount, color, and nature of bleeding (pulsating or nonpulsating)
d. Neurovascular symptoms (see Module 24—Musculoskeletal Injury)
e. Past medical history, e.g., cardiovascular disease, prior vascular surgery, medications (anticoagulants)
2. **Physical examination**
a. Compare one extremity to the other for all parameters
b. Inspection
   (1) Both arms (fingertips to shoulders) and both legs (groin and buttocks to the feet)
      (a) Size and symmetry of extremity
      (b) Color of skin and nailbeds; texture of skin
      (c) Venous pattern
   (2) Hemorrhage or bleeding—estimate blood loss
      (a) Steady flow of dark blood indicates venous injury
      (b) Arterial bleeding
         i) Bright red blood spurting from wound; may cease after period of time
         ii) May lead to exsanguinating hemorrhage or acute pulsatile hematoma
      (c) Skin discoloration—pallor or cyanosis
   (4) Edema
   (5) Skin wounds, e.g., lacerations, contusions, bruises, or penetrating wounds
c. Palpation for signs of interruption of arterial inflow
   (1) Peripheral pulses
      (a) Assess pulse volume
         i) Describe pulses as normal, diminished, or absent
         ii) Numerical classification
            a) 0 = completely absent
            b) 1 = markedly impaired
            c) 2 = moderately impaired
            d) 3 = slightly impaired
            e) 4 = normal

(b) Location of pulses in upper extremities
  i) Radial—flexor surface of the lateral wrist
  ii) Ulnar—flexor surface of the lateral wrist
  iii) Brachial—groove between biceps and triceps muscle above the elbow
  iv) Allen test—test patency of ulnar and radial arteries
    a) Rest patient's hands on his/her lap
    b) Place thumbs over radial artery; have patient clench fists
    c) Compress radial arteries and have patient open hands
    d) Observe color of palms
    e) Repeat, but occlude the ulnar artery
(c) Location of pulses in lower extremities
  i) Femoral—press deeply, below inguinal ligament and midway between anterior superior iliac spine and symphysis pubis
  ii) Popliteal—flex knee; press fingertips of both hands deeply into popliteal fossa, slightly lateral to midline
  iii) Dorsalis pedis—dorsum of foot just lateral to extensor tendon of great toe
  iv) Posterior tibial—place curved fingers behind and below medial malleolus
(d) Clinical appearance is unreliable sign of injury
  i) Peripheral pulses are present in 20 to 25% of arterial injuries (9)
  ii) Patient may be totally asymptomatic with no pulses
    a) Lack of pulses may be due to shock, intense vasospasm, preexisting arterial disease, congenital absence, or arterial injury
    b) Vessel injury may not produce ischemia

(2) Capillary refill
(3) Skin temperature
(4) Determine location and size of surrounding hematoma
  (a) Large, firm, pulsatile hematoma with ill-defined margins surrounding the wound indicates possible arterial injury
  (b) Tense, nonpulsatile hematoma is possible with venous injury
  (c) Swelling or hematoma that increases in size may indicate venous damage in the area
(5) Sensation
  (a) Early sign of peripheral vascular injury is diminished or absent light touch sensation, which is conducted by small nerve fibers very sensitive to ischemia
  (b) Large neural fibers are less affected by ischemia; pain, pressure, and temperature sensations are intact initially
  (c) Peroneal nerve is first to suffer ischemia in lower extremity
    i) Check sensation in the space between the great and second toe
    ii) Check for pain on passive motion of ankle and particularly the great toe

d. Auscultation
  (1) Blood pressure—hypotension associated with a wound near major vessel should raise suspicion of vascular injury
  (2) Use stethoscope or Doppler to listen for presence and quality of pulses, bruits, and/or thrills

(3) Check forearm or pedal pressure bilaterally, and compare to determine the need for angiogram and establish priority of repair
(4) Calculate brachial-ankle pressure difference on each side and document; ankle pressure should be greater than brachial systolic pressure (2)

3. Laboratory studies—trauma profile

4. Radiologic studies

a. Arteriography in resuscitation area, radiologic suite, or OR
(1) Should be done early
(2) Findings indicating vascular injury (1)
(a) Extravasation of dye
(b) Acute pulsatile hematoma
(c) Obstruction or narrowing of vessel
(d) Irregularity of wall of vessel
(e) Early venous filling
b. Digital subtraction angiography
c. Venography is used, rarely, to identify venous thrombosis or pseudoaneurysm
d. Ultrasound or CAT scan

D. NURSING DIAGNOSES, EXPECTED OUTCOMES, AND INTERVENTIONS

1. Fluid volume deficit related to massive hemorrhage

a. Expected outcomes
(1) Vital signs within normal limits
(2) Hemoglobin and hematocrit within normal limits
(3) Skin warm, dry, natural color; good turgor
(4) Urine output greater than 0.5–1.0 ml/kg/hr
(5) Normal serum electrolytes
b. Nursing interventions
(1) Apply direct pressure to site of bleeding
(2) Utilize PASG as temporary vessel tamponade
(3) Administer fluids and blood (see Module 10—Shock—for additional interventions)
(4) Monitor vital signs and urine output
(5) Quickly prepare patient for immediate surgery

2. Alteration of tissue perfusion related to vascular injury, thrombus formation, and/or edema

a. Expected outcomes
(1) Skin warm; capillary refill within normal limits
(2) Peripheral pulses palpable and audible
(3) No decrease in neurosensory status
(4) Edema absent
b. Nursing interventions
(1) Elevate involved extremities; position extremities to optimize blood flow and avoid kinking vessels or grafts

(2) Monitor peripheral pulses for presence and volume; use Doppler to detect blood flow velocity
(3) Monitor edema
(4) Continue to inspect extremity for signs of vascular insufficiency, injury and/or undiagnosed injury, cyanosis, mottling, capillary refill
(5) Auscultate for bruits
(6) Note cross-clamp time of vascular repair to identify potential renal failure due to prolonged ischemia
(7) Administer low molecular weight dextran, if prescribed; lowers viscosity and decreases platelet aggregation
(8) Administer mannitol, if prescribed, to reduce cellular swelling and prevent compartment syndrome, especially if myoglobinuria is present
(9) Monitor for signs and symptoms of compartment syndrome (see Module 16—Medical Sequelae)
(10) Treat diagnosed spasm by local heat; assist with nerve blocks
(11) Monitor hematocrit (Hct), hemoglobin (Hgb), and coagulation studies for signs of hemorrhage, or hemodynamic instability secondary to coagulopathy
(12) Teach patient to exercise extremity; if patient is unable, provide passive ROM
(13) Assess for signs of venous thrombus or arterial obstruction (see Module 16—Medical Sequelae)

3. Potential for infection related to wound contamination and vascular repair

a. Expected outcomes
(1) No purulent drainage, pain, or redness at operative site
(2) Vascular repair intact (infection can disrupt anastomosis)
(3) Normal body temperature and WBC
(4) Negative wound cultures

b. Nursing interventions
(1) Assess and maintain integrity of surgical repair
(2) If graft is exposed, apply wet saline gauze dressing, immobilize extremity to decrease tension on repair site, and elevate to increase venous drainage
(3) Observe wound site for signs of local infection; obtain culture of wound drainage
(4) Measure body temperature; report any elevation
(5) Administer antibiotics and tetanus prophylaxis, as prescribed
(6) Monitor WBC: report any elevations

4. Potential for alteration in skin integrity related to inadequate arterial inflow, or edema secondary to poor venous outflow

a. Expected outcomes
(1) Skin warm; capillary refill within normal limits
(2) Peripheral pulses present
(3) Skin intact

b. Nursing interventions
(1) Protect vulnerable areas
(2) Change patient position frequently
(3) Pad areas of skin-to-skin contact and prevent pressure on skin
(4) Elevate edematous extremity; apply elastic compression wraps
(5) Avoid skin injury by gentle handling (see Module 16—Medical Sequelae, Pressure sores)

5. Additional nursing diagnoses

a. Knowledge deficit related to prevention and/or identification of late complications of vascular repair, e.g., deep vein thrombosis, arteriovenous fistula, pseudoaneurysm

b. Potential alteration of renal perfusion related to hypovolemia and myoglobinuria (see Module 16—Medical Sequelae)

c. Potential decreased cardiac output related to hemorrhage

d. Pain related to ischemia

References

1. Feliciano, D. V. (1989). Peripheral vascular injuries. In E. E. Moore (Ed.), *Early care of the injured patient* (4th ed., pp. 235–240). Philadelphia: B. C. Decker.
2. Schneider, C. (1986). Peripheral vascular trauma. In B. A. Knezevich (Ed.), *Trauma nursing: Principles and practice* (pp. 177–190). Norwalk, CT: Appleton-Century-Crofts.
3. Van Way, C. W., III, & Rutherford, R. B. (1985). Peripheral vascular injuries. In G. D. Zuidema, R. B. Rutherford & W. F. Ballinger (Eds.), *The management of trauma* (4th ed., pp. 631–657). Philadelphia: W. B. Saunders Co.
4. Wiener, S., & Barrett, J. (1986). *Trauma management for civilian and military physicians.* Philadelphia: W. B. Saunders Co.
5. Rich, N. M. (1988). Peripheral vascular injury. In K. Mattox, E. Moore & D. Feliciano (Eds.), *Trauma* (pp. 603–615). Norwalk, CT: Appleton & Lange.
6. Strange, J. M., & Kelly, P. M. (1988). In V. D. Cardona, P. D. Hurn, P. J. Mason, A. M. Scanlon-Schilpp & S. W. Veise-Berry (Eds.), *Trauma nursing: From resuscitation through rehabilitation* (p. 519). Philadelphia: W. B. Saunders Co.
7. Dennis, J. W., Frykberg, E. R., Crump, J. M., Vines, F. S., & Alexander, R. H. (1990). New perspectives on the management of penetrating trauma in proximity to major limb arteries. *Journal of Vascular Surgery, 11*(1), 84–93.
8. Markison, R. E. (1986). Trauma to the extremities. In D. D. Trunkey & F. R. Lewis (Eds.), *Current therapy of trauma* 2. Philadelphia: B. C. Decker.
9. Ernst, C. B. (1976). Vascular injuries. In C. Frey (Ed.), *Initial management of the trauma patient* (pp. 255–273). Philadelphia: Lea and Febiger.

Suggested Readings

Bates, B. (1987). *A guide to physical examination and history taking* (4th ed.). Philadelphia: J. B. Lippincott Co.

Bremer, C. (1982). Promoting healing of trauma wounds. *AORN Journal, 35*(6), 1150–1170.

Campbell, C. (1987). *Nursing diagnosis and intervention in nursing practice.* New York: John Wiley & Sons.

Cass, A. S., & Luxenberg, M. (1987). Management of renal artery injuries from external trauma. *The Journal of Urology, 138*(2), 266–268.

Feliciano, D. V., Mattox, K., Graham, J., & Bitondo, C. (1985). Five year experience with PTFE grafts in vascular wounds. *The Journal of Trauma, 25*(1), 71–82.

Gomez, G. A., Kreis, D. J., Rathner, L., Hernandez, A., Russell, E., Dove, D. B., & Civetta, J. M. (1986). Suspected vascular trauma of the extremities: The role of arteriography in proximity injuries. *The Journal of Trauma, 26*(11), 1005–1008.

Meyer, J., Walsh, J., Schuler, J., Barrett, J., Durham, J., Eldrup-Jorgensen, J., Schwartz, T., & Flanigan, D. P. (1987). The early fate of venous repair after civilian vascular trauma: A clinical, hemodynamic, and venographic assessment. *Annuals of Surgery, 206*(4), 458–464.

O'Gorman, R. B., Feliciano, D. V., Bitondo, C. G., Mattox, K. L., Burch, J. M., & Jordan, G. L. (1984). Emergency center arteriography in the evaluation of suspected peripheral vascular injuries. *Archives of Surgery, 119*(5), 568–572.

Ransom, K. J., Shatney, C. H., Soderstrom, C. A., & Cowley, R. A. (1981). Management of arterial injuries in blunt trauma of the extremity. *Surgery, Gynecology & Obstetrics, 153*(2), 241–246.

Rich, N. M., & Spencer, F. C. (1978). *Vascular trauma.* Philadelphia: W. B. Saunders Co.

Richardson, J. D., Vitale, G. C., & Flint, L. M., Jr. (1987). Penetrating arterial trauma: Analysis of missed vascular injuries. *Archives of Surgery, 122*(6), 678–683.

Roberts, R. M., & String, S. T. (1984). Arterial injuries in extremity shotgun wounds: Requisite factors for successful management. *Surgery, 96*(5), 902–907.

Rose, S. C., & Moore, E. E. (1987). Emergency trauma angiography: Accuracy, safety, and pitfalls. *American Journal of Radiology, 148*(6), 1243–1246.

Ross, S. E., Ransom, K. J., & Shatney, H. S. (1985). The management of venous injuries in blunt extremity trauma. *The Journal of Trauma, 25*(2), 150–153.

White, R. A., Scher, L. A., Samson, R. H., & Veith, F. J. (1987). Peripheral vascular injuries associated with falls from heights. *The Journal of Trauma, 27*(4), 411–414.

Section V
Special Patient Populations

MODULE 28
PEDIATRIC

Judith J. Stellar, MS, RN, CPNP

Prerequisite

Review normal childhood growth and development, including cognitive and psychosocial aspects.

Objectives

1.0 Describe common injuries in the pediatric population.

1.1 Describe major developmental characteristics of each age group which predispose pediatric populations to injury.

1.2 Describe unique anatomy or causative factors that predispose pediatric populations to certain injury patterns.

1.3 Describe pathophysiology of specific injuries unique to the pediatric population.

1.4 State frequent mechanisms of injury for each age group.

2.0 Describe initial assessment of the pediatric trauma patient.

2.1 Identify aspects of the history and physical examination that apply to all pediatric age groups.

2.2 Identify aspects of the history and physical examination specific to particular age groups.

2.3 Describe aspects of the respiratory and circulatory assessment that are unique to the pediatric patient.

2.4 List essential laboratory data for infant assessment.
2.5 List aspects of the psychologic assessment important in the care of each age group.
2.6 List aspects of family assessment necessary in caring for the pediatric patient.
3.0 Anticipate and assist with medical and surgical interventions.
3.1 Given a specific patient scenario, recognize which interventions may be required.
3.2 Identify the correct type and size of equipment required by pediatric patients of specific ages.
4.0 Identify nursing interventions required for the pediatric trauma patient.
4.1 List nursing interventions common to all pediatric age groups.
4.2 List nursing interventions specific to each pediatric age group.
4.3 List nursing interventions that address psychologic considerations and responses in the pediatric trauma patient.
4.4 List nursing interventions utilized in caring for the family of the pediatric trauma patient.
5.0 Evaluate patient response to medical and nursing interventions.
5.1 List desired patient outcomes with measurable criteria for each.
5.2 State rationale for frequent serial assessments and monitoring of the pediatric trauma patient.

A. GENERAL CONCEPTS AND PRINCIPLES

1. Physiological considerations
a. 80 to 90% of childhood trauma is blunt trauma; in most cases, there are no external signs of injury
b. Pediatric trauma victims are usually healthy; most do not present with chronic cardiovascular, pulmonary, or renal diseases
c. Children are smaller organisms than adults, so their clinical status may deteriorate rapidly; children require quick and accurate assessment of injuries, timely treatment, and precise calculation of fluid and drug requirements
d. Children have higher metabolic rates than adults, which results in greater oxygen and caloric requirements
e. Children have a highly reactive vascular system that maintains systolic blood pressure in spite of blood loss; this sympathetic response to injury masks early signs of hypovolemic shock
f. Young children have immature thermoregulating systems thus complicating resuscitation efforts
g. The skeleton of a child is immature and pliable and does not adequately protect internal structures
h. The child is a growing organism; untreated injury may result in progressive or permanent deformity and disability

2. Psychological considerations
a. Pediatric trauma encompasses a variety of age groups and developmental levels
b. Unlike adults, children have not been exposed to life experiences that afford the

development of coping strategies; therefore, they have fewer coping resources in traumatic situations

c. Each age group exhibits unique cognitive abilities, which are used to interpret a stressful event
d. Each age group exhibits unique psychological responses and reactions to stress
e. Each age group possesses unique communication abilities; these must be recognized and interpreted within a developmental framework, in order to effectively interact with and support the child during a traumatic event
f. Every child is an integral part of a family unit, and the family is an essential part of the child's life; in order to holistically treat the child, the family must also be assessed and treated throughout the traumatic event

B. AGE-SPECIFIC PATTERNS OF INJURY

NOTE: In children, injury patterns are often related to specific anatomic and developmental characteristics of the child

1. Infants (birth to 1 year)

a. Developmental characteristics
   (1) Oral motor
      (a) Sucking—reflexive at birth
      (b) Directed hand-to-mouth—5 to 8 months
   (2) Gross motor
      (a) Wriggling—early infancy
      (b) Rolling—by 4 months
      (c) Sits without support—5 to 7½ months
      (d) Crawls—6 to 7 months
      (e) Walks holding on—8 to 12 months
      (f) Walks well alone—11 to 14 months
   (3) Fine motor
      (a) Grasp—reflexive at birth
      (b) Visually directed reaching—3 to 5 months
      (c) Looks for hidden object (object permanence)—8 to 9 months
      (d) Neat pincer grasp of small object—10 to 14 months
b. Mechanisms of injury
   (1) Injuries compromising the airway
      (a) Choking
      (b) Strangulation
      (c) Suffocation
      (d) Foreign body ingestion
   (2) Motor vehicle-related injuries
      (a) Chiefly motor vehicle occupant (MVO) in this age group
      (b) May result from misuse or nonuse of car seats
   (3) Falls
   (4) Burns—scald and flame
   (5) Drownings

(6) Ingestions—usually after 5 months of age
(7) Child abuse—"shaken baby syndrome"
c. Injury patterns
(1) Head, neck
(a) Causative factors
i) Large head in proportion to body
ii) Weak neck muscles; poor head control
iii) Pliable body structures and vessels of head decrease frequency of mass lesions but predispose infants to diffuse head injury
iv) Children exhibit increased vascular response of the brain in the immediate posttrauma phase; this "malignant hyperemia" may mimic a mass lesion
(b) Injuries
i) Skull fractures (abuse, falls)
ii) Subdural hematomas (abuse)
iii) Retinal hemorrhages (abuse, traumatic asphyxia)
iv) Diffuse cerebral swelling (MVO, abuse, falls)
v) High cervical fracture (MVO)
(2) Chest, respiratory
(a) Causative factors
i) Unique anatomy of infant
a) Large tongue in relation to oral cavity
b) Narrow airways
c) Obligate nose breather
d) Short trachea
e) Compliant chest wall; pliable rib cage
f) Mobile mediastinal structures
g) Absence of valves in superior and inferior venae cavae
ii) Mechanisms chiefly center around obstructive and crushing forces
(b) Injuries
i) Respiratory arrest (airway compromise, foreign body ingestion, obstruction)
ii) Traumatic asphyxia (MVO, motor vehicle pedestrian (MVP), crush)
iii) Pulmonary contusions (MVO, falls)
iv) Pneumothorax (MVO, falls, abuse, iatrogenic)
v) Cardiac contusions (MVO, falls)
(3) Abdomen
(a) Causative factors
i) Pelvic girdle is pliable and does not protect internal organs
ii) A portion of the bowel remains fixed to spine
iii) Mechanisms center around crush, direct blow, or pinning of organs between two fixed objects
(b) Injuries
i) Solid organ—liver, spleen, kidney
a) May include laceration, fracture, hematoma, or rupture
b) Caused by high-energy impact, e.g., falls, MVO, abuse
ii) Hollow organ—esophagus, stomach (rare), small and large intestines (duodenum most common)

a) May include hematoma and/or perforation
b) Results from pinning a hollow organ between an object and a bony structure; MVO and abuse cases

(4) Extremities
(a) Causative factors
i) Infants' bones are very pliable, can withstand angulation, and heal quickly
ii) Injuries result from very high-impact, high-energy mechanisms such as falls greater than 15 feet, high speed MVO, and, most commonly, abuse
(b) Injuries
i) Long bone fractures are rare; abuse should be suspected for femur, humerus, radius, ulna, tibia, fibula shaft fractures
ii) Growth plate fractures (Salter-Harris)
a) Type I—epiphysis disrupted or displaced; no fracture in epiphyseal plate
b) Type II—epiphysis displaced and metaphysis fractured
c) Type III—epiphysis displaced and fractured
d) Rare in infants; abuse should be suspected
iii) Dislocations and tendon injuries are rare

2. Toddlers (1 to 3 years) and preschoolers (3 to 6 years)

a. Developmental characteristics of toddlers
(1) Gross motor
(a) Walks well alone—14 months
(b) Stops and recovers—14 months
(c) Walks up steps—20 months
(d) Jumps in place—30 months
(e) Pedals tricycle—34 months
(2) Fine motor
(a) Neat pincer grasp—14 months
(b) Scribbles with pen—15 months
(c) Builds tower of two cubes—18 months
(d) Uses utensils—24 months
(e) Turns doorknobs—28 months
(f) Copies a circle—34 months

b. Developmental characteristics of preschoolers
(1) Gross motor
(a) Masters broad jump—3 years, 3 months
(b) Hops on one foot—4 years
(c) Dresses and undresses—3 years
(d) Throws and catches a ball—5 years
(e) Pedals bicycle with training wheels—5 to 6 years
(2) Fine motor
(a) Builds bridge with blocks—3 years
(b) Buttons clothing—3½ years
(c) Draws man with at least three parts—4 years
(d) Prints letters—5 years
(e) Prints first name—6 years

c. Mechanisms of injury (toddlers and preschoolers)
  (1) Motor vehicle-related
    (a) Occupant
    (b) Pedestrian (MVP)—greater incidence in preschool years
    (c) Bicycle—preschoolers
  (2) Falls
  (3) Burns—scald and flame (toddlers); flame (preschoolers)
  (4) Drownings
  (5) Ingestions—toddlers
  (6) Minor trauma—superficial lacerations, bruises
  (7) Child abuse—both groups but peaks in toddlers
  (8) Firearms—preschoolers
d. Injury patterns (toddlers and preschoolers)
  (1) Head, neck
    (a) Causative factors
      i) Better head control than infant helps prevent high cervical fractures
      ii) Pliable bony structures predispose toddlers and preschoolers to diffuse cerebral injuries
    (b) Injuries
      i) Diffuse cerebral swelling (MVO, MVP, falls)
      ii) Malignant hyperemia (MVO, MVP, falls)
      iii) Subdural hematoma (abuse, falls)
      iv) Skull fractures (abuse, falls, MVP)
      v) High cervical fractures (rare)
  (2) Chest, respiratory
    (a) Causative factors
      i) Short trachea with "natural" cuff
      ii) Compliant chest wall and pliable rib cage
      iii) Major vessels lack valves and predispose toddlers and preschoolers to traumatic asphyxia
      iv) Mobile mediastinal structures
    (b) Injuries
      i) Pulmonary contusions (MVO, MVP, falls)
      ii) Pneumothorax (MVO, MVP, falls, abuse, iatrogenic)
      iii) Cardiac contusions (MVO, MVP, falls)
      iv) Traumatic asphyxia (MVO, MVP)
  (3) Abdomen
    (a) Causative factors
      i) Pelvic girdle is pliable and does not protect internal organs
      ii) A portion of the bowel remains fixed to spine
    (b) Injuries
      i) Solid organ—liver, spleen, kidney, pancreas
        a) Laceration, fracture, hematoma, contusion, rupture
        b) Mechanisms—falls, abuse, MVO, MVP
      ii) Hollow organ—duodenum (common), small and large intestine, esophagus, and stomach (rare)
  (4) Extremities
    (a) Causative factors

i) Bones less pliable than infant but can still tolerate a degree of angulation
ii) Growth plate remains weakest part of bone
(b) Injuries
i) Subluxation of radial head (abuse)
ii) Growth plate fractures—Salter-Harris (MVP, bike, falls, abuse)
a) Types I through III—(see 1.c(4)(b)ii), above)
b) Type IV—fracture through epiphysis, epiphyseal plate, and metaphysis
c) Type V—epiphyseal plate impacted and crushed
iii) Long bone shaft fracture of tibia, fibula, radius, ulna (MVP, bike, falls, abuse)
iv) Distal radial fractures (falls)

3. School age (7 to 12 years)

a. Developmental characteristics
(1) Masters bicycling
(2) Involved in group and competitive sports
(3) Swims well
(4) Increasingly involved in independent activities outside home
(5) Begins risk-taking behavior
(6) Peer group and peer pressure begin to play major roles

b. Mechanisms of injury
(1) MVP or MVO
(2) Bicycle-related injuries
(3) Burns—flame
(4) Drownings
(5) Falls
(6) Penetrating trauma—firearms, GSW, stabbings
(7) Minor trauma—superficial lacerations, contusions
(8) Suicide—ingestions, gunshot wounds

c. Injury patterns
(1) Head, neck (MVP, bike, MVO, falls, sports)
(a) Diffuse cerebral swelling
(b) Malignant hyperemia
(c) Skull fractures
(d) Subdural hematomas
(e) Epidural hematomas
(f) High cervical fractures—rare
(2) Chest, respiratory
(a) Pulmonary contusions (MVO, MVP, bike, falls)
(b) Pneumothorax (MVO, MVP, bike, falls)
(c) Cardiac contusions (MVO)
(d) Rib fractures begin to occur as bones become less pliant (MVP, MVO, bike, falls)
(3) Abdomen (MVP, bike, falls, MVO, sports)
(a) Solid organs—more common than hollow organ injuries
i) Liver—fracture, laceration
ii) Spleen—hematoma, laceration, rupture

iii) Kidneys—hematoma, contusions
iv) Pancreas—contusions, pseudocyst
(b) Hollow organs
i) Small and large intestines
ii) Esophagus and stomach—rare
(4) Extremities
(a) Supracondylar fractures (falls)
(b) Femur, tibia, or fibula shaft fractures (MVP, bike, falls)
(c) Growth plate fractures span Salter-Harris Types I through V (MVP, bike, falls)

4. Adolescents (13 to 17 years)

a. Developmental characteristics
(1) Major physical changes and rapid growth
(2) Increased independence
(3) Peer group plays major role
(4) Risk-taking behaviors peak
(5) Increasing involvement in sports
(6) Increasing involvement in gangs
(7) Experimental behavior (drugs, alcohol, sex, crime)
(8) Begins to operate motor vehicles

b. Mechanisms of injury
(1) MVO
(2) Burns, explosions
(3) Falls
(4) Firearms, stabbings
(5) Assaults
(6) Homicide
(7) Suicide—ingestions, hangings, gunshot wounds
(8) Drowning
(9) Sports-related injuries

c. Injury patterns
(1) Head, neck
(a) Cerebral swelling (MVO, falls)
(b) Epidural hematomas (MVO, falls, assault)
(c) Subdural hematomas (MVO, falls, assault)
(d) High cervical fractures (falls, sports)
(e) Skull fractures (MVO, falls, assault)
(f) Penetrating trauma (firearms, stabbing, assault)
(2) Chest (MVO, falls, sports, assault)
(a) Pulmonary contusion
(b) Hemo/pneumothorax
(c) Great vessel trauma
(d) Rib fracture, flail chest
(e) Penetrating trauma
(3) Abdomen (MVO, falls, sports, assaults)
(a) Liver—fracture, laceration)
(b) Spleen—hematoma, rupture
(c) Perforation of hollow viscus

(d) Kidney—hematuria, contusion
(4) Extremities (MVO, falls, sports, assaults)
(a) Knee injuries
(b) Long bone fractures
(c) Growth plate injuries possible during growth spurt
(d) Tendon injuries and dislocations
(5) External (explosives, assaults, housefires)
(a) Burns—flame, explosive, chemical, electrical
(b) Blast injuries
(c) Deep lacerations

C. MEDICAL AND SURGICAL PRIORITIES AND INTERVENTIONS FOR PEDIATRIC TRAUMA PATIENTS

NOTE: This section specifically addresses those aspects of care which differ from adult care; the reader should refer to the appropriate modules elsewhere in the book for additional information on specific injuries or responses to injuries

1. **Airway and breathing**
a. Administer humidified oxygen; children have higher metabolic rates than adults, so they require higher rates and concentrations of oxygen
b. Intubate airway as needed
(1) Trachea shorter in child than adult; endotracheal tubes should be passed only 2 to 3 cm below vocal cords to avoid bronchial intubation, hypoxia, and perforation; use uncuffed tubes in children younger than 8
(2) Use straight laryngoscope blades to avoid trauma to the larynx and vocal cords; size varies from 0 for newborns to 3 for adolescents
(3) Esophageal obturator airways are contraindicated in pediatric patients
c. Provide manual or mechanical ventilation, as needed
(1) Iatrogenic pneumothorax is the most frequent complication in pediatrics
(2) Use pediatric bags with pop-off valves or pressure manometers to help prevent this
d. Perform needle thoracentesis
(1) In an infant, a scalp vein needle may reduce tension pneumothorax
(2) In an older child, an I.V. catheter is used
(3) Location—fourth intercostal space
e. Perform tube thoracostomy
(1) Use a curved hemostat, not a trochar, to introduce chest tube
(2) Location—fourth intercostal space
(3) Suggested sizes of chest tubes
(a) Infant—12 French (Fr)
(b) Child (less than 30 kg)—12 to 24 Fr
(c) Adolescent (greater than 30 kg)—28 Fr

2. **Circulatory interventions**
a. Obtain intravenous access in recommended order of preference
(1) Percutaneous—arm and leg
(a) Suggested catheter sizes

i) Infant—20 to 24 gauge (g)
ii) Young child—18 to 20 g
iii) Older child—16 to 18 g
(b) Attempt twice in upper and lower extremity, then proceed to cutdown
(2) Saphenous, median, or main cephalic vein cutdown
(3) Proximal saphenous or femoral vein—percutaneous or cutdown
(4) External jugular vein—percutaneous or cutdown
(5) Intraosseous
(a) Insert in one of these sites
i) Proximal tibia—1 to 2 cm below tuberosity
ii) Distal femur
(b) Proceed with caution; avoid growth plate
(c) Indicated for circulatory collapse or cardiac arrest
b. Replace fluid volume
(1) Weigh patient; if not possible, use Broselow tape, team member most experienced in pediatric care estimates weight for calculation of fluids and medications
(2) Estimate total circulating blood volume in children at 80 ml/kg
(3) Recommended algorithm
(a) Give 20 ml/kg of lactated Ringer's solution, I.V. push
(b) Repeat if no clinical improvement
(c) Give 10 ml/kg type-specific or O-negative packed red blood cells, or 20 ml/kg type-specific or O-negative whole blood (1)
(d) Repeat step (c) if no clinical improvement
(e) Apply pneumatic antishock garments
(4) Continue reassessment for possible etiology of shock state
(a) Inadequate ventilation via endotracheal tube
(b) Tension pneumothorax
(c) Pericardial tamponade
(d) Hypothermia
(5) Proceed to operating room for laparotomy and surgical control of source of hypovolemia
(6) Warm all fluids and bloods; maintain normothermia
(7) Anticipate daily fluid maintenance requirements
(a) 0 to 10 kg = 100 ml/kg
(b) 11 to 20 kg = 1000 ml for first 10 kg and 50 ml/kg for each kg over 10 kg
(c) Above 20 kg = 1500 ml for first 20 kg and 20 ml/kg for each kg over 20 kg

3. **Decompress stomach via nasal route; use oral route if basilar skull fracture suspected; gastric distension can impede diaphragmatic excursion and compromise ventilation**
4. **Decompress bladder with indwelling catheter unless urethral trauma is suspected; insert catheter after rectal examination**
5. **Perform pericardiocentesis and/or emergency thoracotomy (rarely done)**
6. **Perform peritoneal lavage (infrequently done); when used, technique is similar to adult, except lavage of 10 ml/kg of warmed normal saline or lactated Ringer's solution is given over 10 min**
7. **Splint extremities, as needed**

8. Obtain blood for laboratory studies

a. Trauma profile (see Module 19—Nursing Assessment)
b. Calcium and glucose for infants
c. Bilirubin (total and direct) for neonates less than 30 days old

9. Obtain radiologic studies in same sequence and priority as in adults

a. Children's bones are translucent, especially at growth plate; portable extremity films are often inadequate and need to be repeated
b. CAT scans used frequently; abdominal CAT scan used in place of peritoneal lavage
c. Contrast material administered with caution; assess for signs of anaphylaxis; oral contrast has high osmolarity and may cause massive fluid shift resulting in dehydration

10. Repair specific injury operatively; less common in children compared to adults with similar injuries

11. Monitor hemodynamic and intracranial pressures, as needed

12. Institute medical protocol for pediatric head trauma, if indicated

a. Elevate head of bed 30°
b. Provide adequate ventilation; maintan PaO_2 at 80 to 100 mm Hg and $PaCO_2$ at 20 to 25 mm Hg; use controlled hyperventilation
c. Provide fluid resuscitation sufficient to maintain systolic blood pressure above (80 + 2 (age in years)) mm Hg
d. Maintain fluid intake restriction per neurosurgeon's directive, usually $\frac{3}{4}$ to $\frac{2}{3}$ of maintenance
e. Administer diuretics as prescribed
   (1) Lasix—1 ml/kg; give prior to mannitol
   (2) Mannitol
      (a) 0.25 mg/kg; administer after child voids
      (b) Use caution in initial resuscitation phase; osmotic diuretic causes initial transient rise in intracranial pressure
f. Sedate (morphine preferred)
g. Insert ventriculostomy and drain cerebral spinal fluid
h. Administer barbiturates and use hypothermia under direction of neurosurgeon
i. Administer steroids (controversial)

13. Provide nonoperative treatment for abdominal trauma, usually blunt injury of solid organs, e.g., spleen, liver, kidney, pancreas

a. Keep NPO; decompress stomach with NG tube
b. Administer I.V. fluids at maintenance or $1\frac{1}{2}$ times maintenance; monitor urine output
c. Frequently monitor vital signs, peripheral perfusion, and sensorium
d. Consistent practitioner, preferably pediatric surgeon, should perform frequent, serial abdominal examinations; avoid sedation and analgesics, as they may mask pain response
e. Monitor hemoglobin and hematocrit frequently; monitor amylase and liver function studies periodically
f. With suspected kidney injury, observe/test urine for hematuria, and monitor BUN and serum creatinine
g. Transfuse with type-specific packed red blood cells, 10 ml/kg, when hemoglobin decreases to 8.5 to 8.0 gm/dl

h. Obtain serial radiographic studies
   (1) Spleen and liver injuries—CAT scan, scintiscan
   (2) Kidney injury—CAT scan, intravenous pyelogram
   (3) Pancreatic injury—ultrasound
i. Resume oral fluids when ileus is resolved and laboratory values are normalized; severe traumatic pancreatitis requires weeks to months of bowel rest and total parenteral nutrition
j. Discharge to home within seven days after normal laboratory values and normal, or significantly improved, radiographs
k. Maintain bed rest with progressive ambulation for liver or kidney injuries; restrict physical activity for six weeks for all injuries
l. Follow-up care includes radiographic studies (CAT scan, ultrasound, scintiscan, intravenous pyelogram) at four to six weeks after injury and p.r.n.; monitor for hypertension after kidney injury
m. Indications for surgical intervention
   (1) Hemodynamic instability
   (2) Blood transfusion of 40 ml/kg or greater than 50% total circulating blood volume
   (3) Multisystem injury requiring exploration, e.g., blunt or penetrating chest trauma
   (4) Splenic injury—multiple splenic fragments noted on CAT scan; attempt splenorrhaphy or partial splenectomy; total splenectomy is last resort
   (5) Liver injury—continued blood loss and deteriorating vital signs
   (6) Pancreas—persistent or unresolved pseudocyst; attempt percutaneous drainage

D. GENERAL NURSING APPROACHES TO PEDIATRIC TRAUMA CARE

NOTE: This section outlines nursing approaches necessary for all pediatric trauma patients, regardless of age; the next section outlines age-specific approaches

1. Assessment

a. Interview parent and/or guardian; interview patient at age-specific level
   (1) Mechanism of injury and accident scenario
   (2) Past medical and surgical history
   (3) Immunization status
   (4) Current medications and allergies
   (5) Review of systems; last meal
   (6) Developmental history
   (7) Family constellation
   (8) Available resources and support systems
b. Physical examination; maintain C-spine immobilization throughout
   (1) Inspect
      (a) Airway patency
      (b) Symmetrical chest excursion and expansion

(c) Color
(d) Respiratory rate and rhythm
(e) Use of accessory muscles; signs of respiratory distress
(f) Abdomen contour
  i) Flat or scaphoid is normal finding
  ii) Distension or fullness may indicate bleeding, especially if child is unconscious and abdominal muscles are relaxed
(g) Capillary refill
(h) Skin for open wounds, lacerations, bruises, contusions, abrasions
(i) Extremity movement
(j) Obvious extremity deformity

(2) Palpate
(a) Airway patency—feel for air flow
(b) C-spine deformity
(c) Tracheal deviation
(d) Subcutaneous emphysema
(e) Carotid pulse
(f) Peripheral pulses—compare side to side
(g) Abdomen—tense vs soft; tender
(h) Pelvic stability
(i) Extremity deformity
(j) Rectal tone

(3) Percuss chest, back, and abdomen
(4) Auscultate
(a) Breath sounds
(b) Heart sounds; apical heart rate
(c) Bowel sounds

(5) Other
(a) Vital signs—frequent assessment and measurement; normal vital signs (1)

	HR (beats/min)	RR (breaths/min)	Sys BP* (mm Hg)
Infants	160	40	80
Children	140	30	90
Adolescents	120	20	100

*(Age-specific BP is calculated as 80 + 2 (age in years) mm Hg)

(b) Temperature documentation mandatory—normal = 36° to 37°C (96.8° to 98.6°F)
(c) Neurologic assessment
  i) Level of consciousness
  ii) Pupillary response; fundoscopic examination
  iii) Extremity movement
  iv) CSF oto/rhinorrhea; hemotympanum
  v) Plantar responses
  vi) Deep tendon reflexes
  vii) Assign Glasgow Coma Scale score
(d) Physiologic signs of pain

i) Increased heart rate
ii) Increased respiratory rate
iii) Flushed skin
iv) Restlessness
v) Pallor
vi) Rigid extremities
vii) Dilation of pupils

c. Psychologic
(1) Cognitive abilities
(2) Psychosocial development
(3) Stress response as influenced by
(a) Developmental age of child
(b) Past traumatic experiences
(c) Communication abilities
(d) Severity of injuries
(e) Pain response

2. Interventions

a. Establish and maintain patent airway
(1) Position—"sniffing," chin lift, or jaw thrust
(2) Insert oral airway with direct visualization; do not rotate airway during insertion
(3) Remove visible foreign bodies; suction secretions
(4) Assist with endotracheal intubation—oral route preferred
(a) Estimate ET tube size by
i) 16 + age (years) ÷ 4 = size, or
ii) Compare with little finger or external nares
(b) Securely tape over upper lip by using benzoin to increase adherence
(c) Mark level to indicate tube length

b. Maintain cervical spine immobilization
(1) Use cervical collar, spine board, sandbags, and tape
(2) Select correct size of cervical collar for child; inappropriate size may cause further C-spine injury

c. Optimize ventilation
(1) Administer 100% humidified oxygen
(2) Use pediatric Ambu bag with pop-off valves or pressure manometer to decrease risk of iatrogenic pneumothorax
(3) Assist with procedures
(a) Needle thoracentesis
(b) Tube thoracostomy; if chest tube suction is needed, use 10 cm H_2O pressure for infants and 20 cm H_2O pressure for children
(4) Place nasogastric tube to adequately decompress stomach
(5) Assess response of respiratory system to above treatment measure

d. Provide adequate circulatory blood volume; recognize and assist in treating shock
(1) Assign and obtain weight estimate
(2) Assess for signs of hypovolemic shock; usual signs seen late due to child's compensatory mechanisms
(3) Obtain I.V. access and administer fluid and blood products, as prescribed
(4) Obtain specimens and monitor results of laboratory studies

(5) Insert urinary catheter if urethral injury is excluded
  (a) Infant—8 Fr
  (b) Child—10 Fr
  (c) Adolescent—14 Fr
(6) Monitor urine output; expected output is 2 ml/kg/hr in infants and 1 ml/kg/hr in children
(7) Assist with peritoneal lavage procedure
(8) Assist with PASG application and decompression; abdominal compartment is used with great caution in all groups except large adolescents
(9) Frequent, ongoing assessment is mandatory in pediatric trauma where nonoperative, conservative management is usually treatment of choice

e. Fully expose child without compromising thermoregulatory status
  (1) Remove all clothing for full physical examination; include inspection of back
  (2) Assess for external signs of trauma; assume internal injury beneath any external trauma (abrasion, contusion, laceration)
  (3) Document any suspicious injuries that could indicate child abuse (see Module 32—Abused/Battered Persons)
  (4) Obtain and document temperature by noting both skin and core temperatures; maintain temperature within normal range
  (5) Conserve body heat
    (a) Administer all fluids and blood through warmers
    (b) Utilize overhead lamps and heating blankets to maintain temperature

f. Prevent disability
  (1) Prevent increased intracranial pressure by correct head positioning, maintaining hyperventilation, etc.; assist with prescribed treatments for closed head injury
  (2) Immobilize fractures with appropriate splints; assist in reduction of fractures
  (3) Collaborate with physiatrist, and physical, occupational, and speech therapists to plan and implement strategies that maintain function and foster normal growth and development

g. Promote comfort
  (1) Assess pain using age-appropriate tools (see Module 14—Pain); pain is most commonly expressed in behavior (2)
  (2) Use nonpharmacologic methods for pain management whenever possible, e.g., age-appropriate preparation for procedures, distraction, parental presence, imagery, cutaneous stimulation, relaxation techniques
  (3) Use analgesics cautiously during early posttrauma period; avoid drugs or dose levels that might mask pain, which provides diagnostic information
  (4) Administer analgesics at weight-appropriate dose, as prescribed; evaluate and document response

h. Provide family-focused care and age-appropriate psychological and emotional support
  (1) Allow parents to see child as soon as safely possible; if child calms down, allow parent(s) to stay (if resuscitation allows); if parent further stresses child, ask parent to leave
  (2) Assign one, or two at most, team member(s) to "talk" child through initial examination, and care and serve as surrogate parent
  (3) Involve social services personnel and chaplain to support parents through resuscitation and hospitalization

(4) Communicate plan of care to family; explain interventions, clinical status, and prognosis

3. **Patient outcomes**

a. Patent airway

b. Optimal ventilatory status
   (1) Normal ABGs
   (2) Normal respiratory rate and volume for age
   (3) Signs of respiratory distress absent
   (4) Activity tolerance at preinjury level

c. Adequate circulation established and maintained as reflected in
   (1) Normal heart rate, blood pressure, and capillary refill
   (2) Adequate urine output

d. Wounds heal with minimal functional or cosmetic impairment

e. Disability prevented and minimized as reflected in
   (1) Glasgow Coma Scale score of 15 to 16
   (2) Neurologic function normal for age
   (3) Cognitive ability at preinjury level
   (4) Motor function at preinjury level
   (5) Resumption of usual activities

f. Temperature within normal limits

g. Verbalizes comfort; functions without pain

h. Family function maintained and optimized
   (1) Parent and sibling roles resumed and maintained
   (2) Parents and siblings exhibit support to child and each other
   (3) Family copes effectively with traumatic event

i. Knowledgeable about injury and follow-up care, and participates in self-care to extent possible according to developmental level; family similarly knowledgeable and able to demonstrate required care

E. AGE-SPECIFIC NURSING APPROACHES TO TRAUMA CARE

1. **Infants (birth to 1 year)**

a. Interview/history
   (1) Include prenatal and birth history
   (2) Development—include milestones, e.g., roll over, sit alone
   (3) Feeding history—include formula type, amount, frequency, last feeding

b. Assessment and interventions based on physiologic characteristics
   (1) Large tongue in relation to oropharynx—utilize sniffing position, chin lift, or jaw thrust maneuvers to open airway
   (2) Little or no neck makes cervical spine immobilization difficult—utilize tape, sandbags, and towel rolls in addition to collar and spine board
   (3) Obligatory nose breathers—suction secretions and debris from nasal passages promptly and frequently
   (4) Breath sounds are easily transferred across chest because of small surface area; assess in midaxillary line bilaterally; assess quality and quantity

(5) Signs of respiratory distress include nasal flaring, grunting, retractions, circumoral cyanosis, paradoxical chest movement, poor chest wall movement
(6) Cricoid ring is narrowest point of infant's airway; utilize uncuffed ET tube and estimate size as follows
  i) Newborn—3.0 to 3.5 mm
  ii) 6 to 12 months—3.5 to 4.0 mm
  iii) Suction catheter size —6.5 to 8.0 Fr
(7) Evaluate vital sign parameters for age
  (a) Normal range—HR = 120 to 160; R = 30 to 60; Sys BP = 60 to 100 (3)
  (b) Stress, fear, pain, and fever increase heart and respiratory rates; may decrease with sleep or vagal stimulation
  (c) Use distraction, music, cuddling; approach with soothing, quiet tone of voice to calm infant and increase accuracy of vital signs
  (d) In the newborn, apnea, bradycardia, and hypothermia may be signs of sepsis
(8) Due to small size, infants require small amounts of fluid during resuscitation; give fluid boluses I.V. push to facilitate rapid but controlled fluid resuscitation
(9) Higher metabolic rates, higher glucose needs, and low glycogen stores result in hypoglycemia; monitor glucose and administer boluses, as indicated
(10) When under stress, infants exhibit increased calcium deposition, which results in hypocalcemia; monitor serum calcium levels
(11) Newborns do not conjugate bilirubin; monitor total and direct bilirubin
(12) Infants less than 6 months do not reflexively shiver and break down body fat to keep warm (nonshivering thermogenesis)
  (a) Provide increased oxygen and calories
  (b) Conserve body heat; transfer to isolette as soon as possible
(13) Abdomen normally full and soft; if scaphoid, suspect diaphragmatic rupture
(14) On verbal portion of Glasgow Coma Scale, assign 5 for normal, vigorous cry

c. Assessment and interventions based on psychologic characteristics
(1) Cognitive development at sensorimotor stage—learning occurs chiefly through reflexes and sensation; landmark is object permanence, i.e., looks for hidden object by 9 months
(2) Psychosocial development at stage of trust vs mistrust
(3) Stress response centers around separation from parents and exposure to strangers
  (a) Minimize separation from parents
  (b) Minimize parental anxiety, which is transmitted to infant
  (c) Provide consistent caretaker
  (d) Minimize number of staff interacting with infant
(4) Pain response
  (a) Infants less than 3 months are unable to localize pain and respond with total body movement
  (b) After 6 months, pain is influenced by past experience and parental anxiety

2. Toddlers (1 to 3 years)

a. Interview/history
(1) Birth history
(2) Developmental milestones—walk, talk, climb stairs

b. Assessment and interventions based on physiologic characteristics
   (1) Use uncuffed ET tube; estimate size as follows
      (a) 18 months—4.0 to 4.5 mm
      (b) 24 to 36 months—4.0 to 5.0 mm
   (2) Estimate size of suction catheters as follows
      (a) 18 months—8 Fr
      (b) 24 to 36 months—8 Fr
   (3) Observe for signs of respiratory distress, including nasal flaring, tugging, grunting, using accessory muscles (substernal, suprasternal)
   (4) Evaluate vital sign parameters for age—HR = 90 to 140; R = 24 to 40; Sys BP = 80 to 112 (3)
c. Assessment and interventions based on psychologic characteristics
   (1) Cognitive development at preoperational stage is characterized by egocentrism, animism, inability to judge action by consequences; little concept of body integrity
   (2) Psychosocial development at stage of autonomy vs shame and doubt
   (3) Stress response centers around separation anxiety and loss of control
      (a) Minimize separation from parents and familiar objects
      (b) Utilize security objects
      (c) Introduce medical play if child is receptive
      (d) Provide explanation immediately prior to procedures
      (e) Prepare for intense reaction to procedures
      (f) Establish routines; create sense of control by allowing child to help or participate
      (g) Give permission to cry; set limits on less desirable behaviors
   (4) Pain response
      (a) Characterized by extreme emotional distress and physical resistance
      (b) Memory, parental separation, and lack of preparation contribute to pain response

3. Preschoolers (3 to 6 years)

a. Interview/history
   (1) Developmental milestone—language
   (2) School and play group performance
   (3) Past experience and response to hospitalization
b. Assessment and interventions based on physiologic characteristics
   (1) Observe for signs of respiratory distress similar to toddlers
   (2) Use uncuffed endotracheal tube size 4.5 mm to 5.5 mm
   (3) Estimate suction catheter size—8 to 10 Fr
   (4) Evaluate vital sign parameters for age—HR = 80 to 110; R = 22 to 34; Sys BP = 82 to 115 (3)
c. Assessment and interventions based on psychologic characteristics
   (1) Cognitive development at preoperational level
      (a) Characterized by egocentrism, animism, and magical thinking
      (b) Child has little concept of time
   (2) Psychosocial development at stage of initiative vs guilt
   (3) Stress response centers around separation, loss of control, and fear of body injury and mutilation
      (a) Prepare child for procedures by using simple explanations and props; give choices if possible

(b) Assure child that painful procedures are not punishment for actions
(c) Be honest regarding painful procedures
(d) Provide consistent caretaker and do not leave child alone
(4) Pain response
(a) Can localize pain
(b) Respond with more control than toddlers
(c) May not verbalize pain; note physiologic signs of pain

4. School age (7 to 12 years)

a. Interview/history
(1) Include school attendance and performance
(2) Social history—involvement with peers, gangs, sports, and other activities
(3) Substance abuse

b. Assessment and interventions based on physiologic characteristics
(1) Use uncuffed endotracheal tubes in children less than 8 years; estimate size of ET tube as follows
(a) 7 to 10 years = 6.0 to 6.5 mm
(b) 10 to 12 years = 6.0 to 7.0 mm
(2) Estimate size of suction catheters
(a) 7 to 10 years = 10 Fr
(b) 10 to 12 years = 10 to 12 Fr
(3) Children less than 6 years old are no longer primarily diaphragmatic breathers; use of abdominal muscles may be a sign of respiratory distress
(4) Evaluate vital sign parameters for age—HR = 75 to 100; R = 18 to 30; Sys BP = 84 to 120 (3)

c. Assessment and interventions based on psychologic characteristics
(1) Cognitive development at concrete operational level
(a) Landmark is conservation by 7 years of age, i.e., conceptualizes objects by more than one characteristic
(b) Begins logical thinking; understands cause and effect, and concept of time
(2) Psychological development at stage of industry vs inferiority
(3) Stress response centers around separation from family and peer group, loss of control, feelings of inferiority, and fear of death and mutilation
(a) Explain all procedures
(b) Give choices, if possible, and honor child's request for parents' presence or absence
(c) Continue to reassure child that procedures are not punishment
(4) Pain response
(a) Pain can be localized and described in terms of onset, location, quality, and intensity
(b) Fear may exaggerate description of pain
(c) Fear may inhibit verbalization of pain; continue to assess for physiologic signs

5. Adolescents (13 to 18 years)

a. Interview/history
(1) School attendance and performance
(2) Involvement with peers, gangs, sports, and other activities
(3) Substance abuse
(4) Sexual history

(a) In females, include age of menarche, pregnancies, abortions
(b) Interview child separately from parents

b. Assessments and interventions based on physiologic characteristics are similar to the adult
c. Assessments and interventions based on psychologic characteristics
   (1) Cognitive development at formal operational level; can think logically and utilize deductive reasoning
   (2) Psychosocial development at stage of identity vs role confusion
   (3) Stress response centers around separation from peer group
      (a) Explain all procedures sensitively and tactfully
      (b) Respect wish to be cared for independent of parents
      (c) Give choices whenever possible; include patient in decisionmaking
      (d) Respect privacy
      (e) Be honest regarding pain and consequences of medical procedures and interventions

F. THE FAMILY OF THE PEDIATRIC TRAUMA PATIENT

1. Family assessment

a. Membership and roles
b. Involvement in traumatic event
   (1) Present at time of injury
   (2) Other family members injured
   (3) Causal agent
c. Other crises within family unit
d. Support systems
   (1) Relatives and friends
   (2) Religious groups and pastoral care
   (3) Community and cultural groups
   (4) Employers
e. Past experiences with trauma and/or sudden death
f. Response to child's hospitalization influenced by
   (1) Guilt regarding injury
   (2) Societal expectations
   (3) Previous experiences
   (4) Culture and ethnicity
   (5) Severity of injury and prognosis
g. Usual coping strategies

2. Role of family

a. Provide emotional support to child
b. Continue parenting behaviors
   (1) Physical care and comfort
   (2) Protection from harm
   (3) Socialization and education
c. Familiarize hospital environment, i.e., provide security objects

d. Anticipatory grieving for loss of "perfect" child or death of child; stages include
   (1) Shock, disbelief—characterized by emotional outbursts
   (2) Reality, acceptance—characterized by sadness, loneliness, feelings of guilt
   (3) Reorganization—resumes tasks of everyday living

3. Nursing support of family

a. Communicate clearly
   (1) Clinical status and prognosis of child; child's response to interventions
   (2) Plan of care
   (3) Interpretation of medical interventions; explanation of equipment
   (4) Listen to fears and concerns
b. Minimize separation
c. Maximize parenting and family functioning
   (1) Allow parents to physically and emotionally care for child whenever possible
   (2) Encourage family to comfort child, minimize fears, provide security objects, familiarize environment and routines
d. Set up family meetings to involve family in mutual care planning with health care team
e. Assist with and facilitate decision making and problem solving
f. Assist with accessing resources; refer to appropriate persons or agencies for social services and home health care needs
g. Be an advocate for the family

References

1. American College of Surgeons, Committee on Trauma. (1989). *Advanced trauma life support student manual.* Chicago: American College of Surgeons.
2. Wong, D. L., & Whaley, L. F. (1986). *Clinical handbook of pediatric nursing* (2nd ed., pp. 372–376). St. Louis: C. V. Mosby Co.
3. Hazinski, M. F. (1984). Children are different. In M. F. Hazinski (Ed.), *Nursing care of the critically ill child* (pp. 1–11). St. Louis: C. V. Mosby Co.

Suggested Readings

Alpert, J. J., & Guyer, B. (Eds.). (1985). Symposium on injuries and injury prevention. *Pediatric Clinics of North America, 32*(1).

Bernardo, L. M., Conway, A., & Bove, M. (1990). The ABC method of emotional assessment and intervention: A new approach in pediatric emergency care. *Journal of Emergency Nursing, 16*(3), 70–76.

Children's Hospital National Medical Center. (1986). *Trauma service manual.* Washington, DC: Author.

Douthit, J. L. (1990). Patient care guidelines: Psychosocial assessment and management of pediatric pain. *Journal of Emergency Nursing, 16*(3), 168–170.

Joy, C. (Ed.). (1989). *Pediatric trauma nursing.* Rockville, MD: Aspen Publishers.

Keen, T. P. (1990). Nursing care of the pediatric multitrauma patient. *Nursing Clinics of North America, 25*(1), 131–141.

Lenehan, G. P. (Ed.). (1988). A fresh look at pediatric emergency nursing. *Journal of Emergency Nursing, 14*(2).

Lewandowski, L. (1984). Psychosocial aspects of pediatric critical care. In M. F. Hazinski (Ed.), *Nursing care of the critically ill child* (pp. 12–62). St. Louis: C. V. Mosby Co.

Mayer, T. A. (Ed.). (1985). *Emergency management of pediatric trauma.* Philadelphia: W. B. Saunders Co.

Moloney-Harmon, P. A. (Ed.). (1989). Pediatric issues in multisystem trauma. *Critical Care Nursing Clinics of North America, 1*(1), 85–95.

Reeves, K. (1989). Assessment of pediatric head injury. *Journal of Emergency Nursing, 15*(4), 329–332.

Schlechter, N. L. (Ed.). (1989). Acute pain in children. *Pediatric Clinics of North America, 36*(4).

St. Christopher's Hospital for Children. (1987). *Trauma manual.* Philadelphia: Author.

U.S. Department of Health and Human Services. (1988). Public health surveillance of 1990 injury control objectives for the nation. *Morbidity and Mortality Weekly Report,* 37, SS-1 (February).

Wong, D. L. (1982). Childhood trauma: Its developmental aspects and nursing interventions. *Critical Care Quarterly,* 5(3), 47–60.

Section V
Special Patient Populations

MODULE 29
OBSTETRIC

Barbara Mankey Henninger, BA, BSN, RN, C

Prerequisite

Review normal anatomical and physiological changes of pregnancy.

Objectives

1.0 List unique characteristics of trauma in the obstetric population.
1.1 State the frequency of obstetric trauma.
1.2 State common mechanisms of injury associated with obstetric trauma.
1.3 Describe patterns of injury in blunt and penetrating trauma in the obstetric patient.
2.0 List physiologic and anatomic changes of pregnancy to be considered during the trauma continuum.
3.0 Describe unique aspects of the primary assessment of a pregnant trauma patient.
3.1 Describe assessment of airway, breathing, and circulation.
3.2 Identify the importance of patient positioning and its relationship to assessment findings.
4.0 Describe the secondary assessment of a pregnant trauma patient.
4.1 Identify the impact of maternal status on viability of the fetus.
4.2 List information obtained during pelvic and abdominal examinations.

4.3 Identify the types of information needed from the medical and obstetrical history.
4.4 Identify the indications for maternal monitoring.
4.5 List critical parameters of fetal status that indicate the need for fetal monitoring.
4.6 Describe signs and symptoms of uterine complications associated with obstetric trauma.
4.7 Discuss the method and indications for peritoneal lavage in the obstetric patient.
4.8 List radiological studies commonly required for definitive diagnosis.
4.9 List laboratory studies used to assess obstetrical trauma patients.
4.10 Identify maternal psychological factors to consider in obstetric trauma.
5.0 Identify medical and surgical interventions specific to obstetric trauma.
5.1 Describe application and benefits of pneumatic antishock garments.
5.2 Describe the importance of venous access and fluid replacement to maternal/fetal well-being.
5.3 List the pharmacologic agents most likely to be used with the obstetric trauma patient; include their effects on the fetus.
6.0 List common nursing diagnoses related to maternal and/or fetal patients.
7.0 Identify nursing interventions, for each nursing diagnosis, commonly implemented for the obstetric trauma patient.
7.1 List the nursing interventions necessary for optimal functioning in the obstetric trauma patient.
7.2 Identify the rationale for nursing interventions.
7.3 Given a patient scenario, prioritize nursing interventions.
8.0 Evaluate maternal and/or fetal response to medical and nursing interventions.
8.1 Identify desirable outcomes with measurable criteria for the obstetric patient.
8.2 Identify desirable outcomes with measurable criteria for the fetal patient.
8.3 Discuss the kinds of data, specific to the obstetric trauma patient, that require nursing documentation.
9.0 For a specific case situation, develop a plan of nursing care for a maternal/fetal unit who experiences trauma and requires care in the various phases of the trauma continuum.

A. GENERAL CONCEPTS AND PRINCIPLES

1. Physiologic and anatomic changes of pregnancy

a. Cardiovascular
   (1) Cardiac output increases from approximately 5 liter/min to 7 liter/min
   (2) Heart rate increases 15 to 20 beats/min
   (3) Blood pressure initially increases, but may actually fall 5 to 15 mm Hg lower than normal in second and third trimester
   (4) Venous pressure increases in lower extremities
   (5) ECG may show left axis deviation with PVCs

(6) Central venous pressure decreases slightly
b. Pulmonary
(1) Tidal volume and minute ventilation increase 50%
(2) Oxygen consumption increases by 15%
(3) Decreased pCO_2 leads to respiratory alkalosis
(4) Functional residual capacity decreases
c. Hematologic
(1) Plasma volume increases by 50%
(2) Red blood cell volume increases only 18 to 32%
(3) Hemoglobin (Hgb) and hematocrit (Hct) are low due to plasma volume/red blood cell volume disproportion (called "anemia of pregnancy")
(4) White blood cell (WBC) count increases to 18,000 to 25,000/mm due to increased circulating neutrophils and polymorphonuclear cells
(5) Fibrinogen increases to 400 to 500 mg%
d. Gastrointestinal—gastric emptying increases
e. Renal and urological
(1) Ureters and renal pelvis dilate
(2) Partial ureteral obstruction possible
(3) Glomerular filtration rate and renal blood flow increase
(4) BUN and serum creatinine fall to approximately one-half normal levels
(5) Bladder becomes intraabdominal organ in second and third trimester
f. Neurological
(1) Preeclampsia, a pregnancy-related disease, is associated with
(a) Altered vascular function
(b) Compromised metabolic function
(c) Significant sodium retention
(d) Reduced renal function
(e) Decreased intravascular volume
(f) Increased central nervous system activity
(2) Eclampsia is a severe progression of preeclampsia that may mimic head injury and is manifested by
(a) Symptoms of severe preeclampsia
(b) Hypertensive crisis or shock
(c) Tonic and clonic convulsions
(d) Possible coma

2. Psychological considerations
a. Maternal concern for her own well-being and fetal well-being
b. Impact of trauma on maternal relationship with significant other(s)

B. PATTERNS OF INJURY

NOTE: In the first trimester, the uterus is a pelvic organ; in the second and third trimesters, the uterus is an abdominal organ

1. Frequency of obstetric trauma
a. Pregnant females are involved in 6.9% of all accidental injuries

b. Each year, an estimated 3 to 4 pregnant patients per 1000 are hospitalized (1)

2. Blunt trauma

a. Most common cause of maternal and fetal injuries
   (1) MVCs are most frequent cause of major injuries
   (2) Falls cause most minor injuries

b. Uterus acts as a shock absorber in the second and third trimesters

c. Bruises anterior abdomen
   (1) Possibility of more serious hidden injuries should be considered
      (a) Uterine injury
      (b) Placental injury
      (c) Fetal injury
   (2) Advanced pregnancy makes abdominal examinations more difficult than in non-pregnant patient; stretching of abdominal wall alters its response to intraperitoneal stimuli

d. May cause ruptured liver and/or spleen
   (1) Pregnancy normally distends, compresses, or displaces these organs and makes them more vulnerable to injury or rupture
   (2) Symptoms are the same as in nonpregnant patients, e.g., upper quadrant pain, referred pain to shoulder, nausea/vomiting, free fluid in abdomen, hemorrhage, and elevated WBC (Reminder: WBC is normally elevated in the third trimester)

e. May cause pelvic fracture, the most common fracture in obstetric trauma patient
   (1) Increased vascularity in the pelvic area increases risk of retroperitoneal hemorrhage and shock
   (2) Ruptured bladder may be a concomitant injury

f. Uterine rupture may occur due to sudden deceleration force tearing uterus away from its fixed point
   (1) Suspect uterine rupture if patient manifests
      (a) Sharp abdominal or suprapubic pain
      (b) Diaphragmatic pain or rapid, shallow breathing
      (c) Absent fetal heart tones or movements
      (d) Vaginal bleeding
   (2) Uterine rupture usually results in fetal death and hysterectomy

g. Abruptio placentae (placental separation) is second most frequent cause of fetal death
   (1) Suspect placental separation if patient manifests
      (a) Vaginal bleeding
      (b) Severe, constant abdominal pain
      (c) Rigid or tender abdomen
      (d) Anxiety and restlessness
      (e) Maternal shock may indicate concealed placental bleeding
      (f) Disseminated intravascular coagulation (DIC)
      (g) Premature labor
      (h) Fetal distress (hypoxia and increased heart rate)

3. Penetrating trauma

a. The uterus acts as a shield in second and third trimesters

b. Gunshot wound to the uterus
   (1) Maternal survival is greater than fetal survival because the uterus shields other maternal organs

(2) Morbidity of both mother and fetus depends on the number of organs damaged and extent of organ damage
(3) Surgery is usually necessary

c. Stab wound to the uterus
(1) Maternal survival is greater than fetal survival
(2) Mother and fetus both have a better chance of surviving a stabbing than a GSW, since a bullet causes more damage
(3) Surgery is necessary; simple uterine laceration can be repaired without affecting the fetus

C. DIAGNOSTIC STUDIES

1. **Trauma profile**
2. **Include Rh factor with type and cross-match**
3. **Radiologic studies**

a. Maternal x-rays should be done with shielding of the fetus, if possible; the more advanced the gestational age, the less harmful the x-rays are to the fetus
b. X-rays should not be withheld, since omission may compromise accurate diagnosis
c. Obtain usual studies required for diagnosis of trauma (same as in nonpregnant patient)
d. Ultrasound of abdomen may be needed to determine
(1) Fetal heart activity
(2) Fetal movement
(3) Fetal position and presentation
(4) Gestational age
(5) Placental separation
(6) Quantity of amniotic fluid

D. MEDICAL AND SURGICAL PRIORITIES AND INTERVENTIONS

1. **General principles**

a. Primary axiom—maternal death is the most common cause of fetal death
b. Every female aged 12 to 50 is considered pregnant unless proven otherwise
c. Emergency care directed toward maternal stabilization increases both maternal and fetal survival rates
d. High-risk obstetrical and neonatal intensive care must be available to increase maternal and fetal survival

2. **Medical and surgical interventions (NOTE: priorities are the same as in the nonpregnant patient)**

a. Obtain and maintain a patent airway

b. Administer high flow humidified oxygen (maternal hypoxia/asphyxia may cause fetal neurological deficits)
c. Control bleeding and maintain optimal blood pressure
   (1) Apply direct pressure
   (2) Apply pneumatic antishock garments
      (a) Apply in prehospital setting to increase systemic vascular resistance and tamponade bleeding
      (b) Inflate leg compartments ONLY, so inferior vena cava is not compressed; could lead to "supine hypotension syndrome"
      (c) When hypotensive patient has possible cervical spine injury, tilt long board to left side to avoid inferior vena cava compression
d. Replace fluids
   (1) Maternal blood loss of 30 to 35% may occur before changes in vital signs are seen, due to the normal increase in plasma volume during pregnancy
   (2) The fetus may be in severe jeopardy due to uteroplacental circulatory shunting and anoxia, while mother's condition and vital signs remain normal
   (3) Establish large bore peripheral I.V.s bilaterally on each upper extremity
   (4) Administer fluid replacement by using 3:1 ratio, i.e., 3 ml crystalloid (lactated Ringer's solution preferred) to 1 ml estimated blood loss
e. Replace blood loss
   (1) Transfuse type-specific blood, if available, or O-negative packed red blood cells to avoid Rh sensitization
   (2) Administer blood component therapy, as required, for severe hemorrhage and coagulation defects
f. Insert urinary catheter and monitor output hourly; maintain urine output at 0.5 to 1 ml/kg/min
g. Peritoneal lavage
   (1) May be necessary to evaluate abdominal injury
      (a) Use supraumbilical approach to avoid enlarged uterus
      (b) Indications of positive lavage are the same as for other patients
   (2) Identify retroperitoneal injuries with intravenous pyelogram, ultrasound, or CAT scan
h. Perform injury-specific surgical procedures as in the nonpregnant patient
i. Prescribe medications
   (1) Oxytocins—used primarily after fetus and placenta are delivered; cause firm contraction of the uterus and decrease postdelivery bleeding
      (a) Methergine, 0.2 mg, I.V. or I.M.
      (b) Pitocin, 20 units, I.V. or I.M.; may also be used in an intravenous drip for the induction of labor
   (2) Antibiotics—in usual doses, as needed
      (a) Aminoglycosides—may cause nerve and renal anomalies in fetus
      (b) Cephalosporins—no demonstrated significant risk to fetus
      (c) Clindamycin and erythromycin—no known effects on the fetus
      (d) Penicillins—no demonstrated significant risk to fetus
      (e) Tetracyclines—cause impaired bone growth and enamel hypoplasia to the fetus and should NOT be used
   (3) Tetanus toxoid—no known effects on fetus; follow usual immunization schedule

(4) Analgesics
  (a) Acetaminophen—may cause nephrotoxicity in the fetus
  (b) Narcotics—may cause neonatal depression and withdrawal; morphine and Demerol cross the placental barrier and should NOT be given initially, as these may compromise the fetus
  (c) Salicylates—cause prolonged labor and possible hemorrhage
  (d) Codeine—no known untoward effects
(5) Anticonvulsants—give as needed; barbiturates may cause central nervous system withdrawal in the fetus
(6) Anticoagulants—give as needed
  (a) Coumadin—may cause nasal hypoplasia, hemorrhage, and stillbirth of the fetus
  (b) Heparin—may cause ophthalmic abnormalities in the fetus
(7) Antiinflammatory agents—give as needed; hydrocortisone may cause cleft palate, adrenal suppression, and enhance pulmonary maturity in the fetus
(8) Dopaminergic agents—use cautiously; vasopressors NOT used to correct hypotension because they further constrict uterine blood flow
(9) Anesthetics—give as needed
  (a) General anesthesia may cause anomalies, abortion, and central nervous system depression in the fetus
  (b) Local anesthesia may cause bradycardia and seizures in the fetus

E. UNIQUE ASPECTS OF THE NURSING PROCESS

1. **Nursing assessment**

a. Primary maternal assessment
  (1) Mechanism of injury
  (2) Signs and symptoms related to injury
    (a) Difficulty breathing
      i) Increased oxygen consumption and decreased functional residual capacity lead to rapid hypoxemia
      ii) Respiratory alkalosis, associated with pregnancy, decreases maternal ability to buffer metabolic acidosis associated with hypovolemia
      iii) Duration and degree of hypoxemia may cause irreversible damage to fetus
    (b) Abnormal blood pressure and pulse rate
      i) Pregnancy normally increases cardiac output and heart rate, and lowers blood pressure; therefore, early diagnosis of shock is difficult
      ii) Supine position causes "supine hypotension syndrome"
        a) Compression of the vena cava by the gravid uterus decreases blood return to the heart
        b) To relieve pressure on the vena cava, place patient in the left lateral recumbent position or elevate right hip

iii) Obstetrical trauma patient may sustain 1500 to 2000 ml blood loss before alterations in vital signs are seen; sympathetic response increases catecholamines, which constrict uterine arteries, leading to fetal hypoxia

(c) Note skin color and mental status—patient who is cool, pale, cyanotic, and/or agitated needs aggressive volume expansion to stabilize herself and her fetus

b. Secondary maternal assessment

(1) Obtain medical and obstetrical history

(a) Past pregnancies and complications

(b) Current medications

(c) Allergies

(d) Rh sensitivity

(2) Examine abdomen

(a) Note size of uterus and its relation to gestational age

i) McDonald's method—measure with tape from symphysis pubic to fundus; 1 cm = 1 week of gestation

ii) Rapid estimate method

a) 0 to 12 weeks—uterus is in the pelvic confines

b) 20 to 24 weeks—uterus at level of the umbilicus

c) 36 weeks—uterus at level of the diaphragm

(b) Assess for uterine contractions or tetany

(c) Monitor uterine contractions, if indicated

i) Palpation may suffice; palpate while listening to fetal heart rate

ii) Electronic monitoring is preferred

(d) Evalutate abdominal pain—differentiate injury-produced pain from pain due to labor, premature labor contractions, or abruptio placentae

(e) Palpate for uterine tenderness or rigidity

(f) Mark fundal height and note any increase during assessment; suspect abruptio placentae if increase noted

(g) Note fetal position, presentation, movements, and heart tones

(3) Examine pelvis for

(a) External vaginal bleeding

(b) Intact or ruptured membranes

(c) Possible presentation of fetal parts

(4) Obtain specimens for laboratory studies

(5) Monitor results of trauma profile and radiologic studies

c. Fetal assessment

(1) Monitor fetus continuously to determine the response of fetus to uterine contractions; mother will maintain homeostasis at the expense of the fetus

(a) Use fetoscope or hand-held Doppler for immediate assessment of fetal heart rate (FHR)

i) Listen to FHR every five minutes

ii) Listen for one full minute each time

(b) Use electronic fetal monitor to continuously monitor FHR and rhythm

(2) Observe for signs and symptoms of injury

(a) Bradycardia (FHR less than 120 beats/min)

(b) Tachycardia (FHR greater than 160 beats/min)

(c) FHR decelerations
i) Early decelerations mirror uterine contractions and do not indicate fetal distress
ii) Late decelerations
a) Begin at the peak of a contraction and persist into the interval after the contraction
b) When persistent, late decelerations indicate fetal hypoxia due to decreased uteroplacental perfusion
iii) Variable decelerations
a) Are transient drops in FHR before, during, or after a contraction?
b) May be due to compression of the umbilical cord
(d) Absent fetal heart tones—notify physician immediately
(e) Decreased fetal movement

2. Nursing diagnoses, expected outcomes, and interventions

a. Ineffective breathing pattern related to pain of injuries, surgical interventions, or fetal size
(1) Expected outcomes—normal respiratory rate, rhythm, tidal volume
(2) Nursing interventions
(a) Maintain patent airway
(b) Assess breath sounds, respiratory pattern, rate, rhythm, and depth
(c) Position patient for optimal chest excursion and deep breathing
(d) Evaluate hemodynamic and pulmonary parameters, and report deterioration to physician
(e) Instruct patient to notify nurse at onset of difficult or ineffective breathing
(f) Reassure patient during periods of respiratory distress and encourage slow abdominal breathing
(g) Instruct patient in relaxation techniques to improve breathing pattern
(h) Provide effective pain relief
(i) Administer humidified oxygen, assist with intubation, and institute mechanical ventilation, if necessary

b. Altered fetal tissue perfusion related to hypovolemia and/or supine hypotension syndrome
(1) Expected outcomes
(a) FHR within normal range
(b) No signs of fetal distress
(2) Nursing interventions
(a) Maintain patent airway
(b) Administer high flow humidified oxygen
(c) Administer fluids and blood components, as prescribed
(d) Position mother to avoid pressure on the vena cava (left lateral recumbent or with right hip elevated) and to increase blood return to the heart
(e) Assess FHR continuously in relation to uterine contractions; report abnormalities to physician
(f) Monitor maternal vital signs
(g) Monitor effects of medications on fetal tissue perfusion

c. Potential for preterm labor related to trauma
(1) Expected outcomes

(a) Absence of premature contractions
(b) Pregnancy continues to full term
(2) Nursing interventions
(a) Administer and monitor pharmacologic agents used to suppress preterm labor (NOTE: administer with supervision of experienced obstetric nurse or obstetrician)
i) Terbutaline (Brethine)
a) Administer 0.25 mg, SC; repeat in 15 to 30 minutes, if needed
b) Side effects of this B_2 receptor stimulant include tachycardia, palpitations, sweating, headache, nervousness, tremors, anxiety, lethargy, drowsiness, tinnitus, dizziness, nausea, and vomiting
ii) Magnesium sulfate
a) Loading dose—4 to 6 gm, I.V., over 20 to 30 min
b) Continuous drip—add 20 gm magnesium sulfate to 500 ml of 5% dextrose in water; infuse at 1 to 3 gm/hr
c) Side effects include flushing, sweating, thirst, hypotension, diminished or absent patellar reflexes
d) Toxic effects include flaccid paralysis, hypothermia, circulatory collapse, depressed cardiac function
e) Antidote—calcium gluconate
iii) Ritodrine (Yutopar)
a) Administered via I.V. infusion
b) Add 100 mg ritodrine to 500 ml 5% dextrose in water; begin infusion at 50 mcg/hr and increase until desired result obtained; maximum rate of 350 mcg/hr
c) Increases blood flow to fetus by maternal vasodilation
d) Side effects of this B_2 receptor stimulant include hypotension, tachycardia, pulse irregularity (NOTE: perform continuous maternal cardiac monitoring)
iv) Betamethasone phosphate, 6 mg I.M.
a) Can be repeated once in 24 hrs
b) Accelerates fetal lung maturity in women with premature labor between 28 and 32 weeks' gestation
(b) Maintain bed rest and position patient to increase blood return to the heart
(c) Assess FHR continuously in relation to uterine contractions; report FHR abnormalities to physician

d. Potential for aspiration related to delayed gastric emptying
(1) Expected outcomes
(a) Patent airway maintained
(b) Patient reports no gastric reflux
(2) Nursing interventions
(a) Position patient with head elevated
(b) Insert nasogastric tube to decompress stomach
(c) Check gastric aspirate for volume and pH
(d) Provide small, frequent meals or feedings
(e) Protect airway in the unconscious patient

e. Anticipatory grieving related to potential loss of fetus

(1) Expected outcomes—patient and family proceed through grieving process normally, and verbalize supportive relationship with nurse
(2) Nursing interventions
(a) Inform patient of any obstetrical complication(s), in relation to gestational age, that may result in fetal demise
(b) Establish trusting relationship with patient to assist with possible loss of fetus
(c) Provide safe, secure, private environment
(d) Encourage patient and significant other(s) to verbalize feelings to facilitate potential grieving process
(e) Discuss with patient and family/significant other(s) the impact of possible fetal loss on the family unit
(f) Provide information about hospital and community resource groups
(g) Acknowledge patient/family grief reactions while continuing with necessary care activities

f. Anxiety related to mother/infant separation due to delivery and continuing health care needs of mother and/or infant
(1) Expected outcomes
(a) Verbal and nonverbal signs of anxiety are minimal
(b) Mother verbalizes knowledge of infant status and communicates with nursery staff
(2) Nursing interventions
(a) Encourage patient to verbalize thoughts and feelings in order to externalize anxiety and express anger; allow patient to cry
(b) Reassure patient during interactions by touch and empathetic verbal and nonverbal exchanges
(c) Keep mother informed of infant's status; establish communications between mother's care unit and the nursery
(d) Establish mother/infant bonding as soon as possible
(e) In the event of infant's death, assist patient/family through the grieving process

g. Knowledge deficit related to self-care needs of continued pregnancy upon discharge from hospital
(1) Expected outcomes—patient verbalizes and demonstrates self-care instructions and activities related to possible sequelae of injury
(2) Nursing interventions
(a) Assess and document patient's level of understanding of prescribed treatment; request return demonstration of specific knowledge or self-care activities
(b) Involve significant other/family in the learning process
(c) Provide written and verbal instructions
(d) Instruct patient to call physician and/or return to hospital if there is
i) Leaking of amniotic fluid
ii) Vaginal bleeding
iii) Sign of preterm or term labor (contractions), or abdominal pain
iv) Decreased or absent fetal movement
v) Difficulty breathing
vi) Change in heart rate
vii) Change in skin condition or mental status

References

1. Schwab, C. W., & Shaikh, K. A. (1986). Shock in the pregnant patient. *Emergency Care Quarterly, 1*(2), 47.

Suggested Readings

American College of Obstetricians and Gynecologists. (1986). Trauma in pregnancy. *ACOG Update Series, 12*(4).

Buchsbaum, H. J. (Ed.). (1979). *Trauma in pregnancy.* Philadelphia: W. B. Saunders Co.

Cardona, V. D., Hurn, P. D., Mason, P. J. B., Scanlon-Schilpp, A. M., & Veise-Berry, S. W. (Eds.). (1988). *Trauma nursing: From resuscitation through rehabilitation.* Philadelphia: W. B. Saunders Co.

Cowley, R. A., & Dunham, C. M. (1982). *Shock trauma/critical care manual: Initial assessment and management.* Baltimore: University Park Press.

Cunningham, F. G., MacDonald, P. C., & Gant, N. F. (Eds.). (1989). *Williams' obstetrics* (18th ed.). Norwalk, CT: Appleton & Lange.

Dees, G., & Fuller, M. (1989). Blunt trauma in the pregnant patient. *Journal of Emergency Nursing, 15*(6), 495–499.

Esposito, T. J. (1988). Pitfalls in resuscitation and early management of the pregnant trauma patient. *Trauma Quarterly, 5*(1), 1–22.

Foster, C. A. (1984). The pregnant trauma patient. *Nursing '84, 14*(11), 58–63.

Gatrell, C. B. (1987). Trauma and pregnancy. *Trauma Quarterly, 4*(1), 67–85.

Sorenson, V. J., Bivins, B. A., Obeid, F. N., & Horst, H. M. (1986). Trauma in pregnancy. *Henry Ford Hospital Medical Journal, 34*(2), 101–104.

Stauffer, D. M. (1986). The trauma patient who is pregnant. *Journal of Emergency Nursing, 12*(2), 89–93.

Section V
Special Patient Population

MODULE 30
ELDERLY

Janet Marie Burns, MSN, RN, CEN
Elizabeth W. Bayley, MS, PhD, RN

Objectives

1.0 Briefly describe physiologic and metabolic changes that occur with aging.
1.1 Identify cellular, organic, and systemic changes that occur with aging.
1.2 Cite how aging may alter effects of drug therapy.
1.3 List common health problems that have synergistic effects on the elderly.
2.0 Describe psychological and social changes that occur with aging.
3.0 Describe common causes of injuries in the elderly client.
3.1 Identify three major types of injuries commonly sustained by the elderly individual.
3.2 Briefly describe mechanisms of injury and defining characteristics of each type of injury.
3.3 Cite environmental hazards that impact upon elder safety.
4.0 Identify specific changes in trauma protocols related to aging.
4.1 List diagnostic tools that help in the diagnosis of elderly patients.
4.2 Describe how medical interventions may be altered in the elderly trauma patient.
4.3 Briefly describe preoperative care considerations for the elderly patient.
5.0 Describe unique aspects of the nursing process in the elderly trauma patient.
5.1 Formulate nursing diagnoses with specific etiologies and supporting signs and symptoms commonly found in the elderly trauma client.

5.2 Briefly describe anticipated nursing interventions appropriate to the management of the elderly trauma client.
5.3 Discuss the elderly trauma patient's needs for safety and information related to self-care during recovery from injury.
6.0 Evaluate patient response to trauma and therapeutic interventions.
6.1 Define expected outcomes for the hospitalized elderly trauma patient.
6.2 List types of data to include in nursing documentation.

A. GENERAL CONCEPTS AND PRINCIPLES

1. Physiological considerations—aging occurs at all levels of body function

a. Cellular
   (1) Cells have a finite life span and do not divide indefinitely; they demonstrate a decreasing capacity for cellular division with age
   (2) Loss of cells and loss of physiologic reserve make up the dominant processes of aging

b. Organic
   (1) There are wide differences in aging from person to person; such differences depend on the individual's health state
   (2) Different organ systems are affected at different rates
   (3) Decreased blood supply to organs and loss of elasticity of collagen fibers cause changes in organ systems

c. Systemic
   (1) Overall effect of aging is seen in altered body functions, usually in the direction of deterioration
   (2) The ability of certain immune cells (lymphocytes) to kill tumor cells decreases markedly, beginning in the fifth decade of life
   (3) Neutrophils (immune cells) that fight acute infection become less efficient with advanced age
   (4) Natural antibodies decline, affecting antibody-antigen responses
   (5) Decrease in dietary nutrients also adversely affects the competency of the immune system

2. Specific physiological alterations

a. Body composition
   (1) Decreased lean body mass and total body water
   (2) Lean body mass is replaced by fat
   (3) Plasma volume increases and extravascular volume decreases; this increases vulnerability to fluid and electrolyte imbalances
   (4) Decreased total plasma albumin

b. Cardiovascular system
   (1) Thickening and sclerosis of heart valves may cause early systolic murmur or S_4
   (2) Decreased elasticity of myocardium as some muscle fibers are replaced by fibrotic collagen, and others become hypertrophied

(3) Decreased muscle tone, pumping effectiveness, stroke volume, and, therefore, decreased cardiac output
(4) Decreased cardiac output results in decreased perfusion of all major organ systems
(5) Decreased response to stress and ß-adrenergic stimulation
(6) Decreased blood vessel resiliency
(7) Thickening of blood vessels
(8) Increased peripheral vascular resistance
(9) Increased systolic and diastolic blood pressures, which may cause misinterpretation of signs of shock

c. Respiratory
(1) Decreased number of functioning alveoli for gas exchange
(2) Decreased elasticity and increased rigidity of lungs with collagen cross-linking
(3) Increased size and stiffening of trachea and bronchi
(4) Increased work of breathing increases oxygen demands
(5) Decreased respiratory muscle strength can impair effectiveness of the cough reflex
(6) Decreased forced expiratory volume
(7) Increased functional residual capacity, residual volume, and dead space
(8) Decreased depth of respirations
(9) Decreased rib cage expansion
(10) Decreased PaO_2 (80 mm Hg or lower); decreased sensitivity to changes in PaO_2 and $PaCO_2$

d. Kidney/bladder
(1) Decreased renal blood flow and lowered glomerular filtration rate (may decline by half by age 90) lead to a decreased effectiveness of the kidneys in ridding body of urea, dangerous toxins, and other substances (1); requires consideration in regulating dosage of drugs excreted by kidney
(2) Decreased number of functioning nephrons
(3) Decreased tubular excretory capacity
(4) Decreased ability to concentrate urine and decreased response to vasopressin may result in hypernatremia
(5) Serum creatinine normal, but urine creatinine clearance is decreased
(6) Decreased muscle tone, which reduces the bladder's capacity for holding urine

e. Liver
(1) Decreases in size but minimal changes in function
(2) May decrease drug metabolism
(3) May decrease synthesis of plasma proteins and clotting factors

f. Gastrointestinal tract
(1) Decreased secretions, e.g., salivary, gastric
(2) Slightly decreased absorption
(3) Decreased intestinal enzymes
(4) Decreased active transport
(5) Decreased peristalsis may result in constipation
(6) Decreased anal sphincter tone
(7) Achlorhydria and delayed gastric emptying
(8) Atrophy of gums with loss of teeth or decay

(9) Dry mouth
(10) Diminished esophageal peristalsis and delayed emptying cause premature feeling of fullness
(11) Diminished gag reflex

g. Endocrine/metabolic
(1) Decreased secretion of glucocorticoids resulting in decreased response to stress
(2) Decreased secretion of other hormones such as aldosterone and estrogen
(3) Delayed insulin release by the pancreas and reduced peripheral sensitivity to insulin produce decreased glucose tolerance
(4) Decrease in body's normal negative feedback system
(5) Decreased thyroid function; however, hypothyroidism is not a common finding
(6) Decreased response of immune system, e.g., by age 60, thymic hormones are completely absent
(7) Shift from anabolic to catabolic activity due to decreased gonadal steroids

h. Nervous system
(1) Decreased cerebral blood flow and brain metabolism; loss of cerebral neurons
(2) Increased fragility of cerebral blood vessels allows minor trauma to cause bleeding with delayed symptoms
(3) Decreased short-term and long-term memory
(4) Motor neurons decline, affecting reaction time and decreasing coordination
(5) Decreased threshold for chemical depressants
(6) Decreased number and sensitivity of sensory receptors in the central nervous system results in reduced pain perception
(7) Slowed reflexes may be partially due to inelastic tendons and other changes in related tissues
(8) Decreased conduction velocity
(9) Decreased central ability to regulate body temperature and adapt to heat and cold
(10) Senile dementia or Alzheimer's disease may occur

i. Musculoskeletal system
(1) Muscle fibers become smaller and fewer; wasting of muscle tissue results in decreased muscle strength
(2) Decreased joint flexibility and range of motion; joint pain due to arthritis
(3) Decreased bone mass and increased bone fragility due to demineralization and osteoporosis; changes are greater in females than males
(4) Thinning of intervertebral discs and vertebrae
(5) Deterioration of cartilage

j. Skin
(1) Decreased sebaceous gland activity results in increased dryness; coupled with thinning, dry skin becomes more vulnerable to trauma
(2) Decreased adipose tissue to cushion bony prominences
(3) Decreased blood supply to the skin results in slower healing, if integrity is interrrupted
(4) Loss of body hair
(5) Less sensitivity to heat and cold

(6) Alterations in appearance affect identity and self-esteem

3. Response to pharmacologic agents

a. Sensitivity to drug actions increases with age
(1) Changes in receptor activity may be responsible
(2) Decline in cellular viability and homeostatic mechanisms may also contribute

b. Increased sensitivity to depressant action of medications such as morphine, diazepam, and chlordiazepoxide

c. Altered absorption results from
(1) Increased gastric pH
(2) Decreased intestinal blood flow (40 to 50%)
(3) Possible decrease in number of absorptive cells
(4) Delayed gastric emptying
(5) Reduced gastrointestinal motility caused by some drugs
(6) Weak acid drugs, e.g., barbiturates, are not well-absorbed

d. Emotional stress and aging can decrease efficiency of gastric emptying, thus decreasing absorption of drugs that are mildly basic, e.g., diazepam, L-dopa

e. Changes in body weight and composition have been associated with changes in drug concentrations and distribution, and, thus, drug action
(1) Total body fluid decreases significantly with age; between ages 30 and 80, total body fluid decreases approximately 20% in males and 15% in females
(2) A change in this volume, coupled with a change in the elimination rate of a drug, can affect drug clearance and result in prolonged drug half-life

f. Metabolically active tissue is replaced by fatty tissue, although there may be no weight change; adipose tissue and lean tissue decrease with age
(1) Such drugs as chlorpromazine, diazepam, and phenobarbital may be stored in fatty tissue to a larger extent in the elderly; if such drugs are prescribed solely on the basis of body weight, the elderly may exhibit increased effects due to existing stores
(2) The volume of distribution for water-soluble drugs decreases

g. Albumin levels fall and gamma globulin levels rise with advanced age; therefore, effects of drugs that bind to protein may be altered

h. Decreased drug metabolism and elimination

4. Altered response to stress

a. Decreased immunocompetence lowers the body's ability to respond to stress, e.g., the elderly have lowered resistance to infection

b. Decreased perfusion of the endocrine organs retards body's normal negative feedback system

c. Epinephrine and norepinephrine secretion is decreased

d. Stress levels remain heightened long after stress is relieved

5. Presence of chronic disease—most persons over 65 are affected by at least one chronic disease that may alter response to trauma; however, the current literature is inconclusive

6. Altered perception

a. Decreased number and sensitivity of central sensory receptors diminishes temperature and pain sensation, and tactile discrimination

b. Visual changes
(1) Decreasing peripheral and night vision
(2) Increased eyelid droop, tearing, and deterioration of blood vessels

(3) Lens yellows and becomes cloudy, which causes problems with color vision (blues and greens may be hard to distinguish)
(4) Pupils become smaller, decreasing the amount of light reaching the retina and reducing visual acuity in dim light
(5) Eyes take longer to accommodate to darkness and glare
(6) Altered depth perception

c. Auditory changes
(1) Decreased number of sensitive cells in cochlea
(2) Thinning of tympanic membrane
(3) Slowed impulse transmission in the auditory nerve
(4) Increased rigidity of small bones of the middle ear
(5) Inability to hear high-frequency sounds often results from degeneration in the cochlea (presbycusis)
(6) Decreased fluid in innner ear may affect balance

d. Gustation and olfaction become less acute
(1) Tastes are diminished, especially salt and sweet
(2) Diminished olfaction decreases awareness of environmental warning signals, e.g., gas or smoke

7. **Psychomotor performance decreases with aging, including slowed reaction time, and decreased speed and accuracy in movement**
8. **Psychological changes**

a. Progressive slowing of response to verbal instruction
b. Learning may be hindered due to decreased short-term memory
c. Depression may be common due to alterations in naturally occurring chemicals and hormones, and changes in levels of neurotransmitters, e.g., monoamine oxidase (MAO) and serotonin increase with age, while norepinephrine decreases
d. Fewer periods of deep sleep in the elderly may predispose them to disorientation when hospitalized
e. Effectiveness of coping mechanisms may decrease
f. Many aged clients have decreased support systems due to loss or distant location of friends and family

B. PATTERNS OF INJURY

1. **Falls are the most frequent cause of injury and the leading cause of death from injury in the elderly**

a. Falls result from a combination of age-related changes, pathological states, and environmental hazards
b. Approximately 30% of elderly persons who live at home fall each year; increased age leads to more frequent falls and more injuries
c. Of those hospitalized for a fall, only half will be alive one year later
d. Women are twice as likely to fall as men
e. Most elderly persons have some type of abnormality in the lower limbs which predisposes them to falls

f. Common injuries associated with falls include fractures (hip, pelvis, rib, proximal humerus, or Colles' fracture of the wrist), head injury with subdural hematoma, and soft tissue trauma

2. Thermal injuries are associated with high mortality in the elderly

a. Scalds from tap water are most common cause
b. Flame burns from clothing ignition associated with the use of cigarettes and matches or lighters, or from cooking, are also common
c. The survival potential for the elderly burn victim is only one-half that of a similarly injured middle-aged person

3. Motor vehicle crashes are the most common cause of death from injury among those aged 65 to 74

a. Injuries occur in all classes of road users, including motorcyclists
b. Serious pedestrian injuries occur frequently among the elderly; older pedestrians often walk directly into the path of oncoming vehicles due to coexisting confusional state, or impairment of visual or auditory acuity

4. Mortality is higher in the elderly for every body region injured

5. Mortality from injury in the elderly increases with age, up to 85 years; after this age, there is a slight decrease

a. Ages 65 to 74 years—50% due to falls, 20% MVC, and 8% burns
b. Ages 75 years or older—33% due to falls, 25% MVC, and 8% burns (1)

C. NURSING ASSESSMENT AND COMMON FINDINGS RELATED TO AGING

1. Cardiovascular

a. Fatigue, dizziness, orthostatic hypotension, and history of falls due to decreased cardiac output and poor vascular response to position change
b. Blood vessels lose elasticity, which increases peripheral resistance; increased systolic and diastolic pressures
c. Hypertension, which may mask volume deficits in early stages of shock
d. Early systolic murmur; S_4
e. ECG alterations due to preexisting cardiac changes; premature beats and arrythmias from conduction deficiencies
f. Peripheral edema
g. Distended neck veins
h. Cardiac monitoring, 12-lead ECG, and hemodynamic monitoring may be used more frequently in the elderly, due to chronic cardiovascular impairment and instability

2. Pulmonary

a. Decreased breath sounds in both bases
b. Decreased chest excursion and depth of respirations
c. Increased anterior-posterior diameter of the chest
d. Decreased ability to mobilize and expectorate secretions due to decreased cough reflex and diminished ciliary effectiveness
e. ABGs reveal decreased PaO_2 (80 mm Hg or lower)
f. Reduced pulmonary function, including vital capacity

3. Neurological

a. Cognitive assessment may be altered due to senile dementia, Alzheimer's disease, or slowed response to sensory overload
b. Delayed signs or symptoms of minor head injury and intracranial bleeding
c. Vague headache or confusion, which may present weeks after injury
d. Altered pain threshold; diminished response to painful event
e. Slowed reaction time
f. Sleep disturbed by wakeful periods; may nap frequently
g. Depressed affect

4. Musculoskeletal

a. Limitation of joint movement and flexibility, and muscle strength
b. Pain on joint movement
c. Preexisting deformity of spine or joints due to osteoarthritis
d. Kyphosis
e. Diminished balance; unsteady gait

5. Renal, metabolism, fluids, and nutrition

a. Modest elevation in BUN and serum creatinine
b. Dehydration
c. Low serum albumin
d. Increased nocturia; frequency and urgency of urination
e. Difficulty initiating urination in males; stress incontinence in females

6. Psychosocial considerations and interview strategies

a. Ask simple questions in straightforward manner; provide sufficient time so client can comprehend and answer without being rushed
b. Consider possible visual and auditory deficits in approach to client
c. Attempt to eliminate noise and other distractions from environment during interview
d. Avoid prejudice and stereotyping of elderly
e. Evaluate reliability as historian; if indicated, interview significant other/family member, as soon as possible, concerning past health history of patient, medications, allergies, social situation

7. Perioperative assessment

a. Shock is a greater risk for the elderly; patient must be monitored frequently
b. Assess for hypothermia due to decreased thermoregulation in the elderly
c. Be alert to untoward effects of anesthetics and analgesics due to altered drug metabolism
d. Assess for sequelae of operative position, e.g., pulmonary, circulatory, and skin complications

D. NURSING DIAGNOSES, EXPECTED OUTCOMES, AND INTERVENTIONS

1. Fluid volume deficit, actual or potential, related to preexisting dehydration

a. Expected outcomes
   (1) Urine output 0.5 to 1.5 ml/kg/hr
   (2) Vital signs within normal limits

(3) Serum electrolytes within normal range
(4) Mucous membranes moist
(5) Skin turgor improved

b. Nursing interventions
(1) Monitor urine output
(2) Assess urine quality, including specific gravity and color
(3) Evaluate laboratory data, including urinalysis, specific gravity, serum creatinine, BUN, and electrolytes, especially sodium
(4) Assess for signs of dehydration; check mucous membranes and skin turgor
(5) Administer oral and/or parenteral fluids, usually 1500 to 2000 ml/day
(6) Monitor weight
(7) Encourage slow movement upon rising, or when changing position, to prevent orthostatic hypotension

2. Fluid volume excess related to ineffective cardiac/renal function

a. Expected outcomes
(1) Vital signs within normal limits
(2) Flat neck veins
(3) CVP less than 15 mm H_2O
(4) Breath sounds clear
(5) Absence of peripheral edema

b. Nursing interventions
(1) Monitor hemodynamic status closely, including apical and peripheral pulses, blood pressure (both arms), CVP, PAWP
(2) Monitor cardiac rhythm and observe for arrythmias
(3) Assess for signs of peripheral edema or distended neck veins
(4) Auscultate lungs for rales and decreased breath sounds
(5) Maintain strict intake and output
(6) Elevate legs to reduce peripheral edema
(7) Teach patient to avoid constricting garters, knee highs, or rolled stockings
(8) Teach patient to do leg exercises or do passive exercises

3. Alteration in nutrition, less than body requirements, related to preexisting inadequate nutritional intake

a. Expected outcomes
(1) Albumin levels within normal limits
(2) Weight within normal limits
(3) Caloric intake meets calculated needs
(4) Wound healing normal

b. Nursing interventions
(1) Assess for dental problems; obtain consultation, as needed
(2) Obtain information on diet and social history
(3) Obtain nutritional consultation to calculate client's nutrient needs
(4) Assist with feeding patient orally, via gastric or enteral tube, or parenterally
(5) Monitor for choking; encourage semisolid foods and small meals; keep patient upright for one hour after meals, if possible
(6) Encourage diet that provides adequate protein and calories to meet energy needs; minimize fat and caffeine, and provide adequate fiber and fluids
(7) Obtain appropriate social service intervention to ensure adequate food availability upon discharge

4. Decreased cardiac output related to ineffective myocardial function and cardiac failure

a. Expected outcomes
   (1) Cardiac output approaches normal
   (2) Vital signs within normal limits
   (3) Patient tolerates progressive activity
   (4) Peripheral pulses palpable
   (5) Skin warm with adequate capillary refill

b. Nursing interventions
   (1) Monitor vital signs; take apical pulse for one full minute; note rhythm on ECG
   (2) Measure cardiac output frequently
   (3) Measure urine output frequently
   (4) Assess peripheral pulses
   (5) Check orthostatic blood pressure
   (6) Auscultate heart sounds
   (7) Assess for signs of peripheral insufficiency, including cyanosis, diaphoresis, decreased skin temperature
   (8) Observe for syncopal episodes

5. Altered physical mobility related to decreased muscle strength, arthritic changes, joint contractures

a. Expected outcomes
   (1) Patient maintains premorbid range of motion
   (2) Patient regains muscle strength sufficient for activities of daily living

b. Nursing interventions
   (1) Assess range of motion of major joints
   (2) Obtain physical therapy consultation
   (3) Encourage active range of motion of joints, several times daily
   (4) Provide muscle strengthening activities in collaboration with physical therapist
   (5) Assist patient to turn in bed and/or sit in chair, as tolerated
   (6) Ambulate as early as possible; provide assistive devices, e.g., cane, walker, as needed
   (7) Protect from injury, e.g., side rails, dry floors, good lighting

6. Potential unrecognized infection due to absence or decrease in usual signs secondary to aging

a. Expected outcomes
   (1) Blood and other body fluid cultures negative
   (2) Wounds appear clean
   (3) Absence of subtle signs of infection
   (4) Lungs clear

b. Nursing interventions
   (1) Be alert to subtle signs of infection, e.g., changes in mental status, increased pulse and respirations, patient complaint of not feeling well, vague complaints of pain
   (2) Auscultate lungs for decreased breath sounds
   (3) Observe urine for cloudiness
   (4) Initiate deep breathing and incentive spirometry; encourage coughing to raise secretions
   (5) Report signs of redness, warmth, tenderness, odor, drainage around wound sites

(6) Closely monitor all culture reports
(7) Administer prophylactic antibiotics, as prescribed

7. **Potential altered thought processes related to slowed cognitive function, unfamiliar surroundings and people**

a. Expected outcomes
(1) Patient provides appropriate responses in conversation
(2) Patient demonstrates orientation to persons, places, things
(3) Patient regains premorbid memory, as confirmed by family and significant others

b. Nursing interventions
(1) Introduce self to patient, speak slowly and distinctly, and stand within patient's visual field
(2) Orient patient to elements in the environment; repeat as needed
(3) Allow patient time for response when queried; eliminate distractions when possible
(4) Utilize memory aids and auditory or visual stimulation, as needed
(5) Have family bring in familiar objects so patient can identify with them
(6) Repeat instructions and questions by using short sentences; allow sufficient time for response
(7) Maintain client safety by using side rails and restraints, as needed
(8) Provide empathy, comfort, and security

8. **Altered sensory perception (auditory, olfaction, visual, tactile) related to physiological changes associated with aging**

a. Expected outcomes
(1) Patient's safety is maintained
(2) Patient interacts with environment and uses appropriate aids, as needed (glasses, hearing aid, cane)
(3) Patient is aware of, and interested in, environment with minimal boredom, confusion, disorientation

b. Nursing interventions
(1) Assess client's perception of sound, smell, sight, touch, pressure, pain, and temperature
(2) Speak clearly and loudly; face the patient
(3) Provide adequate lighting
(4) Provide vision and hearing aids, as needed
(5) Carefully monitor use of cold or warm compresses
(6) If soft extremity restraints are used, assess neurovascular status every hour
(7) Touch patient gently, but firmly, to provide contact and recognition
(8) Be alert to pain indicators such as facial expressions, vocalizations, body movement, decreased activity, changes in speech, and sudden onset of confusion

9. **Additional nursing diagnoses**

a. Sleep pattern disturbance related to new environment, medication effects, premorbid habits, insufficient daytime activity
b. Social isolation related to hospitalization, and lack of support persons and visitors
c. Impaired skin integrity related to immobility, effects of aging on skin, reduced protection over bony prominences, and decreased sensation
d. Self-care deficits (various) related to mental or physical sequelae of injury

e. Potential for injury related to diminished perception and fragile physiologic status
f. Powerlessness related to enforced immobility and dependence on health care providers

References

1. Schwab, C. W. (1987, May). Trauma in the elderly. Address given at Annual Meeting of the American Trauma Society, Washington, DC.
2. Andresen, G. (1989). A fresh look at assessing the elderly. *RN,* 52(6), 32.

Suggested Readings

Blair, K. A. (1990). Aging: Physiological aspects and clinical implications. *Nurse Practitioner, 15*(2), 14–28.

Bobb, J. (1987). Trauma in the elderly. *Journal of Gerontologic Nursing, 13*(11), 28–31.

Bobb, J. (1988). Trauma in the elderly. In V. D. Cardona, P. D. Hurn, P. J. B. Mason, A. B. Scanlon-Schlipp & S. W. Veise-Berry (Eds.), *Trauma nursing: From resuscitation through rehabilitation* (pp. 692–706). Philadelphia: W. B. Saunders Co.

Brunner, L., & Suddarth, D. (1988). *Textbook of medical-surgical nursing* (5th ed.). Philadelphia: J. B. Lippincott Co.

Fulmer, T., Street, S., & Carr, K. (1984). Abuse of the elderly: Screening and detection. *Journal of Emergency Nursing, 10*(3), 131–140.

Hamner, M. L., & Lalor, L. J. (1983). The aged patient in the critical care setting. *Focus on Critical Care, 10*(6), 22–29.

Lomb, K., Miller, J., & Hernandez, M. (1987). Falls in the elderly: Causes and prevention. *Orthopedic Nursing, 6*(2), 45–49.

McCaffery, M., & Beebe, A. (1989). *Pain: Clinical manual for nursing practice.* St. Louis: C. V. Mosby Co.

McCoy, G. F. (1989). Injury to the elderly in road traffic accidents. *Journal of Trauma, 29*(4), 494–497.

Rempsheski, V. F. (Ed.). (1989). Gerontology. *Nursing Clinics of North America, 24*(3).

Schuhman, B., & Acquanina, T. (1987). Falls in the elderly. *Nurse Practitioner, 12*(11), 30–37.

Smith, C. (1985). Trauma in the elderly. *Nursing Mirror, 16*(3), 36–39.

Tinetti, M. E., Williams, T. F., & Mayewski, R. (1986). Fall risk index for elderly patients based on number of chronic disabilities. *The American Journal of Medicine, 80*(March), 429–434.

Section V
Special Patient Populations

MODULE 31
SUBSTANCE USERS AND ABUSERS

Sally Boyle Quinn, MSN, RN, CEN

Prerequisite

Review substance abuse disorders, management, and withdrawal states. Review trauma nursing assessment and resuscitation.

Objectives

1.0 Define and differentiate between substance abuse, and dependence, tolerance, and withdrawal.
2.0 Discuss the relationship of substance abuse and dependence to trauma.
2.1 Discuss the role of alcohol and drugs in society.
2.2 Identify the incidence of drug and alcohol use in trauma patients.
3.0 Describe general medical management of the intoxicated trauma patient.
3.1 Identify the possible substance(s) ingested based on assessment data.
3.2 List antidotes available for specific drugs.
3.3 Discuss controversies in overdose management when the patient has sustained trauma.
3.4 Identify situations in which overdose therapies are contraindicated for the intoxicated trauma patient.
3.5 Describe special needs and considerations in trauma care for the intoxicated patient.
3.6 Develop realistic goals and outcomes for the trauma patient with a substance abuse or dependence problem.
3.7 List referral agencies, organizations, and health providers available to assist this patient.
4.0 Utilize the nursing process to care for specific types of intoxicated trauma patients.
4.1 Identify common nursing diagnoses seen in trauma patients who use drugs and/or alcohol.

4.2 Describe priority nursing measures based on this information.
4.3 Utilize this information to develop a plan of care specific to the alcohol-, opiate-, and/or cocaine-intoxicated patient who has sustained a traumatic injury.
4.4 Evaluate patient response to medical and nursing interventions.

A. OVERVIEW

1. Prevalence of drugs in society

a. United States citizens comprise a small percentage of the world's population, yet consume more than half of all illegal drugs
b. Alcohol remains the most common substance abused
c. Cocaine abuse is the fastest growing drug problem, currently exceeding heroin abuse
d. Substance abuse crosses all socioeconomic barriers

2. Prevalence in trauma

a. Alcohol
   (1) Alcohol plays a role in approximately 20 to 50% of all MVCs and is frequently linked to violent crimes (1)
   (2) Chronic abusers have higher than expected vehicular crash rates, even when sober
   (3) In MVCs, alcohol users have the same survival rate as the nonintoxicated, but tend to be more seriously injured
   (4) Alcoholics are more likely to die from falls than nonalcoholics; alcohol users are prone to falls and head injury and may have chronic subdural hematoma (2)
   (5) Alcohol precipitates more extensive injuries to brain and spinal cord in animal experiments comparing animals given ethanol I.V. vs animals given only saline (3)
b. Relationship of drugs other than alcohol to trauma is not well-established
   (1) Illegal drug use is highly associated with violence and subsequent trauma
   (2) Reports of cocaine-related trauma are increasing
   (3) Behavioral toxicity of PCP (phencyclidine) and altered sensorium associated with hallucinogens (LSD) predispose users to violence and injury to themselves, and those around them
   (4) Suicide is strongly related to alcohol and/or drug use
   (5) Altered judgment and sensorium while one is intoxicated increase risk-taking behavior

3. Mechanisms of injury vary; however, maintain a high index of suspicion with

a. MVC—suspect alcohol, marijuana, or cocaine
b. Accidental drownings—suspect alcohol or PCP
c. Bizarre crimes—suspect PCP
d. Gunshot wounds/stabbings—suspect cocaine or heroin
e. Suicides—suspect alcohol, sedative hypnotics, or hallucinogens
f. Falls/jumps—suspect alcohol, cocaine, or hallucinogens

B. DEFINITION OF TERMS

1. **Tolerance—increased amounts of the substance are required to achieve the desired effect**
2. **Withdrawal—objective and/or subjective symptoms as a direct result of cessation or reduced intake of the drug**
3. **Psychoactive substance abuse vs dependence** (4)

a. Abuse
   (1) Some symptoms have persisted for at least one month, or occurred repeatedly over a longer period of time
   (2) Person has never met the criteria for dependence
   (3) Person meets at least one of the following criteria
      (a) Continues use despite social, occupational, psychological, or physical problems caused or worsened by drug use
      (b) Uses substance recurrently, in physically hazardous situations

b. Dependence
   (1) Symptoms have existed for one month, or have occurred repeatedly over a longer period of time
   (2) Person meets at least three of the following criteria
      (a) Takes substance longer and in larger amounts than intended
      (b) Desires or attempts to cut down or control use
      (c) Spends great deal of time in drug activities (acquiring, using, or recovering from drug)
      (d) Is unable to meet role obligations at work, school, or home due to intoxication or withdrawal
      (e) Experiences social, occupational, or recreational dysfunction (failed marriage, loss of job)
      (f) Develops tolerance
      (g) Experiences withdrawal symptoms
      (h) Takes substance to prevent or relieve withdrawal symptoms

C. CLASSES OF PSYCHOACTIVE SUBSTANCES

Table 31.1

Classes of psychoactive substances

Substance	*Common Names*
Alcohol	Booze, liquor
Amphetamines	Speed, crank
Cannabis	MJ, pot, dope, grass
Cocaine	Coke, crack
Hallucinogens	Acid, LSD, mushrooms
Inhalants	Rush, glue, white-out
Opiates	Heroin (horse), Dilaudid (D's), Darvon
Phencyclidine	PCP, angel dust
Sedatives, hypnotics, anxiolytics	Downers, Valium

D. GENERAL MANAGEMENT OF THE INTOXICATED TRAUMA PATIENT

1. **All trauma patients should be suspected of drug use until proven otherwise**
2. **Golden rule: treat the patient, not the poison**
3. **Few antidotes exist (see Table 31.2)**

Table 31.2

Antidotes used for management of intoxicated patients

Drug	*Antidote*	*Action of Antidote*
Opiates	Naloxone (Narcan)	Reverses narcotic effects
Acetaminophen	N-acetylcysteine (Mucomyst)	Binds with toxic drug metabolites
Anticholinergics	Physostigmine	Reverses effect of anticholinergic agents
Cyanide	Cyanide kit (amyl nitrate, sodium nitrite, sodium thiosulfate)	Provides competitive ferric sites with which the cyanide can bind
Carbon monoxide	Oxygen	Displaces carboxyhemoglobin
	Hyperbaric therapy	Increases rate of carbon monoxide elimination

4. **Initial assessment and resuscitation of intoxicated trauma patients should follow ATLS guidelines (5)**
5. **Management of traumatic injuries may supersede, delay, or be in direct conflict with overdose or intoxication state therapies**
6. **Plan of care requires prioritization of both severity of traumatic injuries and severity of intoxication state**
7. **Adhere to universal precautions**

E. SPECIAL CONSIDERATIONS FOR THE INTOXICATED TRAUMA PATIENT

1. **Primary survey**

a. Assess and maintain airway and C-spine control
   (1) Assess patient's ability to protect airway from aspiration
      (a) Level of consciousness (LOC) may deteriorate during therapy; LOC is particularly important if vomiting is induced
      (b) Gag reflex
   (2) Intubate patients unable to protect airway

b. Assess and maintain breathing
   (1) Rate and rhythm of respirations

(a) Bradypnea common with
i) Depressant agents such as opiates, sedative hypnotics, and alcohol
ii) Carbon monoxide
iii) Cyanide
(b) Tachypnea common with
i) Central nervous system (CNS) stimulants such as amphetamines and cocaine
ii) Salicylate
iii) Theophylline
iv) Withdrawal states
v) Aspiration
(2) Depth of respirations may be inadequate
c. Assess and support circulation
(1) Pulse and blood pressure (BP)
(a) Hypertension and tachycardia common with
i) Amphetamines, cocaine, and PCP
ii) Adrenergics and anticholinergics
(b) Hypotension and bradycardia common with
i) CNS depressants such as opiates and sedative hypnotics
ii) Beta blockers
(2) Aggressively seek source of hypotension; do not make assumptions about the source
(a) If one assumes hypotension is due to drug ingestion, traumatic injury can be overlooked
(b) If one assumes hypotension is due to trauma, intoxication state can be overlooked
(3) Leading cause of hypotension in opiate overdose is volume depletion due to trauma
(4) Patients who have overdosed on sedative hypnotics or barbiturates may be volume depleted, if they have been unconscious for an extended period of time
d. Determine disability by a brief neurologic examination
(1) Assess pupils' size and reactivity
(a) Pupils generally pinpoint with depressant agents
(b) Reaction to light may be absent with barbiturate intoxication
(c) Pupils generally dilate with stimulant drugs
(d) Nystagmus may be present with PCP intoxication
(2) Behavior
(a) Behavior may range from severe agitation and violence to lethargy and coma
(b) Do not assume behavioral abnormalities are either solely drug- or solely trauma-related; may miss traumatic injuries and/or intoxication states
(3) Level of consciousness—assess patient's likelihood of maintaining consciousness throughout therapy

2. Resuscitation phase

a. Administer high flow humidified oxygen, particularly for convulsant or comatose patients
b. Ventilate

(1) Unconscious patient
(a) Establish airway; initiate ACLS/ATLS
(b) Establish I.V. access
(c) Administer Narcan
(d) Administer thiamine, 50% dextrose
(2) Conscious patient
(a) Ensure airway; monitor LOC
(b) Establish rapport; provide support
(c) Obtain brief history
(d) Administer emetic agents such as ipecac to induce vomiting
(e) Protect patient's airway when he/she vomits
(f) Evaluate response; repeat ipecac once, if no vomiting ensues

c. Control hemorrhage
(1) Identify source of hemorrhage
(2) Vital signs of patients in intoxicated states may differ from usual shock indicators
(3) Patient may be tachycardiac and hypotensive, with normovolemia, due to cocaine

d. Provide aggressive shock management
(1) Estimate volume loss
(2) I.V. access often difficult; prepare for cutdowns and central lines
(3) Obtain laboratory specimens for toxicology while starting I.V.; do not use alcohol to prepare skin when obtaining ethanol level
(4) Obtain core temperature
(5) Administer warmed I.V. fluids
(6) If no improvement in BP after 150 to 200 ml, hypotension may be due to
(a) Myocardial depressant ingestion
(b) Potent vasodilator ingestion
(c) Traumatic injuries
(7) Aggressive volume resuscitation may be fatal to the trauma patient who is hypotensive due to intoxication

e. Monitor ECG—12-lead or continous cardiac monitoring

3. Secondary survey

a. Continue to assess body temperature
(1) Hyperthermia common with
(a) CNS stimulants such as amphetamines, cocaine
(b) LSD, PCP
(c) Anticholinergics
(d) Salicylate
(2) Hypothermia common with
(a) CNS depressants such as opiates, alcohol, sedative hypnotics
(b) Carbon monoxide
(c) Cyanide
(d) Antipsychotics

b. Examine patient's personal belongings for clues of drug use

c. AMPLE history (see Module 19—Nursing Assessment)
(1) History often unobtainable
(2) Priority is to determine intent
(a) Accidental
(b) Intentional
(c) Consequential

(3) Intoxication state may mask or minimize pain complaints

4. Diagnostic studies

a. Laboratory specimens

(1) All trauma patients require toxicology screens; obtain urine, blood, and/or gastric specimens

(2) Tests may be quantitative (serum level) or qualitative (type of substance) in nature

(3) Various substances are degraded at different rates; qualitative toxicology results may indicate prior use, not current intoxication

(4) Be familiar with what your institution screens for and what is omitted

b. Radiographic evaluation to diagnose "body packer" syndrome

(1) Cocaine smugglers often package drugs in condoms and store in body orifices (rectum, vagina) or ingest them

(2) Body packers are at risk for massive overdose if condoms rupture or leak

(3) Syndrome is diagnosed by abdominal x-rays

5. Definitive care

a. Continue to evaluate LOC and vital signs

b. Continue supportive management

c. If patient is stable but unconscious, consider the following treatment options

(1) Infuse Narcan

(2) Lavage stomach—may require several liters

(a) Trauma-related contraindications to lavage include abdominal trauma, esophageal trauma, NPO for imminent procedure or surgery

(b) Position patient in left lateral decubitus position, with head lower than feet, for lavage, unless traumatic injuries preclude

(3) Administer activated charcoal via gastric tube

(4) Administer cathartics to empty lower bowel

d. If patient is stable and conscious, consider the following treatments

(1) Repeat ipecac, if second dose has not been given

(a) Trauma-related contraindications to induction of emesis include head injury, abdominal trauma, esophageal trauma, risk of seizures

(b) Lavage stomach if vomiting was not induced with second dose

(2) Give charcoal and/or cathartic p.o.

e. Behavioral management

(1) Protect self first, then protect patient from injury

(2) Provide reassurance and supportive care

(3) Use restraints

(a) Use restraints judiciously with PCP, amphetamines, cocaine, heroin, and marijuana intoxication, due to incidence of rhabdomyolysis

(b) Use restraints properly for intoxicated, uncooperative patients for the purpose of assessment and treatment; usually poses no significant legal issues

(c) Releasing uncooperative, agitated patients, without necessary care (even with signed release), poses significant legal liability

(4) Pharmacotherapy

(a) Administer Valium or similar benzodiazepine; usually effective in controlling patient's behavior

(b) Exercise caution with the use of Haldol or other drugs that decrease seizure threshold for patients at risk for seizures

(c) Paralyzing agents may be indicated for severe behavioral toxicity to
   i) Protect patient from further injury
   ii) Prevent worsening of existing injury (especially if C-spine not cleared)
   iii) Perform necessary procedures and diagnostic studies
(d) Evaluate patient's neurologic status prior to administration of pharmacologic agents
(e) Sedating the patient may increase the need for CAT scan or other diagnostic studies, since patient is not reliable

(5) Manage withdrawal state
   (a) Alcohol withdrawal can be complicated by delirium tremens, a life-threatening condition
   (b) Follow these steps for all withdrawal states
      i) Patient may be combative, destructive, or suicidal; provide safe, protective, supervised environment
      ii) Keep environment well-lighted to decrease sensory illusions
      iii) Keep environment calm
      iv) Lock windows; keep bed in low position
      v) Monitor vital signs for possible decompensation

(6) As traumatic injury improves, management of abuse/dependence problem assumes greater priority

(7) Evaluate for disposition; include psychiatric evaluation for all patients with suspected or known suicide intent

(8) Rehabilitation
   (a) Remember patient accessed system due to traumatic event, not for rehabilitation or detoxification; therefore, goals must be mutual and realistic
   (b) Do not discount the need for teaching or helping the patient to seek rehabilitation
   (c) Help patient identify the relationship between traumatic injury and drug usage (see Module 4—Prevention of Trauma)
   (d) Encourage and involve family and significant other in care of patient
   (e) Initiate appropriate referrals
      i) Social service
      ii) Psychiatry
      iii) Support groups
         a) Alcoholics Anonymous
         b) Narcotics Anonymous
         c) Cocaine Anonymous
      iv) Drug and alcohol treatment programs, both outpatient and residential
      v) Family and child welfare services
      vi) Public assistance services

F. NURSING DIAGNOSES, EXPECTED OUTCOMES, AND INTERVENTIONS

1. Potential for injury related to altered sensorium, seizure activity, behavior abnormalities, withdrawal syndromes, thermal abnormalities, and/or drug toxicity

a. Expected outcomes
  (1) No secondary injuries occur while patient is hospitalized
  (2) Acute withdrawal symptoms are absent while patient is hospitalized
  (3) Intoxication state is identified; plan of care reflects injury prevention methods
b. Nursing interventions
  (1) Maintain high index of suspicion for drug use
  (2) Protect self and patient
  (3) Monitor lab data (electrolytes, glucose, magnesium, calcium, ABGs, toxicology results) for abnormalities that may cause or increase risk of seizures
  (4) Monitor neurological status—should improve over time, not deteriorate
  (5) Protect patient during seizures, especially C-spine and fracture sites
  (6) Monitor renal function (due to incidence of rhabdomyolysis)
  (7) Obtain core body temperature; implement cooling measures or rewarming, as indicated
  (8) Do not administer aspirin for fever, if patient is at risk for coagulopathy or actively bleeding (alcohol user)
  (9) Anticipate and administer pharmacologic therapy
    (a) If patient is unconscious or exhibits decreased LOC, and traumatic injuries do not preclude pharmacologic therapy, administer
      i) Narcan
        a) Opiate reversal may produce hypertension, tachycardia, nausea, and vomiting
        b) Use with caution in the head-injured patient
      ii) Thiamine
      iii) Dextrose—administer thiamine prior to dextrose, if patient is a known or suspected alcohol user, to prevent Wernicke-Korsakoff syndrome
    (b) If patient is conscious and traumatic injuries do not preclude, administer emetic agent, e.g., ipecac
    (c) Charcoal, cathartics
    (d) Valium
    (e) Antiepileptics
    (f) Paralyzing agents (avoid succinylcholine in cocaine user—may precipitate cocaine toxicity)
    (g) Antidotes
  (10) Protect patient's airway during episodes of vomiting and gastric lavage
  (11) Assess patient for risk of withdrawal and implement plan as appropriate (anesthesia and pain management can delay onset of withdrawal)
  (12) Protect patient from falls
  (13) Restrain as necessary
  (14) Administer Haldol and/or Ativan with caution (lowers seizure threshold)
  (15) Decrease patient's anxiety and agitation by reassuring and providing clear explanations of happenings (intoxicated patients may not recall events or understand why they are now hospitalized)
  (16) Administer medications to prevent withdrawal, i.e., methadone

2. **Fluid volume deficit related to volume loss due to trauma and/or effects of substance use (nausea, vomiting, decreased p.o. intake, vasodilation)**

a. Expected outcomes

(1) Normovolemic state
(2) Etiology of fluid volume deficit known and treated

b. Nursing interventions
(1) Employ universal precautions
(2) Evaluate volume status; determine classification of shock (see Module 10—Shock)
(3) Assess for hidden sources of volume loss; if patient is intoxicated, complaints of pain may be minimal and patient's history unreliable, which makes assessment difficult
(4) Ensure I.V. access; prepare for cutdowns (I.V. access may be difficult)
(5) Obtain core body temperature prior to administration of warmed fluids or utilization of fluid-warming devices
(6) Administer appropriate fluids, including blood components as required
(7) Assess patient for signs and symptoms of pulmonary edema prior to and during fluid resuscitation (seen in opiate and cocaine intoxication)
(8) Evaluate patient response to fluid resuscitation (aggressive fluid resuscitation, without ongoing evaluation, may be harmful if hypotension is due to intoxication, or in the chronic alcoholic with cardiomyopathy)
(9) Monitor CBC and coagulation profile
(10) Administer phosphate, as prescribed (alcohol users may be phosphate depleted)

3. Infection, actual or potential, related to preexisting infection, e.g., AIDS, hepatitis, endo- or myocarditis, and/or immunosuppression

a. Expected outcomes
(1) Preexisting infectious states identified and treated
(2) No signs or symptoms of new infection posttrauma
(3) Afebrile with normal WBC
(4) Normal wound healing
(5) Negative cultures

b. Nursing interventions
(1) Assess patient for signs and symptoms of infection
(2) Use sterile technique for invasive procedures and dressing changes
(3) Isolate patient as appropriate; follow CDC recommendations
(4) Use universal precautions (even if patient is not an intravenous drug abuser (IVDA), substance abuse places patient at risk)
(5) Provide maximum nutrition (see Module 11—Nutrition)
(6) Additional interventions (see Module 13—Wound Healing—and Module 12—Infection)

4. Potential decreased myocardial tissue perfusion and dysrhythmias secondary to drug toxicity, endocarditis, or ischemia

a. Expected outcomes
(1) Normal sinus rhythm
(2) Dysrhythmias promptly identified and treated

b. Nursing interventions
(1) Assess for myocardial contusion; increased mortality is reported with alcohol intoxication (6)
(2) Assess patient's ability to identify and/or report chest pain
(3) Obtain 12-lead ECG and evaluate cardiac rhythm; lethal dysrhythmias are common (7)

(4) Prepare for administration of Valium for adrenergic crisis (cocaine toxicity)
(5) Monitor patient closely if beta blockers or nitrates are utilized, due to the hypotensive properties of these agents

5. **Additional nursing diagnoses**
a. Ineffective individual coping related to inadequate stress management skills, dependence on drugs, and/or low frustration tolerance
b. Potential for violence, self-directed or directed at others, related to CNS effects of chemicals, lack of impulse control, and/or impaired judgment, perception, and mental ability
c. Altered self-concept related to effects of alcohol, guilt, and/or depression
d. Altered nutrition, less than required, secondary to inadequate nutritional intake
e. Ineffective family coping related to alcohol and/or drug abuse
f. Ineffective thermoregulation related to intake of CNS stimulants or depressants
g. Potential for aspiration related to decreased LOC, emetic therapy, and/or noxious effects of alcohol and/or drugs

References

1. The National Committee for Injury Prevention and Control. (1989). *Injury prevention: Meeting the challenge* (pp. 119, 197). New York: Oxford University Press.
2. Hingson, R., & Howland, J. (1987). Alcohol as a risk factor for injury or death resulting from accidental falls: A review of the literature. *Journal of Studies on Alcohol, 48*(3), 212–219.
3. Brodner, R., Van Gilder, J., & Collins, W. (1981). Experimental spinal cord trauma: Potentiation by alcohol. *The Journal of Trauma, 21*(2), 124–129.
4. American Psychiatric Association. (1987). Psychoactive substance use disorders. In *Diagnostic and statistical manual of mental disorders* (rev. ed., pp. 165–185). Washington, DC: Author.
5. American College of Surgeons, Committee on Trauma. (1989). *Advanced trauma life support student manual.* Chicago: Author.
6. Nicholas, G., & DeMuth, W. (1980). Blunt cardiac trauma: The effect of alcohol on survival and metabolic function. *The Journal of Trauma, 20*(1), 58–60.
7. Stein, P., Sabbah, H., Przybylski, J., Goldberg, D., Hamid, M., & Viano, D. (1988). Effect of alcohol upon arrhythmias following nonpenetrating cardiac impact. *The Journal of Trauma, 28*(4), 465–471.

Suggested Readings

Boyle, S., & Strange, J. (1990). Practical management of the cocaine-intoxicated patient. *Trauma Quarterly, 6*(2), 27–37.

Cooper, K. (1989). Drug overdose. *American Journal of Nursing, 89*(9), 1146–1148.

Goldfrank, L., Flomenbaum, N., Lewin, N., Weisman, R., Howland, M., & Kulberg, A. (1986). *Toxicologic emergencies.* Norwalk, CT: Appleton-Century-Crofts.

Higgins, R. (1989). Cocaine abuse: What every emergency nurse should know. *Journal of Emergency Nursing, 15*(4), 318–324.

House, M. A. (1990). Cocaine. *American Journal of Nursing, 90*(4), 41–45.

Izor-Povenmire, K., & House, M. A. (1989). Acute crack cocaine intoxication: A case study. *Focus on Critical Care, 16*(2), 112–119.

Knezevich, B. A. (1986). Substance abuse. In B. A. Knezevich (Ed.), *Trauma nursing: Principles and practice* (pp. 387–403). Norwalk, CT: Appleton-Century-Crofts.

Rea, R., Bourg, P., Parker, J., & Rushing, D. (1987). *Emergency nursing core curriculum*. Philadelphia: W. B. Saunders Co.

Strange, J. M. (1987). Substance abuse in the trauma patient. In J. M. Strange (Ed.), *Shock trauma care plans* (pp. 204–205). Springhouse, PA: Springhouse Corp.

MODULE 32
ABUSED/BATTERED PERSONS

Elizabeth M. Blunt, MS, RN, CEN, EMT
Judith J. Stellar, MS, RN, CPNP

Objectives

1.0 **Identify specific factors that put individual at risk for abuse.**
1.1 List social, economic, and environmental factors that put an individual at risk for abuse.
1.2 Identify specific risk factors for particular patient populations.
2.0 **Describe common injuries found in battered persons.**
2.1 Explain the necessity of identifying injuries at various stages of healing.
2.2 Describe common patterns of injury resulting from abuse in children, adults, and the elderly.
3.0 **List factors that lead health care providers to suspect abuse.**
3.1 Explain the rationale behind being suspicious of injuries that are inconsistent with the patient history.
3.2 Recognize patient behaviors that lead health care providers to suspect nonaccidental trauma.
3.3 Identify patterns of injury that cause health care providers to suspect abuse.
4.0 **Describe the legal responsibilities of health care providers in reporting suspected abuse in specific patient populations.**
4.1 Identify state requirements for reporting suspected abuse.
4.2 List the responsibilities of the health care provider in filing abuse reports for each of the identified populations.

4.3 Explain the steps necessary to document suspected abuse.
4.4 List situations where "protected" custody is appropriate.
5.0 Describe procedures for recording and documenting physical, and emotional, signs and symptoms of abuse.
5.1 Briefly explain the rationale for documenting injuries.
5.2 Describe special considerations for photographing injuries resulting from suspected abuse.
5.3 Explain the need for informed consent for photography of adults.
5.4 Differentiate between objective and subjective findings in abusive injuries.
5.5 Recognize the importance of using a body map diagram for documenting injuries.
6.0 Identify the role of the multidisciplinary team in caring for the abused person.
6.1 List members of the multidisciplinary team.
6.2 Briefly describe the role of each team member.
6.3 Describe reporting procedures for each member of the team.
7.0 List prevention strategies for each specific population at risk for injury due to abuse/battery.
7.1 Explain the nurse's role in case finding through early identification of suspicious injuries and behaviors.
7.2 Explain the role of family counseling in abusive situations.
7.3 Explain the violence escalation theory and its role in early detection.
7.4 Describe strategies that aid prevention of abuse in each identified target population.
8.0 List appropriate assessment and intervention strategies for each segment of the abused population.
8.1 Given specific patient data, recognize which medical/surgical interventions may be required in the care of abused persons.
8.2 Given specific patient data, list equipment necessary for medical interventions.
8.3 Identify treatment goals related to optimal function.
9.0 Identify nursing diagnoses commonly found in trauma patients who have been abused.
10.0 Identify and prioritize nursing interventions required for patients who have injuries resulting from abuse.
11.0 Discuss the evaluation of patient response to treatment of injuries resulting from abuse.
11.1 Define expected patient outcomes with measurable criteria for each outcome.
11.2 List nursing activities required for continuous monitoring and evaluation of patient status.
11.3 List types of data to include in nursing documentation that contribute to evaluation of patient response to care.
12.0 Identify community resources that may be helpful to persons at risk for, or who have experienced, injuries from abuse.
12.1 List local, state, and national organizations involved in abuse prevention and education.
12.2 Cite trends in state and national efforts to prevent abuse.

A. GENERAL CONCEPTS

1. **Definition of abuse**
a. Children
(1) Physical abuse—nonaccidental injury of a child by a caretaker
(2) Neglect—acts of omission that affect the child's health and/or well-being
(3) Sexual abuse—sexual exploitation of a child by an adult caretaker
(4) Emotional abuse—severe verbal abuse and/or rejection of a child by an adult caretaker
b. Adults (including elderly)
(1) Physical abuse
(a) Inflicting physical harm
(b) Restraining an individual against his/her will
(c) Withholding basic physical care
(2) Emotional/verbal abuse
(a) Humiliation
(b) Intimidation
(c) Threats to leave and/or remove others
(d) Insults aimed at self-worth, religious beliefs, sex, race
(3) Sexual abuse
(a) Forcing unwanted sex acts
(b) Withholding sex or affection
(4) Destruction or withholding of property
(a) Personal possessions
(b) Money or goods
2. **Demographic characteristics of abuse**
a. Children
(1) Abuse occurs in all geographic areas, socioeconomic classes, and ethnic groups (1)
(2) Reporting is incomplete—case finding is more common in lower socioeconomic classes, while underreporting is more common in the more affluent sector
(3) Estimated cases per year in the U.S.—500,000 to 4,000,000
(a) Children under 3 years are most frequently abused
(b) Peaks of abuse occur at 6 months and 18 to 36 months, due to the demanding developmental tasks the child is accomplishing at these ages
(c) 10% of injuries in children under 5 years are presumed to result from abuse (2)
(4) Both sexes experience physical abuse; sexual abuse is reported to occur more frequently in girls
(5) Morbidity
(a) Neurologic damage occurs in 15% of abused children (1)
(b) 15 to 20% of abused children are rebattered, even if supervised (1)
(6) Mortality rate is reported at 2 to 11% of all abused children (1), or 1000 to 4000/year (3)
b. Adults
(1) 6,000,000 wives and 280,000 husbands are beaten each year in the U.S. (4)

(2) 16 to 30% of emergency department visits by women are abuse-related (5)
(3) In 53% of all spouse abuse families (male or female victims), children are also abused (6)
(4) Half of all rapes in women over 30 years old are part of an abusive episode (7)
(5) In the U.S., every 74 sec, a woman is beaten by her male partner (5)
(6) 4000 women die each year from battering (6)

c. Elderly
(1) Approximately 500,000 to 1,000,000 senior citizens are believed to be victims of domestic abuse each year (8)
(2) It is estimated that only one in six episodes of elder abuse is reported (9)
(3) "Benign neglect" is the most prevalent form of physical abuse (10)
(4) The typical abused elder is female, over 70 years of age, physically or mentally impaired, or both, and lives in the community with an adult child or other family member (10)
(5) Elder abuse is a nationwide problem, as signficant as child abuse (9)

3. Theoretical frameworks

a. Violence theory—phases are cyclical
(1) Tension building—characterized by verbal harassment, threats of abuse, and minor abusive incidents; victim often compliant or tries to stay out of the batterer's way, hoping that avoidance will prevent the batterer's anger from escalating
(2) Explosion or acute abusive episode—despite victim's efforts to maintain peace, small incidents escalate to an acute battering episode; most severe injuries occur during this period and police may be called
(3) Calm, loving respite—acute attack is followed by initial shock, denial, and disbelief; tension is gone and both batterer and victim try to rationalize what has happened—both minimize the seriousness of the injuries, genuinely believing that the attacker will never repeat the violence (11)

b. Power and control cycle (6)
(1) Physical abuse or threat of physical abuse is always present
(2) A cycle begins, including emotional abuse, sexual abuse, abusing children and pets, threats, economic abuse, intimidation, and isolation; can start at any point in the cycle (see Figure 32.1)

c. Stress/pathology model (12)
(1) Violence is a family affair, learned and transmitted in childhood, culturally supported, and provoked by stressors such as poverty and unemployment
(2) Violence circulates from family member to family member, until all domestic life is affected by the violence
(3) Assailants and victims are distinguished by a common profile—dependence, hostility, inability to communicate or empathize, and low self-esteem
(4) Alcoholism, depression, and drug addiction may both cause and/or result from abuse

4. Causative or risk factors (13)

a. Environmental stress factors
(1) Economic difficulty
(2) Poor housing
(3) Unemployment
(4) Illness

Figure 32.1

Power and control wheel. From E. Pence & M. Paymar, *Power and control: Tactics of men who batter.* Duluth, MN: Minnesota Program Development, Inc., Domestic Abuse Intervention Project. Reprinted with permission.

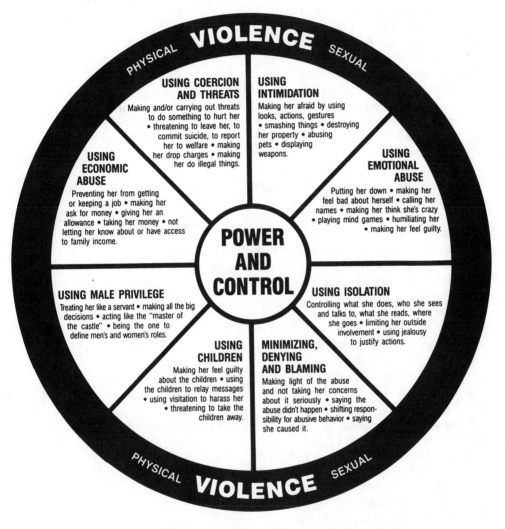

(5) Crowding

b. Psychological factors (caretaker)
   (1) Impulse disorder
   (2) Depression
   (3) Drug/alcohol abuse
   (4) Psychosis
   (5) Retardation

c. Parenting factors
   (1) Lack of preparation
   (2) Poor role models; abused as a child
   (3) Unrealistic expectations of child
   (4) Use of corporal punishment
   (5) Unsupportive spouse
   (6) Inconsistent parenting
d. Child-related factors
   (1) Premature birth
   (2) Chronic illness
   (3) Mental retardation; developmental delay
   (4) Triggering behaviors, e.g., crying of a "colicky" baby, incontinence in a toddler
e. Social factors
   (1) Social isolation
   (2) Distant or absent extended family
   (3) High societal expectations of parents
   (4) Domestic violence
   (5) Children in foster care
f. Cultural factors
   (1) Belief that violence is an acceptable way to attain goals
   (2) Belief that women and children are subservient

5. Barriers to leaving an abusive situation

a. Situational
   (1) Economic dependency, e.g., of woman on spouse
   (2) Fear of physical injury
   (3) Lack of knowledge or fear of judicial system
   (4) Fear of losing custody of children
   (5) Lack of affordable, available housing
   (6) Lack of job skills
   (7) Social isolation
   (8) Lack of knowledge about, and access to, available resources
b. Emotional
   (1) Helplessness and powerlessness
   (2) Fear other family members cannot survive alone
   (3) Guilt about failed relationships
   (4) Belief that abuser will change
   (5) Fear of physical or emotional harm to self or others
   (6) Anger at self for being too weak to leave

6. Reporting of abuse

a. Children
   (1) Since 1970, all states have had child abuse reporting laws
   (2) Since 1974, all states have had child abuse treatment acts
   (3) Teachers, social workers, and all health professionals, including physicians and nurses, are required to report suspected child abuse
      (a) These individuals are held liable for failing to report child abuse
      (b) Penalties vary from fines to criminal indictment
b. Adult

(1) Many states have some form of mandatory reporting
(2) Adults may choose to return to a potentially unsafe environment

c. Elderly
(1) 17 states have specific elder abuse laws
(2) 34 states include elder abuse as part of a more general protective services statute (14)

B. PATTERNS OF INJURY

1. Skin

a. Bruises, contusions
(1) Normal bruises tend to be peripherally located, e.g., knees, shins, forehead, elbows, over bony prominences
(2) Inflicted bruises have characteristic locations; injury patterns are significantly different from those whose injuries are from nonabusive causes; body map provides framework for assessment of abuse
(a) Children—centrally located
i) Buttocks, genitals
ii) Lower back
iii) Abdomen
iv) Face (cheek)
v) Neck (circumferential bruising or rope burns from choking)
vi) Upper lip and frenulum (lacerations from forced feeding)
(b) Adults and elderly
i) Face and neck
ii) Head
iii) Arms
iv) Breasts
v) Back and buttocks
vi) Abdomen
vii) Legs
viii) Genitals
(3) Bruises at various stages of healing may indicate a repeated pattern of abuse
(a) Red or reddish-blue—bruise is not more than 24 hrs old
(b) Dark purple or blue—bruise is 5 to 7 days old
(c) Yellow, brown—bruise is 7 to 10 days old
(d) Skin may clear (no bruise apparent) within 1 to 3 weeks

b. Burns
(1) Sharply demarcated scald burns indicate a patient has been forcefully held in water
(2) Water temperature above 54°C (130°F) causes a full-thickness burn in 30 sec
(3) Degloving scald burn of lower extremities (called "stocking feet effect") is characteristic of abuse; may also occur in upper extremities
(4) Contact or pattern of burns from iron, lighter, cigarette also common

c. Bizarre or unusual marks

(1) Human hand or bite marks
(2) Pattern marks—belt buckles, straps, wooden spoons
(3) Circumferential neck marks or friction burns
(4) Skin breakdown—decubiti inconsistent with other physical signs
(5) Marks caused by restraints at wrists, ankles, chest, arms

d. Skin injuries account for over 50% of injuries in child abuse

2. Head injury—leading cause of death in child abuse; accounts for 15% of injuries in children

a. Children
(1) External injuries
(a) Scalp bruises
(b) Subgaleal hematomas
(c) Traumatic alopecia
(2) Skull fractures
(a) Etiology—a direct blow
(b) Highly suspicious in children under 1 year old; bone of skull is pliable and not yet fused; requires a great deal of energy to fracture skull bones
(3) Intracerebral injury
(a) Subarachnoid hemorrhages
(b) Epidural hematomas (rare)
(c) Subdural hematomas (common)
i) Etiology—direct blow
a) Occurs with skull fractures
b) Associated with external trauma—scalp swelling, bruising
c) May exhibit concomitant retinal hemorrhage
ii) Etiology—violent shaking ("shaken baby syndrome") (15)
a) No skull fracture
b) No external trauma
c) Diagnostic indicator—retinal hemorrhage in all children
d) Concomitant long bone fractures in 25%
e) Bilateral rib fractures in some
f) Grasp marks on upper arms and/or chest in some patients
g) Usual presentation
(i) Lethargy, seizures, signs of sepsis
(ii) Negative physical examination in most patients, except for retinal hemorrhages
(iii) Gross blood on lumbar puncture
(iv) CAT scan of head shows occipital contusion and intrahemispheric blood

b. Adult and elderly
(1) External injuries
(a) Scalp bruises
(b) Subgaleal hematomas
(c) Traumatic alopecia
(2) Skull fractures
(a) Etiology—direct blow
(b) Basilar fractures manifested by raccoon's eyes and Battle's sign
(3) Intracerebral injuries

(a) Subarachnoid hemorrhages
(b) Epidural hematomas
(c) Subdural hematomas
i) Etiology—direct blow
a) Occurs with skull fractures
b) Associated with external trauma—scalp swelling, bruising
ii) Usual presentation
a) Lethargy, seizures, signs of sepsis
b) CAT scan of head shows occipital contusion and intrahemispheric blood

3. **Skeletal injuries**
a. Children—8% of injuries in abused children are skeletal
(1) Types of fractures
(a) Transverse fractures—from a direct blow
(b) Spiral fractures—from torsion or twisting; suspicious in nonambulatory child
(c) Metaphyseal chip fractures—most commonly due to abuse in form of violent pulling, yanking
(d) Subperiosteal hematomas—from direct trauma to bone
(2) Location of fracture
(a) Accidental—clavicle, dislocation of radial head
(b) Inflicted
i) Sternum
ii) Scapula
iii) Long bone fracture in very young children, especially under one year old
iv) Bilateral rib fractures—result from squeezing, crushing
b. Adults and elderly—no discernible fracture pattern
c. Age of fracture (all groups)
(1) Soft tissue injury—first 2 to 3 days after traumatic event
(2) Callous formation of long bone—7 to 10 days after injury
(3) Complete healing—varies with age; may take a few weeks in young child and months in adult
(4) A suspicious fracture indicates the need for a total body survey to rule out other earlier fractures

4. **Abdominal injuries**
a. Etiology—usually a direct blow (blunt trauma)
b. Account for 2% of inflicted injuries in children; second leading cause of death
c. Solid organ injuries (liver, spleen, kidney, pancreas)
(1) Fracture
(2) Laceration
(3) Contusion
(4) Hematoma
(5) Rupture
d. Hollow organ injuries (small and large bowel)
(1) Perforation—occurs when bowel is pinned between two fixed objects, i.e., striking agent and the spine
(2) Hematoma of bowel wall—almost exclusively seen in children

(a) Duodenum most common site
(b) Results in acute or chronic obstruction; patient usually afebrile with persistent bilious vomiting

e. Abdominal vessels and mesentery may also be injured
f. Presentation
  (1) Children and elderly—frequently delayed in seeking care; may present in acute shock, sepsis, or with peritonitis due to complications of abdominal trauma, rather than from the trauma itself
  (2) Adults—do not delay seeking treatment; complain of abdominal trauma but may not give accurate account of mechanism of injury

5. Genital trauma

a. Children
  (1) Rarely complain or present with physical findings
  (2) When present, physical findings include
    (a) Bruising, tenderness, bleeding, lacerations/tears
    (b) Vaginal, urethral, and/or rectal discharge
    (c) Venereal disease
    (d) Pregnancy in young adolescent
  (3) Emotional manifestations are more common
    (a) Sleep disturbances
    (b) Fear
    (c) Behavioral problems
    (d) Withdrawal, depression
    (e) Guilt

b. Adult and elderly
  (1) Adults usually present with multiple physical findings
    (a) External
      i) Bruises, scratches, other marks, and skin wounds
      ii) Blood, edema, lacerations, visible secretions, foreign objects in genital or rectal area
    (b) Internal
      i) Lacerations, semen, lesions, and foreign objects in vagina, cervix, or vault
      ii) Injuries or foreign bodies in rectum
    (c) Associated oropharyngeal injury possible
  (2) Emotional manifestations
    (a) Suicide attempts
    (b) Depression or hysteria
    (c) Drug and alcohol abuse
    (d) Powerlessness

C. MEDICAL AND SURGICAL PRIORITIES AND INTERVENTIONS

1. Perform primary assessment
2. Resuscitate and treat life-threatening injuries
3. Perform secondary assessment

4. Obtain diagnostic studies (13)

a. Laboratory
   (1) Blood studies—based on specific injuries
      (a) CBC, platelets, prothrombin time, partial thromboplastin time, and albumin—to rule out anemia and bleeding disorders, and assess nutritional status
      (b) BUN, electrolytes—to assess hydration
      (c) Creatinine phosphokinase—reflects muscle damage
      (d) Amylase, liver function studies—when abdominal injury is suspected
      (e) Toxicology screen—in suspected poisoning
      (f) Calcium, phosphorus, alkaline phosphatase—to rule out bone disease
      (g) Cultures—to diagnose sepsis
   (2) Urine
      (a) Blood—may be found in renal or genital trauma
      (b) Specific gravity—indicates hydration
      (c) Ferric chloride—significant in poisonings
   (3) Other
      (a) Oropharynx cultures
      (b) Vaginal cultures
      (c) Rectal cultures

b. Radiographic
   (1) X-rays for suspected skeletal injury
   (2) Full skeletal survey to rule out multiple fractures or fractures at different stages of healing
   (3) Bone scan—assesses stages of healing
   (4) Upper GI—to diagnose duodenal hematoma
   (5) Head or abdominal CAT scan—to detect central nervous system or abdominal trauma

c. Procedural
   (1) Peritoneal lavage—in adult with suspected abdominal trauma
   (2) Lumbar puncture—in children with suspected central nervous system trauma or to rule out sepsis
   (3) Internal pelvic examination for sexual assault (see hospital protocol for special considerations and specimen collection)
      (a) In prepubescent children without external signs of sexual abuse, internal examination is not indicated
      (b) Children with suspected sexual abuse may have internal examination performed under general anesthesia because resisting the examination may cause further trauma
      (c) In young children, vaginal and rectal lacerations may extend into the peritoneal cavity, resulting in intraabdominal bleeding

5. Documentation

a. Complete appropriate state/local child abuse form

b. Additionally, the medical record must contain a detailed written description of injuries, impression of medical care providers, and recommendations for the plan of care

c. Diagrams (body maps)—assist in describing the injuries objectively

d. Photographs
   (1) Children—consent not needed in suspected abuse
   (2) Adults—signed consent required
   (3) Elderly—signed consent required; if senility has impaired patient's mental competency, follow institutional policy regarding administrative consent
   (4) Photograph all injuries with identifying information visible in the picture (patient's name, date, medical record number); patient's face need not be visible

e. Physical evidence
   (1) Examine clothing; document tears, blood, or body fluids
   (2) Save and label all clothing in individual paper bags

6. **Reporting procedures**

a. Children—file a report of child abuse whenever suspicion exists; definitive proof not required; reporting is mandatory in all states
   (1) Make telephone report of suspected abuse to authorized investigative agency
   (2) Utilize language that is objective, concise, and avoids libeling a suspected perpetrator
   (3) Notify caretaker of report
      (a) Emphasize concern for child
      (b) Stress responsibility of health professional to report suspected abuse
      (c) Provide honest, open approach, which may gain trust of caretaker

b. Adults
   (1) Competent adults may refuse police or Department of Human Services' assistance in reporting or prosecuting assailants
   (2) Most local jurisdictions require reporting of violent attacks involving firearms or stabbings

c. Elderly
   (1) Reporting is mandatory in 47 states (14)
   (2) Individual state statutes vary widely in scope, purpose, reporting requirements, and mandatory investigation or service components
   (3) Existing statutes address responsibility of nurses to report suspected abuse and provide immunity from prosecution for "good faith" reporting (9)

d. Suspected sexual assault and/or homicide
   (1) Preserve the chain of evidence (a process to secure objective data that reflects the sequence of events from the time of assault, until presentation of data and evidence in a court of law; assures that specimen or evidence is directly connected to the victim)
   (2) Procedure
      (a) Police will obtain written list of all individuals who collected, handled, or stored specific specimens relating to a criminal case
      (b) Nurse must clearly identify all specimens, clothing, objects, and photographs; include data and time obtained, victim's name and identification number, and signature of person handling specimen
      (c) Follow institutional policy and procedures for handling evidence; usually provide for direct observation, hand-to-hand transfer, and specific format for records

D. MULTIDISCIPLINARY TEAM APPROACH

1. General principles

a. Team composition changes from institution to institution; some teams may have only a physician and a nurse, while others are quite comprehensive

b. Team must work cohesively to gather and exchange vital data elements; team members' roles may overlap

c. Mandatory information for team to collect
   (1) Past medical history of patient, including records review
   (2) Family social history
   (3) History of present injury from perspectives of patient, family, and witnesses
   (4) Environmental assessment—usually done by Department of Human Services or other public health agency

2. Role of team members in care of abused/battered person

a. Physician—develops and implements medical treatment plan; documents injuries via written reports, photographs, and/or videotapes; interprets diagnostic study results; plans follow-up medical care; consults with other disciplines

b. Nurse
   (1) Assesses and documents patient's physical and emotional status
   (2) Assesses and documents family history and social interactions
   (3) Assists physician during diagnostic procedures, treatments, and photography
      (a) Documents in nursing record any pictures taken and indicates number of photographs
      (b) Places all clothing items, individually, in paper bags sealed with staples and marked with data, time, patient's name, and identification (medical record) number; signs each bag
      (c) Assists in obtaining appropriate specimens from patients who have been sexually assaulted
      (d) Preserves the chain of evidence when handling specimens
   (4) Implements medical orders
   (5) Develops nursing diagnoses and implements nursing interventions
   (6) Initiates discharge planning in collaboration with other services and team members

c. Social worker
   (1) Provides social service referral information to patient and family
   (2) Assesses family situations in regard to other children, elderly relatives, and other individuals in the home
   (3) Coordinates and provides for alternative living arrangements, if available

d. Psychiatrist—evaluates mental/emotional status; implements diagnostic and therapeutic interventions; prescribes appropriate medications

e. Psychologist—performs formal psychological testing and evaluation to assess special educational and functional learning needs of the patient

f. Pastoral counselor—provides religious comfort and support to patient and family; often able to assist with community-based support systems such as baby-sitting, elder respite services, recreational and group activities

3. **Rehabilitation team—used when injuries require rehabilitation services to return patient to his/her original or optimal state of physical health; often provides physical, cognitive, and speech testing required for appropriate placement**
4. **Family counseling—team approach to assessing family dynamics that lead to violence, and assisting the family to change behaviors that result in crises**
5. **Public health agencies—complete environmental assessment of the home to identify risks to patient, family, and community from physical and/or situational dangers**

E. UNIQUE ASPECTS OF THE NURSING PROCESS

1. **Assessment**

a. Interview
- (1) Interview guidelines
  - (a) Interview victim in a private, secure environment, separately from caretaker, if possible
  - (b) Avoid having victim repeatedly recall traumatic events by using tape recorder or video recorder
    - i) Serves as evidence in court
    - ii) Patient consent may be required
  - (c) Interview child at appropriate level of understanding; may use drawings, dolls, puppets
- (2) History of injury—significant findings
  - (a) Discrepancy or inconsistency in caretaker's description of injury when described to various staff members or discussed among family members
  - (b) Delay in seeking care
  - (c) Patient brought for care by someone other than primary caretaker
  - (d) Absent history, i.e., injury occurred, but no one knows how or why
  - (e) Repeated injuries or hospitalizations
  - (f) History of injuries does not reflect injuries presented
  - (g) Patient blamed for injuries although developmentally or physically incapable of causing presenting injuries
  - (h) In sexual assault, obtain history of event prior to physical examination, if possible
    - i) Date and time of attack
    - ii) Events of the attack, including whether or not orifices were penetrated
    - iii) Past obstetrical/gynecological/medical history, as appropriate
- (3) Past medical history
  - (a) Noncompliance with primary care visits
  - (b) Poor nutritional status; failure to thrive
  - (c) Repeated injuries or hospitalizations
  - (d) Rule out history of bleeding disorder or bone disease
  - (e) Note mental retardation, chronic illness, prematurity, developmental delay

(f) Medications; pattern of use/misuse
(g) Frequent episodes of leaving emergency department before being seen or evaluated; leaving against medical advice
(h) Lag in immunization status (children)
(i) Suicide attempts

(4) Family and social history
(a) Assess for risk factors (see section A.4.)
(b) Crisis event in household
(c) Domestic violence
(d) Caretaker with history of abuse as a child
(e) Substance abuse in household
(f) Absenteeism—from work or school
(g) Other possible caretakers or sources of housing—extended family

(5) Physical symptoms related to abuse/battering
(a) Headaches
(b) Insomnia; sleep disturbances
(c) Anxiety; palpitations; hyperventilation
(d) Anorexia; feeding intolerance
(e) Irritable bowel; gastrointestinal symptoms
(f) Irritability; short attention span

b. Review previous written, radiographic, photographic, and videotaped medical records

c. Physical examination
(1) Fully expose patient and perform complete physical examination; key areas include skin, central nervous system, abdomen, skeleton, and genitourinary system (see Module 19—Nursing Assessment)
(2) Assess general hygiene; note if caretaker is clean and well-groomed, but patient exhibits poor hygiene
(3) Growth and nutrition status
(a) Measure height (or length), weight, and, in children, head circumference; plot on growth chart
(b) Assess hydration
(c) Note signs or symptoms of failure to thrive
i) Decreased muscle mass and subcutaneous fat
ii) Sensory deprivation

d. Observe interactions between patient and caretaker
(1) Children and elderly
(a) Caretaker appears overly concerned about patient, or caretaker appears unconcerned
(b) Caretaker and patient maintain eye contact or attempt to be in view of each other to extent possible
(c) Caretaker exhibits touch and comforting behaviors toward patient
(d) Patient appears to be comforting the caretaker, i.e., the "parental child"
(2) Adults
(a) Victim frequently presents for treatment alone
(b) When present, however, the perpetrator
i) Remains close to patient and is often overly solicitous
ii) Answers questions for patient

iii) Frequently refuses to leave patient's side

e. Note significant patient/caretaker behaviors in interactions with staff
   (1) Hostile, defensive
   (2) Disinterested
   (3) Clinging, passive, or withdrawn
   (4) Nervous and fearful; flinches when approached by staff
   (5) Poor eye contact with staff
   (6) Hesitant, reluctant to answer questions
   (7) Appropriately concerned
   (8) Relieved that someone has "found out" and now services can be made available to family

f. Assess development and related behavior in children
   (1) Milestones—perform mini-developmental examination
      (a) Gross motor
      (b) Fine motor
      (c) Language
      (d) Toilet training
   (2) Appropriateness of behaviors for child's age and developmental stage, e.g., does child cling to unfamiliar staff when he/she should be afraid of strangers? Is child complacent, when separated from caretaker, when protesting due to separation anxiety is the norm?
   (3) Isolation—is child a "loner"?
   (4) Does child respond appropriately to painful medical procedures?

2. **Nursing diagnoses, expected outcomes, and interventions**

a. Altered parenting related to unmet social, emotional, or maturational needs of parents, multiple socioeconomic stressors, and/or lack of knowledge
   (1) Expected outcomes
      (a) Parent verbalizes appropriate role functions and expectations of child
      (b) Parent accesses resource persons and agencies to assist with parenting responsibilities
      (c) Parent conveys concern and realistic expectations for child, and uses strategies for discipline according to child's developmental level
   (2) Nursing interventions
      (a) Collaborate with multidisciplinary team members to treat patient and family unit
      (b) Notify appropriate agencies of suspected abuse, verbally and in writing
      (c) Provide emotional support to parents/family and patient
      (d) Educate parents
         i) Child development issues
         ii) Realistic expectations of child
         iii) Alternative methods of discipline
         iv) General child-rearing principles
         v) Setting consistent limits
         vi) Role modeling—"reparenting the parent"
      (e) Refer family to appropriate community support groups, health and education classes

b. Chronic or situational low self-esteem related to pattern of abuse/battering
   (1) Expected outcomes
      (a) Patient verbalizes progressively improved self-esteem

(b) Patient takes steps to ensure own safety; removes self from abusive situation if unable to change behaviors of self, or perpetrator, which trigger abuse

(2) Nursing interventions

(a) Discuss patient's perception of self related to abuse situation

(b) Support patient's identity and self-worth through therapeutic communication, and positive reinforcement of appropriate behaviors and patient strengths

(c) Educate patient about

i) Rights under judicial system

ii) Alternative methods of coping

iii) Use of, or access to, support systems that may help overcome specific barriers to leaving a dysfunctional situation

iv) Potential for vocational training

(d) Involve patient in planning for discharge, and encourage patient to make decisions that may improve quality of life

(e) Collaborate with other members of health team and community agencies to help patient achieve personal growth and wellness

c. Potential for injury related to return to abusive situation and/or caretaker

(1) Expected outcomes

(a) Patient free of physical/emotional abuse

(b) Coping strategies are used effectively to avoid abusive episodes

(c) Social service and judicial agencies are accessed, as needed, to provide patient safety

(d) Patient pursues daily activities without fear of injury from caretaker or other perpetrator

(2) Nursing interventions

(a) Through assessment of factors discussed above, determine whether it is safe to return patient to home

(b) Consider alternatives such as discharge to home with supervision of Department of Human Services or home health services; alternate housing with another family member or in an emergency shelter; foster care or adult protective services

(c) Document history and injuries objectively and concisely; use diagrams, photographs, direct quotes, and videotape, as appropriate

(d) Collaborate with other members of health team to ensure that necessary supports and physical care are provided during all phases of the trauma continuum

(e) Teach patient self-protective behaviors, including rights under judicial system, use of, or access to, appropriate agencies to overcome barriers to leaving abusive situations, and specific coping strategies to prevent episodes of battering

(f) Educate patient and family as in nursing diagnoses 2.a (2)(d) and 2.b.(2)(c), above; provide information regarding community resources that may assist the abusive person to modify unacceptable and potentially harmful behavior

(g) Notify judicial system of threats or need for protective services

d. Rape-trauma syndrome related to sexual assault

(1) Expected outcomes

(a) Emotional sequelae are minimized

(b) Patient resumes daily activities
(c) Patient verbalizes safety measures to reduce risk of future assaults
(d) Patient uses effective coping strategies to deal with emotional and physical aftermath of rape
(e) Physical injuries heal

(2) Nursing interventions
(a) Assess patient's physical and emotional status
(b) Treat physical injuries as indicated
(c) Maintain supportive, nonjudgmental attitude; listen and remain with patient
(d) Document history and injuries objectively and concisely; use diagrams, photographs, direct quotes, and videotape appropriately
(e) Assist with collection of evidence according to rape protocol
(f) Collaborate with rape center or crisis intervention and mental health staff, as needed, for initial evaluation and ongoing counseling
(g) Educate patient regarding rights under judicial system and strategies for coping with situation
(h) Assist patient with concerns resulting from rape event—preventing pregnancy or disease, legal matters, relationship with spouse or significant other, disclosure of traumatic event, various fears, and anger

e. Additional nursing diagnoses (see Module 15—Psychosocial Response to Trauma—and Module 28—Pediatric)
(1) Social isolation related to absence of supportive significant others and/or inadequate personal resources
(2) Potential for violence related to rage and/or panic
(3) Pain related to injuries from battering
(4) Disabling, ineffective family coping related to parent/spouse/caretaker with unresolved history of abuse and impoverished personal resources
(5) Fear related to inability to remove self from abusive caretaker/significant other
(6) Knowledge deficit related to parenting and disciplinary skills, and/or social resources for protection and personal growth
(7) Alteration in nutrition, less than body requirements, related to neglect by caretaker
(8) Alteration in health maintenance related to neglect by caretaker, knowledge deficit, and/or unachieved developmental tasks
(9) Alteration in role-relationship patterns related to knowledge deficit, role denial, or physical or psychological inability to perform role
(10) Powerlessness related to situational anxiety, knowledge deficit, perceived inaccessibility of resources, low self-esteem

F. COMMUNITY RESOURCES FOR COUNSELING AND CONTINUING CARE OF VICTIMS OF ABUSE AND/OR THEIR ABUSERS

1. Children

a. Local/state child abuse reporting agencies: statewide child abuse registry
b. Local Child Abuse Hotline
c. National Child Abuse Hotline (1-800-422-4453)

d. Parents Anonymous
e. Emergency foster care; private foster care agencies
f. Crisis nurseries
g. Therapeutic day care programs
h. Lay home visitors
i. Social services for home supervision and ongoing monitoring
j. Religious organizations, e.g., Catholic Charities, chaplains, neighborhood clergy
k. Local chapters of National Committee for the Prevention of Child Abuse
l. Primary care agencies/practitioners for ongoing supervision of nutrition and health

2. Adolescents
a. Home Run (1-800-543-9198)
b. The Vanished Children's Alliance (1-800-VANISHE)
c. Runaway Hotline (1-800-231-6946)
d. National Runaways Switchboard (1-800-621-4000)

3. Adults
a. Women Organized Against Rape (WOAR)
b. National Coalition Against Domestic Violence
c. Women Against Abuse
d. Salvation Army
e. Community Legal Services
f. Adult Protective Services
g. Action Alliance
h. Local women's and children's shelters

4. Elderly
a. Gray Panthers
b. Coalition of Advocates for the Rights of the Infirm and Elderly (CARIE)
c. Elderly Victims' Assistance Program
d. Elder Abuse Task Force
e. American Association of Retired Persons
f. Social Security Hotline

References

1. Parkes, D., & Sylvestre-Simon, C. (1981). The care of the abused and neglected child. In A.R. Oakes (Ed.), *Critical care nursing of children and adolescents* (pp. 320–321). Philadelphia: W. B. Saunders Co.
2. Holter, J. C., & Friedman, S. B. (1968). Child abuse: Early case finding in the emergency department. *Pediatrics, 42*(1), 128.
3. National Center on Child Abuse and Neglect. (1988). *Study findings: Study of national incidence and prevalence of child abuse and neglect.* Washington, DC: U.S. Department of Health and Human Services.
4. U.S. Department of Justice. (1985). *Crime and justice facts.* Washington, DC: U.S. Bureau of Justice Statistics.
5. McLeer, S. V., & Anwar, R. (1987). The role of the emergency physician in the prevention of domestic violence. *Annals of Emergency Medicine, 16*(10), 107–113.
6. Battered Women Training Project for Hospital Emergency Departments. (1987). *Course curriculum.* Philadelphia: Philadelphia Health Management Corp.

7. Stark, E., Flitcraft, A., & Zuckerman, D. (1981). *Wife abuse in the medical setting: An introduction for health personnel* (Domestic Violence Monograph Series, No. 7). Rockville, MD: National Clearinghouse on Domestic Violence.
8. Siegel, M. A., Plesser, D. R., & Jacobs, N. R. (Eds.). (1985). *Domestic violence—No longer behind the curtains* (pp. 101–102). Plano, TX: Instructional Aides, Inc.
9. Sayles-Cross, S. (1988). Profile of familial abuse: A selected review of the literature. *Journal of Community Health Nursing, 5*(4), 209–217.
10. Pollick, M. F. (1987). Abuse of the elderly: A review. *Holistic Nursing Practice, 1*(2), 45–53.
11. Walker, L. E. (1979). *The battered woman.* New York: Harper Colophon.
12. Flitcraft, A. H., & Stark, E. (1983). Women battering: A prevention-oriented approach. In D. Finkelhor, R. J. Gelles, G. T. Hotaling, & M. A. Straus (Eds.), *The dark side of families.* Beverly Hills, CA: Sage.
13. Ludwig, S. (1983). Child abuse. In S. Ludwig & G. Fleisher (Eds.), *Textbook of pediatric emergency medicine* (pp. 1027–1062). Baltimore: Williams & Wilkins.
14. Brewer, R., & Jones, J. (1989). Reporting elder abuse: Limitations of statutes. *Annals of Emergency Medicine, 18*(11), 127–131.
15. Caffey, J. (1974). The whiplash shaken infant syndrome: Manual shaking by the extremities with whiplash induced intracranial and intraocular bleedings, linked with residual permanent brain damage and mental retardation. *Pediatrics, 54*(4), 396–403.

Suggested Readings

Campbell, J. C., & Sheridan, D. J. (1989). Emergency nursing interventions with battered women. *Journal of Emergency Nursing, 15*(1), 12–17.

Danis, D. M., Halper, S. J., Mian, P., Gatzert-Snyder, S., Kane, L., & Sheridan, D. J. (1989). Battered women handout and referral card. *Journal of Emergency Nursing, 15*(1), 49–51.

Fontana, V. J. (1971). *The maltreated child: The maltreatment syndrome in children.* Springfield, IL: Charles C. Thomas.

Kauffman, C. K., & Neill, M. M. (1979). The abusive parent. In S. Hall-Johnson (Ed.), *High risk parenting: Nursing assessment and strategies for the family at risk.* Philadelphia: J. B. Lippincott Co.

Keil, M. (1989). Child abuse. In C. Joy (Ed.), *Pediatric trauma nursing.* Rockville, MD: Aspen Publishers.

Kemp, C. H., Silvernman, F. N., Steele, B. F., Droegemeuller, W., & Silver, H. K. (1962). The battered child syndrome. *Journal of the American Medical Association, 181*(1), 17–24.

Marmon, L., Stellar, J., & Vinocur, C. (1989). The problem of child abuse. *Trauma Quarterly, 6*(1), 1–6.

Straus, M., Gelles, R., & Steinmetz, S. K. (1980). *Behind closed doors: A survey of family violence in America.* New York: Doubleday.

Wolf, R. S. (1988). Elder abuse: Ten years later. *Journal of American Geriatrics Society, 36*(4), 758–762.

MODULE 33
PERSONS WITH SUICIDAL/SELF-INFLICTED INJURIES

Joanne Michener, MSN, RN

Prerequisite

Review principles of psychosocial nursing and crisis interventions.

Objectives

1.0 Discuss common patterns of self-inflicted injuries.
2.0 Describe general physiological considerations in caring for patients with self-inflicted injuries.
3.0 Describe general psychological considerations in caring for patients with self-inflicted injuries.
4.0 List unique aspects of the nursing process for patients with self-inflicted injuries.

A. DEFINITION OF SUICIDE

Suicide is an active or passive act of self-destruction; the person who attempts suicide and incurs traumatic injury is the focus of this module.

B. COMMON PATTERNS OF INJURY

1. **Incidence (1)**
   a. Causes 25,000 to 30,000 deaths per year in the U.S.
   b. Common in elderly and adolescents; second leading cause of death in those aged 15 to 24 years, after MVCs
   c. 5th leading cause of potential years of life lost; 10th leading cause of death
   d. Percent of unreported cases estimated at 25% to 50%
   e. Ratio of attempted to completed suicides is about 8:1 (1)
   f. Although females attempt suicide three times more often than males, white males complete suicide three times more often than females
   g. Cultural factors also play a role; age-adjusted rate for whites is almost twice that of blacks and other races
2. **Mechanisms of injury**
   a. Firearms (60% of suicides) (1)
      (1) Most common sites are head, chest, and abdomen
      (2) Powder burns at the site may be apparent
   b. Hanging (14% of suicides) (1)
      (1) Usually occurs at home or work
      (2) Produces deep neck injuries
         (a) Fracture of thyroid cartilage, approximately 50% (2)
         (b) Hyoid and laryngeal injuries in about 50%; hyoid fracture in 20% (2)
         (c) Carotid injuries, 5%, may increase with age and atherosclerosis (2)
         (d) Cervical spine injuries in hangings with long drops (2)
      (3) External compression causes
         (a) Autonomic reflex activity, resulting in cardiac arrest, occurs due to parasympathetic discharge from vagal pressure, or sympathetic discharge from pericarotid pressure
         (b) Airway compromise due to upward displacement of tongue and epiglottis
         (c) Occlusion of veins and arteries (3)
      (4) Death is usually due to interrupted cerebral blood flow and ischemia; asphyxia uncommon (3)
   c. Poisoning
   d. Jumping from high building, roof, etc.
   e. Carbon monoxide inhalation
   f. Drowning
   g. Other methods include self-inflicted wounds, self-immolation, and alcohol or drug intoxication
   h. Single-car accidents, often a collision with stationary object, may be unrecognized suicide attempts; incidence unknown
3. **Suicide is a symptom, not a disease entity**
4. **Common myths about suicide (see Table 33.1)**

Table 33.1

Common myths and facts about suicide. Adapted from E. Henderson & M. G. Hill, Psychotrauma. In E. Howell, L. Widra & M. G. Hill (Eds.), *Comprehensive trauma nursing.* Glenview, IL: Scott, Foresman & Co., 1988, pp. 760–761. Adapted with permission.

Myth	*Fact*
1. People who attempt suicide are mentally ill	Suicial people are usually in emotional turmoil, not necessarily mentally ill
2. Good circumstances (home, job) prevent suicide	Suicide cuts across class, race, age, and gender; frequency varies among different groups
3. People who talk about suicide rarely attempt it	People who succeed at suicide usually talk about it or give clues about intentions; these behavioral warnings may not be recognized
4. People who talk about suicide, or do not succeed initially, are not at risk for suicide	Most people who attempt suicide eventually succeed; all threats and self-injury must be taken seriously
5. Discussing suicide with a person who is upset will put the idea into his/her head	Suicide is a complex process; many factors other than inquiry regarding suicidal intent must be present
6. People who are severely depressed lack the energy to commit suicide	Energy levels are difficult to assess; people may commit suicide when they are depressed, or when their condition improves; frequent assessment is important

C. MEDICAL AND SURGICAL INTERVENTIONS

1. Physiological considerations

a. Priorities of physical treatment do not differ from that of other trauma patients

b. Specific injuries and interventions

- (1) Firearms injuries
  - (a) Treated as any other GSW
  - (b) Note any powder burns at site and, if burns present, document color and size; photograph, if possible
  - (c) The hands of the patient may show powder residue
    - i) Police may test this to determine if the injury was self-inflicted
    - ii) Protect area with paper bags
- (2) Hanging (2, 3)
  - (a) Possible clinical manifestations
    - i) Observe for hemorrhage at site of injury
    - ii) Observe for respiratory distress
    - iii) Note severe hoarseness and stridor secondary to traumatic edema of larynx and supraglottic tissue; monitor for at least 24 hrs
    - iv) Subconjunctival hemorrhages and petechiae on skin

v) ARDS or pulmonary edema may occur; may be due to central neurogenic problem (2)
vi) Neuropsychological sequelae are most significant aftermath; anoxia may cause minor to major effects, some of which may be reversible
(b) Stabilize neck
(c) Aggressive pulmonary management—intubation, ventilation, and PEEP
(d) Monitor cardiovascular status with PCWP, CO, arterial line
(e) Neurological effects from increased intracranial pressure—use hyperventilation, oxygen (PaO_2 above 100), osmotic agents, hypothermia

2. Psychological considerations

a. The entire trauma team should be aware that the patient's injury was self-inflicted since he/she may attempt to harm him/herself again
b. A qualified psychiatric team member should be involved immediately to interview the patient, and/or the family, and obtain a thorough psychosocial history

3. Hospitalize patient to prevent further harm

4. Establish communication and rapport with patient

5. Help patient express guilt, anger, and hostility

6. Help patient identify resources, support systems, and coping skills

7. Utilize pharmacological therapy to manage patient's anxiety or other psychological problems

D. NURSING ASSESSMENT

1. Suicidal intent is not always obvious at the time of injury or during early care; therefore, a careful assessment and interview of patient and family is essential

2. Interview

a. Family composition and roles
b. Patient's emotional state, prior to traumatic injury, and expectations about event
c. Level of preoccupation with self and disengagement from others
d. Past or current psychiatric history
(1) Severe depression—signs and symptoms
(a) Loss of appetite
(b) Weight loss
(c) Insomnia
(d) Apathy or dependence
(e) Social withdrawal
(f) Emotional and physical fatigue
(g) Slowed movement and/or speech
(2) Psychosis, particularly with auditory command hallucinations
(3) Acute severe paranoid state
(4) Manic depressive disease
(5) Personality disorder
e. Precipitating events that could have contributed to the patient's suicidality
(1) Loss of loved ones

(2) Divorce or breakup of relationships
(3) Loss of job (especially if sole provider for family); change in employment (retirement)
(4) Severe, chronic, debilitating disease
(5) Social disgrace (arrest, bankruptcy)
(6) Loss of reason to live (real or perceived)

f. One or more prior suicide attempts
g. Plan for suicide event; assess lethality, availability of means, degree of detail in plan, and plan for rescue
h. Perceived support system and resources
i. Interaction with immediate family and/or significant others
j. Substance abuse
k. Coping abilities
l. Is this an anniversary of a loss?
m. Family history of suicide (family members of suicide victims are believed to have greater risk for physical and mental health problems than other bereaved persons) (4)

3. Patients at high risk for suicide often have the following

a. History of prior attempts—65% of those who make very serious attempts have made prior attempt (5)
b. Disorganized thoughts
c. Limited or nonexistent support systems
d. Feeling of physical isolation; unexplained change in behavior, depression, or mental illness
e. A definite plan for suicide and the means to carry out the plan, e.g., patient states, "I want to throw myself out of the window," and room is on 12th floor with easily accessible and unlocked window
f. Feelings of helplessness or hopelessness
g. Emotional disorganization; inability to adapt
h. History of substance abuse—may increase suicide potential due to decreased inhibition, decreased ability to reason, and increased impulsive behavior
i. Recent history of specific activities—giving away belongings, "settling affairs," or writing a "good-bye" note

4. Guidelines for assessing suicide potential in adults are listed in Table 33.2

5. Acronyms to guide assessment

a. MA'S SALAD (6)
(1) M = mental state
(2) A = attempt
(3) S = support system
(4) S = sex
(5) A = age
(6) L = loss
(7) A = alcohol
(8) D = drugs

b. SAD CHILDREN (7)
(1) S = support system
(2) A = alcohol/drugs
(3) D = depression

Table 33.2

Guide for assessing suicide potential in adults. From S. G. Fought & A. N. Throwe, *Psychosocial nursing care of the emergency patient,* p. 139. Copyright © 1984 John Wiley & Sons, Inc. Reprinted by permission of John Wiley & Sons, Inc.

Low Suicide Risk	*High Suicide Risk*
Problem	
No significant problem or stress associated with job decline or promotion	Significant loss (death, divorce, marital separation, job, money, status)
Plan	
No suicide plan, or some possible consideration but no definite plan	Has a definite plan (time, method, and availability), and has made one or more previous attempts
Feelings	
Expresses feelings of anger, hostility, rage; appears agitated, anxious	Despondent, hopeless, and sees no change in future; loss of appetite; declining job performance
Symptoms	
No medical problems or minor illness complaints	One or more previous suicide attempts using highly lethal methods; impotence, weight loss, declining social interests
Resources	
Has available economic, social, family, or agency resources	Limited or no available resources; does not know how or where to seek help
Attitudes	
States good reasons for living; suicidal thoughts are upsetting to the individual	Denies he/she has a reason for living; does not attempt to control suicidal ideation
Significant Others' Reactions	
Supportive, concerned; reactions may alternate from anger and rejection, to acceptance and receptiveness, to offers of help	Defensive, rejecting, or displaying no concern or understanding
Strengths	
Has demonstrated attempts to solve problems; has a history of seeking help or is now attempting to seek help	Has not sought out help; feels that the problem is unsolvable
Alcohol	
Does not use alcohol or uses alcohol only in social situations	Uses alcohol as a medicine to ease pain and escape from stress; has history of alcohol use and impulsive acting out; has history of combined use of barbiturates and alcohol
Cognitive Function	
Is in contact with reality; affect appears appropriate for situation or crisis at hand	Demonstrates disturbed thought processes; thoughts are illogical and irrational; psychotic and out of touch with reality; hallucinates; affect is lowered

(4) C = communication
(5) H = hostility
(6) I = impulsiveness
(7) L = lethality
(8) D = demographics
(9) R = reaction of evaluator—if patient makes evaluator depressed or angry, patient probably deserves more thorough evaluation)
(10) E = events—why now?
(11) N = no hope

6. **Physical examination**
a. Follow guidelines for primary/secondary survey in Module 19—Nursing Assessment
b. Make observations and gather evidence related to specific methods of attempted suicide

7. **Diagnostic indicators**
a. Laboratory studies
(1) Trauma profile
(2) Toxicology screens and levels
b. Radiologic evaluation specific to predicted injury

E. NURSING DIAGNOSES, EXPECTED OUTCOMES, AND INTERVENTIONS

1. **Potential for violence, self-directed, as evidenced by recent self-inflicted injury**
a. Expected outcomes
(1) Patient communicates needs, concerns, and feelings with staff and significant others
(2) Patient asks for, or cooperates with, mental health resources
(3) Patient is protected from harming him/herself and makes no further suicide attempts
(4) Patient is future oriented in discussions
(5) Patient communicates plan for continuing psychiatric care
b. Nursing interventions
(1) Continue to assess patient's mental status and potential for further suicide attempts
(2) Take all threats seriously
(3) Initiate suicide precautions (according to hospital policy) while waiting for mental health professionals
(a) Lock windows
(b) Remove sharp objects (knives, scissors, nail files, glass objects)
(c) Remove matches, cigarette lighters, belts, etc.
(d) Use paper or plastic meal service
(e) Observe patient to prevent pill hoarding when giving medications; use liquids if possible

(4) Restrain patient's arms to avoid removal of ET tube, etc.
(5) May require 1:1 staffing, constant sight observation, or observations every 15 min
(6) Increase surveillance in early morning hours, Sundays, holidays, visiting hours, and during increased unit activities (shift change) (8)
(7) Consult with appropriate mental health professionals, e.g., psychiatric clinical nurse specialist or psychiatry staff, even if suicidality of patient is vague
(8) Observe and document degree of isolation, frequency of crying, verbalizations, tone of voice, facial expressions, eye contact, and mental status exam
(9) Continue to assess for ongoing suicidal ideation—morbid thoughts, hopelessness, decreased self-esteem, flat affect with no participation in care, and/or depressive symptoms may indicate active risk
(10) Use kind, sympathetic manner and straightforward communication
(11) Accept suicidal behavior as logical from patient's point of view—do not pass judgment
(12) Reinforce individual's self-esteem by interacting in such a manner as to accord dignity
(13) Reinforce positive aspects of patient's self-concept—assist him/her in identifying strengths
(14) Encourage verbalizations of feelings; offer support about impulses of self-harm, e.g., "We will not let you hurt yourself"
(15) Assist patient to reestablish supportive relationships with those whom he/she chooses
(16) Support significant others so they can support the patient
(17) Be aware of, and seek support for, your own feelings regarding the patient and suicide in general
(18) Contrary to myth, discussing suicide with a person who is upset will not put the idea into his/her head; rather, an honest, direct approach is usually a relief to patients, who will generally discuss their feelings when given the opportunity and compassion

2. **Additional nursing diagnoses**

a. Ineffective individual coping related to mood disturbances, and feelings of worthlessness or helplessness
b. Ineffective family coping related to suicidal event
c. Hopelessness related to situational events
d. Potential for violence, directed against others, related to frustrated suicide attempts
e. Social isolation related to inadequate personal resources, depression, or altered self-concept
f. Chronic or situational loss of self-esteem related to family dynamics, loss of support system, or loss of meaningful quality of life
g. Powerlessness related to low self-esteem, and feelings of hopelessness and worthlessness
h. Dysfunctional grieving related to actual/perceived losses of significant other, or chronic disease

References

1. The National Committee for Injury Prevention. (1987). Suicide. In *Injury prevention: Meeting the challenge* (pp. 252–260). New York: Oxford University Press.
2. Iserson, K. V. (1984). Strangulation: A review of ligature, manual, and postural neck compression injuries. *Annals of Emergency Medicine, 13*(3), 179–185.
3. McHugh, T. P., & Stout, M. (1983). Near-hanging injury. *Annals of Emergency Medicine, 12*(12), 774–776.
4. Jones, M. B., & Peacock, M. K. (1988). Loss. In E. Howell, L. Widra & M. G. Hill (Eds.), *Comprehensive trauma nursing: Theory and practice* (pp. 223–246). Boston: Scott, Foresman & Co.
5. Henderson, E., & Hill, M. G. (1988). Psychotrauma. In E. Howell, L. Widra, & M. G. Hill (Eds.), *Comprehensive trauma nursing: Theory and practice* (pp. 747–775). Boston: Scott, Foresman & Co.
6. Pellitier, L. C., & Cousins, A. (1984). Clinical assessment of the suicidal patient in the emergency department. *Journal of Emergency Nursing, 10*(1), 40–43.
7. DiVasto, P. V., West, D. A., & Christy, J. E. (1979). A framework for the emergency evaluation of the suicidal patient. *Journal of Psychiatric Nursing, 17*(6), 15–20.
8. Knezevich, B. A. (1986). Psychiatric trauma. In B. A. Knezevich (Ed.), *Trauma nursing: Principles and practice* (pp. 299–327). Norwalk, CT: Appleton-Century-Crofts.

Suggested Readings

Alspach, J. G. (Ed.). (1991). *Core curriculum for critical care nursing* (4th ed.). Philadelphia: W. B. Saunders Co.

Kay, S. (1987). Oh, no: Another suicide. *Nursing Life, 7*(3), 30–32.

Lewis, S., McDowell, W. A., & Gregory, R. J. (1989). The patient with suicidal ideation. In S. Lewis, R. D. Grainger, N. A. McDowell, R. J. Gregory & R. J. Messner (Eds.), *Manual of psychosocial nursing interventions: Promoting mental health in medical-surgical settings* (pp. 173–185). Philadelphia: W. B. Saunders Co.

Stuart, G., & Sundeen, S. (Eds.). (1983). *Principles and practice of psychiatric nursing* (2nd ed.). St. Louis: C. V. Mosby Co.

Section VI
Professional Perspectives in Trauma Nursing

MODULE 34
LEGAL CONCEPTS

Jacqueline M. Carolan, BSN, JD, RN, CCRN

Objectives

1.0 **Appraise the legal impact of Nurse Practice Acts on the scope of professional practice and/or responsibility.**
2.0 **Discuss the legal responsibility of the professional nurse regarding documentation.**
3.0 **Discuss several implications of current highway safety legislation on professional nursing practice.**
4.0 **Determine the legal accountability of the professional nurse regarding informed consent.**
5.0 **Describe the legal implications of disclosure of patient information.**
6.0 **Discuss several implications of current living will legislation on professional nursing practice.**
7.0 **Discuss new trends in defining and determining death.**
8.0 **Determine the legal accountability of the professional nurse in common situations related to trauma nursing, including**
8.1 Arriving first at the scene of an accident.
8.2 Caring for a potential organ donor.
8.3 Participating in evidence collection.
8.4 Caring for a patient with a reportable injury.

A. INTRODUCTION

1. Law is the body of rules and regulations that govern all of society and protect the health, safety, and welfare of citizens
2. Each state, and the federal system, has its own structure and rules resulting in a large and complex set of laws
3. Laws are dynamic and responsive; laws change as nursing changes
4. Trauma nurses should be familiar with the specific language of pertinent laws in their states and tailor approaches to practice to current law

B. SOURCES OF LAW

1. U.S. Constitution
2. Common law—made by a judge; derived from earlier court decisions (legal precedent), custom, and tradition
3. Statutory law—enacted (codified) by legislature; published in United States Code (federal), or individual state codes
4. Administrative regulations

a. Some statutes delegate authority to administrative agencies to promulgate (publish) regulations that will implement a particular statute
b. Agency adopts regulations according to a specific process
c. Allow legislature to delegate administrative authority to an administrative agency that has expertise in a particular area of law, e.g., rules and regulations for EMS may be developed by Department of Health

C. NURSE PRACTICE ACTS

1. Define standards established by state boards of nursing
2. Protect the public by broadly defining the legal scope of nursing practice
3. The nurse who gives care beyond defined practice limits becomes vulnerable to charges of violating the Nurse Practice Act
4. Lag time between changes in these statutory laws and commonly accepted expectations of professional nurses may cause nurses to violate Nurse Practice Acts, e.g., nurses commonly make nursing diagnoses, although some Nurse Practice Acts do not indicate whether they may legally do so
5. Reliance on education, training, and knowledge of institutional policies and procedures is helpful when Nurse Practice Acts do not address specific practice concerns
6. Upon request, the state board may issue interpretations of the act to clarify whether or not specific practices are within the scope of professional nursing, e.g., arterial puncture, intubation

7. **Nurses must educate their legislators and the public, and support lobbying by their professional organizations to effectively impact and update the language of Nurse Practice Acts**

D. DOCUMENTATION

1. **Patient record**
   a. Intended to be a complete and accurate reflection of contact with the health care system
   b. Chief means by which nurses and other trauma team members communicate
   c. Used to plan care, educate and train health care professionals; used for research, statistical data, and in legal proceedings to determine malpractice
   d. Legal proof of the quality of care provided; attests to whether or not standards of care have been met
   e. As a written record, captures events that may be forgotten by the time a malpractice suit is filed
2. **Governed by rules, including federal regulations (e.g., Medicare), state laws, professional organization standards (more stringent than state), voluntary accreditation bodies (Joint Commission on the Accreditation of Healthcare Organizations), and hospital policies**
3. **Flowsheets**
   a. While useful, may lead to habit of routine checkoffs without thorough observation
   b. Should not be only source of documentation; nurses' notes needed to document patient response
4. **Guidelines for documentation to ensure compliance with legal standards**
   a. Document accurately, completely, and in a timely manner
      (1) Record date and time of each entry; time should reflect, as closely as possible, the time the action actually occurred (especially in emergencies)
      (2) Include normal, as well as abnormal, findings
      (3) Be specific; avoid generalities or vague terms
      (4) Document symptoms in patient's own words
      (5) Be objective; record facts and describe signs and symptoms that support conclusions concerning patient's condition
      (6) Record all observations, responses to therapy, and any safeguards used in patient care
      (7) Include procedures, incidents, and communications with family and physicians; attempts to reach a physician should be described
      (8) Indicate that the nursing care plan and physician's orders have been carried out, or describe the reason for omitting any prescribed treatments
   b. Never falsify a record to cover up a negligent act
   c. To avoid attempts to falsify records, sign entries immediately following the last word in the entry; do not skip lines between entries
   d. Write legibly with unerasable ink

e. If an error is made in documentation, cross out the incorrect section with a single line, mark it "error," and initial

5. **Documentation can protect the trauma nurse whose care is called into question in a lawsuit**

E. EMERGENCY MEDICAL SERVICES LEGISLATION

(see Module 5—Emergency Medical Services Systems)

1. **Federal Emergency Services Act of 1972 established over 300 EMS regions throughout the country**

a. Grants and contracts provided support for
   (1) Education of emergency medical technicians
   (2) Development of hospital-to-ambulance communications systems
   (3) Regional categorization of hospital facilities and services

b. Continued through 1970s but repealed in 1981 with subsequent loss of federal funding

2. **States enacted similar legislation and linked EMS development to Highway Safety Acts to ensure that persons involved in highway accidents receive prompt emergency medical care**

a. State legislation can include provisions for a dedicated funding source, and educational and treatment standards

b. Funding sources are derived from fines levied on traffic violations

3. **Specific legislation to develop standards for accreditation and operation of trauma centers has been enacted in some states, e.g., Pennsylvania (see Module 6—Trauma Care Systems)**

4. **The Trauma Care Systems Planning and Development Act of 1990 is expected to establish comprehensive trauma systems through state trauma plans, based on national standards, and to help trauma systems defray a portion of uncompensated costs**

5. **Additional federal trauma bills have been introduced to address radio communication between ambulances and hospitals, appropriations to trauma centers affected by violence related to drug trafficking, and compensation to trauma centers who care for uncompensated and undercompensated aliens**

F. HIGHWAY SAFETY LEGISLATION

1. **Federal law requires each state to have a highway safety program approved by the secretary of transportation, and designed to reduce traffic accidents and deaths, injuries, and resultant property damage**

2. **Such programs are under uniform guidelines to improve driver and pedestrian performance, and bicycle safety**

3. **Guidelines include provisions for**

a. An effective record system for accidents, injuries, and deaths
b. Vehicle registration, operation, and inspection
c. Highway maintenance and traffic control
d. Vehicle codes and laws
e. Surveillance of traffic for detection and correction of high, or potentially high, accident locations
f. Emergency services

4. **Federal funds are authorized to aid states in conducting highway safety programs; may be used to develop and implement manpower training, or demonstration programs that will contribute directly to reducing accidents and resultant injuries and deaths**
5. **The federal government provides incentive programs for states to encourage safety practices such as the use of safety belts by motor vehicle occupants**
6. **Federal funding of research and development**

a. Available for independent research or studies in cooperation with other federal departments and agencies; may include grants to state or local agencies and individuals
b. Study areas include use of safety belts and motorcycle helmets, and the relationship between the use of controlled substances and highway safety
c. Funding also supports training or education of highway safety personnel, research fellowships in highway safety, development of improved accident investigation procedures, emergency service plans, demonstration projects, and related activities deemed worthy by the secretary of transportation

7. **Drunk driving**

a. Grants are available to states that adopt and implement effective programs to reduce traffic safety problems caused by persons driving while under the influence of alcohol or controlled substances
   (1) Programs include mandatory license suspension and either an assignment of 100 hrs of community service, or a minimum sentence of imprisonment for 48 consecutive hrs; used for first conviction for driving under the influence of alcohol
   (2) A second violation requires a mandatory minimum 10-day prison sentence and license revocation for not less than one year
   (3) Conviction of a third or subsequent violation, within five years after a prior conviction for the same offense, carries a mandatory minimum imprisonment for 120 days and revocation of driver's license for not less than three years
   (4) Programs for mandatory blood alcohol concentration testing also may be funded
b. Some states have developed innovative programs such as Accelerated Rehabilitation for first offenders

8. **Most states set speed limits of 55 mph in urbanized areas (population 50,000 or greater) and 65 mph in less urbanized areas (population less than 50,000); may benefit citizens economically and reduce trauma**

G. GOOD SAMARITAN STATE STATUTES

1. **Encourage health professionals to volunteer their services at an accident or an emergency scene**
2. **Provide for immunity from civil liability for any act, or omission, of a person who, in good faith, renders care at the scene of the emergency**

3. **In almost every state, except Vermont, a health professional has no legal duty to assist in a rescue**
4. **If a health professional does decide to render assistance, he/she incurs a legal duty to stay with the victim until he/she is being cared for by another health professional with at least as much training, or until ordered from the scene by the police**
   a. By offering assistance, one gives the appearance to potential rescuers that one will care for the victim
   b. At that point, one establishes a nurse-patient relationship and owes the injured individual the normal duty owed to any patient, i.e., treatment that meets the standard of care of a reasonably prudent nurse in a similar situation
5. **Good Samaritan Acts do not protect the health professional who is grossly negligent, i.e., demonstrates flagrant and inexcusable failure to perform a legal duty in reckless disregard of the consequences**

H. INFORMED CONSENT

1. **Defined as a person's agreement to allow something to happen, such as surgery, that is based on a full disclosure of facts needed to make the decision intelligently, i.e., knowledge of risks and alternatives**
   a. Serves to protect the individual's right of self-determination
   b. Based on premise that the individual's freedom to decide what shall be done with his/her body may be paramount to preservation of the patient's health
2. **Information disclosed to patient should include**
   a. A description of the treatment or procedure
   b. The name and qualifications of the person who will perform the treatment or procedure
   c. An explanation of the potential for death or serious harm, or discomforting side effects during or after the treatment or procedure
   d. An explanation and description of alternative treatments or procedures
   e. An explanation of the possible effects of not having the treatment or procedure
3. **In most states, a signed consent form is evidence of informed consent; however, it is not conclusive proof and may be challenged in court if a patient claims he/she did not understand the information, or was not given the relevant information**
4. **The responsibility for obtaining a patient's informed consent is with the person who will be performing the treatment or procedure**
   a. The nurse may witness the patient's signature
   b. The nurse's signature indicates that the nurse saw the patient sign the consent form and that the patient was awake, alert, and aware of what he/she was signing; preanesthetic drugs, narcotics, barbiturates, or anesthesia may alter the patient's ability to give informed consent
5. **The nurse is required to take action to prevent any harm to a patient and should independently ensure that informed consent has been freely given**
   a. A patient's uncertainty about the proposed treatment should be reported to the involved physician and the appropriate administrator

b. Mere documentation is not sufficient; a nurse may be held liable for another health care provider's failure to disclose material information

6. **Emergency situations**

a. A physician can legally treat a patient, without getting consent, if the patient needs immediate treatment to save his/her life, or to prevent loss of an organ, limb, or function, and consent cannot be obtained because the patient is unconscious, or the family (guardian) cannot be reached
   (1) The law assumes that if a patient could decide, he/she would choose to receive treatment rather than risk the consequences of no treatment
   (2) This privilege does not apply if the patient previously refused the procedure, or the physician can wait for the proper consent from the patient, or family, without increasing the patient's risk

b. Physicians must document reasons for proceeding without consent, and the specific risks the patient faces without treatment

I. EVIDENCE

1. **Laws requiring nurses to participate in obtaining samples of body fluids for evidence may vary according to laws in each jurisdiction**

a. Law enforcement officers may request health professionals to remove a sample of a patient's blood or urine for evidentiary purposes, e.g., in the investigation of an MVC

b. If a patient agrees to the removal of a bodily substance (usually blood or urine), there is no issue of liability

c. If the patient refuses to consent to a blood test, and the nurse or physician proceeds to extract blood on the request or order of the police officer, the issue of holding the nurse or physician liable for civil battery may arise

d. Generally, health care providers are insulated from liability when performing a nonconsensual procedure at the request or order of the police; some state laws grant immunity to physicians, nurses, and their employers in such situations

2. **Search requested by police**

a. Requires a warrant unless the patient is under arrest

b. Evidence in plain view can be confiscated

c. If a nurse finds a gun, knife, drug, or other item that the suspect could use to harm him/herself or others, the nurse has a right to remove it
   (1) Notify hospital administration
   (2) Maintain control over the evidence until it is given to an administrator or law officer

3. **Documentation of possible evidence**

a. Record item description and name of person to whom evidence is given (courts require guarantee of where and how evidence was gathered before it is admissible in court)

b. Never leave evidence, for which you are responsible, unattended

c. Follow hospital procedure for labeling evidence and comply with chain of evidence protocol; before marking evidence, check with police to ensure that evidence is not destroyed by the process of handling and labeling

4. Zeal of police to obtain evidence must not interfere with efforts to treat and stabilize a patient; refer to hospital policy manual, or call administrator if conflict occurs

J. DISCLOSURE

1. Right to privacy

a. Defined as the right to be left alone and to make personal choices without outside interference

b. In many jurisdictions, a physician (and in some cases, a nurse) is foreclosed (barred) from divulging, in judicial proceedings, information that he/she acquired while attending a patient in a professional capacity and that was necessary to enable the physician (nurse) to act in his or her professional capacity

2. ANA Code for Nurses holds nurses responsible for safeguarding the client's right to privacy by "judiciously protecting information of a confidential nature" (1)

a. Code allows limited exceptions to the rule that disclosure of patient information requires the patient's consent

b. Exceptions
   (1) Disclosure to other members of the health team for purposes of patient care
   (2) Disclosure for quality assurance purposes
   (3) Disclosure in a court of law when a patient waives or lacks a statutory nurse-patient privilege of communication

3. Hospital records

a. Owned by the hospital, i.e., they are the hospital's business records

b. Health care record is unusual because while it physically belongs to the hospital (which must exercise considerable control over access), patients and others have an interest in the information the record contains

c. Patients and others have a right to access the information contained in the patient record, but not possess the original records
   (1) Most state laws impose on hospitals a duty to disclose certain information from a patient's medical records without patient consent or authorization
   (2) Hospitals cannot, then, be held liable for such disclosure, even if a disclosure is made against the patient's express wishes

4. Reporting laws

a. Child abuse
   (1) Most states require health professionals to report any case of suspected child abuse or neglect to the appropriate public agency, e.g., police, welfare, public health
   (2) Only a "reasonable cause to believe" is required of health professionals in most states
   (3) The health professional who fails to report abuse may be held liable

b. Drug abuse
   (1) Some states require physicians and hospitals to report the names of patients who have been prescribed drugs that are subject to abuse

(2) Justification is based on the state's interest in controlling drug abuse

c. Communicable disease

(1) All states require hospitals to report cases of infectious diseases such as syphilis and AIDS

(2) The report statute commonly requires the patient's name, age, address, sex, and details of the illness to be reported

(3) Failure to report a communicable disease may result in liability if a patient is discharged and infects others

d. Sexual assaults, rape, gunshot wounds, stabbings—most states require hospitals to report cases involving victims of violent crimes to authorities

e. Threats to an identified person—some states have ruled that there is a duty to warn an identified person whom a patient has made a credible threat to kill

f. Other disclosures required may include animal bites, poisonings, MVCs, suicides and suspicious deaths, and radiation contamination

5. **Confidentiality of patients treated or referred for treatment of chemical abuse and federally enacted laws (which preempt state laws) may forbid disclosure of patient information (even of the patient's admission to the facility) without the patient's full consent in writing**

6. **Guidelines for disclosure**

a. Know both federal and individual state laws concerning the duty to report and privilege laws

b. Report only required information to the proper governmental agency, and ensure that others who have a duty to disclose health-related information do so promptly

c. Reporting must be done in good faith; civil and criminal liability may be incurred for failure to report, if disclosure is required by law

d. Carefully follow hospital policy regarding access to medical records

e. Breach of confidentiality is usually considered unprofessional conduct and grounds for disciplinary action by a state board of nursing

f. Report only the information that is required; no freedom from liability exists for information that was not required, or for information that is given to other than the proper governmental agency

K. LIVING WILL

(also see Module 35—Ethical Issues)

1. **Also known as "right to die" or "natural death" legislation**

2. **Living will statutes have been enacted by many states to formally recognize certain forms of written statements requesting that some kinds of medical care be discontinued under specific circumstances**

a. The courts in most states will not order a physician to discontinue treatment to meet the written requests of a patient, but will attempt to make it easier for physicians in hospitals to honor those requests

b. Statutes differ in several respects

(1) In some states, the living will may be executed by any person, at any time; in other states, living wills require a waiting period and may not be executed during a terminal illness

(2) In some states, adults are authorized to make a living will for minor children
(3) Some laws permit living wills of indefinite duration; in other states, they expire after a determined number of years
(4) Statutes may address only the terminally ill or may include those in irreversible coma; some provide for different conditions to trigger the substantive provisions of the document
(5) The formalities of a will may be required in some states; other states require alternative formalization of the living will

c. Physicians and other health care providers are generally relieved of any civil or criminal liability, if they properly follow the requirements of the statute and implement the desires expressed in a legally executed living will
(1) Some statutes require that any physician who cannot, in good conscience, carry out those provisions, transfer the patient to a physician who can carry out the patient's wishes
(2) In states without a living will statute, immunity is not assured
(3) Nurses should be familiar with hospital policy and state laws, and seek advice from the institution's legal department when a living will appears on a patient's record

3. In several situations, a living will need not be honored

a. A state without a living will law may, but need not, honor a living will that was executed in another state
b. A living will need not be honored if
(1) It is out of date
(2) The patient asks that it be disregarded
(3) It has been revoked
(4) The patient asks for treatment that disagrees with statements in the living will

4. Relationship to family's wishes

a. In a state with a living will law, the patient's family cannot contradict the will unless they can prove it is invalid
b. In a state without a living will law, the health team or a court will consider both a patient's living will and his family's wishes before deciding on treatment or nontreatment
c. In 1990, the U.S. Supreme Court ruled that states have the right to prevent family members from taking permanently unconscious patients off life support systems in cases where there is no clear and convincing proof that the patients want treatment ended

5. Guidelines for the living will

a. Must be written, signed, and witnessed
b. States with living will laws specify the execution requirements
c. In states without living will laws, a person may use a standardized form or have his attorney design one
d. Although not always required, an individual may want to file a copy of the living will with his medical records, his doctor, and his family

6. Patient rights legislation

a. The Federal Patient Self-Determination Act requires Medicare and Medicaid providers to establish procedures to inform patients of their rights under state law to control health care decisions that affect them

b. The Department of Health and Human Services is required to evaluate compliance with the Act and to develop a national campaign informing the public that it has the option to execute advance directives

L. ORGAN DONATION STATUTES

(See also Module 18—Organ Donation)

1. **All states have adopted the Uniform Anatomical Gift Act, which allows anyone over age 18 to sign a donor card, in the presence of two witnesses, willing some or all of his/her organs after death; may also be recorded on back of a driver's license**
   a. Legally, the decision to donate organs is binding on the family after a person's death; in reality, most hospitals will comply with the wishes of the decedent's family
   b. In some states, consent is not necessary where a donor card authorizing a gift of the donor's eyes has been validly executed
2. **A family member may authorize donation of a decedent's organs by signing an appropriate document**
3. **If death occurs within 24 hrs of the patient's admission to a hospital, or results from an accident, homicide, or other unnatural cause, a medical examiner must also consent to organ donation; for donation to occur, death must be legally established**
4. **Required request legislation**
   a. Many states have enacted statutes that require hospitals to request consent to a donation of all or any part of the decedent's body, for any purpose specified under the act
      (1) The request and its disposition must be noted in the medical record
      (2) Acute care hospitals must develop a protocol for identifying potential organ and tissue donors
   b. Nurses have an important role in assisting clients and families in the decisionmaking process, implementing required request protocols, educating people about organ donation, and encouraging people to sign donor cards

M. LEGAL RESPONSIBILITIES RELATED TO PATIENT DEATH

1. **The health care institution in which a person dies has a duty to inform an appropriate family member of a death; information regarding deaths should be confirmed prior to notification to avoid upsetting a family and increasing the risk of a lawsuit**
2. **Failure to make reasonable efforts to notify the appropriate family member within a reasonable time can also result in liability; in some institutions and circumstances, nurses assist with notification of death and must be familiar with local procedures and required documentation**

3. All states have laws providing for legal investigation of certain suspicious deaths by a legal officer such as a medical examiner or coroner

a. Most laws require a physician in attendance at a death, known or suspected to be of the type requiring investigation, to report it to the medical examiner or coroner

b. Deaths that usually come under the jurisdiction of the coroner or medical examiner include those with violent or suspicious circumstances, e.g., suspected homicides and suicides, and deaths following abortions, surgery, or hospital stays of less than 24 hrs

  (1) When in doubt as to whether or not a patient is a coroner's case, report it and let the medical examiner determine if further investigation is required

  (2) All health care providers have a duty to cooperate with the investigation; the body should not be disturbed without permission of the medical examiner, e.g., all lines, catheters, etc., should be kept in place

4. Determination of death

a. The inadequacy of traditional criteria, i.e., the cessation of circulation and respiration, has become apparent with organ transplantation and legal situations related to inheritance, survivorship, insurance claims, wrongful death, and homicide

b. Brain death statutes are an attempt to resolve this awkward problem

c. The legal criteria adopted by legislatures and courts are based on four basic models—a two-tiered model, the Capron-Kass model, the Uniform Brain Death Act, and the Uniform Determination of Death Act (see Module 18—Organ Donation)

N. ACCOUNTABILITY OF THE PROFESSIONAL NURSE

1. **Health care is a dynamic enterprise; therefore, all trauma nurses must keep informed of changes in federal and common law, and the statutes (including Nurse Practice Acts) of the states in which they perform nursing activities**
2. **In addition, trauma nurses must practice, in compliance with appropriate job descriptions, institutional or agency policies and procedures, and professional nursing standards**

Reference

1. American Nurses' Association. (1985). *Code for nurses with interpretive statements* (p. 1). Kansas City, MO: Author.

Suggested Readings

Feutz, S. A. (1989). Legal implications of institutional standards for nurses. *Journal of Nursing Administration, 19*(7), 4–7.

Furrow, B., Johnson, S., Jost, T., & Schwartz, R. (1987). *Health law.* St. Paul, MN: West Publishing Co.

George, J. E., & Quattrone, M. S. (1988). Malpractice insurance. *Journal of Emergency Nursing, 14*(4), 242–243.

Guido, G. (1988). *Legal issues in nursing.* Norwalk, CT: Appleton & Lange.

Joint Commission on Hospital Accreditation. (1985). *JCAH manual for hospitals.* Chicago: Author.

King, J. (1986). *The law of medical malpractice.* St. Paul, MN: West Publishing Co.

Lewis, S., & McCutchen, J. (1987). *Emergency medicine malpractice.* New York: John Wiley & Sons.

McCafferty, M., & Meyer, S. (1985). *Medical malpractice: Bases of liability.* New York: McGraw-Hill.

Northrup, C., & Kelly, M. (1987). *Legal issues in nursing.* St. Louis: C. V. Mosby Co.

Potter, D. (1984). *Practices.* Springhouse, PA: Springhouse Corp.

Rhodes, A., & Miller, R. (1985). *Nursing and the law.* Rockville, MD: Aspen Publishers.

Taylor, J. E., Taylor, J. P., & Sieh, M. K. (1988). Emergency nurses' knowledge of legal liability. *Journal of Emergency Nursing, 14*(4), 225–229.

Section VI
Professional Perspectives in Trauma Nursing

MODULE 35
ETHICAL ISSUES

Steven Frantz, MSN, RN, CCRN

Prerequisite

Review Module 18—Organ Donation.

Objectives

1.0 Define basic ethics terminology.
2.0 Explain the differences and similarities between beneficence and autonomy.
3.0 Describe an ethical dilemma.
4.0 Differentiate between brain death, coma, and persistent vegetative state.
5.0 Describe a decisionmaking process that may be used to address ethical issues.
6.0 Use a specific model to address a typical ethical dilemma encountered in trauma care.

A. DEFINITION OF TERMS

1. **Ethical dilemma—situation in which either the knowledge of what is good is confused, contradictory, or absent, or the justification for choosing one option over the other is not convincing or clear (1)**
2. **Informed consent has four essential components**
   a. Person is competent to make the decision

b. Person receives information, including risks, based on the magnitude of harm for each risk, and the probability that it will occur
c. Person comprehends relevant information
d. Person voluntarily grants consent without coercion or duress

3. **Decisional capacity—ability to understand options and relevant consequences of acting on them**
4. **Morals—reflection of society via the rules and customs of its people; relates especially to the concepts of right and wrong behavior**
5. **Values—reflect an individual's beliefs freely chosen throughout life; values are incorporated into life by socialization, even if those values are not congruent with morals or society**
6. **Values clarification—process by which an individual chooses a set of standards; an ethical and moral guide on which to base actions**
7. **Autonomy—self-determination; person's ability to make his/her own decisions, including those affecting his/her medical care**
8. **Beneficence—seeking the greater balance of good over harm; locus of control originates with the physician or health care system**
9. **Good—health; what the patient wants; what the physician thinks is best; prevention, elimination, or control of disease; relief from unnecessary pain and suffering; prolonging life**
10. **Justice—impartiality; fairness; equal distribution of resources**

B. MODELS FOR ETHICAL DECISIONMAKING

(NOTE: The models presented here are to be used as a guide or framework for approaching problems; no model can be used in isolation—ethical decisions must be viewed from multiple perspectives)

1. **Autonomy**

a. Philosophical origins
   (1) Self-governance—determining directions through adequate knowledge and understanding; free from the controlling interference of others or personal limitations
   (2) Freedom of choice
   (3) One is autonomous only if capable of controlled deliberation and free action (2)

b. Legal origins
   (1) Self-determination—sovereignty over one's life; protects privacy, as well as rights to control what happens to one's person
   (2) Developed as a check or limit on the control of government or one person over another
   (3) Sovereignty limits the sphere into which others may legitimately intrude
   (4) Legal rights limit the physician's power and protect the patient from unwarranted intrusion, e.g., surgery without consent—unless an emergency exists and consent is not possible (2)

c. Related concepts
  (1) The moral goal of medicine is to promote the patient's best interest, as determined by the patient's autonomous decision
  (2) The basic moral principle of autonomy requires the physician and health care team to respect a patient's autonomous decision and actions regarding medical care
  (3) Derived moral obligations include disclosure of medical information to the patient, confidentiality, and fidelity
  (4) Derived moral virtues are based on truthfulness and faithfulness (2)

d. Operationalizing the model of autonomy
  (1) One interprets the best interests of the patient exclusively from the perspective of the patient
  (2) One takes the values and beliefs of the patient to be of primary moral consideration in determining the health care provider's moral responsibility in patient care
  (3) If a physician and a patient are in conflict, the fundamental responsibility is to facilitate, within reason, a patient's self-determination (autonomy) about his/her medical fate
  (4) Conflict may develop between a physician's understanding of the patient's best interests and the patient's understanding of those interests
  (5) Physicians do not have the right to treat patients as they see fit; this may violate equal standing of the patient/physician relationship

2. Beneficence (above all, do no harm)

a. Philosophical origins
  (1) Hippocrates was committed to a distinct moral goal or purpose as the basis of medical practice—to keep one's patients from harm and injustice
  (2) John Gregory added the concepts of sympathy, truthfulness, moral judgments, telling the truth to the dying, and feeling what the patient is feeling

b. Legal origins
  (1) There is a fiduciary (trusting) relationship between physician and patient
  (2) When trust is broken, issues of battery and neglect arise

c. Related concepts
  (1) Physician is obligated to seek the cure of disease and injury, if there is reasonable hope of cure
  (2) Pain and suffering from disease and injury are to be avoided, prevented, or removed
  (3) Medically, good is balanced over harm
  (4) The general moral goal of medicine is to promote a patient's best interests from the medical perspective

d. Operationalizing the model of beneficence
  (1) Provides for an understanding of a patient's best interest exclusively from the medical perspective
  (2) Decisions are based on tested knowledge, skill, and experience
  (3) Patient input into decisionmaking is considered but not paramount, as in the model of autonomy

C. PROCESS OF ETHICAL DECISIONMAKING

(See reference (3))

1. Data collection

a. Diagnosis
b. Prognosis
c. Current condition
d. Patient's values and goals
e. Identification of the decisionmakers

2. Identification of options/wishes

a. What is real
b. What is possible

3. Evaluation of options based on

a. Moral knowledge
b. Rules
c. Values
d. Laws

4. Decision—selection of a justified option

5. Action—based on decision

6. Reflection

D. EXAMPLES OF ETHICAL DILEMMAS

1. Patient refuses treatment against medical advice

a. All informed, competent individuals have the right to refuse treatment, or have treatment halted
b. Informed patients
   (1) Have a reduced sense of uncertainty
   (2) Develop an enhanced trust of health care providers
   (3) Have increased ability to act
   (4) Have a greater sense of control
   (5) Meet above essential criteria for informed consent
c. Principles
   (1) Right to refuse treatment is granted under principles of autonomy and self-determination
   (2) It is implied that a patient, when properly informed, knows what is in his/her best interest
   (3) Patient's decision should be based on his/her values, beliefs, and understanding surrounding health care
   (4) Patient's expectations and decisions will be based on the information provided from the health care team, and presented in terms of its relevance for the patient
d. Potential barriers to decision based on autonomy
   (1) Historically, physicians have acted paternalistically

(2) Health care providers may protect patient with optimism that does not reflect the reality of the patient's condition; hinders patient from making a truly informed decision
(3) Health care is fraught with uncertainty
(4) Health care team frequently waits too long to initiate a dialogue with the patient
(5) It may be difficult to know what a patient believes to be in his/her best interest
(6) Patient's situation and health status may change very rapidly

e. Legal considerations
(1) When patients refuse treatment, the courts have ruled by considering four state interests
(a) Prevention of suicide
(b) Preservation of life
(c) Third-party interests
(d) The integrity of the medical profession (4)
(2) Generally, courts have ruled that health care providers deliver, within reason, the level of care requested by a patient's family
(3) Family requests for discontinuation of care must be carefully examined to ensure that the family's motives are in the patient's best interest, and reflect what the patient would have wanted for him/herself, if he/she were able to voice an opinion
(4) Other principles or maxims that guide decisions include
(a) The "Golden Rule"—do unto others as you would have them do unto you
(b) Do what a reasonable person would do or would want done
(5) In the future, the courts may rule against families who insist on continued care, basing the decision on the physician's belief that treatment would be futile

f. Questions to consider
(1) Is the patient's decisionmaking capacity intact?
(2) How much information is required for informed consent in a given situation?
(3) Can a patient's decision be overridden if the family disagrees with his/her decision?

2. Health care providers withhold life-preserving treatment in situations when (5)

a. Treatment will not save a life
(1) In the face of futility, health care providers must weigh the burdens entailed in providing care against its potential benefits
(2) Burdens may include providing a variety of resources for care of the patient (equipment, personnel, etc.), availability of resources, and costs to society, family, and patient
(3) Questions to be addressed include
(a) How is futility determined and by what criteria?
(b) At what point does one establish futility?
(c) What will the patient's outcome be with and without treatment?
(d) Should time be a factor in the decision?

b. Intervention will result in an unacceptable quality of life
(1) Although patient survival may be achieved, the question arises, will the resulting quality of life be acceptable to the patient?

(2) Some believe that treatment is pointless if the patient will survive in a persistent vegetative state (PVS)
(3) Related questions that arise include
(a) Who determines acceptable quality of life if the patient has provided no clear directives, and his/her wishes are unknown or in dispute?
(b) How does the trauma care team evaluate expected outcomes from the treatments/resources invested in the patient's care?
(c) What qualifies as purposeless intervention?

c. Intervention consumes too many resources—either because society does not want resources wasted, or because resources needed by other individuals might be consumed by the patient with PVS
(1) Society no longer has, or is willing to allocate, the resources needed to provide all possible health care to everyone, e.g., there are only so many units of blood available or only so many specialized hospital beds
(2) A highly disproportionate amount of Medicare funding is spent on sustaining patients for the last few days or weeks of their lives (6)
(3) Relevant questions include
(a) Should the bedside clinician be both gatekeeper and caregiver for health care services?
(b) What responsibility do bedside clinicians have toward the distribution of resources?
(c) Should limits on the amount of health care and/or the amount spent for health care be set?
(d) What role should the cost of care have in decisions made regarding the amount of care to be given in specific situations?
(e) If care is to be limited, how can this be done in a society that has grown accustomed to high levels of health care?
(f) If care cannot be limited, what are the options, given present public opinion about health care costs?
(g) How do we, as a society, decide how much care for what quality of life is worth how much money?
(h) How certain can one be that care provided presently can be withheld at a later time?

3. Brain death (also see Module 18—Organ Donation)

a. Cerebral function ceases and brain stem functions are lost
(1) Semiautonomous functions such as heartbeat and digestion may continue
(2) Shortly after brain death, the heart begins to lose its intrinsic rhythm

b. The cause of underlying unresponsiveness must be identified; potentially reversible conditions must be determined and ruled out

c. Once brain death is diagnosed, the patient is clinically and legally dead

d. Ethics questions that may occur include
(1) Can family members insist on continued treatment despite brain death?
(2) How long should a brain dead individual be maintained for organ donation?
(3) If discontinuation of life support for brain dead individuals is accepted by society, will other types of patients, i.e., those in coma or PVS, also become candidates for discontinuation of life support?

4. Persistent vegetative state (PVS)

a. Differs from brain death; brain stem, including the ascending reticular activating system, is intact

(1) Neurologic insult, usually secondary to ischemia or hypoxia, is limited to cerebral hemispheres
(2) Cerebral hemispheres are very sensitive to low flow and low oxygenation states; brain stem, less active metabolically, is less sensitive to oxygen or flow deficits

b. Coma also differs from coma
(1) Coma is characterized by extensive damage to the ascending reticular activating system, cerebral hemispheres, or both
(2) Coma results in a state of sleep-like unarousability and severely impairs protective reflexes, e.g., gag, cough, swallow
(3) Ability to clear secretions is decreased in coma; may result in fatal pneumonia

c. Manifestations of PVS
(1) Various brain stem functions may be intact
(2) Eyes may open at times but do not display sustained visual pursuit (wander)
(3) Periods of wakefulness and sleep present
(4) Gag and cough are normal; long-term survival can occur
(5) Patient is completely unconscious and unaware of self or surroundings
(6) Voluntary reactions or behavioral responses, reflecting consciousness, emotion, or volition, at the cerebral cortical level are absent
(7) Patient may react to painful stimuli but will not feel pain

d. Ethical questions presented by patients in PVS
(1) Quality of life
(a) Is PVS a lifestyle that a reasonable person would want?
(b) If a patient is unable to interact with his/her environment, is he/she still considered a "person"?
(c) Should institutional policy address futility of care in some situations?
(d) Does limiting treatment for patients with PVS border on active euthanasia?
(2) Cost/resource allocation
(a) Should cost of care be a factor in treatment decisions?
(b) Who should decide how health care dollars are allocated?
(c) Can a primary physician be both a caregiver and a fiscal monitor?
(d) If families insist on care, is the health care provider obligated to comply?
(e) Is the health care system obligated to treat patients in the face of futility?
(f) When resources are limited, should access to aggressive treatment be limited?—who should decide?

e. Additional considerations/ethical concerns
(1) A fine line exists between the moral rule against killing and senselessly prolonging life
(2) The etiology of PVS must be carefully considered before making an attempt to alter the plan of treatment
(3) Patients in a PVS secondary to injury, or toxic or metabolic insults, have a potentially better outcome than those whose insult was anoxia
(4) The level of care for PVS patients may range from minimal/supportive to complete/aggressive
(5) With vigorous care, individuals in PVS may live for years
(6) Hospital ethics committees have few, if any, policies for withholding or withdrawing therapy from PVS patients

(7) Ethicists vary with regard to their views on aggressive treatment for patients in PVS

(8) Each patient's situation must be considered on an individual basis

5. **Nurses may find the following framework useful for decisionmaking on ethical issues** (7)

a. To determine whether an ethical dilemma exists, identify

(1) People involved, their histories, and their previous involvement with a similar situation

(2) Proposed action(s)

(3) Setting or context of the proposed action(s)

(4) Intention or purpose of the proposed action(s) and the values being expressed

(5) Alternatives or choices available

(6) Probable implications or consequences of proposed action

b. Address the following questions

(1) Who should decide and why?

(2) For whom is the decision being made?

(3) What criteria should be used to make the decision?

(4) What degree of consent is needed from the patient to implement the decision?

(5) What, if any, moral principles are enhanced or negated by the proposed course of action?

c. Consider moral, clinical, and legal perspectives

6. **Conclusion**

a. Ethical issues will increasingly enter decisions regarding trauma care

b. Limited financial and personnel resources, an increasing geriatric population, and advances in medical technology are but a few of the factors that will require nurses to utilize models for making ethical decisions

c. Bioethics committees, clergy, legal counsel, health professionals with postgraduate expertise, ethical standards published by professional nursing organizations (8), and a growing body of literature are helpful resources for nurses confronted with ethical dilemmas

References

1. Olowski, J. P. (1986). Ethical principles in critical care medicine. *Critical Care Clinics,* 2(1), 13–25.
2. Beauchamp, T. L., & McCullough, L. B. (1984). *Medical ethics: The moral responsibilities of physicians.* Englewood Cliffs, NJ: Prentice-Hall.
3. Kanoti, G. A. (1986). Ethics and medical-ethical decision-making. *Critical Care Clinics,* 2(1), 2–12.
4. Delaware Valley Ethics Committee Network. (1989, March). Presentation on ethics. *DVECN Newsletter* (4), 1–3.
5. Lo, B., & Jonsen, A. R. (1980). Clinical decisions to limit treatment. *Annals of Internal Medicine,* 93(5), 764–768.
6. Zook, C. J., & Moore, F. D. (1980). High cost users of medical care. *New England Journal of Medicine,* 302(18), 996–1002.

7. Aroskar, M. A. (1980). Anatomy of an ethical dilemma: The theory. *American Journal of Nursing, 80*(4), 658–660.
8. American Nurses' Association. (1985). *Code for nurses with interpretive statements.* Kansas City, MO: Author.

Suggested Readings

Brody, B. B. (1988). Ethical questions raised by the persistent vegetative patient. *Hastings Center Report, 18*(1), 33–37.

Cassell, E. J. (1986). Autonomy in the intensive care unit: Refusal of treatment. *Critical Care Clinics,* 2(1), 27–41.

Cranford, R. E. (1988). The persistent vegetative state: The medical reality—getting the facts straight. *Hastings Center Report, 18*(1), 27–32.

Engelhardt, H. T., Jr. (1984). Shattuck lecture: Allocating scarce medical resources and the availability of organ transplantation: Some moral presuppositions. *New England Journal of Medicine, 311*(1), 66–71.

Engelhardt, H. T., Jr., (1986). *The foundations of bioethics.* New York: Oxford University Press.

Engelhardt, H. T., Jr., & Rie, M. A. (1986). Intensive care units, scarce resources, and conflicting principles of justice. *Journal of the American Medical Association, 255*(9), 1159–1164.

Fleetwood, J. (1989). Solving bioethical dilemmas. *Nursing, 19*(3), 63–64.

Fowler, M., & Levine, J. (1987). *Ethics at the bedside.* Philadelphia: J. B. Lippincott Co.

Fromer, M. J. (1981). Ethical issues in health care. St. Louis: C. V. Mosby Co.

Fry, S. T. (Ed.). (1989). Part I: Ethics in nursing. *Nursing Clinics of North America,* 24(2).

Fry, S. T. (Ed.). (1989). Part II: Ethics in nursing. *Nursing Clinics of North America,* 24(4).

Hannegan, L. (1987). Brain death: Diagnosis and dilemma. *Critical Care Nursing Quarterly, 10*(3), 83–91.

Iverson, K. V., Sanders, A. B., Mathieu, D. R., & Buchanan, A. E. (Eds.). (1987). *Ethics in emergency medicine.* Baltimore: Williams & Wilkins.

Jonsen, A. R. (1984). What is extraordinary life support? *Western Journal of Medicine, 141*(3), 358–363.

LaPuma, J. (1987). Consultations on clinical ethics—Issues and questions in 27 cases. *Western Journal of Medicine, 146*(5), 633–637.

Lisson, E. L. (1987). Ethical issues related to pain control. *Nursing Clinics of North America,* 22(3), 649–659.

Roy, D. J., Verret, S., & Roberge, C. (1986). Death, dying, and the brain. *Critical Care Clinics,* 2(1), 161–172.

Thompson, J. B., & Thompson, H. O. (1983). *Bioethical decisionmaking for nurses.* Norwalk, CT: Appleton-Century-Crofts.

Veatch, R., & Fry, S. (1987). *Case studies in nursing ethics.* Philadelphia: J. B. Lippincott Co.

Walleck, C. A. (1988). Ethical concerns in trauma care. In V. D. Cardona, P. D.

Hurn, B. J. B. Mason, A. M. Scanlon-Schilpp, & S. W. Veise-Berry (Eds.), *Trauma nursing: From resuscitation through rehabilitation* (pp. 63–70). Philadelphia: W. B. Saunders Co.

Widra, L., & Pence, G. (1988). Ethical considerations. In E. Howell, L. Widra & M. G. Hill (Eds.), *Comprehensive trauma nursing* (pp. 887–902). Glenview, IL: Scott, Foresman, & Co.

Wikler, D. (1987). Not dead, not dying? Ethical categories and persistent vegetative state. *Hastings Center Report, 18*(1), 41–47.

Younger, S. J. (1986). Patient autonomy, informed consent, and the reality of critical care. *Critical Care Clinics, 2*(1), 41–52.

Younger, S. J., (1987). Do not resuscitate orders: No longer secret, but still a problem. *Hastings Center Report, 19*(1), 24–33.

Younger, S. J., & Bartlett, E. T. (1983). Human death and high technology: Failure of the whole-brain formulations. *Annals of Internal Medicine, 99*(2), 252–258.

Section VI
Professional Perspectives in Trauma Nursing

MODULE 36
STRESS MANAGEMENT

Lynn Kennedy-Ewing, MA

Objectives

1.0 Identify sources of vulnerability to stress in trauma nursing.
1.1 Describe how nursing care creates the potential for stress to develop among care providers.
1.2 Recognize personality trait strengths and weaknesses.
1.3 Recognize the role of an expanding technological knowledge base as a cause of stress.
2.0 Identify sources and causes of intrinsic stress.
2.1 List some types of intrinsic stress.
2.2 Increase awareness of when the impact of stress may be evident.
2.3 Discuss alternative solutions in the management of intrinsic stressors.
3.0 Develop an awareness of critical incident stress and its management.
3.1 Define critical incident stress.
3.2 Identify the types of events that may produce critical incident stress.
3.3 Identify the role of a critical incident stress management (CISM) program.
3.4 Demonstrate an understanding of the debriefing process.
3.5 List some typical reactions to critical incidents.
3.6 Describe how debriefing services are effective as a CISM technique.
3.7 Describe why staff clinicians and those not trained in CISM may not be effective.
4.0 Define the mechanism of cumulative stress.
4.1 Identify ways in which cumulative stress develops.
4.2 List common symptoms of cumulative stress.

4.3 Explore ways to eliminate or prevent cumulative stress.
5.0 Develop an understanding of the role of daily personal stress management.
5.1 Identify the need for good nutrition.
5.2 Describe ways exercise may be used for stress management.
5.3 Identify the need for a support system in stress management.
5.4 List ways in which interests outside professional work can help control stress.
5.5 Discuss ways in which personal priorities can be arranged to promote wellness.
5.6 Identify how stress can influence job performance.
5.7 Identify the benefits of adequate sleep.
5.8 Discuss relaxation methods.
5.9 Describe how daily stress management can enhance personal and professional life.

A. INTRODUCTION

1. Trauma nurses are vulnerable to stress for many reasons, including
a. Rapid advances in knowledge and technology
b. Complex skills required
c. Being in a job that is difficult for others to understand
d. Necessity for rapid decisionmaking
e. Little margin for error in daily work
f. Seeking situations with high potential for stress reaction
g. Situations when patients cannot be helped strike at nurse's need for control, idealism, and goal orientation
h. Psychological support services have been unavailable or inadequate until recently; when available, services may not be used (1)
i. Personality traits common to EMS providers (1)
(1) Action oriented
(2) Detail oriented
(3) Desire for control
(4) Tendency to be idealistic and goal oriented
(5) These traits are helpful in emergency situations; enable one to respond quickly and perform efficiently

2. Rendering trauma care has the potential to create stress reactions of significant proportions (2)
a. Stress response can interfere with job performance and personal life
b. Workers may not be able to resolve stress reaction with their own resources (1, 3, 4)
c. Stress reactions may be ongoing
d. Stress contributes to marked attrition, family/marital strife, and substance abuse in care providers

3. Stress is a highly personal phenomenon

a. Stress is perceived and experienced differently by different persons, even though related to a common event

b. One cannot predict when someone may suffer stress reaction; the same situation may cause a severe response in one person and no reaction in another (1, 3, 4)

c. Self-understanding is an important defense in coping with stress

B. INTRINSIC STRESSORS IN TRAUMA NURSING

(See reference (5))

1. Defined as stress that is directly associated with, and integral to, one's job

2. Types/sources of intrinsic stress

a. Administrative—frequent complaint among nurses (1); includes
   (1) Insensitivity on part of administrators
   (2) Constant performance evaluation
   (3) Policies and dictates, e.g., excessive paperwork, "red tape," staffing shortages, reimbursement policies, which may reduce time for quality patient care (6)
   (4) Increased patient acuity with increased needs for care in shorter length of stay (6)
   (5) Concerns for cost-effectiveness and efficiency

b. Environmental
   (1) Noises
      (a) Often integrated into daily routine without realization
      (b) Medical equipment relies on auditory stimuli as signals to perform a task, e.g., beepers, buzzers, bells
      (c) Vocalizations of people in pain
   (2) Odors
      (a) Malodorous stimuli from by-products of patient's condition, e.g., excretions, secretions
      (b) Disinfectants and other noxious products
      (c) Although one adapts by focusing away from the olfactory insult, a psychologic effect remains; may result in olfactory hallucination later
   (3) Viewing grotesque situations may affect the nurse in an unconscious manner by causing
      (a) Inability to watch movies that depict blood or violence
      (b) Nightmares or unusual dreams
      (c) Other effects, specific to the individual

c. Shift rotation can lead to
   (1) Problems with "biological clock" adjustment
   (2) High levels of fatigue
   (3) Low nutritional levels
   (4) Possible family/interpersonal difficulties due to frequent changes in schedule

d. Lack of recognition

(1) Duration of patient contact may be short in some phases of the trauma continuum, resulting in lack of recognition for the nurse's initial efforts on patient's behalf
(2) Those with power to reward, i.e., administrators, may be insensitive to the value and work of caring vs task accomplishment
(3) Nurses may not be recognized by other team members as significant participants or collaborators in patient care (6)
(4) Financial compensation may be inadequate

e. High social and personal expectations
(1) Public assumes that emergency/trauma care will correct all medical and, sometimes, social problems
(2) Nurse may expect that with increased training and special skills she/he will not fail or make mistakes; feels invincible
(3) Routine exposure to emergencies may lead to assumption of immunity to emotional effect
(4) Emotional effect may result in guilt or feelings of inadequacy (1)
(5) Ineffective coping with emotional effects of stressful situations can lead to "burnout"

f. Variable activity level
(1) Anticipation of emergencies results in some degree of satisfaction when emergency occurs and disappointment when emergency does not occur
(2) Nurse may be required to perform alternative, less stimulating duties while awaiting emergency call/situation
(3) Work flow may be erratic and require frequent change in pace and activity level
(4) Results in fatigue and inability to relax after work is over

C. STRATEGIES TO COMBAT INTRINSIC STRESSORS

1. **Increase nurse input to development of EMS/health care agency philosophy, mission, and goals (6)**
2. **Provide sufficient support staff and services**
3. **Increase nurse's recognition as integral part of patient care team; resolve interrole conflicts**
4. **Control undue exposure to noxious sights and sounds**
5. **Eliminate short time intervals between shift rotations**
6. **Adapt personal routine to ease adjustment to new shift**
7. **Reward clinical practice through performance appraisals, awards, publicity in institutional or community media**
8. **Introduce self and explain role to patient and family when providing care**
9. **Monitor and maintain realistic personal expectation level**
10. **Commend other team members on a regular basis; support peers and be available to listen to them, if needed**
11. **Remember that every EMS/trauma team member will, at some time, experience emotional effects of stressful situations (3)**

D. CRITICAL INCIDENTS AND EVENTS

(See also reference (1))

1. **Defined as incidents and events with the potential to create acute emotional distress, which may be severe enough to result in a worker's inability to perform professional and home responsibilities (1, 2, 3, 5)**
2. **Critical incidents first recognized in prehospital disaster situations; now known to occur in other emergency and trauma-related settings (1)**
3. **Common forms of critical incidents (1)**

a. Death, injury, or suicide of a co-worker
   (1) Trauma/emergency care is a team effort
   (2) The team becomes a "family" as common bonds form, and team members depend on each others' skills for task achievement
   (3) When a team member dies or is injured, grief of team members is similar to that experienced in a biological family
   (4) Typical reactions
      (a) Team becomes fragmented
      (b) Team struggles to reorganize
      (c) Self-doubt, fear, and self-blame also emerge due to loss of control
      (d) If event occurs on the job, effect is intensified
   (5) Effects may also be seen in adjunct team members, e.g., police officers, paramedics, and trauma/emergency care providers at another institution

b. Death or injury of a child (7)
   (1) Interrupts societal norm for life progression from birth to death at old age
   (2) Care providers are naturally more invested in children, under normal conditions
      (a) Resuscitative efforts often last longer with children than adults
      (b) Added effort is usually put into many aspects of care
      (c) Injuries resulting from abuse, neglect, or carelessness produce more anger than other causes (1, 7)
   (3) Fear-producing situations
      (a) Include caring for individuals with communicable diseases such as AIDS or hepatitis B; hazardous conditions; abusive patients; urban violence
      (b) Cause care providers to recall fears encountered in similar situations; renew anxiety
      (c) If fears and anxieties are not relieved by effective coping strategies, performance and well-being are affected; may result in attrition from profession
   (4) Mass or multiple casualties
      (a) Often cause feelings of being overwhelmed
      (b) Interrupting or withholding care for one patient in order to attend to patients with more severe injuries can result in feelings of dereliction in fulfilling one's duty
      (c) Inability to control the situation causes psychological distress
   (5) Knowledge of victim or identification with victim
      (a) Personal knowledge of victim can produce same effect as injury to an EMS/trauma team member

(b) Victim may remind worker of similar life situation of self or loved one; results in transference to own situation of fear for self or loved one

(c) May interfere with normal interpersonal relations, job performance, and other tasks

(6) Prolonged rescue/resuscitation attempts that end in death of victim

(a) Feelings of inadequacy arise

(b) Anger often surfaces and may be directed at patients or co-workers

(c) Raises self-doubts regarding personal abilities and performance

4. Critical incident stress reactions may be physical, emotional, cognitive, or behavioral (4)

a. Common physical reactions

(1) Nausea; diarrhea

(2) Fatigue

(3) Rapid heart rate

(4) Chest pain; difficulty breathing

(5) Shock-like symptoms

(6) Muscle cramps; headaches; body aches

b. Common emotional reactions

(1) Apprehension; anxiety

(2) Fear

(3) Grief

(4) Guilt

(5) Denial

(6) Depression

(7) Panic

(8) Anger

(9) Vague, uncomfortable feelings

c. Common cognitive reactions (4)

(1) Memory problems

(2) Inability to concentrate or be attentive

(3) Poor problem solving

(4) Disorientation

(5) Time distortion

(6) Intrusive images

(7) Hyperalertness

(8) Sleep disturbance

(9) Nightmares

d. Behavioral reactions

(1) Avoidance or withdrawal

(2) Restlessness

(3) Increased startle reflex

(4) Emotional outbursts

(5) Blaming others

(6) Change in eating habits

(7) Increased use of chemical substances; substance abuse

5. Critical incident stress intervention (1, 2)

a. Critical incident stress debriefing teams

(1) Team role—provide intervention and support services to EMS/trauma workers who have encountered a critical incident

- (2) Team membership
  - (a) Mental health workers
  - (b) Peer support personnel—nurses, physicians, paramedics, etc.
- (3) All team members are trained to apply specific interventions for critical incidents and to mitigate manifestations of stresses common in EMS/trauma care providers
- (4) Teams are part of an organized system dedicated solely to specialized critical incident services; intervention outside of the system is discouraged

b. Services provided include
- (1) On-scene support—assists obviously distressed individuals during critical incident and serves as resource for administrative/command personnel during the event (5)
- (2) Defusing—rapid intervention held shortly after conclusion of the event; allows for the initial ventilation of emotion and provides education on measures for minimizing stress effects (2)
- (3) Debriefings—usually follow a specific structure and process suggested by psychologist J. T. Mitchell, Ph.D. (1)
  - (a) Seven-phase sequence—introduction, fact, thought, reaction, symptom, teaching, and reentry (1, 2, 3)
  - (b) Take approximately 3 hrs
  - (c) Conducted 24 hrs to one week after critical incident
  - (d) Debriefings involve (1)
    - i) A meeting between persons involved with critical event and critical incident stress debriefing (CISD) team members
    - ii) A nonevaluative discussion of the incident, i.e., operation and procedure are not critiqued
    - iii) Discussion of personal involvement, reactions, and thoughts of participants
    - iv) Via psychological and educational strategies, debriefings help to reduce the fallacy of uniqueness in experience, assert the stress experience as a normal reaction to an abnormal situation, identify those who may need further counseling, and assist in restoring group cohesiveness and recovery
  - (e) Confidentiality is strictly maintained; no notes or rolls are taken; only those directly involved are admitted
  - (f) CISM activities should only be performed by qualified personnel
  - (g) Participation by clinicians on staff who work regularly with the involved EMS/trauma care providers is discouraged
  - (h) Participation by unqualified clinicians may result in
    - i) Less than optimal effectiveness
    - ii) Mislabeling of content due to lack of understanding of CISM and inappropriate planning/help for dealing with care providers' stress
    - iii) A critical incident for the staff clinicians
    - iv) Participants' fear of breach of confidentiality
- (4) Follow-up services are suggested following initial debriefing and may take several forms (4, 5)
  - (a) A second debriefing or follow-up meeting
  - (b) An informal visit by a CISM team member

(c) Referral for more in-depth educational or psychological support/ intervention

(5) Educational/informational programs for health care providers
(6) Spouse/loved one support services
(7) Resources and referral services for stress management related to stressors other than critical incidents
(8) CISM teams are available 24 hrs a day, 7 days a week

E. CUMULATIVE STRESS AND BURNOUT

1. **Defined as events, demands, and changes that are allowed to build over time, without resolution**
2. **Can lead to total physical and emotional deterioration**
3. **Common symptoms include**
   a. Denial or suppression of emotions
   b. Ignoring problems
   c. Extreme activity levels
   d. Little rest or relaxation
   e. Difficult to work with and get along with
   f. Extreme need to control; unwilling to be flexible or adapt
4. **Management of cumulative stress requires a change in lifestyle and adjustment of priorities**
5. **Many resources for stress management are available**

F. SUGGESTIONS FOR STRESS MANAGEMENT

1. **Eat a well-balanced diet; avoid excessive caffeine and sugar**
2. **Exercise on a regular basis**
   a. Select a desirable activity
   b. Make exercise a three-times-a-week habit
   c. Strive to elevate heart rate for 15 to 20 minutes at each session
   d. Exercise at work by parking farther from the door and walking (in safe areas), taking the stairs instead of elevators, and doing relaxation mini-exercises during breaks
3. **Increase your support system**
   a. Interaction with others can yield positive effects
   b. Good interpersonal relations offer a cushion for difficult times
   c. Share with and listen to co-workers
   d. Share your feelings when necessary, i.e., say "ouch"; do not suppress your emotions
4. **Rest and relax**
   a. Determine your adequate sleep requirement

b. Obtain needed sleep each 24 hrs
c. Find an enjoyable method for relaxation; practice relaxation and make it part of your daily routine

5. **Develop interests outside of your profession**
a. Learn a new hobby and meet new people to feed your need for action
b. Outside interests can serve as a remedy for boredom and a method for relaxation, offer a clearer definition of work vs free time, and provide a "vacation" from work in the off-hours

6. **Examine your list of priorities**
a. Eliminate excess activities and obligations
b. Say "no" when your schedule is full
c. Remember what is truly important to you
d. Look out for "Number One;" taking care of your own needs first is essential to accomplish other priorities

7. **TAKE TIME FOR YOURSELF**

G. CONCLUSION

1. **A healthy nurse experiences the most professional and personal satisfaction**
2. **Stress management increases wellness and happiness, provides a clearer world view, makes stressful work more tolerable, decreases the need to self-medicate, escape, or avoid, and enhances the opportunity to reach optimal potential**

References

1. Mitchell, J. T. (1988). *CISD team training.* Media, PA: Delaware County Department of Human Resources.
2. Mitchell, J. T. (1983). When disaster strikes. *Journal of Emergency Medical Services,* 8(1), 36–39.
3. Kennedy-Ewing, L. (1987). *The development and implementation of CISM services.* Media, PA: Delaware County Department of Human Resources.
4. Kennedy-Ewing, L. (1989, May). *Research findings on CISDs.* Paper presented at the Surviving Emergency Service Stress International Conference, Baltimore.
5. Kennedy-Ewing, L. (1988). *Delaware County, Pennsylvania critical incident stress management program operational guidelines.* Media, PA: Delaware County Department of Human Resources.
6. Perry, L. (1989). Best way to keep RNs: Treat them as professionals. *Modern Healthcare* (February).
7. Dyregrov, A. (1989, May). *Psychological effect of working with traumatized children.* Paper presented at the Surviving Emergency Service Stress International Conference, Baltimore.

Suggested Readings

Epperson-Sebour, M. (1985). *Role stressors and supports for emergency workers.* Washington, DC: U.S. Department of Health and Human Services, Center for Mental Health Studies of Emergencies.

Lachman, V. D. (1983). *Stress management for nurses.* New York: Grune and Stratton.

Mitchell, J. T. (1986, Fall). Critical incident stress management. *Response: The Magazine of Emergency Management,* pp. 24–25.

Notowidlo, S. J., Packard, J. S., & Manning, M. R. (1986). Occupational stress: Its causes and consequences for job performance. *Journal of Applied Psychology, 71* (November).

Rubin, J. G. (1990). Critical incident stress debriefing: Helping the helpers. *Journal of Emergency Nursing, 16*(4), 255–258.

Taylor, A. J. W., & Frayer, A. G. (1982). The stress of postdisaster body handling and victim identification work. *Journal of Human Stress, 8*(12), 4–12.

Section VI
Professional Perspectives in Trauma Nursing

MODULE 37
PROFESSIONAL DEVELOPMENT

Helen Noyes Downey, MSN, RN
Elizabeth W. Bayley, MS, PhD, RN

Objectives

1.0 Describe the purposes and functions of national nursing organizations that have an interest in trauma nursing.

2.0 Identify the benefits of membership and active participation in professional organizations.

3.0 Identify community organizations that welcome or collaborate with trauma nurses in community education efforts.

4.0 Discuss the role of continuing education in the professional development of the trauma nurse.

4.1 Cite the goal of continuing education.

4.2 Identify the purpose of participation in educational programs that have formal contact hours granted by a nationally recognized organization.

4.3 Cite strategies for informal and independent learning in the professional development of trauma nurses.

4.4 List journals that publish articles pertinent to trauma nursing.

5.0 Discuss the role of graduate education as preparation for advanced nursing practice.

6.0 Relate the purposes of specialty certification in nursing.

6.1 Define certification.

6.2 Differentiate between certification and skills verification by employers.

7.0 Describe the role of the professional nurse in the research process.

7.1 Define research.
7.2 List the steps in the research process.
7.3 Differentiate between "nurse" and "nursing care" as the subject of nursing research.
8.0 Discuss the roles and opportunities for trauma nurses as contributors to professional publications.
8.1 Define "refereed journal."
8.2 Describe the steps in writing for publication.
9.0 Describe a plan for lifelong learning and career development as a trauma nurse.

A. OVERVIEW

1. **Professional development as a trauma nurse involves identifying career-related goals, and programming work, education, and related experiences to provide direction, timing, and sequencing of steps toward specific career goals (1)**
2. **Phases of professional development include professional identification, maturation, and mastery (2)**
3. **Career development is enhanced by participation in professional organizations, continuing education and skills development, and activities such as speaking to professional and community groups, engaging in various aspects of the research process, and writing for publication**

B. PROFESSIONAL NURSING ORGANIZATIONS

1. **General organizations**

a. American Nurses' Association (ANA)
2420 Pershing Road
Kansas City, MO 64108
(816) 474-5720
  (1) Purposes
    (a) Work for the improvement of health standards
    (b) Promote the availability of health care services to all people
    (c) Promote the professional development of nurses
    (d) Promote and protect the economic and general welfare of nurses
    (e) Represent and speak for the nursing profession with other health groups and the public
  (2) Functions/goals
    (a) Expand the scientific and research base for nursing practice
    (b) Clarify and strengthen the education system for nursing
    (c) Develop a coordinated system of credentialing for nursing

(d) Restructure the organizational arrangements for delivery of nursing services
(e) Develop comprehensive payment systems for nursing services
(f) Achieve effective control of the environment in which nursing is practiced and services offered
(g) Enhance organizational strength of the ANA
(h) Maintain and strengthen nursing's role in client advocacy

b. National League for Nursing (NLN)
350 Hudson Street
New York, NY 10014
(800) 669-1656
(1) Purpose
(a) Promote quality nursing service
(b) Foster effective educational preparation of nursing practitioners
(2) Functions
(a) Publish criteria for the evaluation of nursing education programs
(b) Provide consultative services to schools of nursing
(c) Provide standardized tests relevant to nursing
(d) Collect data relevant to nursing
(e) Accredit schools of nursing
(f) Accredit agencies that provide home health care

2. Specialty organizations of interest to trauma nurses

a. American Association of Critical Care Nurses (AACN)
101 Columbia
Aliso Viejo, CA 92656-1458
(800) 899-AACN
(1) Purposes (missions)
(a) A not-for-profit service association dedicated to the welfare of people experiencing critical illness or injury
(b) Advance the art and science of critical care nursing
(c) Promote environments that facilitate comprehensive professional nursing practice for those experiencing actual or potential critical illness or injury
(2) Functions (pledges)
(a) Provide leadership and leadership development within critical care nursing
(b) Demonstrate responsiveness to issues and concerns raised by members and interested parties
(c) Promote means to enhance affiliations and support networks for members and colleagues
(d) Operate effectively and efficiently with respect to human and financial resources
(e) Provide value and quality in all programs, activities, and products
(3) Values—education, research, and collaboration

b. American Association of Neuroscience Nurses (AANN)
218 N. Jefferson Street, Suite 204
Chicago, IL 60606
(312) 993-0043
(1) Purpose—foster health, welfare, and education of the general public through education, research, and high standards of practice in neuroscience nursing

(2) Functions
  (a) Represent nurses throughout the neuroscience continuum
  (b) Provide educational programs at local, national, and international levels
  (c) Provide for growth in the specialty
  (d) Provide mechanisms for communication among neuroscience nurses

c. American Association of Spinal Cord Injury Nurses (AASCIN)
75–20 Astoria Boulevard
Jackson Heights, NY 11370-1178
(718) 803-3782
  (1) Purpose—promote excellence in meeting the health care needs of individuals with spinal cord injury
  (2) Functions
    (a) Advance, foster, encourage, promote, and improve nursing care of spinal cord injured individuals
    (b) Develop and promote education and research related to spinal cord injury nursing
    (c) Provide educational opportunities for spinal cord injury nurses
    (d) Increase communication and maintain liaison with other nursing and health care organizations and consumer groups
    (e) Recognize nurses whose careers are devoted to the problems of spinal cord injury

d. American Society of Post Anesthesia Nurses (ASPAN)
11512 Allecingie Parkway
Richmond VA 23235
(804) 379-5516
  (1) Purpose (mission)—maintain and upgrade the standards of the specialty and promote the professional growth of its members
  (2) Functions
    (a) Provide education, with respect to all phases of postanesthesia care, through a variety of formats
    (b) Develop standards of nursing practice
    (c) Promote public awareness and understanding of the care of pre- and postanesthesia patients
    (d) Enhance professional knowledge
    (e) Facilitate cooperation among postanesthesia nurses, physicians, and other members of the health care team concerned with the care of the patient in the immediate pre- and postanesthesia period
    (f) Encourage specialization and research in all phases of postanesthesia nursing
    (g) Promote interest and professional growth of nurses engaged or interested in the care of patients in the immediate pre- and postanesthesia nursing period
    (h) Cooperate with universities, government agencies, or any organizations in matters affecting the purposes of the society

e. Association of Operating Room Nurses (AORN)
10170 E. Mississippi Avenue
Denver, CO 80231
(303) 755-6300
  (1) Purposes

(a) Enhance the professionalism of perioperative nurses
(b) Improve the performance of perioperative nurses to serve the needs of society better
(c) Provide a forum for interaction and exchange of ideas among perioperative nurses

(2) Functions
(a) Facilitate research in nursing care of surgical patients
(b) Provide opportunities for continuous learning through diversified educational activities
(c) Develop and promote professional and administrative standards and technical recommended practices
(d) Collaborate with other health care professionals, agencies, associations, and industry

f. Association of Rehabilitation Nurses (ARN)
5700 Old Orchard Road, 1st Floor
Skokie, IL 60077
(708) 966-3433
(1) Purposes
(a) Advance the quality of rehabilitation nursing service throughout the community
(b) Offer educational opportunities that promote awareness of and interest in rehabilitation nursing and improve expertise of personnel on all levels
(c) Facilitate exchange of ideas in rehabilitation programs

(2) Functions
(a) Provide educational programs for nurses
(b) Publish a journal, a core curriculum, and audio-visual materials
(c) Develop standards of rehabilitation nursing practice
(d) Promote certification in rehabilitation nursing

g. Emergency Nurses Association (ENA)
230 E. Ohio Street, Suite 600
Chicago, IL 60611
(312) 649-0297
(1) Purpose—a voluntary association committed to excellence in emergency care and dedicated to the advancement of emergency nursing practice
(2) Functions
(a) Definitive authority on emergency nursing
(b) Define the standards of excellence for emergency nurses
(c) Promote the specialty of emergency nursing
(d) Promote quality emergency care through continuing education activities
(e) Resource for emergency nursing practice, professionalism, education, research, and consultation
(f) Identify and address emergency care issues
(g) Work collaboratively with other health-related organizations toward the improvement of emergency care
(h) Affirm the ENA Code of Ethics

h. National Flight Nurses Association (NFNA)
6900 Grove Road
Thorofare, NJ 08086
(609) 384-6725

(1) Purpose—to support the unique expanded role of the professional flight nurse
(2) Functions
(a) Seek out and develop close working relationships with all available supportive services to ensure maximum support to the patient
(b) Establish national standards of care during flight
(c) Disseminate new knowledge
(d) Guide change toward the improvement of health care standards in emergency nursing
(e) Offer educational programs and services
(f) Serve as a medium for communication and exchange of information

i. National Association of Orthopaedic Nurses (NAON)
N. Woodbury Road, Box 56
Pitman, NJ 08071
(609) 582-0111
(1) Purposes—promote, in cooperation with all members of the health team, the highest standards of nursing practice
(2) Functions
(a) Educate practitioners
(b) Promote research
(c) Maintain effective communications between orthopaedic nurses and other external interested persons and groups

j. Society of Trauma Nurses (STN)
888 17th Street, N.W., Suite 1000
Washington, DC 20006
(301) 328-3930
(1) Purpose—to provide a forum for nurses involved in all facets of trauma care, from prevention through rehabilitation
(2) Functions
(a) Communicate trauma nursing information
(b) Recognize excellence and innovations in trauma nursing
(c) Facilitate nursing research and publication
(d) Develop a coalition to address legislative issues on all levels
(e) Facilitate the development and dissemination of trauma nursing standards
(f) Serve as an expert resource for policymakers, professional organizations, and other agencies

3. Other organizations

a. American Burn Association (ABA)
c/o Andrew M. Munster, M.D., Secretary, ABA
Baltimore Regional Burn Center
Francis Scott Key Medical Center
4940 Eastern Avenue
Baltimore, MD 21224
(800) 548-2876
(1) Purpose—a multidisciplinary organization dedicated to burn care education, research, and patient care, and the prevention of burn injuries
(2) Functions
(a) Promote the burn team concept, i.e., the collaboration of physicians, nurses, physical and occupational therapists, social workers, nutritionists, and other health professionals dedicated to the care of individuals with burn injuries

(b) Inform members of the burn team of significant advances in burn prevention, research, education, delivery of acute care, and rehabilitation
(c) Provide a forum for presentation of new scientific findings regarding treatment and prevention of burn injuries
(d) Facilitate communication for special interest groups related to burn care
(e) Increase community awareness of burn hazards and knowledge of burn prevention
(f) Provide expertise and liaison to other organizations in regard to issues such as disaster planning, injury control, standards, and health care policy

b. American Trauma Society (ATS)
8903 Presidential Parkway, Suite 512
Upper Marlboro, MD 20772-2656
(800) 556-7890
(1) Purpose—a nationwide, voluntary health organization of professionals and lay individuals, institutions, and corporations dedicated to the prevention of trauma and the improvement of trauma care
(2) Functions
(a) Increase public awareness of the term "trauma" so that it becomes a household word
(b) Initiate and coordinate national prevention programs aimed at reducing the incidence and severity of trauma
(c) Promote the use of trauma systems throughout the nation

4. **Additional activities and benefits of membership in professional organizations**
(a) Collaborate with certification boards to test and certify nurses; nurses may recertify by retest or verification of continuing education activities
(b) Network with peers who share common interests and needs
(c) Develop standards for nursing practice
(d) Monitor state and national legislation that impacts on the members, or the patient population of interest to the association
(e) Provide educational programs and leadership development opportunities
(f) Publish journals, books, audiovisual media, and consumer education brochures
(g) Develop and publish curricula
(h) Sponsor scholarships and awards
(i) Collaborate with other professional organizations to solve common problems and represent unity in nursing and the health care community
(j) Offer discounted insurance (including professional liability) and reduced travel rates

C. VOLUNTARY COMMUNITY ORGANIZATIONS RELATED TO TRAUMA

1. **American Red Cross**
17th and D Streets, N.W.
Washington, DC 20006
(202) 737-8300

a. Purpose—assist individuals and communities to prevent, prepare for, and cope with emergencies
b. Functions
   (1) Provide emergency services, including immediate help for disaster victims, worldwide communications, emergency services for military families, and other veterans' services
   (2) Provide services to older adults
   (3) Present health and safety courses
   (4) Provide services to community youth, including service opportunities, health and safety education, and leadership training
   (5) Maintain a safe and adequate blood supply

2. Mothers Against Drunk Driving (MADD)
669 Airport Freeway, Suite 310
Hurst, TX 76053
(817) 268-6233

a. Purpose—mobilize victims and their allies to establish the public conviction that impaired driving is unacceptable and criminal, in order to promote corresponding public policies, programs, and personal accountability
b. Functions
   (1) Provide victim assistance
   (2) Increase public awareness
   (3) Monitor the criminal justice system
   (4) Increase youth awareness of the problem
   (5) Lobby for legislative reform
   (6) Promote activities of Students Against Drunk Drivers (SADD)

3. National Coalition Against Sexual Assault (NCASA)
The Sexual Violence Center
1222 W. 31st Street
Minneapolis, MN 55408
(612) 824-2864

a. Purpose—to develop a network for members of the antirape movement in order to share expertise, experience, and information
b. Functions
   (1) Advocate for and on behalf of rape victims
   (2) Disseminate information on sexual assault
   (3) Bestow awards
   (4) Compile statistics
   (5) Initiate and support related legislation

4. National Committee for Prevention of Child Abuse (NCPCA)
332 S. Michigan Avenue, Suite 1600
Chicago, IL 60604-4357
(312) 663-3520

a. Purpose—eliminate child abuse
b. Functions—primary and secondary prevention of child abuse activities through education of parents regarding child growth and development

5. National Head Injury Foundation (NHIF)
333 Turnpike Road
Southborough, MA 01772
(800) 444-NHIF

a. Purposes—to improve the quality of life for persons with head injuries and their families, and to develop and support programs to prevent head injuries
b. Functions
   (1) Increase public, family, and professional awareness of the silent epidemic
   (2) Advocate recognition of the problem of head injury and the needs of head-injured people
   (3) Create an information and resource center for head injury
   (4) Develop a unifying structure to provide support for the head-injured and their families
   (5) Assist in the establishment of rehabilitation programs for the head-injured—from coma to community
   (6) Raise monies to support research
   (7) Prevention

6. **National SAFE KIDS Campaign**
   111 Michigan Avenue, N.W.
   Washington, DC 20010-2970
   (202) 939-4993

a. Purpose—to promote public awareness of childhood injury prevention; a national organization with local coalitions
b. Functions
   (1) Promote education
   (2) Emphasize local community-based action
   (3) Change public policy
   (4) Work with the media to promote awareness
   (5) Target a specific injury each year, e.g., bicycle safety (1989), prevention of scald injuries and house fires (1990); car seat use (1991)

7. **Other organizations that support trauma prevention and may welcome speakers on trauma-related topics include**

a. Alcoholics Anonymous
b. Elks
c. Kiwanis
d. Rotary International
e. Shriners
f. Lions Club International

D. CONTINUING EDUCATION (CE)

1. **Definition: "Continuing education includes learning activities intended to build upon varied educational and experiential bases for the enhancement of practice, education, administration, research, or theory development, to the end of maintaining and improving the health of the public"** (3)
2. **Didactic and clinical activities are included**
3. **Emphasis may be on learning new or more advanced skills, learning about patient populations new to the practitioner, developing role-related knowledge**

and skills, e.g., management, education, keeping abreast of research findings, and/or learning about innovations in practice and technology

4. **Nurses may gain credit, in the form of contact hours, for participating in approved continuing education programs**
   a. Approval of continuing education programs may be granted by professional nursing organizations, e.g., ANA, through a process designed to assure quality of programs offered
   b. Providers, including individuals, institutions, agencies, and organizations that meet specific standards, may be accredited to award approved contact hours
5. **CE is mandatory in 26 states for relicensure as a registered nurse (4)**
   a. Trauma nurses must be aware of CE requirements for relicensure in the states in which they practice, as well as CE standards related to institutional accreditation as a trauma center
   b. Development of an adequate system for personal recordkeeping regarding CE is a professional nursing responsibility
6. **Trauma nurses can continue their education independently and informally by**
   a. Reading books and journals, including
      (1) *AORN Journal*
      (2) *Critical Care Nurse*
      (3) *Critical Care Nursing Clinics of North America*
      (4) *Dimensions of Critical Care Nursing*
      (5) *Emergency*
      (6) *Focus on Critical Care*
      (7) *Heart and Lung*
      (8) *Journal of Burn Care and Rehabilitation*
      (9) *Journal of Emergency Nursing*
      (10) *Journal of Emergency Medical Services*
      (11) *Journal of Head Trauma Rehabilitation*
      (12) *Journal of Neuroscience Nursing*
      (13) *Journal of Postanesthesia Nursing*
      (14) *Journal of Trauma*
      (15) *Nursing Clinics of North America* (issues on trauma topics)
      (16) *Orthopaedic Nursing*
      (17) *Prehospital and Disaster Medicine*
      (18) *Rehabilitation Nursing*
      (19) *SCI Nursing*
      (20) *Topics in Acute Care and Trauma Rehabilitation*
      (21) *Topics in Emergency Nursing*
      (22) *Trauma Quarterly*
   b. Completing independent study modules published in journals, or developed by individuals or institutions
   c. Learning from other professionals
      (1) Identify learning needs
      (2) Identify professionals who possess in-depth knowledge and/or skills needed
      (3) Arrange for individual or group tutorial
      (4) Contract with an experienced individual to act as a clinical preceptor to help with meeting specific learning objectives

E. ACADEMIC EDUCATION

1. **Nurses who wish to prepare for advanced practice roles as clinical nurse specialists, trauma program coordinators, nurse managers, or staff development educators will benefit from graduate education; faculty and research positions frequently require a doctorate**
2. **A listing of master's degree programs, accredited by the National League for Nursing, is available from the NLN (see address in section B., 1., b.)**
   a. The list identifies areas of specialization
   b. More than a dozen programs in the U.S. offer a master's degree in trauma nursing

F. PROFESSIONAL CERTIFICATION

1. **A process that attests to one's knowledge and/or skill in regard to a specific area of nursing practice; protects the public**
2. **The amount of experience required for taking certification examinations varies across programs, as does the duration of certification status**
3. **May be based on nationally recognized continuing education programs**
   a. Examples
      (1) BCLS—Basic Cardiac Life Support
      (2) ACLS—Advanced Cardiac Life Support
      (3) PALS—Pediatric Advanced Life Support
      (4) APLS—Advanced Pediatric Life Support
      (5) PHTLS—Prehospital Trauma Life Support
      (6) BTLS—Basic Trauma Life Support
      (7) ATLS—Advanced Trauma Life Support
      (8) TNCC—Trauma Nurse Core Course
      (9) ABLS—Advanced Burn Life Support
   b. Course length varies from 8 to 24 hrs
   c. Successful completion of written and clinical skills tests provides certification for a specified time period
4. **May be based on a nationally recognized curriculum developed by a nursing specialty organization**
   a. Independent study or review courses help nurses to prepare for a testing process that is carefully developed and regulated by the certification boards associated with major nursing organizations
   b. Recertification may be accomplished by retesting, or a combination of continuing education and dossier review; usually required every three to five years
5. **Certification differs from verification of skills by an employer, which indicates competence in specific skills needed in the work environment, i.e., drawing arterial blood gases**

G. RESEARCH ROLE OF THE TRAUMA NURSE

1. **Research may be defined as "all systematic inquiry designed for the purpose of advancing knowledge" (5)**
2. **The subject of research may be the nurse (personal characteristics) or nursing care (clinical aspects of patient care)**
3. **Steps in the research process**
   a. Formulate and delimit a problem
   b. Review related literature
   c. Develop a theoretical framework
   d. Identify variables of interest
   e. Formulate hypotheses
   f. Select a research design
   g. Collect data
   h. Analyze data
   i. Interpret results
   j. Communicate/disseminate findings
4. **Trauma nurses can participate at any step of the research process and have a critical role in the identification of researchable problems**
5. **Trauma nurses also need to be active consumers of research**
   a. Evaluate the study for scientific merit
   b. Assess findings for relevance to practice
   c. Determine the potential for clinical evaluation

H. WRITING FOR PUBLICATION

1. **Essential to communicate expertise and experience to large numbers of practitioners**
2. **Beginners may start with a short article for a professional journal; more experienced nurses may contribute a chapter to a book, or edit or author a book**
3. **Acting as a reviewer for a journal or book publisher is another way to learn more about publishing while sharing one's expertise**
4. **Steps to publishing an article**
   a. Identify the topic of interest
      (1) Review related literature
      (2) Select an approach for organization of content, i.e., case history, "how to," opinion, etc.
   b. Select a journal relevant to your target audience
      (1) Consider advantages of a refereed (reviewed by experts) vs nonrefereed journal
      (2) Review the content and format of articles previously published by the journals under consideration
   c. Write a query letter requesting information regarding
      (1) Desired format for materials published

    (2) Policy regarding unsolicited manuscripts
    (3) Interest in the topic to be addressed (optional)
d. Prepare the manuscript
    (1) Use correct grammar, spelling; credit borrowed sources, references
    (2) Ask one or more colleagues familiar with topic, or who have successfully published, to review the manuscript
    (3) Follow the format regulations the journal has provided
    (4) General suggestions
        (a) Proofread carefully
        (b) Check length of article
        (c) Include required material, i.e., abstract, curriculum vitae
e. Submit manuscript; keep a copy
f. Expect to respond to need for revisions; do not be discouraged by the need for this as even experienced authors frequently prepare several revisions before a manuscript is accepted for publication

References

1. Lucas, L. (1984). Career development programs: Part I—An overview. *TORCH* (St. Louis Metropolitan ASTD) 9(11), 4.
2. Sovie, M. D. (1982). Fostering professional nursing careers in hospitals: Part I. The role of staff development. *Journal of Nursing Administration, 12*(12), 5–10.
3. American Nurses' Association. (1984). *Standards for continuing education in nursing* (p. 15). Kansas City, MO: Author.
4. Weiss-Farnan, P., & Willie, R. (1988). Mandatory continuing education: The discussion a decade apart. *The Journal of Continuing Education in Nursing, 19*(2), 73.
5. Kelly, L. Y. (1985). *Dimensions of professional nursing* (5th ed., p. 256). New York: Macmillan.
6. LoBiondo-Wood, G., & Haber, J. (1986). *The role of research in nursing* (p.24). St. Louis: C. V. Mosby Co.

Suggested Readings

American Journal of Nursing Company. (1990). Directory of nursing organizations. *American Journal of Nursing, 90*(4), 143–151.

Barr, N. J., & Desnoyer, J. M. (1988). Career development for the professional nurse: A working model. *The Journal of Continuing Education in Nursing, 19*(2), 68–72.

Camilleri, R. (1988). On elegant writing. *Image, 20*(3), 169–171.

Coleman, B., Stanley, M., Chenevey, B., Sullivan, S., & Cardin, S. (1988). CCRN certification: Exclusive or expensive. *Focus on Critical Care, 15*(5), 23–27.

Collins, H. L. (1987). Certification: Is the payoff worth the price? *RN, 50*(7), 36–44.

Fickeissen, J. L. (1990). 56 ways to get certified. *American Journal of Nursing, 90*(3), 50–57.

Greenwood, E. (1957). Attributes of a profession. *Social Work,* 2(3), 45–55.
Hagemaster, J. N., & Kerins, K. M. (1984). Six easy steps to publishing. *Nurse Educator,* 9(4), 32–34.
Massoni, M. (1987). How to do your best on a certification exam. *RN,* 50(7), 38–39.
National League for Nursing. (1986). *Patterns in specialization: Challenge to the curriculum.* New York: Author.
Peplau, H. E. (1986). Internal vs external regulation. In *Credentialing in nursing: Contemporary developments and trends.* Kansas City, MO: American Nurses' Association.
Soiken, K. L. (1985). Critiquing research: Steps for complete evaluation of an article. *AORN Journal,* 41(5), 882–893.
Styles, M. M. (1978). Why publish? *Image,* 10(2), 28–31.
Styles, M. M. (1986). USA within a world view. In *Credentialing in nursing: Contemporary developments and trends.* Kansas City, MO: American Nurses' Association.
Swanson, E., & McCloskey, J. C. (1982). The manuscript review process of nursing journals. *Image,* 16(3), 72–76.
Tanner, C. (1987). Evaluating research for use in practice: Guidelines for the clinician. *Heart and Lung,* 16(4), 424–430.

INDEX